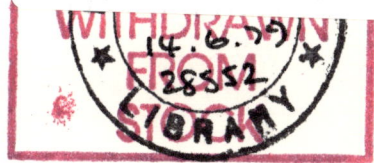

Epidemiology of Diabetes and Its Vascular Lesions

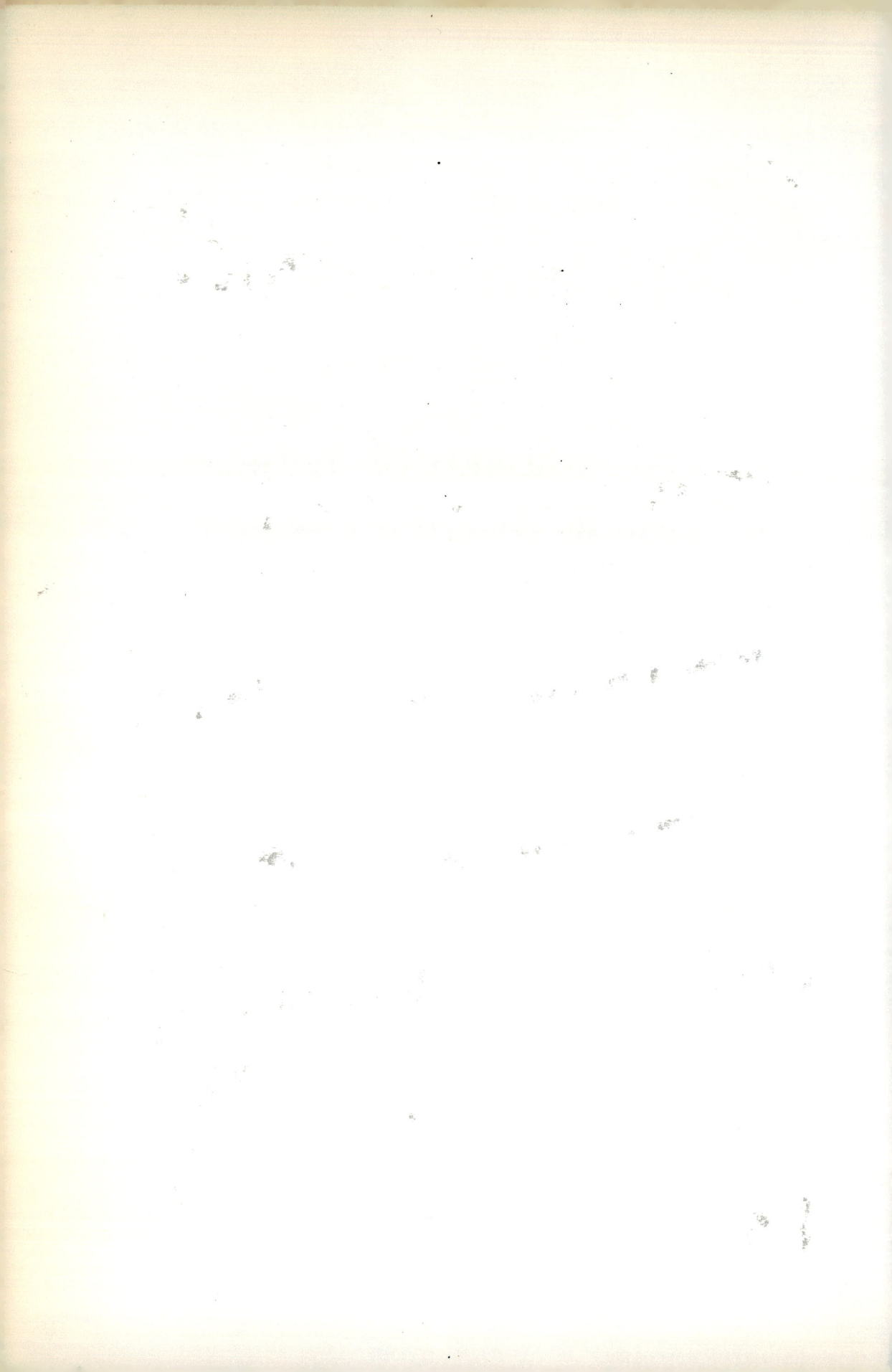

Epidemiology of Diabetes and Its Vascular Lesions

Kelly M. West, M.D.

Professor of Biostatistics and Epidemiology
Clinical Professor of Medicine
University of Oklahoma Health Sciences Center

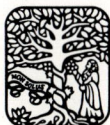

ELSEVIER · NEW YORK
NEW YORK · OXFORD

Elsevier North-Holland, Inc.
52 Vanderbilt Avenue, New York, NY 10017

Distributors outside the United States and Canada:
THOMOND BOOKS
(A Division of Elsevier/North-Holland Scientific
        Publishers, Ltd.)
P.O. Box 85
Limerick, Ireland

Library of Congress Cataloging in Publication Data
West, Kelly M.
  Epidemiology of diabetes and its vascular lesions.

  Bibliography: p.
  Includes index.
  1. Diabetes. 2. Diabetic angiopathies. 3. Epi-
demiology. I. Title. [DNLM: 1. Diabetes mellitus—
Occurrence. 2. Diabetic angiopathies—Etiology.
WK810.3 W518e]
RC660.W45   616.4'62   78-5980
ISBN 0-444-00254-5

Manufactured in the United States of America

CONTENTS

CONTENTS

PREFACE

Diabetes mellitus has become one of the most important of human problems. It is a significant cause of disease and death in all countries and all major races. In the past quarter-century diabetes has killed more people than all wars combined.

In most affluent societies diabetes is one of the major causes of coronary disease, the main cause of amputation, and a leading cause of blindness and kidney disease. Among the other factors suggesting the importance of diabetes is the extraordinary diversity of its morbid effects that require attention from endocrinologists, cardiologists, neurologists, microbiologists, pathologists, biochemists, pediatricians, obstetricians, urologists, nephrologists, vascular and orthopedic surgeons, ophthalmologists, gastroenterologists, nutritionists, and public health specialists. In many countries more than 5% of the older segment of the population has diabetes. This book describes several societies in which present incidence rates suggest that a majority may expect to become diabetic!

Few have recognized the great potentialities for preventing diabetes, mainly because of the common but erroneous notion that disorders having a genetic or "constitutional" basis are not likely to be influenced substantially by environmental factors. Evidence outlined here indicates that this widely prevalent fatalism has not been justified. On the contrary, epidemiologic studies are now yielding many exciting facts and clues applicable to the prevention and treatment of diabetes. In affluent societies a substantial majority of diabetics are or have been fat. In lean populations rates of diabetes are typically only one-third to one-tenth as great as in genetically-related societies where corpulence is common. It is insufficiently understood that much of the familial aggregation of diabetes is secondary to the familial aggregation of obesity. While obesity is widely believed to be only a "precipitating" factor in those persons genetically disposed to diabetes, the epidemiologic evidence now available strongly suggests that obesity alone is quite capable of producing diabetes, and often does.

The synergism of epidemiologic and laboratory investigations is increasingly apparent. Epidemiologic studies linking diabetes and obesity have been followed up by insulin-secretion studies at the bench. These investigations confirm that beta-cell function often returns to normal in diabetics in whom long-term control of obesity is achieved. Recent epidemiologic and laboratory studies reviewed in this book show that a preventive and a cure are *already* at hand for most diabetes. The cause is usually obesity; the preventive, and often the cure, is leaness. In the minority of diabetics who have never been fat, cures are rarely feasible, and preventive measures are not well developed. Even in this group, however, epidemiologic data are beginning to suggest some prospects for research that could lead to the development of preventive measures.

One of the newest and potentially most productive applications of epidemiology in the study of diabetes is the investigation of its specific manifestations or "complications." More evidence is needed, but it now appears that these complications, previously thought by many to be the inevitable concomitants of diabetes, are to a considerable degree preventable. In several populations of several races, rates of coronary disease are low in diabetics. Preliminary evidence suggests that environmental factors are responsible for this, and that a substantial potential exists for mitigating the vast toll exacted by these lesions.

For centuries observations relating to diabetes had been made from time to time which were in a sense "epidemiologic". But systematic epidemiologic studies were very few prior to 1960. In the past two decades, however, epidemiologic methods have been used with rapidly increasing frequency in the study of diabetes. Rather suddenly, considerable body of literature of worldwide scope has developed. The nature of these developments is described in some detail in the section on history in Chapter 1. It has become evident that many factors contribute in an important way in increasing or decreasing susceptibility to diabetes, and that systematic epidemiologic study has great potential for elucidating mechanisms by which both diabetes and its various specific manifestations are caused or prevented. These circumstances prompted the U.S. National Institutes of Health to sponsor the preparation of this book as a special project of its National Library of Medicine. A grant was made to the author in 1975, of which this book is the product.

One of the major deterrents in this field has been that pertinent publications have arisen from widely diverse and sometimes obscure sources in many countries. A major purpose of this book is to facilitate scholarship in this discipline by compiling a comprehensive bibliography. The collaboration of the University of Oklahoma Health Sciences Library and the international network of the National Library of Medicine made possible the retrieval and review of approximately 5,000 publications from which a selected list of about 2,500 was developed for presentation here as an alphabetized bibliography. More than 90% of these are recent publications, but publications of historical interest are also included.

This book is designed to serve the wide range of disciplines concerned with the diabetes problem. It will be of particular interest to scientists in diabetes and epidemiology, but also to several related disciplines. For example, Chapters 7 and 8 review the profound effects of nutrition and obesity on the pathogenesis of diabetes. Important obstetric aspects of diabetes are discussed in Chapters 7 (parity) and 9 (fetal morbidity). Chapter 7 also reviews the genetics of diabetes. Chapter 8 will be of interest to pediatricians, since it contains the most comprehensive review yet published on the epidemiology of childhood-onset diabetes, including discussion of the roles of infection and immunopathy. The section on screening in Chapter 4 is intended to assist public health specialists in designing and conducting screening programs. The section on diagnostic procedures in Chapter 5 has direct relevance for practicing physicians. Finally, Chapter 10 on the morbid effects of diabetes reviews subjects of concern to surgeons, cardiologists, neurologists, ophthalmologists, and nephrologists. Another major objective of the book is to bring these epidemiologic observations to the attention of scientists in basic and clinical research who will be in a position to exploit these clues.

This book is dedicated to my mentors, colleagues, and students, from whom I have learned so much, and particularly to Elliot P. Joslin (1869–1963). Joslin was not regarded as an epidemiologist, but in a sense he was the first epidemiologist in the field of diabetes. As early as 1921, amidst a general nihilism about this "constitutional" disorder, he was stressing that most cases were preventable and describing the need for systematic studies of the diabetes "epidemic".

Kelly M. West

ACKNOWLEDGEMENT

*Preparation of this book was made possible by a grant
from the Special Scientific Project Program
of the National Library of Medicine,
National Institutes of Health, U.S.A.*

1
CHAPTER

Epidemiologic Approaches in the Study and Control of Diabetes

HISTORY

The Appendix to this chapter lists some landmarks in the history of the epidemiology of diabetes. Details concerning most of these events and a discussion of their significance appear in the various sections of this volume to which they apply. Specific bibliographic citations are not provided in the Appendix, but these are given in subsequent discussions of these landmark publications. Many other observations of historical importance are also mentioned in these other sections. Before 400 BC Hindu physicians had recognized the importance of both genetic and environmental factors in the etiology of diabetes (Ajgaonkar, 1972).

The utility of epidemiologic approaches became apparent when they provided important clues to the causes and prevention of infectious diseases such as cholera and yellow fever. But as early as the eighteenth century the potentialities of epidemiologic observations in noninfectious diseases had also been demonstrated. In 1775 Sir Percival Potts showed that cancer of the scrotum was much more common in chimney sweeps than in the general population, thereby providing an important clue concerning one of its causes. Since that time epidemiologic studies have become a powerful weapon in the attack on

Doctors Lewis Kuller and Nabih Asal made helpful suggestions concerning this chapter.

cancer. Indeed, the demonstration by epidemiologists that smoking causes cancer of the lung greatly enhanced the recognition of the potentialities of this discipline. Another important example of the practical application of epidemiologic methods in the control of noninfectious disease was the observations of Goldberger (1914) that led to the discovery of the cause of pellagra and to its virtual eradication in the United States.

The recent success of epidemiologic approaches in the investigation of cardiovascular diseases served as an important stimulant to the application of epidemiologic methods in the study of diabetes. It became evident that susceptibility to most of the major cardiovascular diseases is strongly affected by environmental factors that are subject to identification, measurement, and control. Large-scale cardiovascular studies initiated in the 1950s and 1960s were emulated with profit by diabetologists in the 1960s and 1970s.

Important landmarks in the discipline of epidemiology itself are not cited in the Appendix. Nor does this historical summary cite the many important events in the science of diabetes (eg, the discovery of insulin). The history of epidemiology and of diabetes have been well covered in many other publications.

Systematic epidemiologic studies in diabetes were few prior to 1960. Although Joslin applied the term "epidemic" as early as 1921, his famous diabetes textbook did not mention the term epidemiology in its 1959 edition, and this term was quite rare in other diabetes literature of the time. In fact, the author of this book did not even realize his own work constituted epidemiology until he was informed of this by a "real" epidemiologist in 1966! Very little of the work on the epidemiology of diabetes was done by persons with formal training in epidemiology. Much of the early work on the epidemiology of diabetes, including that of the author, suffered from this shortcoming. Joslin and his associates were, however, greatly helped by the collaboration of professional statisticians, especially Dublin and Marks, whose work is repeatedly cited below. It is now clear that the most effective designs are developed when there is competence and experience in both epidemiology and diabetes. In very recent years epidemiologic studies in diabetes reflect an increasing sophistication, as diabetologists learn from epidemiologists and vice versa.

OBJECTIVES, POTENTIALITIES, AND METHODS

There is no standard definition of the term *epidemiology*. Many definitions have been offered, differing more in language than in concept or meaning. One of the better brief descriptions has been formulated by D. D. Reid (1973): "The immediate aim of epidemiologic research is to seek the sources of disease in the variation of its frequency according to time or season, geography or the habits and characteristics of those affected by it". A distinctive feature of the epidemiologic approach is the study of populations and subpopulatons. Clues to prevention are sought by systematically examining the circumstances under which susceptibility to the disease is high or low. A major objective of epidemiologic work is disease prevention.

Epidemiologic approaches useful in the study of diabetes are quite similar to those employed in the epidemiologic investigation of other chronic diseases. Since these approaches have been well described elsewhere (eg, McMahon and Pugh, 1970; Lilienfeld, 1976), this dicussion will not restate these principles or discuss their application in detail. Rather, some examples and explanations will be given concerning their application in the study of diabetes. Many other examples will be given in subsequent chapters. Kessler and Levin (1970) have published a good summary on epidemiologic studies in communities, much of which has application to diabetes-related investigation.

Epidemiology is basically a research discipline, but some of its operational methods make possible achievement of other objectives. Epidemiologic studies in populations, for instance, frequently serve also as instruments for case detection. Screening and detection have become a traditional element of the epidemiology of diabetes (Chapter 4). Another potentiality of the application of epidemiologic methods in diabetes is the assessment of the costs of diabetes and the evaluation of effectiveness in relation to cost of alternative approaches in attacking this problem (Chapter 2). Rather little diabetes-related work of this type has been done, but this method has considerable potential (White, 1976). Another potentiality of epidemiologic approaches is the further definition, classification, and characterization of the various special types of diabetes (eg, fat and lean maturity-onset diabetes, insulin-dependent and insulin-independent diabetes, ketosis-prone and ketosis-resistant types, and the like). These matters are discussed in detail below, particularly in Chapters 3 and 8. It is now clear that diabetes has many causes and that multiple etiologic factors are often present in individual cases. This indicates the applicability of the "risk factor" concepts so widely employed in the study of vascular disease. The section on heredity in Chapter 7 outlines the many potentialities of epidemiologic approaches in determining the importance and characteristics of genetic influences in the etiology and manifestations of diabetes.

The epidemiologic approach to the study of diabetes has four main elements:

1. Studies designed to define diabetes or its characteristics or manifestations (eg, "ketosis", "hyperglycemia"); a closely related aspect of this function of definition is the development of standards of classification and methods;

2. Descriptive epidemiology, including appraisal of the distribution of diabetes or its manifestations in relation to time, place, person, and the natural history of the disease;

3. Analytic epidemiology, including the study of the relationships of certain "risk factors" and host characteristics to the likelihood of developing the disease, and the evaluation of the etiologic significance of these relationships;

3

4. Experimental epidemiology and clinical trials, including evaluation of the efficacy of various approaches to prevention and treatment, and the development and execution of experimental designs to test specific hypotheses.

The Need for Definition and Standardization

Standardization of definition and technique is crucial to interpretation. The following examples will illustrate this need. Rates of diabetes differ as much as threefold depending on its definition (West, 1975). Rates may also differ several fold depending on methods of ascertainment. In Bedford, England (Keen, 1964) rates of impaired glucose tolerance were more than six times the rates of known diabetes, and also more than six times the rates of confirmed diabetes as determined by follow-up diagnostic tests in all glycosurics. In the United States roughly 4% of middle-aged adults say they have diabetes, but about 15% have imparied glucose tolerance by certain traditional standards (West, 1971). The same need for standardization of definition and procedure exists in the study of the manifestations of diabetes. For example, rates of neuropathy vary tremendously, depending on methods of appraisal and criteria. An important accomplishment of the epidemiologic study of diabetes has been to show the imprecision of definition that had often prevailed concerning terms such as "diabetes" and "abnormal glucose tolerance". Epidemiologic evaluations have helped to reveal the great waste that results when data are collected in the absence of such definitions. Certain aspects of the need for standardization are dicussed in some detail in Chapter 3 under definition and classification, and receive further review in other sections. Techniques for measuring sensitivity and specificity of tests for diabetes are reviewed in Chapter 4 in the section on screening.

Descriptive Epidemiology

Mortality statistics have been a major focus of previous work on the epidemiology of diabetes. Many valuable clues concerning the nature of diabetes and its causes have come from this source. It is now evident, however, that further improvement and refinements of method will be required in order to exploit further the potentialities of death registration data. These matters receive attention in Chapter 6 on mortality.

A prime epidemiologic instrument is the measurement of rates of occurrence and their relationship to such variables as the factors of time, place, and person. Occurrence may be measured by determining prevalence or incidence. Chapter 5 discusses prevalence and incidence in detail. *Incidence* is the frequency of new cases in a certain fixed period of time, and has usually been expressed as a proportion of the population at risk (eg, 132 per 100,000). With a chronic disease such as diabetes this rate is usually most appropriately expressed in a unit of considerable duration (eg, 132 per 100,000 per year). *Prevalence* is the rate of disease as measured at one point in time. For chronic diseases such rates are often expressed as number of cases per 1,000 of the population at risk. In this book rates are frequently expressed as a percentage of the population at risk (cases per 100).

Newill (1963) has reviewed methods of ascertaining and expressing incidence and prevalence of diabetes and problems relating thereto. In some circumstances the number of hospital inpatients and outpatients with diabetes reflects fairly well the actual rate of diagnosed cases. This is particularly true if numbers can be counted in all hospitals or clinics serving an area and if practice is largely confined to these clinics. Data on sales or distribution of insulin and oral hypoglycemic agents, as well as counts of those requiring diabetic diets have also been used in estimating prevalence. Methods of this kind were used in some of the pioneer surveys in Scandinavia as described in Chapter 5 on prevalence. Of the very few special registries that have been developed, prime examples are the registries in Denmark and Britain for childhood-onset cases as described in Chapter 8. Another method of measuring occurrence is to select a representative sample of physicians and then count the number of diabetics they observe. Some of the estimates of the U.S. National Diabetes Commission (1976) were based on that approach.

One of the better methods for estimating prevalence is to administer screening tests to a representative sample of a population, and to follow up with definitive testing on all available positive screenees and on a subsample of negative screenees. Among the advantages of this approach is the ability to ascertain rates of both known and occult diabetes. An example of this was the survey in Bedford, England (Sharp, 1964; Butterfield, 1964; Keen, 1964). In a very few instances glucose-loading tests have been performed on whole populations (eg, Hayner, et al, 1965; Welborn et al, 1968) or in a large representative sample (eg, Gordon, et al, 1964). Probably the most frequent mistake made in previous epidemiologic studies of diabetes has been the computation of prevalence rate under the erroneous assumption that the prevalence of diabetes in negative screenees was zero. This and other methodologic problems are explained further in Chapter 5 on prevalence and incidence. Chapter 5 also discusses the sensitivity and specificity of the various methods of ascertainment.

Studies of incidence (not prevalence) of diabetes have been rare, but would be quite useful. The few data available are reviewed in Chapter 5. Among the best data of this type are those of Bennett el at (1976a). Of particular utility would be studies of the incidence of the particular manifestations of diabetes in whole populations or representative samples thereof. Examples of this approach include the studies of Garcia, et al (1974) and Bennett, et al (1976a). Studies of incidence and prevalence of diabetes or its complications in clinic populations have been common and useful. But patterns of these manifestations in clinics may be different in some respects from patterns of morbidity in the general population of diabetics. The more famous the clinic, the greater the potential for certain kinds of bias.

Typical illustrations may be given of the value of incidence data. If one studies the prevalence of blindness or of amputation in a group of diabetics, rates of these vascular complications are usually modest, but only because diabetics who have these lesions also have very high death rates. In such circumstances rates of prevalence of blindness or amputee status reflect very incompletely the occurrence of these problems, while incidence rates reveal the profound excess of these problems in diabetics. Most studies show that among patients with acute myocardial infarction, diabetics are more likely to die than nondiabetics. For this reason the importance of myocardial infarction in diabetes is better reflected by its incidence than by its prevalence.

The best way to determine the incidence of diabetes is to perform glucose-tolerance tests or fasting blood glucose determinations in a whole population on a periodic basis. This is rarely feasible. The program of studies in the Pima Indians is probably the only current study of this kind (Bennett, et al, 1976a). It is usually necessary to use less optimum methods of ascertainment that are less expensive and more feasible. Other sections of this volume describe recent evidence that differences in rates of diabetes as great as fivefold are not uncommon among populations and subpopulations. This suggests very great potential for preventive measures, particularly because these differences are not mainly the results of genetic influences.

In most populations prevalence of diabetes varies greatly with age. Interpretation of comparative data from populations or subpopulations requires that this be fully taken into account. In well-fed societies prevalence rates in the seventh decade of life are typically more than ten times rates in the second decade. For this reason, apparent differences in rates of diabetes as great as twofold may not be significant after age corrections; moreover, similar rates may actually be quite different after age correction. Fortunately, there are standard methods available to perform such adjustments when data are available on age distribution. Many examples are cited below of age-distribution patterns of diabetes that are quite different than in the United States and Western Europe. There are also interpopulation differences of considerable degree in the distribution of diabetes between the sexes. In Belgium, for example, diabetes is considerably more frequent in women, while in Korea it is much more frequent in men. For these reasons, the most informative approach is usually an analysis of age-specific rates by sex. This permits interpopulation comparisons of prevalence of diabetes for each of several age levels. The same applies for incidence data, but they are available for very few populations. Other factors that are often matched or corrected for before making comparisons include fatness, race, and social or economic status.

Experience has shown that well-collected data on diabetes in representative samples of modest size usually provide more useful information than large-scale studies on samples that are not representative. The excellent data on diabetes gathered in the US National Surveys were obtained by testing less than 0.1% of the population. It is, of course, not always easy to select and recruit a representative sample. The technical and logistic problems of sampling are well covered in standard books on epidemiology and biostatistics. Often it is necessary to make compromises with the ideal; to the extent feasible, these compromises should be identified and acknowledged. Sometimes it is possible to compare systematically the characteristics of the subjects in the sample with known characteristics of the general population from which they are drawn. In diabetes-related studies requiring such compromises, it is well to keep in mind the major factors that influence rates of diabetes. These include family history of diabetes, age, fatness, and the many factors that may determine or be associated with adiposity (eg, sex, occupation, age, social and economic status, race, indolence). Substantial bias in respect to these factors often yields misleading results when estimates of diabetes prevalence are based on studies of samples.

A special potentiality that has received little attention until recently in epidemiologic studies of whole populations is the study of the different "complications" of diabetes. It is increasingly evident that manifestations of diabetes are greatly influenced by measurable environmental influences. In some affluent societies, for example, most diabetics die of coronary disease, while in other populations coronary disease is much less common as a manifestation of diabetes. The World Health Organization (WHO) is coordinating a multinational study on the vascular lesions of diabetes in which standardized methods are being employed. Results of studies of this kind will be helpful in determining the nature and degree of these interpopulation differences in the various vascular lesions, and in learning more about the factors that account for these variations.

Direct measurements of incidence or prevalence of diabetes have seldom been performed over time. The reasons for this are discussed in other sections of this book. Yet this approach has considerable potential. The studies in Pimas (Bennett, et al, 1976a) may be unique in this respect, although a few other studies permitted some degree of comparison over time (eg, O'Sullivan, et al in Oxford and Sudbury, Massachusetts). Changes in incidence and prevalence over time have often been crudely estimated by indirect means (eg, changes in diabetes mortality rates); in most such comparisons, however, methods and circumstances of measurement have not been well standardized over time.

Studies showing seasonal variations in the incidence of diabetes are discussed in some detail in the section on juvenile diabetes (Chapter 8). These observations are providing important leads concerning the possibility that certain infections may play a significant etiologic role in this type of diabetes.

Using techniques described above, occurrence can be related to place. The study of migrant populations has been a valuable approach in assessing the effects of environment in the etiology of diabetes. In several sections below examples will be cited illustrating the profound effects of environment on susceptibility to diabetes. It has often been difficult to determine the significance of apparent differences among countries or geographic regions in the prevalence of diabetes. But these differences will be discussed in some detail in this book because they have provided many important clues. This discussion includes a section on geography in Chapter 7.

Diabetes-related factors specific for person include birth weights of babies and parity. Among the other factors to which rates of diabetes have been related are occupation, diet, exercise, economic status, and race. These factors of time, place, and person are discussed in considerable detail in the chapters that follow.

Analytic Epidemiology

Until quite recently almost all epidemiologic studies of diabetes were mainly "descriptive". Typically, prevalence has been measured and related to certain traditional variables such as age, sex, obesity, or family history of diabetes. With increasing frequency, diabetes-related studies have included analytic elements as well. These have included appraisals of the strength of risk factors in diabetes or its complications, and systematic analyses of the interrelationships of these factors. Some of these analytic methods will be described below in this chapter and in other chapters to which they apply.

As in investigations of other chronic diseases, both prospective and retrospective approaches have been used in the study of diabetes. The characteristics, advantages, and disadvantages of these two methods have been well described in the standard epidemiology texts (eg, Lilienfeld, 1976). In general, prospective data are much to be preferred but such investigations are usually more expensive, less feasible, and may require several or many years of study before results are available. Retrospective studies are usually cheaper and more feasible. Results are available more promptly but are sometimes difficult to evaluate. If well-designed and interpreted with caution, retrospective studies are often useful. For example, in a group of diabetics the frequency of obesity or coronary disease may be compared with a nondiabetic control group whose other characteristics match as well as possible those of the diabetics (eg, matching for age, sex, geographic location, economic status). These controls may be patients with other diseases; or they may be spouses, relatives, friends, or neighbors of the diabetics. Many of the shortcomings and difficulties of interpretation with previous studies have been the result of inadequate matching of the samples of diabetics and the controls. Problems and techniques of matching are well covered by standard works in epidemiology and biostatistics, including the books of Susser (1973) and McMahon and Pugh (1970). The analytic methods to be employed must be carefully selected in light of the particular character of the data being appraised. Susser (1973) has published an excellent discussion of strategies for establishing or excluding cause-effect relationships.

There are also some applicable generalizations in determining whether associations are causal. These have been well summarized by Lilienfeld (1976). The degree of the association is relevant and important, but not decisive. The consistency of the association between the risk indicator and the disease is a useful clue. Is the association regularly observed among different populations in varying circumstances? Does the association prevail in intrapopulation studies as well as interpopulation comparisons? In our own interpopulation studies to be described in Chapters 5 and 7 we found an excellent correlation of income and frequency of diabetes. But within the United States population the association is exactly opposite; poor people have higher rates of diabetes (Bennett, et al, 1976). In ten countries where we studied diabetes, poor people were leaner than their middle-class countrymen; but in the United States poor people are now fatter than their more affluent countrymen (US Dept. of HEW, 1972). In several circumstances a strong association has been found between mean sugar consumption of populations and rates of diabetes. On the other hand, several intrapopulation studies have been negative in this respect. Details relating to these illustrations are provided in Chapter 7. When two variables have a causal relationship it is usually possible to demonstrate a relationship between the level or degree of the causal factor and risk of disease. As shown in Chapter 7, for example, increased risk of diabetes is much greater in persons who are very fat than in those who are only slightly obese.

Another approach is to examine the correspondence of the epidemiologic evidence with other scientific evidence and with common sense. There is good correlation between the number of bathtubs per country and rates of diabetes, yet it hardly seems appropriate to pursue this clue. There is no evidence from other types of scientific investigation to suggest that diabetes is caused by bathing. In contrast, consider the association by country between rates of diabetes and the use of electric power or automobiles. In evaluating the significance of the latter associations, it is relevant that exercise expends calories, promotes leanness, lowers blood glucose; and that physical conditioning appears to make possible the disposition of carbohydrate at considerably lower levels of insulin (Bjorntorp, et al, 1977).

Even strong associations may be indirect or coincidental as well as causal. And sometimes it is not obvious whether A is the cause of B, or B the cause of A. The degree of association between a factor and a disease do not necessarily reflect the extent to which that factor is causal. For example, the very strong relationship between age and risk of diabetes is to a considerable extent incidental to the relationship of age to degree and duration of adiposity. It has been suggested, therefore, that the expression "risk indicator" be used rather than "risk factor", because the latter expression is usually understood to mean causal factor. Some analytic instruments have been developed in recent years that are useful in examining the character, degree, and significance of associations. Several that have been employed in studying the causes and risk indicators in vascular disease are also applicable in diabetes-related studies. These include multiple linear regression analyses, multiple logistic regression analyses, and discriminate function analyses. These and related methods have been explained and discussed by Truett, et al (1967), Feinstein (1973), and Moss (1975). None of these sophisticated methods is a panacea for determining the extent to which associations are direct or independent; and they do not in themselves establish or exclude causal relationships.

The analytic approaches applicable in the study of diabetes are quite similar to those employed previously in the study of the epidemiology of other chronic diseases. These methods are well described in the standard texts. Among the methods for doing this is the measurement of *relative risk* (eg, rate of liver cirrhosis in diabetics in relation to rate of this disorder in nondiabetics or in the general population). *Attributable risk* is a measurement of the degree to which risk of a disease can be attributed to a specific factor either in a person or a population. Attributable risk in a population is affected by the frequency of the risk factor as well as its strength. Lilienfeld (1976) provided a good succinct summary on relative risk and attributable risk, together with references on details of computing and of ascertaining the statistical significance of differences observed.

A determination of correlation coefficient is often appropriate and useful in estimating degree of association. Indeed, this procedure is so frequently applicable that there is a tendency to employ it and interpret it mindlessly. An example will illustrate a circumstance in which this method of analysis would not be appropriate. In some urban communities of poor countries, obesity is a fairly common cause of diabetes, but many such persons later lose weight because of diabetes. There are also other persons of normal weight in these communities who become emaciated because of inadequately treated diabetes. A determination of the correlation coefficient between fatness and diabetes in such a population at one point in time might show little if any association between fatness and diabetes, even though fatness was an important cause of diabetes in that community. Chi-square tests and related procedures are sometimes applicable in determining whether differences among populations of diabetics are significant with respect to the frequency of various complications, or whether complication rates are significantly different in diabetics and nondiabetics of the same population.

Experimental and Theoretical Epidemiology

Unanimity does not exist concerning the bounds of epidemiology. Some would classify the famous studies of the University Group Diabetes Program (1970,1976) as "experimental epidemiology", while others would consider this as primarily a "clinical investigation". This Program had several aspects, some of which were well within even a narrow definition of epidemiology, but the main element was an intervention study. Groups of patients taking different forms of therapy were followed to compare many indexes of outcome with type of treatment. Enterprises of this kind have very important potentialities. They receive limited attention in this book only because they constitute a rather special type of "epidemiologic" research distinct from the major thrust of this volume.

In this study of the dynamics of infectious disease the construction of theoretical models has sometimes been helpful in developing or examining hypotheses. This technique has been little used in diabetes, but it would appear to have some application (eg, in examining some of the possible interrelationships of the factors that protect against or induce retinopathy, such as age, duration of diabetes, degree of hyperglycemia).

SOME LANDMARKS
IN THE EPIDEMIOLOGY OF DIABETES

1850   Gathering of death certificate information on diabetes was beginning in Europe and America. Followed in 1900 by development of international standardization and, after World War II, the mortality data system of World Health Organization.

1875   Bouchardat notes profound reduction and mitigation of diabetes during Prussian seige of Paris. Followed by confirmation in several societies of marked effects of deprivation during World Wars I and II.
Great nineteenth century clinicians and experimentalists of Europe make observations fundamental to epidemiology. These include Naunyn, Kulz, Frerichs, Von Noorden, Kussmaul, Hofmeister, Lancereaux, Trousseau, Bernard, and Bouchardat.

1885   August Hirsch cites geographic differences in the prevalence of diabetes.

1886   Cheevers reports on marked differences in rates of diabetes among various subpopulations of India. Followed by reports of Sen (1893) and Bose (1895) on this subject.

1907–
1909   Symposium on Diabetes in the Tropics (Havelock Charles, et al, 1907) shows the dramatic differences among and within societies in rates of diabetes.
Futcher (1907), Saundby (1908), Williamson (1909), and Lepine (1909) identify and report interpopulation differences. Barringer (1909) shows the potentialities of life insurance data, and that diabetes had become common in America.

1913   Frederick Allen's monumental book further elucidates the importance of epidemiologic factors.
Bang describes procedures for measuring blood glucose.

1916   First of 11 editions of Joslin's books.
LeGoff translates book of Iwai on diabetes in Japan.
Gottstein and Umber report on a pioneer prevalence study in a German community.

1921   Joslin applies the term "epidemic" to diabetes and demonstrates the utility of the epidemiologic approach in establishing the profound influence of fatness on risk of diabetes.

1924   First publication using the expression "epidemiology of diabetes", by Emerson and Larimore.

1930 Mills presents and analyzes data on associations between diabetes rates and variables such as geography, occupation, race, and diet.

1933–
1936 Series of classic papers of Joslin, Dublin, and Marks on the factors to which diabetes relates.
First US National Health Survey (1936) estimates prevalence of diabetes, and relates prevalence to a few variables such as age and sex.
Himsworth (1935–1936) publishes epidemiologic observations on diet and diabetes.

1940s Comprehensive countrywide and community surveys of known cases begin in Scandanavia: Vartiainen and Vartiainen (1944), Hanssen (1946), Dryer and Hey (1946), Dahlberg (1947), and Engel (1950).

1947 Wilkerson and Krall report on a comprehensive survey in a whole community (Oxford, Mass.), in which pioneer screening methods are employed. Followed by East Berlin studies of 1951 by Schliack; and by those of O'Sullivan, et al in Massachusetts.

1952 First Congress of International Diabetes Federation.

1954 S. M. Cohen on marked differences in diabetes rates among American Indian tribes.

1955 Hugh-Jones reports on some peculiar characteristics of diabetes in the tropics.
Zuidema describes diabetes in young patients with pancreatic fibrosis and calcification; followed by publications of Geevarghese.
Population surveys begin in Britain. Projects of Burns, Andrews, Redhead, Walker; followed by epidemiologic studies of Pyke, FitzGerald, Stowers, and others.

1957 Cosnett reports high prevalence of diabetes in Indians of South Africa, with a more detailed report in 1959. Followed by many other studies of migrants from India to countries of Africa, Asia, and Latin America.

1958 Silwer publishes results of a model comprehensive study of diabetes in a whole community (Kristianstad, Sweden).

1961 Observations of A. M. Cohen on diabetes in different groups of Israelis showing profound effects of environment on risk of diabetes.

1962 Landmark book of Tulloch on diabetes in the tropics. Followed by works on diabetes in Africa of Seftel, Campbell, Greenwood and Taylor, Osuntokun, Wicks, Gelfand, Jackson, and others.

1962–
1963 College of General Practitioners studies in Birmingham, England (Malins, et al).
Reports on high rates of diabetes in Polynesians of New Zealand (Prior) and Hawaii (Sloan).

1964 US National Center for Health Statistics (Gordon, et al) reports on blood glucose levels in a representative population sample.
First reports from Bedford, England on extensive and excellent studies of Keen, Jarrett, Butterfield, et al (1964–77).

1965 Hayner, et al report on blood glucose levels in a whole community (Tecumseh, Michigan).
Organization of the European Diabetes Epidemiology Study Group.
Entmacher and Marks publish a review on worldwide diabetes.

1966 First report by West and Kalbfleisch (1966–1975) on prevalence by country in international studies using standardized methods and criteria.

1967 US National Center for Health Statistics reports on characteristics of persons with diabetes in a representative sample (Bauer, MacDonald, et al).
Beginning of a series of important publications on diabetes in Pima Indians (Bennett, Miller, et al).
O'Sullivan, et al continue reports on studies in Sudbury, Boston, and Oxford.
Epidemiologic studies in Sweden of Nilsson, et al and Grönberg, et al.

1969 Reports of Goodkin, et al (1969–1975) on long-term follow-up of large numbers of insured diabetics.

1970 Publications on diabetes in Asia (Tsuii, Wada, et al), Japan (Mimura), and worldwide (Jackson) demonstrate marked effects of environment on both prevalence and manifestations of diabetes.

1971 Falconer, Duncan, and Smith on incidence of diabetes in Edinburgh and on methods in the study of incidence.

1976 Report of US Commission on Diabetes.
Publication of Bennett, et al summarizing unique and important epidemiologic studies in Pima Indians.

2

SCOPE, MAGNITUDE, AND COSTS

Only a summary is presented here; details appear in other chapters (eg, prevalence [5], mortality [6], and morbidity [10]). Arguments set forth in the Preface suggest that diabetes is now one of the major human problems, affecting all societies and all races. Although still rather uncommon in some populations, it is very common in most. Evidence described below suggests that in the more privileged societies constituting about half the world's population, roughly 10% of the inhabitants may be expected to develop diabetes. Indeed, in several populations a majority can expect to become diabetic if present trends continue (West, 1974).

Only a few systematic studies have estimated the priority and cost of diabetes as a public health problem. These costs include direct expenses of treatment such as physicians' services, drugs, and hospital care. The major cost of diabetes is the morbidity and mortality associated with its complications. This includes the tremendous costs of disability and of loss of productivity and earnings. Particularly, the toll includes blindness, amputation, and disability related to excessive rates of heart disease, stroke, and kidney failure. In Chapter 10 on morbid effects, some specifics are given on morbidity and mortality associated with each of these conditions. The significant costs difficult to measure include pain of neuropathy, discomfort of diabetic diarrhea, and the tragedy of sexual impotence, a common manifestation in men. Another very major cost is premature death from diabetes-related factors; details on mortality are set forth in Chapter 6. Suffice it to mention here that average life expectancy of childhood-onset cases is about half the normal, and, in adult-onset cases, roughly two thirds of standard. There is some evidence that, with particularly good therapy, average life expectancy of youth-onset cases is also about two thirds of normal.

Another cost of diabetes is the expenditure on programs of research and prevention (eg, screening, detection, and education). In relation to total costs these expenses are relatively trivial, roughly 1% of the costs of diabetes.

The National Diabetes Commission estimated the monetary cost of diabetes in the United States, very conservatively, at $5 billion per year (Entmacher, et al, 1976). This estimate did not include costs of undiagnosed diabetes, nor was an attempt made to compute and include full costs of the complications in those with known diabetes. Table 1 summarizes some of the estimates of the Commission concerning various elements of these costs.

Entmacher and Marks (1971) summarized data on certain of the costs of diabetes. In this, they drew upon the data of the US National Center for Health Statistics (Bauer, 1967). These latter studies provided information on rates of

TABLE 1   Costs of Diabetes in the United States (Estimated 1975)

Costs		Dollar Amounts (in Millions)
Direct Costs		
Hospital care		1,050*
Physicians' services		590†
Drugs		300‡
Nursing home care		520
Other medical professional services		60
Total direct costs		2,520 (2.5 billion)
Indirect Costs		
Earnings loss for employed diabetics		461
Morbidity	$397	
Mortality (annual)	63	
Imputed earnings loss for housewives		65
Morbidity	47	
Mortality (annual)	17	
Imputed earnings loss for institutionalized diabetics		235
Imputed earnings loss for disabled (noninstitutionalized) diabetics		996
Lifetime earnings loss from mortality of diabetics		1,066
Total indirect cost		2,823 (2.8 billion)
GRAND TOTAL (direct plus indirect)		5,343 (5.3 billion)

Source: These data are crude estimates of Entmacher, et al (1976) for National Commission on Diabetes. These costs do not include all elements of the cost of complications of diabetes.

Note: Excludes expenditures for dentists' services, eyeglasses and appliances, prepayment and administration, government and other health services, research and medical facilities construction.

*Based on days of care in short-stay hospitals.
†Cost of patient visits to physicians.
‡Cost of patient visits to physicians for which drugs were prescribed.

hospitalization, as well as work loss, frequency and degree of limitation of activity, and "bed disability". Those data also made possible rough estimates of the extent of disability from some of the major manifestations of diabetes, such as amputation and heart conditions. Details of these findings are recounted in some detail in other sections of this book as they apply to specific complications of diabetes. Although the National Center data on disability are in many respects the best available, their interpretation is in some respects difficult because control data from the general population, although gathered, were not matched with those for the diabetics with appropriate corrections for age and other characteristics. In diabetics all the types of disability mentioned above were greater than in the general population, but the diabetics were considerably older than the general population.

The excellent publication of Entmacher and Marks (1971) also reviews data of the United States Social Security Administration on disability in diabetics, and results of studies in industry of the work records of diabetics. Among the more informative of these was the study of Pell and D'Alonzo (1967). In the United States, industrial surveys of this kind have usually shown (a) that most diabetics have good records of attendance and performance, and (b) that absenteeism is slightly to moderately higher in the total group of diabetics than in nondiabetics. In some circumstances, however, rates of absenteeism for diabetics have compared very favorably with those in nondiabetics (Moore and Buschboom, 1974). In the United States and probably elsewhere there is a variable degree of discrimination against the employment of diabetics. This is another cost of diabetes. Diabetics usually pay higher rates for life insurance and face some additional restrictions; for example, those who take hypoglycemic agents cannot be licensed as aircraft pilots.

A work group of the United States National Diabetes Commission chaired by Puckett (1976) reviewed the psychosocial costs of diabetes. The most detailed account of the economic costs is also contained in the Commission Report. The section on economic impact was written by Entmacher, et al (1976). They point out the need for more complete and satisfactory data on the costs of diabetes. This review also cites some of the literature on methods of ascertaining costs of care, morbidity, and mortality relating to a specific disease. One of the major problems has been that it is often difficult to determine in individual cases whether a specific cost, disability, or death of a diabetic should be attributed to diabetes or not. This is particularly true if the diabetic himself is making this determination (eg, Was your visit to the hospital primarily for diabetes?). But this is a problem even when physicians or epidemiologists are evaluating individual cases. Often the best way to estimate costs of diabetes will be to ascertain a cost or costs in a sample of diabetics, without attempting to describe whether each of the costs is due to the diabetes or other diseases. These costs in diabetics can then be compared to those in a group representing the general population in which age and other characteristics are similar to those of the diabetics. If, for example, hospitalization is twice as common in diabetics, the excess attributable to diabetes can be estimated and a cost assigned.

17

Data on costs of diabetes are quite incomplete, but it seems likely that they constitute roughly 1% to 5% of disease costs in industrialized societies. This crude guess assumes that such costs for diabetics are excessive by a factor of about 1.5, and that the prevalence of diabetes is typically between 1% and 3%. More systematic study is warranted of each of the major elements of these costs. Data of Entmacher, et al (1976) suggest that care of diabetes accounts for about 3% of health care costs in the United States; but they point out that their estimates did not include a large segment of the costs of certain complications of diabetes.

Few data are available on diabetes-related hospital costs. In a rare study of this kind, Rabkin and Field (1962) measured costs of treating diabetics at the Massachusetts General Hospital (MGH) during the year 1957. The percentage of patients with diabetes in this institution is probably limited to a modest degree by the presence nearby of another renowned institution specializing in diabetes (New England Deaconess Hospital—Joslin Clinic). Of patients on the public wards at MGH, 6.4% were diabetics, and 2.1% of private inpatients had diabetes. The costs per patient were higher for diabetics. Costs of care of diabetics represented 8.0% of all costs for ward services, and 2.3% of costs for private services. About 15% of the costs of care of diabetic patients were for treatment of peripheral vascular disease. This heavy burden appeared to be the main reason that hospital care of diabetics was more expensive than that of nondiabetics. In a general hospital of Israel, where diabetes seems to be less common than in the United States, only 2.5% of patients were diagnosed diabetics Lender and Menczel (1977). But 13% of patients over 40 years of age were diagnosed diabetics.

Ranofsky (1977) found that in 1975 about 533,000 of the patients discharged from short-stay US non-federal hospitals had a primary diagnosis of diabetes (1.5% of all cases). There were, however, 1,893,000 cases in which diabetes was one of the diagnoses (5.6 of all patients). In patients over 44 years of age diabetes was mentioned in 10%. Average hospital stay was 7.7 days for all patients, but 10.2 days for those with a primary diagnosis of diabetes.

Almost no data are available on the relationship of cost to effectiveness of various preventive or therapeutic methods. What, for example, is the cost of dietary instruction? And what measurable benefits are achieved by different approaches to dietary instruction? A major need is for data relating subsequent expenditures for hospitalization to the quality, quantity, or character of instruction of diabetics.

18

3

CURRENT CONCEPTS,
NATURAL HISTORY, CLASSIFICATIONS, AND DEFINITIONS

DEFINITION AND BRIEF DESCRIPTION OF DIABETES

No widely accepted definition exists. Diabetes mellitus is a disease in which there is an excess of glucose in the plasma. Frequently there are other metabolic aberrations, including qualitative and quantitative abnormalities of carbohydrate and lipid metabolism, characteristic pathologic changes in small blood vessels and in nerves, and intensification of atherosclerosis.

The classical symptoms of diabetes, excessive urination (polyuria) and thirst (polydipsia) are the direct result of the elevated blood glucose levels. These cardinal symptoms are not present with mild hyperglycemia. Polyphagia (excessive food intake) is also a classical symptom, but it occurs only with severe diabetes. The primary controlling influence on the level of blood glucose is insulin secreted by the pancreas. Diabetes is thus the result of inadequate circulating insulin. This lack may be either absolute or relative. In obese subjects with mild diabetes, for example, rather generous amounts of insulin are often secreted; but because of the resistance to insulin that characterizes obesity, these amounts are inadequate to meet the raised requirements.

The major deterrent to the development of a relatively simple standard definition is the reluctance of many scholars to accept a definition in which the sole criterion is the excessive blood glucose. This reluctance is based on several considerations. Some have thought that certain of the manifestations of diabetes may be the direct result of a fundamental genetic defect or defects, and not

19

attributable to hyperglycemia itself. Moreover, evidence is not yet conclusive that correction of hyperglycemia mitigates or prevents all of the several patho- logic changes observed with diabetes. Also, there have been a few instances in which characteristic complications of diabetes have been observed before hyperglycemia was apparent. These matters are discussed in some detail below, and the conflict of evidence and opinion is reviewed. The arguments against hyperglycemia as the sole diagnostic criterion deserve attention, but this writer does not find them persuasive.

Taking into account all available evidence, the most useful and appropriate short definition of diabetes mellitus is simply "too much glucose in the blood". With monotonous regularity characteristic complications have attended long- standing hyperglycemia in man irrespective of its cause. It is not yet clear to what extent these pathologic changes are the result of hyperglycemia itself or of related factors such as insulin insufficiency, changes in osmolality of plasma or tissues, aberrations of serum lipids, etc. But there is increasing evidence (Cahill, et al, 1976) that the elevated blood glucose levels are of truly funda- mental importance. Chapter IV on diagnostic methods discusses criteria for determining the level at which blood glucose concentration should be deemed excessive.

PATHOPHYSIOLOGY, SYMPTOMS, AND PHYSICAL FINDINGS

When serum insulin levels reach or approach zero, as in typical cases of untreated juvenile diabetes, hyperglycemia and other metabolic aberrations become severe. These complex changes are well covered in standard textbooks. Some of the better short summaries are in *Diabetes Mellitus*, edited by Suss- man and Metz (1975), including the succinct review of Felig on pathophysiol- ogy. When blood glucose values reach levels that are about twice normal, the kidney tubules can no longer reabsorb all of the glucose presented to them and glucose begins to appear in the urine. At plasma glucose levels of 200 to 300 mg/100 ml, substantial amounts of glucosuria are usually observed. This pro- duces an osmotic effect that increases urinary flow and causes excessive thirst. When glycemia and glycosuria are severe, calories are lost from two major sources. Glucose is lost in the urine, and body protein is also depleted. This is because insufficiency of insulin enhances gluconeogenesis in liver from amino acids derived from muscle. Thus, with severe uncontrolled diabetes there is weight loss and weakness. With mild hyperglycemia, however, there are usually no symptoms.

One of the most grave manifestations of severe untreated diabetes is ketosis. The difficulty in utilization of glucose leads to a series of physiologic events producing ketones as the prime substitute fuel. These ketones have considera- ble utility as a nutrient, but their production in large amounts also leads to metabolic acidosis (ketoacidosis). Severe ketoacidosis causes coma that is sometimes fatal. As will be pointed out below, the frequency of the propensity to ketosis varies considerably among groups of diabetics. The findings of Silwer (1958) in a Swedish population are typical of those usually observed in well-fed societies. Thirteen percent of diabetics had had ketosis and an additional 10% had exhibited a tendency to develop ketosis. Thus, about 77% were "ketosis-resistant". In fatter populations the proportion who are ketosis-prone is smaller. In Oklahoma Indians it is less than 5% (West, 1974). In general, this propensity is related to the degree of insulinopenia. A very high percentage of patients with childhood-onset diabetes have little or no insulin in the blood and a marked tendency to develop ketosis, if treatment is suboptimal.

A common symptom of uncontrolled diabetes is blurring of vision. This is often secondary to reversible changes in configuration of the lens produced by osmotic effects of hyperglycemia. Another common symptom is itching of the vagina and its orifice. This "pruritis vulvae" is primarily the result of contamination of gential tissues by urine glucose. In some circumstances it is the most common symptom of diabetes in females.

Prevalence of Symptoms

Surprisingly few studies have determined systematically the frequency of various symptoms and their relationship to factors such as age, sex, and degree of glycemia. One problem is that most clinic groups of diabetics are not representative samples of the entire population of diabetics. Also, the frequency of most symptoms is quite different in previously undiscovered diabetes, as contrasted with diabetics who have been under treatment for months or years. Frequency of the different symptoms is also affected by factors such as intensity of treatment, degree of acceptance of recommended therapy, and age of onset.

One of the most informative assessments of the frequency of symptoms was a study by Bauer and her associates (1967) from the United States National Center for Health Statistics. They interviewed a large group of diabetics drawn from a sample of 134,000 that was representative of the United States general population, except that persons in institutions were not included. Responses were recorded from approximately 1,700 diabetics. Table 2 summarizes the results. To varying degrees, all of these symptoms lack specificity for diabetes. No data were gathered in this study on the frequency of these symptoms in the general population or in nondiabetics. Fifty-two percent of the diabetics had none of these "diabetic" symptoms. One of the few controlled studies on symptoms was that of Welborn, et al (1968) in Bussleton, Australia. They compared rates of symptoms in known diabetics and in those found to be either diabetic or nondiabetic in a survey. Increase of thirst was reported by 12% of the new "screenee" diabetics, 13% of known diabetics, and 5% of nondiabetics. Polyuria was reported by 28% of new cases, 13% of known diabetics, and 11% of nondiabetics. "Visual deterioration" was reported by 35% of new diabetics, 31% of known diabetics, and 25% of nondiabetics. A history of pruritis vulvae was reported by 29% of both groups of diabetic females and 15% of nondiabetic

21

TABLE 2 Percent of Diabetics in Each Age Group Who Had Selected Diabetic Symptoms in Month Preceding Interview, by Sex: United States, July 1964 to June 1965

SEX AND AGE	EXTREME TIREDNESS	LEG PAIN	EYE TROUBLE	SUDDEN WEAKNESS	FREQUENT URINATION	THIRST	ITCHING	LOSS OF WEIGHT	LARGER APPETITE	SMALLER APPETITE
					PERCENT					
BOTH SEXES										
All ages	26.5	22.5	20.1	18.6	18.0	14.3	14.0	9.0	8.9	7.4
Under 45 years	23.7	11.2	14.8	17.6	11.5	13.7	11.2	5.3	8.1	3.3
45–64 years	26.1	22.7	19.1	18.6	17.1	14.5	14.6	7.8	9.3	6.5
65 years and over	28.1	27.1	23.5	19.0	22.1	14.1	14.6	11.9	8.8	10.2
MALE										
All ages	21.7	18.2	15.6	14.1	16.2	11.5	9.7	6.9	7.4	5.7
Under 45 years	17.5	8.5	10.6	12.7	*7.4	11.6	*4.2	*2.6	*6.9	*4.2
45–64 years	23.1	19.0	15.7	15.7	15.7	10.6	11.1	5.8	7.0	5.8
65 years and over	22.3	22.1	18.2	13.4	21.5	12.6	10.9	10.3	8.1	6.4
FEMALE										
All ages	29.8	25.6	23.3	21.8	19.4	16.2	17.1	10.5	10.0	8.6
Under 45 years	29.4	13.7	18.1	22.5	15.2	15.7	17.2	7.4	9.3	*2.5
45–64 years	23.0	25.3	21.5	20.6	18.0	17.5	17.2	9.3	10.8	6.9
65 years and over	31.9	30.3	27.0	22.8	22.5	15.0	17.0	12.9	9.4	12.7

Source: Bauer, 1967 (National Center for Health Statistics).
*Data to be evaluated with caution because of small numbers.

women. Higher rates of symptoms would be expected in new diabetics discovered by means other than glucose tolerance tests.

In the Bedford, England survey, symptoms of diabetes were only slightly more common in those with two-hour blood glucose levels over 120 mg/100 ml than in those with lower values (Keen, 1964). Beaser (1948) studied the frequency of various symptoms at the time of discovery of diabetes in a group subsequently treated in a large diabetic clinic. Only 34% had had classical symptoms of diabetes, and 23% had had no symptoms deemed suggestive of diabetes. In Rochester, Minnesota, the prevalence of polyuria and thirst was determined at the onset of diabetes in 1,099 cases (Palumbo, et al, 1976). These classical symptoms were found to be present in 31%. In patients with discovery after age 30 only about one quarter had these symptoms, as compared to three quarters of the younger patients. A history of weight loss was recorded in only 24%, even though 47% of those with onset under 30 years of age had had weight loss.

No standard conventions exist with respect to the form of questions intended to elicit information about symptoms. Note, for example, that the National Survey Questionnaire asked about "frequency of urination", not polyuria (amount) of urine. Nor has there been any standardization of the time frame to which the questions apply. The frequency of positive answers would, of course, be different if the subject were asked whether the symptoms had occurred during the past days, weeks, months, or years. None of the three leading textbooks on diabetes lists the term "symptoms" in its index. There is need to evaluate more fully effectiveness in relation to cost of interview methods in the detection of diabetes in both the general population and in special elements such as children, close relatives of diabetics, and obese people. Development of standard conventions would make possible such studies and comparisons. Standardization would also make it possible to compare data from different populations of diabetics. It would also be helpful to evaluate more fully the sensitivity and the specificity of each of the different symptoms in various circumstances, age groups, etc, by applying standard questions in both diabetics and nondiabetics.

Here is suggested some standard nomenclature for determining presence and degree of symptoms relating to diatetes. They might serve as a basis for developing later an improved revision to be promulgated by an official body such as the International Diabetes Federation or the World Health Organization.

In the past two months have you:

> been unusually thirsity?
> been passing more urine than usual?
> been unusually hungry?
> lost weight?
> been unusually tired?

been unusually weak?
had blurred vision?

Quantitation can be determined if desired by applying three grades of degree to any of the symptoms when present: "Would you say that this symptom or problem (eg, thirst) is of slight, moderate, or severe degree?" Weight loss might be further specifically quantitated by asking whether it is estimated to exceed 2 kg or 5 lb ("yes", "no", "don't know").

This language with very slight modification could be applied in assessing previous status during the two-month period just before discovery of diabetes.

Physical Findings

The clinically detectable stigmata associated with the major complications of diabetes will be reviewed in detail below. Among the findings that sometimes suggest the diagnosis are the following: carbuncles, gangrene, retinopathy, inflammation of the vaginal labia, balantitis and xanthomata. None of these has both a high degree of sensitivity and specificity for diabetes.

NATURAL HISTORY AND MAJOR COMPLICATIONS

In sections below, details will be provided on mortality, on morbidity, and on mortality by complication. The classical symptoms of diabetes (polyuria and polydipsia) are usually easily controlled with standard therapeutic measures. Patients with no endogenous insulin usually have blood glucose levels that are labile as well as high. Aggressive attempts to lower blood glucose levels with insulin therapy in such instances often lead to "insulin reactions", particularly if treatment is clumsily applied. When such hypoglycemic episodes are mild or of short duration they produce unpleasant symptoms, sometimes even unconsciousness, but no permanent damage to nervous tissue. Rarely, with severe prolonged hypoglycemia, permanent brain damage occurs, resulting in decreased mental accuity or death. Risk of serious brain injury is negligible with skillful therapy, but significant with clumsy insulin therapy. Death from diabetic coma (hyperglycemia) is much more common, and death from the vascular complications of diabetes is in most circumstances about 100 times more common than death from hypoglycemia secondary to overtreatment with insulin.

Many diabetic children survive more than forty years, but averge life expectancy is about half the normal. Expectancy is better with optimal therapy. Death and severe complications are now very uncommon in the first decade of childhood-onset diabetes. In this first decade of diabetes the main cause of these infrequent deaths is diabetic coma (ketoacidosis). Severe kidney failure often occurs in the second or third decade of diabetes. The main culprit is usually glomerulosclerosis. In the third and fourth decade of childhood-onset diabetes the main causes of death are coronary disease and glomerulosclerosis.

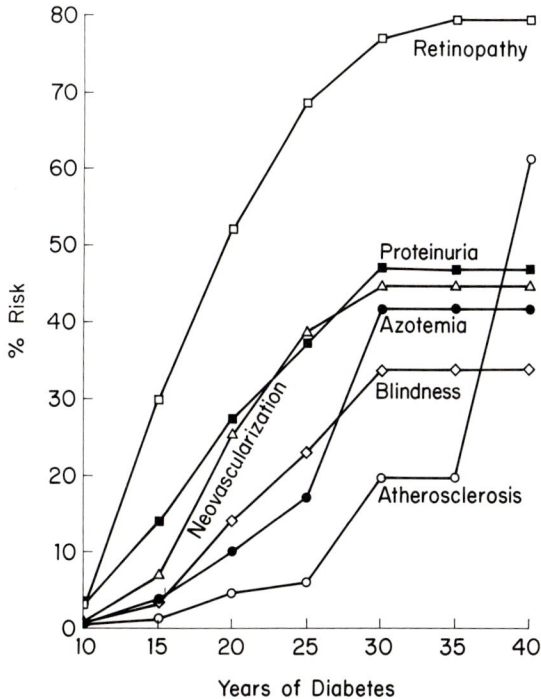

FIGURE 1. Cumulative risks of complications in juvenile diabetes. These observations of Knowles, et al (1971) yielded results typical of those of other investigators.

An excellent account of the natural history of diabetes appears in the 11th edition of Joslin's book (Marble, et al, 1971). Figure 1 summarizes a typical experience in a group of childhood-onset diabetics (Knowles, et al, 1971).

In adult-onset cases longevity is highly variable, averaging about two thirds of normal. In most affluent societies of the West the main cause of death in diabetics is coronary disease. This is discussed below in detail. In diabetics over 60 years of age of Western societies, gangrene of the foot is common, usually requiring amputation of the leg. Both young and old diabetics more commonly develop cataract than age-matched nondiabetics. A major problem for both young and old diabetics is retinopathy, now the major cause of new cases of blindness in American adults under the age of 70.

The major "complications" of diabetes are summarized here:

1. *Large-vessel disease* (mainly atherosclerosis);

> Coronary disease (myocardial infarction, congestive heart failure, angina)
>
> Leg vessel disease (gangrene, ulceration, and infection of feet)
>
> Cerebrovascular disease (cerebral thrombosis).

25

2. *Small-vessel disease:*

>   Glomerulosclerosis (uremia, hypertension)
>
>   Retinopathy (blindness)

3. *Neuropathies:* pain, numbness, paralysis; sexual impotence (in men)

4. *Ketoacidosis:* diabetic coma

5. *Cataract*

6. *Increased susceptibility to certain infections:* eg, tuberculosis, carbuncles

7. *In diabetic mothers:* increased rates of fetal and neonatal death, increased birth weights of babies

Some have with good reason questioned the propriety of using the expression "complications" in this sense. Indeed, the terms "manifestations" or "effects" are probably more appropriate, because these morbid changes are for the most part direct effects of the disease. The term "complications" was applied widely because many diabetics did not have evidence of some or any of these stigmata. It is now evident that most with long-standing diabetes have these pathologic changes to some degree. Certain of these manifestations appear to be an integral element of the disease. Most patients with long-standing diabetes, who do not have clinically evident microvascular or neuropathic diseases, do exhibit morbid changes when more sensitive methods are applied, such as biochemical analyses of nerves, biopsy of capillaries, and retinal examination after fluorescein injections.

It is generally held that diabetes is seldom curable or reversible. Indeed, neither cure no substantial mitigation of severity is very common. But potentialities for reversal are considerably greater than is generally recognized. The very great potentialities for reversing diabetes in obese patients are documented in detail in the section on obesity (Chapter 7). In severe juvenile diabetes temporary remission of severity is common with aggressive therapy. Spontaneous remission is uncommon in diabetes, but not so rare as most physicians believe. Patel, et al (1966c) have observed 24 cases. Long-term complete remission is particularly rare in well-established insulin-dependent diabetes, but occurs occasionally (Peck, et al, 1958).

CLASSIFICATION, NOMENCLATURE, AND CONVENTIONS

Problems

Chapter 8 discusses further the classification of special types of diabetes. Several different classification schemes have been proposed (eg, WHO, 1965; Lawrence, 1951; Marble, 1971; Danowski, 1975; Irvine, 1977). None has received general acceptance as a means for standardization, description, or data collection, due to several difficulties. One was that older schemes did not have the advantages of more recent knowledge and methods such as the measurement of insulin secretion. Another problem has been that classifications can and have been based on several *different* indexes or mixtures thereof, including etiology, age of onset, severity of hyperglycemia, presence or absence of ketonemia, type of treatment required or employed, degree of adiposity, and other clinical characteristics.

Attempts to simplify also created problems. Since in affluent societies most youth-onset cases are lean, insulin-dependent, and ketosis-prone, it was suggested that these cases be called juvenile-type diabetes. We now know, however, that insulin-independent diabetes is not rare in young, that occasionally youth-onset cases may be fat, that insulin-dependent diabetes is not uncommon in adults, and that it may constitute a substantial portion of adult-onset diabetes in some societies. Moreover, diabetes is sometimes mild in lean diabetics, and in some societies a majority of young insulin-dependent diabetics are not ketosis-prone. Thus attempts to simplify by grouping the four parameters (severity, age of onset, adiposity, and susceptibility to ketosis) inevitably leads to formidable problems. Many etiologic agents, both genetic and enviromental, may produce either mild or severe diabetes. Thus classifications by etiology are not appropriately mixed with classifications by severity or clinical characteristics. Listed below are some indexes of classification that have been traditionally employed.

1. Etiology (genetic, pancreatic, steroid, etc)
2. Age of onset (juvenile or growth-onset, adult or maturity-onset, senile, etc)
3. Adiposity (obese and nonobese)
4. Severity of expression or therapy required
   a. presence or absence of classical symptoms (clinical, symptomatic, or chemical diabetes)
   b. degree of hyperglycemia (mild, moderate, severe)
   c. presence or absence of ketonemia (ketosis-prone or ketosis-resistant)
   d. presence or absence of complications (eg, Kimmelsteil-Wilson syndrome)
   e. type of therapy required (insulin-dependent, insulin-independent, diet-controlled)
   f. sensitivity to insulin (sensitive or resistant)
5. Other concomitants (hyperlipoproteinemia, gestational diabetes, lipodystrophy, liver disease), or specific combinations of concomitants ("J" or Jamaica diabetes, syndromes of Zuidema and of Tattersall, presence of immunologic indices, such as islet-cell antibodies or certain histocompatibility antigens, etc)

One of these indexes of classification has been sensitivity to insulin (Falta and Boller, 1931; Himsworth, 1936, 1939). This index has much to recommend it, but there are problems in developing and applying this criterion of definition. Degree of insulin sensitivity may often be correctly deduced on clinical grounds. For example, fat subjects are usually resistant, and most lean patients are sensitive, but there are exceptions to these generalizations. Furthermore, the relationship of insulin sensitivity to severity of hyperglycemia is not predictably inverse. Even with simultaneous measurement of serum insulin and glucose it may be difficult to measure sensitivity to endogenous or exogenous insulin with precision, and sensitivity to endogenous and exogenous insulin do not always correspond.

The simplified classification of diabetes shown below is based only on clinically measurable responses to therapy with insulin or diet. It explains the usual relationships between this index of classification and other factors such as age of onset, adiposity, endogenous insulin secretion, severity of hyperglycemia, and susceptibility to ketosis.

1. Type of I-D (insulin-dependent)

   a. *IDc (insulin-dependence complete or nearly conplete)*:
   ketosis-prone. Endogenous insulin absent or grossly inadequate. Ketonemia and severe hyperglycemia despite optimal diet therapy. Patients usually, but not invariably, lean. Onset typically in youth, but not rare in maturity. If duration short, may sometimes be reversible for months or years with aggressive insulin therapy;

   b. *IDp (insulin-dependence partial)*:
   hyperglycemia and attendant symptoms in the absence of insulin treatment despite otherwise optimal therapy. Under basal conditions ketosis does not occur even in the absence of insulin therapy;

2. Type I-I (insulin-independent):

   If present, classical symptoms can be reversed without insulin therapy. Endogenous insulin is relatively inadequate but usually considerable. In affluent societies these patients are usually obese but may be lean. Not ketosis-prone unless beta-cell function later deteriorates. Optimal diet therapy usually greatly improves beta-cell function in fat patients.

A disadvantage of this system is that it does not specifically list many of the type of diabetes that have either a peculiar etiology (eg, lipotrophic diabetes) or special manifestations (eg, hypertriglyceridemia). On the other hand, all known types of diabetes can be accommodated within the general framework of this simplified system.

There is, however, no generally accepted definition of "insulin-dependence"; developing a standard definition would be very difficult, perhaps impossible. The line between insulin-dependence and insulin-independence must be an arbitrary one, and the difference among cases in this respect is only one of degree. One possible criterion of insulin-independence is whether classical symptoms secondary to hyperglycemia, such as polyuria, can be relieved in a given period of time by standard therapeutic procedures other than insulin. It could be argued, however, that even asymptomatic patients should be regarded as insulin-dependent unless normal or near-normal fasting glucose levels are achieved without insulin. On the other hand, this line of reasoning could lead to the argument that all diabetics are insulin-dependent unless therapy without insulin is capable of restoring normal fasting glucose values, or even normal or nearly normal postpradnial levels. Indeed, it would be highly desirable to have these or some other indexes of degree of reversibility without insulin as part of the classification system, but the information required is rarely available. Normal body weight has been achieved permanently only rarely in typical obese maturity-onset diabetics. Thus it is seldom possible in fat diabetics to determine with certainty the long-term effects of optimum therapy.

Another difficulty in the great variation among clinicians in their criteria of "satisfactory" control. Some physicians would classify almost all diabetics as "insulin-dependent" from a clinical standpoint, while others would classify as insulin-dependent only the small minority who are symptomatic despite optimum therapy with diet and oral agents. Another problem of classification is that some patients, who would not require insulin after long-term optimum diet therapy, will require insulin at first, even with optimum diet treatment.

An alternative criterion of insulin-dependence would be whether, in fact, the patient is taking insulin, rather than whether he or she appears to need insulin. This system, however, introduces even greater heterogeneity within classes. This heterogeneity is the result of factors such as differences among physicians in criteria in discerning whether treatment with insulin is needed, the lack of any standard epidemiologic conventions for need of insulin therapy, and intergroup differences in rates of patient acceptance of advice to take insulin.

With optimal diet a substantial portion of those who take insulin would not need it (Mahler, 1974a). Probably more than half of American diabetics take oral agents, but this group is divided between the substantial majority who with adequate weight reduction would not require medication, and a significant minority who would need medication despite optimal diet.

Type of therapy does reflect roughly the degree of insufficiency of endogenous insulin. Beta-cell decompensation is greatest in those who take insulin, least in those treated with diet alone, and intermediate in those to whom oral agents are administered. But type of therapy is not a highly reliable index of residual beta-cell capacity. One reason for this is the very substantial differences in the criteria used by physicians in advising therapy of the various types.

From 13 published studies, Silwer (1958) reviewed information on the percentages receiving insulin in different groups of diabetics. Most of these surveys were performed before the introduction of oral agents. The proportion taking insulin ranged from 21% to 83%. Mimura (1970) cited some figures from Asian countries on the percentage of diabetics who were treated with insulin: in Japan 23% were receiving insulin, in Hong Kong 46%, and in Korea 41%. Bauer (1967) found that about 28% of American diabetics took insulin (see Table 3 for details). It appeared that to a considerable degree these differences

29

TABLE 3 Percent of Diabetics in Each Age Group, by Medication at the Time of the Survey: United States, July 1964 to June 1965

AGE	INSULIN ONLY	ORAL DRUGS ONLY	NEITHER MEDICATION
		PERCENT	
All ages	25.7*	48.4	24.0
Under 25 years	67.6	7.2	23.4
25–44 years	30.2	31.3	35.9
45–54 years	24.9	48.8	23.9
55–64 years	21.1	55.7	21.2
65–74 years	23.4	53.1	21.6
75 years and over	20.7	54.7	23.0

Source: Bauer, 1967 (US National Center for Health Statistics).
*Total on insulin was 28% because 3% took both insulin and oral agents.

are attributable to differences in criteria of insulin-dependence. For these reasons, classifications based on the type of therapy actually being applied leave much to be desired. This formidable list of problems in defining insulin-dependence is not an exhaustive one. Some other means of classification would be preferable, but the use of the terms insulin-dependent and insulin-independent is so ingrained that departure from this concept is difficult.

In diabetes clinics there is often considerable bias in distribution of types of cases. For example, physicians in general practice may treat mild cases, while referring more severe cases to a diabetes clinic. Another problem is that type of diabetes may change with time. Obese mild diabetics, for example, occasionally develop complete decompensation with severe ketosis (Drenick and Johnson, 1975). Nilsson, et al (1967) showed that in Kristianstad, Sweden, the percentage of diabetics taking insulin increased with duration of diabetes.

Recently, Irvine (1977) has suggested a system of classification an important element of which is the presence or absence of islet-cell antibodies at the time of diagnosis. But some problems with the latter system have been emphasized by Barbosa (1977) and by Cudworth and Woodrow (1977). Among the difficulties in developing a simple system of classification are the heterogeneity of etiology and the rather considerable limitations of our present knowledge of these causes of diabetes.

Some Suggestions

Standardization of classification and nomenclature would do much to enhance the collection and interpretation of epidemiologic data (Baumslag, et al, 1970). Standardization would also be helpful in teaching current concepts of diabetes to students and practitioners. The classification systems given above and below suggest many of the factors that ought to be defined and reported in epidemiologic studies (eg, fasting plasma glucose, relative weight, presence of ketonuria, age and age of onset of diabetes, type of therapy, and duration since discovery).

For reasons cited above it is clear that classifications based on insulin dependence or independence will be very difficult to design and implement. An alternative system is shown in Table 4. This system is by no means problem-free, but is probably is a more feasible instrument for epidemiologic comparisons than others that have been employed. The main index of classification is level of fasting hyperglycemia. Cases would be classified by degree of hyperglycemia in the absence of antidiabetic medication. It would seldom be necessary to withdraw such medications to permit classification, because most of these patients have had blood glucose values measured during trial periods in which the sole therapy was diet. Most of the others are patients who have had grossly elevated values of known degree before antidiabetic therapy was started. In a small percentage it would be necessary either to estimate the effects of withdrawing medication or to withdraw medication briefly to discern status of classification.

This system also contains a subclassification for fatness, because it is seldom practicable to standardize for dietary intake. Degree of glycemia is the result not only of degree of beta-cell decompensation, but also of caloric intake. In estimating degree of "diabetes", it is therefore necessary to know both degree of hyperglycemia and fatness. To enhance simplicity, fatness is not expressed

TABLE 4   Classification of Diabetes by Degree of Hyperglycemia

DEGREE OF HYPERGLYCEMIA	FASTING PLASMA GLUCOSE*
Possible (hyperglycemia) (glucose tolerance abnormal)	Normal (<130 mg/100 ml)
Mild	130–199 mg/100 ml Obese† Nonobese
Moderate	200–299 mg/100 ml Obese Nonobese
Severe	>299 mg/100 ml Obese Nonobese

Note: This classification is based on level of fasting hyperglycemia and fatness in the absence of antidiabetic drugs under basal conditions. The subclassification by fatness is necessary because degree of glycemia is related not only to degree of beta-cell decompensation, but also to caloric intake and fatness. Since caloric intake can seldom be controlled adequately for long periods in obese subjects, it is necessary to include information on fatness in order to interpret information on degree of glycemia properly.

*On a venous specimen. For determining comparable levels with other methods and types of specimens, see Cooper (1973) and Chapter 4.

†Obesity is defined as relative weight greater than 119% of standard by criteria of the NIH conferees (Bray, et al, 1976), based on the Metropolitan Insurance Company standard. Because relative weight occasionally reflects fatness inaccurately (eg, in muscular athletes), status of classification may be determined by other indexes when relative weight is deemed misleading. For example, persons with subscapular skinfolds of less than 21 mm (about 13/16 in) may be considered nonobese irrespective of weight. Another index of leanness is waist girth less than 79 cm (31 in) in women or less than 94 cm (37 in) in men.

quantitatively; rather, cases are classified as obese or nonobese by the standard criteria suggested in Table 4. Whenever possible it would be desirable to gather and report more detailed information on frequency distribution of fatness. This might include, for example, the number of diabetics who are exceptionally lean (less than 90% of standard weight), lean (90% to 109%), slightly overweight (110% to 119%), moderately obese (120% to 139%), very obese (150% to 199%), and massively obese (more than 199%). Other indexes might be used (eg, "mass index", which is weight over square of height).

Also of interest would be data on frequency distribution of fasting blood glucose levels in treated diabetics. Additional information on type of therapy would enhance the utility of such data. Degree of hyperglycemia has frequently been used as an index of severity, but few data have been presented on frequency distribution of blood glucose in populations of treated diabetics. Among these few are those of John (1950) and Mimura (1970). In the Japanese cases of Mimura only 14% had fasting values greater than 200 mg/100 ml. These levels seem lower than those prevailing in Europe and America, but it is difficult to find data with which to compare. Bennett, et al (1976a) have published data on the two-hour values of Pima Indians. More observations are needed on the frequency distribution of fasting glucose levels in representative samples of treated diabetics. It will be appropriate to exclude blood glucose data obtained at the time of acute illness since these values are not representative. This raises the problem of a need for a definition of *basal conditions* or *acute illness.*

Data for age and age of onset can be grouped by ten- or twenty-year intervals (ie, 0–19, 20–39, 40–59, 60–79, and over 79). In studies of youth-onset diabetes, however, data are sometimes needed on onset by intervals of one or two years. In this case important information may be missed by lumping of five- to ten-year periods. Data on duration of diabetes can usually be grouped by five- or ten-year intervals.

Other more elaborate measurements useful in classification exist that will not be feasible in many circumstances. These include levels of serum or plasma insulin and ratios of insulin to plasma glucose under standardized conditions such as the fasting state, or one hour after oral glucose. Another index of classification and definition is the stage of diabetes. This is based mainly on a chronology of progression. Here is a classification of this type, promulgated by the British Diabetes Association (FitzGerald and Keen, 1964). The language of the original presentation has been editorially modified slightly, but the definitions were not materially altered. In general, these conventions are in accord with those employed in the United States and elsewhere, although differences of opinion still prevail among experts.

1. *Potential diabetes:* Persons with a normal glucose-tolerance test (GTT) but a potential risk of developing diabetes
   a. an identical twin of a diabetic;

    b. a person with one diabetic parent whose other (nondiabetic) parent has or had either a diabetic parent, sibling, or offspring, or a sibling having a diabetic child;

    c. a woman who has given birth to a live or stillborn child weighing 4.5 kg (10 lb) or more at birth, or a stillborn child showing hyperplasia of the pancreatic islets not due to rhesus incompatibility.

2. *Latent diabetes*

    a. a person with a normal glucose tolerance test who is known to have had a diabetic glucose tolerance test at some time during pregnancy, infection, other stress, or when obese;

    b. a person who has abnormal blood glucose responses (similar to those found in diabetes mellitus) to provocative tests, such as the cortisone-augmented GTT or the intravenous sodium-tolbutamide test.

3. *Asymptomatic diabetes:* sometimes referred to as subclinical or chemical diabetes

    a. a person with a diabetic response to the GTT whose fasting blood sugar is below 130 mg/100 ml (capillary) or 125 mg/100ml (venous);

    b. as above, but with fasting blood sugars above the stated values.

4. *Clinical diabetes*

    a. a person with an abnormal GTT with the symptoms or complications of diabetes;

    b. the term "prediabetic" is reserved for the period in the life of a diabetic before glucose tolerance becomes abnormal.

Expert committees of the World Health Organization and the American Diabetes Association have also promulgated classifications and definitions in the past, but objections to some aspects of these can be raised on several grounds including subsequent insights based on recent research progress. Table 5 presents a classification by etiology.

Other Terms of Classification

Among the designations previously suggested and used but not universally accepted or understood are the following:

Type 2 or II has been used by some to apply to milder diabetes; but information has seldom been provided in its application with respect to whether the critical criteria are degree of glycemia, age of onset, degree of fatness, or combinations thereof.

Type 1 or I has been used to designate "juvenile-type" diabetes but there is little uniformity of convention as to how to apply criteria such as age of onset, degree of glycemia, presence or absence of ketosis, or of islet-cell antibodies.

The expression *J-type* tends to be confusing. It is discussed in some detail in

TABLE 5   Some Causes, Suspected Causes, and Risk Indicators of Diabetes

GENERALLY ACCEPTED

Obesity
  Caloric excess, indolence
Heredity (many mechanisms)
Destruction or damage of beta cells
  Cancer
  Pancreatectomy
  Pancreatitis from many causes
  Viral infections
  Beta cytotoxic drugs
    (streptozotocin, alloxan, certain thiazides, eg, diazoxide)
Diabetogenic hormones (exogenous or endogenous)
  Growth hormone (acromegaly)
  Epinephrine (pheochromocytoma)
  ACTH or glucocorticoids (adrenal corticism or Cushing's syndrome)
  Hyperaldosteronism
  Hyperglucagonemia (probably rare)
Hemochromatosis
Disorders of insulin receptors (eg, ancanthosis nigricans)
Factors of immunity and autoimmunity

WIDELY SUSPECTED OF CAUSING OR PRECIPITATING DIABETES

Pregnancy (but some challenge this)
Excessive serum iron (eg, thalassemia)
Cassava (manioc or tapioca) consumption when combined with protein malnutrition
Some drugs (eg. diphenylhydantoin, colchicine, lithium carbonate, l-asparaginase)
Cirrhosis
Potassium deficiency (eg, excess of powerful diuretics)
Certain brain lesions (uncommon)
Affluence in some circumstances and poverty in others
Myotonic dystrophy

SUSPECTED BY SOME SCIENTISTS BUT DOUBTED BY OTHERS

Dietary fat
Dietary sugars
Refined carbohydrates
Insufficient dietary fiber
Some drugs with mild hyperglycemic effects (eg, phenothiazines, hydrochlorothiazides, caffeine, sympathomimetics, marijuana)
Contraceptive steroids
Male sex in some societies,
  female sex in others
Deficiency states
  chromium, iron, zinc, pyridoxine
Severe protein malnutrition
  in some circumstances
Psychologic stress
Stress of prolonged or severe illness
Temperate climate
Coxsackie viruses
Hypertriglyceridemia
Specific racial susceptibility (eg, Jews, Indians, American Indians, Polynesians)

Chapter 8 on special types of diabetes. This expression, coined by Hugh-Jones (1955), refers to lean cases with onset in youth that are resistant to ketosis despite high insulin requirements. The first cases were described in Jamaica; thus, the designation "J". The term does have some utility and is probably here to stay, despite the unfortunate coincidence of the letter "J" in designation of both the ketosis-resistant and typical juvenile diabetes (usually ketosis-prone). The designations K-R and K-P have been used to designate presence or absence of propensity to ketosis. I suggest a convention to the effect that K-P cases have persistent ketonuria in the absence of insulin even under basal conditions, while K-R cases do not, although they may have ketosis during periods of stress when they may decompensate to K-P status. At present there is no convention with respect to the classification of cases that have had one or more episodes of ketosis despite the absence of ketonuria under basal conditions. Moreover, there is no uniformity in the classification of cases that have marked hypergly-cemia but no ketosis on suboptimal amounts of insulin, and ketosis only when insulin is completely withdrawn for long periods. Finally, no convention exists concerning the definition of *ketosis* or *ketonemia*. One possible definition might be persistent ketonuria in the absence of deprivation of dietary carbohy-drate (at least 150 gm/day).

The old French terms *diabete maigre* and *diabete gras* (Lanceraux, 1890) served a useful function in the past but were never well defined and are not useful epidemiologic terms today. Shaper (1958) suggested the term "K-type" for cases of a certain kind of diabetes observed in Uganda. The characteristics of this type were similar to those of the J-type, except that they were sensitive to insulin. But the designation K-type has not been widely used or understood.

No agreement exists concerning the definition of the widely used term *juvenile diabetes*. The need for a definition has become more apparent with the realization that mild cases of diabetes are not rare in childhood and that ketosis-resistant childhood diabetes is very common in some societies. In the United States and Europe most cases with onset in the first two decades of life eventually develop insulin-dependent ketosis-prone diabetes. Sometimes the designation juvenile-type is applied to ketosis-prone cases with onset much later in life. There has been no uniformity of categorization in reporting and analyzing cases of "juvenile" diabetes with respect to age of onset. Among the more common upper limits employed have been ages 14, 15, 16, 17, 18, 19, and 20. There is a disinclination to refer to persons from 16 to 29 years of age as "juveniles"; yet the type of diabetes observed in cases with onset at this time of life is usually typical of that seen in younger people. It would be better to classify according to clincial type rather than social conventions concerning the upper age limit of childhood. The term growth-onset has several disadvan-tages: the disparity between the sexes in the average age at which growth ends; the lack of uniformity of age of completion of growth; and the lack of distinc-tion between the type of diabetes in cases with onset during growth and those with onset in the first several years after growth has ended. These are among the reasons that the classification nomenclature given above—ie, Types I-D (insulin-dependent) and I-I (insulin-independent)—does not use in its key designations the terms, juvenile or growth. Yet it would be difficult to discourage the well-entrenched term, juvenile diabetes. There is little hope of replacing it soon despite all the problems its use creates. In epidemiologic reporting, however, it would be preferable to abandon it as a classifying term. Rather, separate information on age of onset should be included (by year, five-year period, or decade), type of therapy required, susceptibility to ketosis, and some index of fatness prior to onset of the disease, such as relative weight.

The term *senile diabetes* has been used occasionally (Burch and Meallie, 1967), but not standard definition exists. The term *genetic diabetes* has been used commonly, but its utility is limited. It can be used with considerable confidence only in unusual circumstances (eg, lean diabetic identical twins). The term *idiopathic diabetes* has been employed occasionally, but it has rather limited utility. It should probably not be applied in obese subjects. The term *pancreatic diabetes* is widely used but is subject to misinterpretation as explained below in the section on secondary diabetes. A preferable term would be *diabetes associated with disease of the exocrine pancreas.* Designation by etiology, when such is evident, is desirable; but because there are scores of causes, a classification based on etiology would be quite long and complex as shown in Table 5. Furthermore, only a small percentage can be etiologically classified except for those with obesity. Finally, multiple etiology in single cases is common.

Use of the Type I-D or I-I classification scheme proposed above will be greatly facilitated when methods are widely available to measure endogenous insulin in patients who are taking insulin. This can be done now, but the methods are not yet available in most laboratories.

The term *prediabetes* has been well defined but has often been misused. Asymptomatic patients with occult hyperglycemia do not have prediabetes; they have early diabetes. Only persons with normal glucose tolerance can be said to have prediabetes, and prediabetes can only be comfirmed retrospectively after diabetes develops. A substantial portion of identical twins of juvenile diabetics and offspring of two diabetic parents probably do *not* have prediabetes.

The term *clinical diabetes* has been frequently used but not with uniformity. Generally accepted definitions do not exist for either "clinical" or "diabetes"! Conceivably this category could include only patients with classical symptoms, or it could include those with other findings detectable by physical examination (eg, retinopathy), by laboratory procedures (eg, hyperglycemia), or by history (eg, symptoms suggestive of neuropathy). Problems in defining hyperglycemia are discussed elsewhere in this volume. Another widely used but poorly defined term, *chemical diabetes,* is often employed in describing asymptomatic cases with mild hyperglycemia. But the specific limits of this category have not been standardized; for example, do asymptomatic diabetics with retinopathy have "chemical" diabetes? Another major problem is that the size of this group can be greatly contracted or enlarged by changing the definition of diabetes. The term *gestational diabetes* is often mistakenly used to include all cases with discovery in pregnancy. It should include only those cases in whom glucose tolerance returns to normal after pregnancy. This and related problems of nomenclature and definition have been discussed by Sutherland, et al (1974).

Another major problem is the lack of uniformity in definition of obesity; this will be discussed at some length in other sections of this book. No recognized conventions exist for "mild", "moderate", or "severe" diabetes, but these designations generally refer to degree of hyperglycemia and its attendant symptoms. By these criteria an amputee blinded by retinopathy, paralyzed by neuropathy, and killed by diabetic coronary disease might be classified as having "mild diabetes"! Quantitation of degree of hyperglycemia is desirable and useful both in the absence and the presence of treatment, but the terms mild and severe hyperglycemia are usually preferable to mild and severe diabetes.

Brittle diabetes is a term used to describe cases in which the blood glucose is unusually labile. When such cases are given insulin in amounts adequate to mitigate hyperglycemia, hypoglycemic episodes are often a problem. This lability is often a feature of childhood-onset diabetes, but also occurs in insulin-dependent cases of later onset. It seems likely that many factors may, to varying degrees, be responsible for this lability, but a prime determinant is the degree of insufficiency of endogenous insulin. *Labile hyperglycemia* is a less ambiguous expression than "brittle" diabetes. The degree of this lability is measurable by special and elaborate methods (Service, et al, 1970), but no conventions exist for its precise quantitation under usual conditions. In patients treated with insulin, the number and severity of hypoglycemic reactions is a product of many factors, so the propensity to insulin reactions is only a crude index of the inherent lability of the blood glucose.

Some other problems and considerations relating to classification are discussed in several of the sections below, particularly in Chapter 8 on special types of diabetes.

Secondary Diabetes

The term *secondary diabetes* has been widely used when diabetes is associated with a specific and identifiable inciting factor (other than obesity or heredity). Such factors are of two types. One type includes conditions that directly destroy or impair function of beta cells (eg, pancreatitis, cancer of the pancreas, pancreatectomy, administration of alloxan or streptozotocin). Usually hemochromatosis is also included in this group because it is associated with pancreatic fibrosis. However, it is probable that other factors also contribute to development of diabetes in patients with hemochromatosis. Another type of factor produces "secondary" diabetes by increasing resistance to insulin. At first insulin insufficiency is only relative, but later it may become absolute as beta-cell exhaustion ensues. This group of factors includes acromegaly (excess of growth hormone) and the several circumstances that lead to excessive quantities of circulating glucocorticoids (Cushing's syndrome). These latter compounds are now widely and frequently administered to suppress severe inflammation, so that this mechanism has become a fairly common cause of diabetes.

Excessive epinephrine secretion resulting from pheochromocytoma leads to diabetes by a combination of untoward effects. Glucose release by liver is increased, peripheral action of insulin is antagonized, and beta-cell function is suppressed. A very rare cause of diabetes is glucagonoma. Diabetes is sometimes precipitated by hyperthyroidism. When hyperaldosteronism leads to low levels of extracellular potassium, glucose tolerance may be impaired and diabetes produced. Alcoholism may sometimes cause diabetes indirectly when it leads to pancreatitis. Virus infections as a cause of diabetes will be discussed below, as will the special type of diabetes observed in the tropics in which diabetes in young persons is associated with calcification of the pancreas (Chapter 8).

A good argument can be made for abandoning the term "secondary" diabetes, since all diabetes is in a sense secondary. Also, genetic factors often play a role in persons considered to have secondary diabetes. For example, some persons with mild pancreatitis become diabetic while others with rather extensive pancreatitis do not. Moreover, some types of secondary diabetes (ie, those associated with obesity and hemochromatosis) have strong hereditary features. The term secondary diabetes was introduced at a time when the extent and importance of environmental influences on etiology were not fully appreciated, and when it was widely held that the vast majority of cases of diabetes were attributable to a single specific genetic defect. It is now clear that a great number of environmental and genetic factors influence susceptibility and resistance to diabetes. Sophisticated scientists are no longer looking for *the* cause of diabetes. It is, of course, possible that in some societies a certain single specific genetic mechanism may play the major role in producing either insulin-dependent or typical maturity-onset diabetes. Even if this is so, it is not at all clear whether the deleterious effect is a result of a direct and "primary" failure of beta-cell function or whether the pancreatic failure is secondary to a deficit at another site or sites. It has been argued that certain vascular lesions are less frequent or absent in secondary diabetes and that a genetic "primary" type of diabetes leads directly to vascular and neurologic lesions independent of its effect on beta-cell function, insulin insufficiency, or glycemia. If this were so, the distinction between "secondary" and "primary" diabetes would be relevant, appropriate, and highly useful. Most of the evidence, however, suggests that patients with "secondary" diabetes of sufficient duration are susceptible to most, if not all, of the vascular and neurologic lesions that plague patients with "primary" diabetes. The term secondary diabetes probably ought to be abandoned, but this discussion is necessary because abandonment does not seem imminent.

Table 5 lists many of the factors that have or may have etiologic significance in diabetes. Several of the "secondary" types of diabetes, including diabetes associated with gross lesions of the pancreas, are discussed in Chapter 8, under special types of diabetes. The relative frequency of these "secondary" types of diabetes has seldom been measured with precision, even in societies with sophisticated scientific resources. In affluent populations they usually constitute less than 10% of all cases of diabetes. Perhaps the best estimate available is one based on the observations of Palumbo, et al (1976) in Rochester, Minnesota residents. In this comprehensive community study of diabetes, 3% of diabetics appeared to have had diabetes of the "secondary" type. In a cooperative autopsy study of the Japanese Pathological Society (Goto and Fukuhara, 1968), 122 of 933 cases (13%) were deemed to be of secondary type. Fifty-one had liver cirrhosis, 27 cancer of the pancreas, 22 drug-induced steroid diabetes, 7 hemochromatosis, 7 acromegaly, and 3 Cushing's disease.

4
CHAPTER

SCREENING, DETECTION, AND DIAGNOSIS

SCREENING AND DETECTION

Screening and detection are functions of clinicians as well as epidemiologists and public health specialists. This section will concern itself mainly with the types of mass screening that are traditionally collaborative enterprises involving diabetologists and public health specialists or epidemiologists. Fortunately, these mass screening and detection surveys have often yielded information applicable to clinical practice, such as data on the sensitivity and specificity of screening tests and their relationship to the characteristics of the subjects tested. Some of these clinical implications will be mentioned, but the main thrust of the discussion below will relate to the epidemiologic or public health aspects of screening. It should be stressed here, however, that a prime mechanism for screening is the testing performed by individual physicians in their day-to-day care of patients and families. High-priority screenees in clinical practice include patients who are fat as well as those with a strong family history of diabetes.

History

Mass screening for diabetes began only recently. Prior to World War II, large-scale screening enterprises had been confined to special population groups such as military inductees, employee groups in industry, and life insurance applicants. Among the earliest data of the latter type were those of Barringer, who reported in 1909 the results of urine sugar tests on 71,729 persons by the medical departments of life insurance companies in New York. It is not clear what percentage of those with glycosuria had diabetes, but these results provided the best evidence then available that diabetes was a common condition in the United States. In men, the rate of glycosuria was 2.8%, and a urine glucose concentration of 1% or greater was present in 0.9% of men.

Pioneer surveys included those summarized in publications of Joslin (1923) and Emerson and Larimore (1924) on rates of diabetes in United States military inductees and military personnel of World War I. Marble (1949) published similar data for World War II personnel, in which he reviewed earlier data of Blotner and Hyde (1943), of Blotner (1946), and of Spellberg and Leff (1945) on glucosuria and diabetes in inductees and volunteers for military service. These early studies revealed some interesting epidemiologic findings, some of which are discussed in other sections of this volume. Glycosuria was, for example, much more common in Boston (Blotner, 1946) than in New Orleans (Spellberg and Leff, 1945). Other special groups surveyed included University of Minnesota students (Watson, 1939) and DuPont Company employees of Niagra Falls, New York (Gates, 1942).

In Europe, surveys of the frequency of clinical cases were common in various population groups even prior to World War II, but mass screening was rare before 1950. Some of the important early European surveys are described in the section on the history of the epidemiology of diabetes in Chapter 1.

Wilkerson and Krall published in 1947 the results of the first of the modern series of mass screening and detection enterprises. Postprandial urine and blood glucose levels were measured in a whole community. This population of Oxford, Massachusetts has been the subject of a series of studies by the late Hugh Wilkerson, and associates including Leo Krall and John O'Sullivan. Oxford is the birthplace of E. P. Joslin, who sponsored and encouraged these studies. Joslin had suggested in a publication of 1921 the need for community screening of this type, to evaluate and contend with what he called "epidemics" of diabetes. Other pioneer screening and detection programs included those described by Ford in Florida (1949), by Kenny, et al in Canada (1951), Sharkey in Dayton, Ohio (1950), and Schliack in East Berlin (1952).

In North America the screening and detection effort was initiated and led by the American Diabetes Association and its affiliate elements. The early work in St. Louis was typical (MacBryde, 1949; Olmstead, et al, 1953). Subsequently, screening programs were developed in a substantial portion of state and local health departments (Ford, 1949; US Public Health Service, 1967). Initially, most screening programs were an intermittent activity, often once yearly for a few days. More recently, many have been conducted on a continuing basis. Some of the most successful programs have involved collaboration of public and private agencies (health departments, diabetes associations, hospitals, medical societies, civic clubs, etc).

The feasibility of mass screening was greatly enhanced by the development in the 1950s of automated methods for accurately measuring concentration of blood glucose at low cost.

Among the first to incorporate diabetes screening as part of multiphasic screening were Canelo, et al (1949), Breslow (1950), and Petrie, et al (1952). In Britain some of the first multiphasic studies that included diabetes testing were those reported by Burn in 1956. In Bergen, Norway, chest radiography and diabetes screening were combined in 1956 (Jorde, 1962).

The present extent of mass screening has not been well quantitated. Reports to the American Diabetes Association suggest that about 1 million tests annually are performed by its affiliates. State Health Departments in the United States and their subelements also perform about a million tests yearly. According to the 1967 edition of the *USPHS Diabetes Source Book*, the largest program was that of the Michigan State Health Department where tests were being performed at the rate of about 150,000 annually. The Pennsylvania Department of Health has sponsored one of the largest screening programs. In fiscal year 1965, for example, 100,183 persons were screened and at least 923 new cases were discovered (Millington and Tinsman, 1966). Perhaps the largest program was that described by Petrie, et al (1954); more than 500,000 were screened in this Georgia program. State Health Departments in Missippi and North Carolina also conduct large screening programs. Between 1965 and 1970 the Cleveland Diabetes Association screened more than 300,000 (Genuth, et al, 1976). Very large numbers of screening tests are performed in America by industry and the insurance companies.

Objectives and General Approaches

Some of the purposes and strategies of screening programs have been reviewed by Marble and Blotner (1951) and, more recently, by Butterfield (1968), Proust and McCracken (1968), Keen and Jarrett (1969), West, et al (1970), Orzeck, et al (1971), Welborn, et al (1972), and by Genuth, et al (1976). Multiphasic screening systems that incorporated diabetes screening have been described by Collen, et al (1969) and by Wilson and Jungner (1968). The United States Public Health Service issued in 1969 a *Program Guide for Diabetes Control*, which describes screening procedures. Screening of hospital patients has been reviewed by Danowski, et al (1966a). Jackson and his associates (1968,1970a) have reported on their wide experience in South Africa on screening tests and strategies. The studies of Sullivan, et al (1967) in Sudbury, Massachusetts, are instructive with respect to screening processes. The American Diabetes Association supplies instructional materials on organizing and conducting screening and detection programs.

DETECTION

The central purpose of most screening and detection programs is to discover diabetes at an early stage so that these persons will have the advantage of early treatment. But screening and detection programs have several other potentialities (West, et al, 1970). The discussion below under evaluation includes a review of positive and negative evidence concerning the utility and priority of early detection.

43

Public Education

Screening and detection programs may further public education in several ways. The need for early detection can be emphasized. Public understanding can be enhanced concerning the symptoms of diabetes and the characteristics of those in special need of testing (eg, obese persons, those with a family history of diabetes, mothers of large babies). The need for intensified private and public action against diabetes can be shown. In some special circumstances it has been feasible to combine screening and detection activities with fund raising to support either screening itself or other antidiabetes enterprises such as research or education of diabetics. The value of screening of high-risk groups through their regular channels of health care can be emphasized.

Methods for public education have included providing written materials to screenees or prospective screenees, use of the mass media (eg, radio, television, newspapers), circulation of information to high-risk groups (eg, to relatives of diabetics through diabetes associations or public health departments), and providing information to "accessible" groups (eg, mailings or verbal presentations to employee groups, civic clubs, church groups).

Professional Education

Screening programs represent an excellent opportunity to teach health professionals about screening and diagnosis and also about objectives, methods, and priorities of treatment. Sending information to busy physicians seldom produces changes in the ways they do things. Unsolicited material of this kind is not likely to be read, understood, or remembered. Prospects for a significant educational impact are considerably better when such information is made an integral part of the process of referring a specific positive screenee for diagnosis or treatment. The best time to show physicians the difference between glucose levels in whole blood and in plasma is, for example, when they are deciding how to design or interpret a test in their own patient. The central purpose of this effort to further professional education is to improve treatment of patients, but another possible objective is to demonstrate potentialities for the prevention of diabetes and its complications.

Research and Other Epidemiologic Objectives

It is often possible to design and conduct screening programs in a manner that will yield useful epidemiologic information. This may include an assessment of rates of diabetes or occult diabetes, and their relationship to factors such as age, sex, and fatness. Two excellent programs in Australia illustrated well these potentialities (Smithurst, 1969; Welborn, et al, 1968). Data of these kinds may also be helpful in establishing the priority of diabetes-related public health programs. Other epidemiologic by-products in screening enterprises may include investigations of operational methodology (eg, evaluations of the sensitivity and specificity of alternative screening and diagnostic methods, and of their effectiveness in relation to cost).

A simple mechanism that has rarely been applied, but can often greatly enhance the epidemiologic utility of a screening program, is simply to perform diagnostic tests on a sample of the negative screenees. This sample should be at least crudely representative of the total group of negative screenees, but often it can be quite small (eg, every 10th negative). Most estimates of rates of diabetes have been based mistakenly on the assumption that there was no diabetes in the negative screenees. This is probably the most frequent and important defect in the early surveys that purported to yield information on prevalence. Unfortunately, the error is still being made in designing and interpreting modern surveys. Another approach that adds epidemiologic information in a screening enterprise is to do diagnostic testing with a standard method on a sample of the positive screenees that are to be referred to their physicians for follow-up. This makes possible not only an estimate of rates of diabetes in the positive screenees using any one of several diagnostic criteria, but also an evaluation of the sensitivity and specificity of the information later provided by physicians to whom positive screenees are referred.

Methods

The applicability and justification of some of the traditional screening methods and strategies are now open to question. The cost of blood glucose determinations is now under many circumstances quite low, particularly when large batches of specimens are involved. Under some conditions the best method of detection is probably to perform a loading test without the traditional preliminaries (MacDonald, et al, 1963; Kent and Leonards, 1968; Welborn, et al, 1968). Several techniques have been used to load screenees. They may be asked to report one to two hours after a meal or large meal. The characteristics of the meal may or may not be prescribed. A standardized meal (eg, rice, candy) or sweet drink may be administered, or a glucose load given. Leonards developed a special testing solution now marketed by Ames Company as Glucola. It is a partial hydrolysate of cornstarch. Glucola produces effects on blood glucose and insulin secretion very similar to those of glucose (Kent and Leonards, 1965; Genuth, 1969). Its osmotic effect in the small intestine is less than that produced by glucose, and rates of nausea and vomiting are probably less than with glucose (Kent and Leonards, 1965). On the other hand, Murray, et al (1969) observed only two cases of vomiting when 2,500 subjects were given 50-gm loads of glucose. We have observed marked differences among cultures in frequency of nausea and vomiting after oral glucose. In all poor countries we found these untoward effects much less common than in American whites. These findings deserve further study.

There is also a need to reexamine traditional approaches to staging procedures in the screening process. A very common approach in the past has been to perform simple tests on blood or urine in the field and to refer positive screenees to their own physicians for definitive testing. Several recent developments suggest that other approaches may sometimes be preferable. Costs of

45

blood glucose tests have declined and personnel costs have risen. It is now clear that in most circumstances mishandling by individual physicians is common. The possibility of diabetes is often dismissed on the basis of insensitive tests, and the diagnosis is not infrequently made on the basis of inadequate evidence. In general, the automation of laboratory determinations by the multi-channel process has decreased the relative priority of uniphasic screening programs (eg, diabetes screening alone) and increased the feasibility and priority of multiphasic screening. It has been found that the traditional follow-up process is somewhat costly with respect to the time required of positive screenees, their physicians, and the personnel of the screening program. Thus, the staging strategies selected should be less bound by tradition and based more on the conditions and priorities of particular screening programs. Under some circumstances this may lead to an approach in which definitive follow-up tests are performed immediately at the site of the screening procedure.

Future approaches will be affected greatly by how diabetes is defined. The discussion below and that under diagnostic tests suggest some possibilities of "revolutionary" proportions. It is being argued by some, for example, that "abnormalities" of glucose tolerance, when unaccompanied by fasting hyper-glycemia, do not in themselves warrant a diagnosis of diabetes. To the extent that this and similar views gain acceptance, the main screening strategy will be to identify fasting hyperglycemia. In this approach, a one-stage process would often be applicable. In my judgment the present evidence does not justify mass screening to find persons who have normal fasting glucose levels together with abnormal glucose tolerance as defined by traditional standards. Reasons for this conclusion are set forth in discussions above and below (eg, in section on diagnostic methods). But the views expressed above are still in the minority among specialists in diabetes. Most still believe that glucose tolerance tests have utility both as clinical instruments and as definitive tests in screening programs. So long as this view prevails, there will be loading tests at some stage of the process of screening and follow-up. One of the advantages of giving glucose loads in the first stage is that a single cut-off point can sometimes be used irrespective of the circumstances of testing. For example, all those with one-hour plasma glucose values over 230 mg/100 ml might be considered positive and referred for further testing. Another advantage is that loading tests may be given at any time of day, at a time convenient to the screenee and those who perform the tests. In interpreting such tests it may be appropriate to take into account the effects of time of day and duration of pretest fasting (see section below on diagnostic methods). Even if one believes with the minority that glucose tolerance tests are poor diagnostic instruments, one may advocate them in screening on the grounds that almost all positive screenees will eventually be advised by their physicians to have such tests, at greater expense on an individual basis than on a mass basis. One possible compromise in this matter is to employ screening loading tests, but very conservative criteria of interpretation (high cut-off points).

Table 6 summarizes first-stage screening procedures that have been employed in large-scale screening projects.

TABLE 6   Methods Used in Screeni...

	S... ...city	Cost and Comments
Fasting urine*	Very	Inexpensive. Requirement for fasting may increase cost of recruitment and reduce number recruited. Requirement for toilet facilities may also be disadvantageous.
Postprandial urine*	Fair	Inexpensive. Requirement for timing of specimen collection may increase cost of this approach.
"Random" urine (neither time of day nor relation to meal is standardized)	Poor	Very inexpensive and usually convenient.
Fasting plasma glucose	Fair (but some be... it is good; se... text)	...ost intermediate. Necessity ...r fasting state is often disad... ...ntageous to recruitment. An ...ernative is to require only ...e hours of fasting.
Postprandial plasma glucose* (usually one or two hours; timing standardized or unstandardized)	Good	...cificity and sensitivity are ...nced by standardization ...al characteristics and of ...g of interval between ...nd specimen collection, ...t is usually increased ...creased ...lization
Plasma glucose after measured load (eg, candy, cola drink, glucose; often at one or two hours)	Very good	...stly to perform but ...ost of follow-up
Random blood glucose (neither time of day nor relation to meal are standardized)	Fair F	...her inexpensive
Semiquantitative blood glucose (eg, Dextrostix)		...d specificity ...tors such as rela... ...ut in general, ...n of the method ...mewhat. A ...of this is the ...ability of ...es much cler-

Note: The generalizations expressed in this Table are subject to ...strated in the discussion below, depending on the characteristics of the populatio... ...es of testing. Sensitivity and/or specificity of postprandial tests are improved when (1) ...eg, more than 70 gm of carbohydrate), (2) timing of specimen collection is standardize... ...er eating, (3) characteristics of the meals are standardized. Sensitivity of postprandial ...bjects empty bladders before the meal.

*Much of the lack of sensitivity and specificity of urine tests is because traditional methods are only semiquantitative. As shown by Davidson, et al (1975), sensitivity and specificity are greatly improved when quantitative methods are used.

URINE TESTING

Laboratory procedures for urine testing have been well reviewed by Marble (1971) and Pyke (1966). Probably the most common screening approach used previously (worldwide) has been a test of urine glucose followed by referral of positive screenees for further testing with a more sensitive and specific procedure such as a glucose tolerance test. Examples of this approach have included the Trinidad program of Poon-King, et al (1968) and the English surveys in Birmingham (Birmingham Working Party, 1963) and Bedford (Sharp, et al, 1964). Because of the apparent lack of sensitivity and specificity of urine glucose tests as traditionally performed, the American Diabetes Association has for two decades discouraged the use of urine glucose tests as the main screening instrument in mass screening projects. The World Health Organization expert Committee on Diabetes (1965) also cited the shortcomings of urine testing as a screening instrument. Some, including the author, have thought these official indictments of urine testing too broad, for reasons set forth below. Malins (1974a) also recommended postprandial urine testing as a routine screening method in subjects under 65 years of age. But the point is well taken that urine testing is in many circumstances a decidedly suboptimal screening instrument (Keen, 1964). Details are reviewed below under sensitivity and specificity; the same section also reviews data showing the greater sensitivity of urine tests in men than in women.

There has been little enthusiasm for mass screening of children in which blood tests are done as the initial screening procedure. When children are screened most programs have used urine tests as the stage one procedure. The advisability of mass urine testing in children has, however, been challenged by Rosenbloom and Allen (1973). Criticisms of this approach in children are based on the rarity of disorder as well as the limitations of the usual types of urine tests in reflecting blood glucose concentrations. On the other hand, children with early diabetes are more likely to have glycosuria than are adults with early diabetes. Moreover, severe ketoacidosis rather commonly occurs before the discovery of childhood-onset diabetes. Thus, early discovery of diabetes is highly desirable in children.

Normally, there is a very small concentration of glucose in the urine (usually 0.001% to 0.03%), but this level is not detectable by standard semiquantitative methods (Fine, 1965). When the concentration reaches 0.02% to 0.04%, glucose is detected by these traditional methods in some specimens but not in others. When concentration reaches 0.1%, glucose is regularly detectable by the standard simple methods. As concentration rises, crude quantitation is possible with these simple methods. For example, by the Clinitest method, specimens having 2% or more usually produce a color that is read as 4+ (on a scale of 1 to 4). Not surprisingly, specificity of the result for the presence of diabetes increases considerably as glucose concentration rises. Most people with moderate to heavy (3 or 4+) postprandial glycosuria have diabetes, while most with minimal glycosuria (trace or 1+) do not. However, those persons with slight glycosuria are much more likely to have diabetes than those with no detectable urine glucose.

Unfortunately, the different popular methods do not correspond exactly with respect to the relationship of concentration to number of pluses. But their sensitivities in detecting glucose are similar. Quantitation is somewhat better with the Clinitest method than with the enzyme-strip methods, but the Clinitest procedure is not specific for glucose and is somewhat more likely to yield false positives; and under some conditions it has been less sensitive than the enzyme-strip methods. Details on these urine testing methods may be found in the publications of Moran, et al (1957), Ackerman, et al (1958), Chertack and Sherrick (1959), O'Sullivan, et al (1962), Dobson, et al (1968), and James and Chase (1974). Among the most informative publications on urine glucose is that of Fine (1965).

Recently a method has been introduced that is capable of rapidly measuring glucose concentration of both blood and urine with precision (Kadish and Sternberg, 1969). A disadvantage is that the machine is moderately expensive. It is very simple to operate but is not a self-testing method. Using this more precise procedure, Davidson, et al (1975) found that urine glucose concentration corresponded closely with glucose tolerance. Developments of this kind will increase the effectiveness of urine testing as a screening instrument and will require reassessment of urine testing as a screening procedure. Apparently much of the poor sensitivity and specificity has been attributable to the lack of precision of the laboratory methods for its quantitation. Even if this impression is confirmed there will remain the problem of the high renal threshold for glucose in the elderly (Butterfield, et al, 1967).

Most of the expert consultants of the American Diabetes Association have not been favorably impressed with the effectiveness of self-testing as a screening procedure. However, it may be kept in mind that this method is technically feasible, and that under certain circumstances it may be an alternative worth considering. It is possible to distribute testing units at very low cost, but one should not underestimate considerable numbers who do not test, do not test properly, or do not report for follow-up when the test is positive. Dr. Joslin strenuously advocated urine screening by diabetics of their relatives. This approach has great potential although it is seldom used.

The role of urine testing is further reviewed below under sensitivity and specificity; that section also includes discussion of the effects of race, age, and sex on the relationship of glucosuria to blood glucose levels. Knowles (1975a) has published an excellent summary on follow-up procedures on patients with positive urine tests.

SEMIQUANTITATIVE BLOOD GLUCOSE METHODS

In several countries semiquantitative blood glucose methods have come into wide use as screening procedures (Keen and Jarrett, 1969; West, et al, 1966,-1970). "Dextrostix" are enzyme-impregnated strips prepared by the Ames Company. When exposed to a drop of blood obtained either by lancet or venipuncture, the degree of color change is proportional to the concentration of blood glucose (Rennie, et al, 1964; Alberti and Caird, 1965). The accuracy of this method has varied considerably by circumstances. Some of this variation was probably due to inattention to technical details. Kent and Leonards found only minimal variations between results with this method and control determinations with a precise quantitative method. Others have experienced a less precise correspondence (Pawliger and Shipp, 1965; McKay, et al, 1965; Keet, et al, 1969; Junker and Ditzel, 1972). We (West, et al, 1966) found the error of this method to be quite appreciable but not sufficient to exclude its utility as a screening instrument in some circumstances. It does appear, however, that the newer reflectance meters have increased the precision of this method (Jarrett, et al, 1970; Balazs, et al, 1970; Mazaferri, et al, 1970). These instruments, such as the "Eyetone" colorimeter, determine more precisely the degree of color development on the strips than was possible when estimates were made visually with the use of color chart standards. Even so, the method is still only semiquantitative (Junker and Ditzel, 1972; Teuscher, 1975).

Since many factors influence the degree and character of the error, it is usually desirable to determine this error by control procedures carried out under circumstances approximating the field conditions of the screening procedures (eg, testing 50 to 100 specimens with both the semiquantitative and the quantitative methods). In screening programs the degree of error at the bottom and top of the scale of values is usually of little importance. For example, a specimen read as 250 mg/100 ml, even though it contains 340 mg/100 ml, is still correctly classified as positive. Thus, in screening programs the need for examining the error of the method is greatest in the borderline range of glucose values. In most circumstances, moderate degree of error does not diminish greatly the utility of the method as a screening procedure, provided that the degree of this error is well understood and taken into account.

Fluoride is commonly present in collecting tubes. It interferes with this glucose oxidase reaction. Care should therefore be taken to avoid exposure to this substance in specimens to be tested by the Dextrostix method. The reaction is temperature sensitive, so chilled specimens should be warmed before testing.

The greatest advantage of this method is the immediate availability of the result, which often saves considerable clerical time, and also makes possible immediate follow-up advice or testing. Theoretically, a result can also be made available as promptly as five minutes using automated quantitative methods, but in actual practice this is seldom feasible. Under most conditions, costs of semiquantitative testing materials approach or exceed costs of performing quantitative determinations. In mass screening the decision to use a semiquantitative method usually reflects the advantage of having a result immediately available rather than an advantage of cost of the laboratory procedure.

When semiquantitative methods are used in screening, typical criteria of classification are as follows. Capillary blood levels over 130 mg/100 ml may be regarded as positive in subjects who have not eaten in the two-hour period before testing. In persons who have not fasted for at least two hours, values over 150 may be considered positive. Positive screenees are tested with more definitive procedures or referred for such testing. All values over 200 can be considered strongly suggestive of diabetes irrespective of relationship of time of testing to previous feeding. It should be made clear to negative screenees that this inexpensive procedure does not rule out very mild diabetes.

QUANTITATIVE BLOOD GLUCOSE METHODS

The development of automated methods has made it feasible under many circumstances to determine blood glucose levels precisely in the initial stage of the screening process. A good example was the screening program in Rangiora, New Zealand (Murray, et al, 1969). There was a very good correlation between the screening blood glucose level and the results of the definitive glucose tolerance test. In the mass screening project in Cleveland, sensitivity was increased by giving the screenees a drink containing 75 gm of simple carbohydrates two hours before the test (Kent and Leonards, 1965; Genuth, et al, 1976). Other exemplary detection surveys in which loading tests were used as first-stage screening instruments included the project of Welborn, et al (1968) in Busselton, Australia and that of MacDonald, et al (1963) in which United States federal employees were tested after ingesting a standardized amount of candy.

The educational brochure available from the American Diabetes Association (1974) recommends that screening be done by measuring plasma or serum glucose levels. The brochure recognizes that the first-stage procedure may be a fasting value, a "random" value, or a postprandial test according to local circumstances. The term *random* in this sense describes circumstances in which subjects are tested whenever they are available with no attempt to control the relationship to feeding or time of day. Sometimes, however, it is appropriate to relate the screening level to the duration of fasting prior to the test. In this and other situations there is need to define the term, *meal* or *eating*. We have sometimes classified eating or drinking as negligible when it is obvious that less than 15 gm of carbohydrate had been consumed (eg, 1 tsp of sugar in coffee). Under some conditions it is appropriate to relate screening criteria to size of the meal by rough quantitation of the feeding. For example, meals containing less than 50 gm of carbohydrate may be classified as "snacks", while larger feedings may be designated as "meals". On the other hand, such distinctions are often unfeasible. More commonly, subjects are simply divided into those who have, in the two- to three-hour period preceding the test, fasted completely or not. A common error is to ask explicitly about eating but not about drinking of nutrients.

Table 6 summarizes some of the advantages and disadvantages of using the fasting blood glucose, the random glucose, the postprandial glucose, and the blood glucose after a standard load. These are also discussed below under evaluation and comparison of methods. Laboratory methods for measuring blood glucose are discussed below under diagnostic tests. In screening either capillary or venous blood may be used. Some advantages are described below

51

for using plasma or serum rather than whole blood, but whole blood may also be effectively used. It is very important, however, that physicians to whom screening results are referred know which type of specimen was analyzed, and that they understand the relationships between glucose concentration in whole blood and in plasma or serum. This is also discussed under diagnostic tests.

When loading tests have been used as screening procedures, the most popular interval before determining blood glucose has been two hours, although the one-hour specimen has also been used. This alternative has the advantage of shortening the test. It is rather generally believed that the two-hour value has greatest ratio of sensitivity to specificity, but there is no conclusive evidence that it is better than the one-hour value. This is discussed more fully below under diagnostic tests.

SCREENING LEVELS

Screening levels commonly employed for the fasting *plasma* glucose value on venous blood range from 120 to 130 mg/100 ml; for random glucose the dividing line between negative and positive is usually placed in the range of 130 to 170; and for values one to two hours after eating the cut-off point is usually set in the range of 150 to 200. When whole blood is used screening levels are about 15% (not mg %) lower. When capillary blood is used in fasting subjects the screening levels are about the same, but postprandial levels are typically about 25 mg/100 ml higher at one hour and approximately 10 mg/100 ml higher at two hours. Postloading levels and screening criteria relating thereto may be affected by the size and character of the load. For example, when all subjects are given 100 gm of oral glucose, screening levels should be different from those employed when all are tested one to two hours after their ordinary breakfasts. The circumstances and objectives of some screening programs require considerable specificity in the results of screening, while high sensitivity has priority under other conditions. This should be taken into account in determining the screening criteria to be used. Criteria should not be matched mindlessly to tradition, but should rather be specifically tailored to local priorities and circumstances. In some circumstances it may be appropriate to relate blood glucose screening levels to age. The effects of age and type of load on the normal range of blood glucose are discussed later in this chapter under diagnostic tests.

OTHER METHODS

It is easy to estimate crudely the concentration of glucose on the surface of the skin (Miller and Ridolfo, 1960; Parker, 1962; Botros, 1966; West, et al, 1963). Concentration of glucose in skin is usually proportional to the concentration of blood glucose, and under certain conditions skin-surface glucose reflects fairly well the concentration in skin and blood. On the other hand, the practical utility of the skin-surface glucose as a screening procedure is very limited. An enzyme-impregnated strip such as Testape (Lilly) may be used. The

strip is moistened and gripped between the thumb and index-finger and read after one minute of exposure. When blood glucose levels are very high the skin test is usually positive, but people with decidedly elevated blood glucose values usually have symptoms of diabetes. Subjects who have blood glucose levels that are slightly or moderately elevated are also more likely to have positive skin glucose tests than nondiabetics, but many do not, and the sensitivity and specificity of this method leaves much to be desired. False-positive tests are also fairly common (West, et al, 1963). When contaminated by glucose on the outer surface of the skin, sweat may contain small amounts of glucose, but usually sweat and saliva contain no measurable glucose even in the presence of substantial hyperglycemia (Allen, 1913).

Under some conditions, gingival blood has served well as the screening specimen (Stein and Nebbia, 1969). This enables the dentist to perform screening procedures using the semiquantitative enzyme-impregnated strips. Piercing the finger is a convenient way to obtain capillary blood, but this usually produces more discomfort than similar trauma at other sites such as the earlobe. In persons with severe diabetes, ketones can be easily detected in breath samples, but these persons usually have glucosuria, ketonuria, and characteristic symptoms.

According to a recent report, absence of corneal reflex is especially common in persons with occult diabetes (Daubs, 1975). Other neurologic abnormalities are also more common in those with early diabetes than in nondiabetics, but none of these aberrations has sufficient specificity and sensitivity to suggest routine employment in mass screening.

There are a few other physical stigmata that are fairly common in early diabetes. Search for these stigmata is, however, seldom a part of the process of mass screening for diabetes. It is not feasible to examine for some of these on a mass basis, and all have poor sensitivity or poor specificity as indicators of diabetes. In some groups of positive screenees, rates of retinopathy have been negligible, but in other populations the rate of retinopathy at discovery of diabetes has been as high as 5%. Carbuncles not infrequently bring diabetes to attention, as does gangrene or ulcers of the feet. In women who have cytologic screening tests for cancer of the uterine cervix, those who have inflammation of the vaginal labia should be tested for diabetes. This particular potentiality has seldom been exploited routinely, but it should be. Pruritis vulvae is the most common symptom of diabetes in some groups of women. All patients with evidence of coronary disease or tuberculosis should be screened for diabetes.

Symptoms of diabetes have been discussed in Chapter 3, including their frequency in those with early diabetes and in nondiabetics. Patients with classical symptoms of diabetes have substantial elevations of urine and blood glucose levels. For this reason the asking of questions about symptoms adds little to sensitivity of mass screening programs in which these laboratory tests are performed. Moreover, many nondiabetics complain of these same symptoms (Jorde, 1962; Welborn, et al, 1968). On the other hand, the discovery of

53

these cases with symptoms has a particular priority. Their symptoms can be relieved, and, in the absence of treatment, risk of certain complications is higher in symptomatic than in asymptomatic patients. It is thus desirable in some circumstances to ask these questions on a mass basis as part of the process of selectively recruiting screenees who are at high risk.

In the section below on sensitivity and specificity, studies of Jorde on symptoms in positive and negative screenees are summarized. Symptoms of diabetes in undiagnosed diabetics were only slightly more common than in the general population. It has been suggested that persons with symptoms relating to the oral cavity are particularly likely to have occult diabetes (Chinn, et al, 1966). But few control data are available to evaluate the sensitivity and specificity of such symptoms.

Comparative Sensitivity and Specificity of Methods

The sensitivity of a screening test is computed by determining the percentage of cases it identifies. If, for example, the test is positive in 45 of the 50 diabetic screenees, the sensitivity of the test is 90%. Specificity is defined as the percentage of normals correctly classified as such by the screening test. If, for example, 196 of 200 nondiabetics have negative tests, the specificity of the test is 98%. The ideal test would, of course, have a sensitivity of 100% and a specificity of 100%. Typically, tests approaching the ideal are expensive. Often more cases can be found per dollar invested by employing cheaper tests with less optimal sensitivity and specificity. Specificity and sensitivity of test results are strongly affected by the screening levels employed. Lowering screening level increases sensitivity but usually decreases specificity, while raising the screening level usually decreases sensitivity and raises specificity.

The traditional way of expressing specificity has some limitations as it applies to diabetes screening, and sometimes may be misleading to those who think of specificity in a broader sense to include also the specificity of positive tests. Suppose, for example, a group of 1,000 young adults are tested in whom the actual rate of occult diabetes is 1%. Suppose the rate of positive tests is 5% (50 positive tests). Of the 50 positive tests, five are true positives and 45 are false positives. By application of the standard definition the sensitivity of the test is 50% (half of the diabetics were identified). The specificity of the test is 96% because 950 of the 990 nondiabetics are correctly identified as negative. Note, however, that the "specificity" of a positive test is poor: only 10% are true positives and 90% are false positives. The best index of the effectiveness of diabetes screening test is provided by determining not only sensitivity and specificity employing traditional standards, but also by appraising the specificity of positive tests. A convenient measurement of this is the percentage of positive tests that are true positives (West and Kalbfleisch, 1971a). Galen and Gambino (1975) have called this figure the "predictive value". They have suggested a formula for measuring the "efficiency" of a diagnostic test. In this computation the number of true positives and true negatives are added. This sum is then divided by the total number of tests to yield an efficiency (E) percentage:

$$E = \frac{TP + TN}{N} \times 100$$

Among the earliest systematic studies of sensitivity and specificity of diabetes screening tests were those of Harting and Glenn (1951) and of Kurlander, et al (1954). This was followed by related pioneering work of Remein and Wilkerson (1961). Some criticisms can be made of this latter publication, but in some respects it represented a model for future attempts to measure systematically the effectiveness of various alternative methods for screening. One of the chief problems then (and now) was the lack of a truly definitive test for diabetes to use as a measuring instrument. Remein and Wilkerson used what was considered by most the best index available, the oral glucose tolerance test interpreted by diagnostic standards of the United States Public Health Service. Their subjects were 580 adult outpatients, 70 of whom were found to have occult diabetes. These investigators examined systematically the sensitivity of urine and blood glucose tests before, and at various intervals after, a stadardized test meal containing 74 gm of carbohydrate. This was done by comparing in all subjects the results of full glucose tolerance tests with the results of various screening procedures. Some of their results are shown in Table 7 and 8.

TABLE 7   Somogyi-Nelson Blood Test (Venous) Sensitivity and Specificity for Diabetes at Different Screening Levels, by Hours After Test Meal

BLOOD SUGAR LEVEL CONSIDERED POSITIVE (MG PER/ 100 ML)	BEFORE TEST MEAL		AT ONE HOUR AFTER TEST MEAL		AT TWO HOURS AFTER TEST MEAL		AT THREE HOURS AFTER TEST MEAL	
	SENS. % POS.	SPEC. % NEG.	SENS. % POS.	SPEC. % NEG.	SENS. % POS.	SPEC. % NEG.	SENS. % POS.	SPEC. % NEG.
70	95.7	11.0	100.0	8.2	98.6	8.8	94.3	8.6
80	91.4	36.3	97.1	22.4	97.1	25.5	91.4	34.7
90	82.9	65.7	97.1	39.0	94.3	47.6	82.9	67.5
100	65.7	84.7	95.7	57.3	88.6	69.8	70.0	86.5
110	54.3	92.7	92.9	70.6	85.7	84.1	60.0	95.3
120	50.0	96.7	88.6	83.3	71.4	92.5	51.4	98.2
130	44.3	99.0	78.6	90.6	64.3	96.9	48.6	99.8
140	37.1	99.6	68.6	95.1	57.1	99.4	41.4	100.0
150	30.0	99.8	57.1	97.8	50.0	99.6	32.9	100.0
160	25.7	99.8	52.9	99.4	47.1	99.8	28.6	100.0
170	25.7	99.8	47.1	99.6	42.9	100.0	28.6	100.0
180	22.9	99.8	40.0	99.8	38.6	100.0	28.6	100.0
190	21.4	100.0	34.3	100.0	34.3	100.0	24.3	100.0
200	17.1	100.0	28.6	100.0	27.1	100.0	20.0	100.0

Source: Remein and Wilkerson (1961).
Note: See text for further explanation.

TABLE 8   Sensitivity and Specificity Ratings of Four Urine Tests for Diabetes at Different Screening Levels, by Hours After Test Meal

SCREENING TEST AND LEVEL ASSUMED TO BE POSITIVE	BEFORE TEST MEAL		AT ONE HOUR AFTER TEST MEAL		AT TWO HOURS AFTER TEST MEAL		AT THREE HOURS AFTER TEST MEAL	
	SENS. % POS.	SPEC. % NEG.	SENS. % POS.	SPEC. % NEG.	SENS. % POS.	SPEC. % NEG.	SENS. % POS.	SPEC. % NEG.
Clinitest								
Trace	34.4	88.3	37.7	83.5	54.1	80.6	45.9	86.6
1+	29.5	98.7	31.1	96.9	44.3	96.5	36.1	98.5
2+	23.0	100.0	27.9	98.9	37.7	98.7	34.4	99.3
3+	19.7	100.0	24.6	99.3	31.1	99.1	29.5	100.0
4+	9.8	100.0	21.3	99.8	24.6	99.3	2.2	100.0
Galatest-								
Trace	37.7	83.3	47.5	73.8	54.1	66.1	50.8	72.9
1+	29.5	95.0	37.7	90.3	47.5	87.2	44.3	90.7
2+	24.6	98.7	29.5	97.4	39.3	96.9	34.4	97.1
3+	18.0	99.6	26.2	99.1	34.4	98.7	31.1	98.7
4+	11.5	99.8	23.0	99.6	29.5	99.3	21.3	99.6
Benedict's								
Trace	42.6	73.6	68.9	54.4	88.5	34.6	80.3	51.1
1+	32.8	92.1	49.2	84.6	59.0	79.3	49.2	86.3
2+	21.3	99.8	34.4	97.4	41.0	97.4	34.4	99.3
3+	19.7	100.0	24.6	99.3	34.4	99.8	29.5	99.8
4+	4.9	100.0	11.5	100.0	13.1	100.0	9.8	100.0
Dreypak								
Trace	41.0	85.0	62.3	71.4	62.3	63.2	54.1	77.5
1+	27.9	97.8	39.3	93.4	45.9	90.3	39.3	95.8
2+	23.0	99.6	27.9	97.8	39.3	98.0	34.4	99.3
3+	13.1	100.0	24.6	99.3	32.8	99.3	24.6	100.0
4+	3.3	100.0	6.6	100.0	16.4	100.0	8.2	100.0

Source: Remein and Wilkerson (1961).
Note: See text for further explanation.

It should be kept in mind that their standardization of the meal probably increased its ratio of sensitivity to specificity. Indeed, there is no certainty that response to a standardized meal is a less definitive test for diabetes than a glucose-loading test. It is also relevant to interpretation of data of these kinds that reproducibility of results of oral glucose tolerance tests leave much to be desired. It is possible, for example, that the ratio of sensitivity to specificity of a two-hour value obtained in the course of a duplicate oral glucose tolerance test would not have been any better than that of the two-hour postprandial value. Postglucose values tend to be greater than postprandial values, but this does not necessarily mean that the postglucose test is more sensitive. Both dietary fat and protein intensify the insulinogenic effect of carbohydrate. It is not surprising, therefore, that blood glucose values are somewhat higher after glucose alone. It is not known whether persons whose blood glucose levels rank at the fifth percentile after a standardized large meal are any less likely to be or become diabetic than those whose blood glucose values are at the fifth percentile after oral glucose.

Subsequent studies have confirmed in a general way the results of Remein and Wilkerson. On the other hand, it is now evident that the sensitivity and specificity of screening tests are highly variable in differing circumstances. The factors that affect them are several, including especially the diagnostic criteria employed in the "definitive test". If older traditional criteria are applied, the urine glucose in most circumstances is a very insensitive instrument. In many societies, about 15% of older adults have "diabetes" by these blood glucose criteria, and only a small percentage of these "diabetics" have glycosuria (Keen, 1964). On the other hand, when criteria now recommended by other scientists are used (Siperstein, 1975; West, 1975; Andres, 1976), rates of "diabetes" are very much lower and the sensitivity of the urine glucose is much greater. Table 9 shows the very substantial effects on sensitivity and specificity in a urine test with changes of modest degree in diagnostic criteria.

In Bedford, England, even though the subjects were asked to collect the urine specimen one to two hours after a meal, only 4% had glycosuria; and of glycosurics two thirds had clearly normal glucose tolerance (Keen, 1964). But in a subsample in which all subjects had glucose loading tests, the sensitivity of urine tests was much better in subjects whose two-hour values were greater than 160 mg/100 ml. Four of ten had postprandial glycosuria and nine of ten had glycosuria after 50 gm of oral glucose. It is also important to recognize that the sensitivity and specificity of urine tests vary greatly depending on the concentration of glucose used as the index of positivity. Under most conditions urine glucose concentrations of 1% or greater (3 to 4+) are highly specific for diabetes, while trace amounts usually have weak specificity. Sensitivity and specificity of urine tests are also affected by their relationship to feeding and the precision of the methods used (see above).

Studies by the Birmingham Working Party (1970), and in Bedford, England (Butterfield, et al, 1967; Keen, 1964) provided some of the most useful information on the sensitivity and specificity of urine tests and their relationship to various factors.

In several populations it has been shown that men have greater glycosuria than women at comparable glucose levels. These populations include Minnesota college students (Watson, 1939), Americans from many sites (Gordon, 1964), Swedes (Nilsson, et al, 1964), the English (Fine, 1965; Butterfield, et al, 1967), New Zealanders (Beaven, 1974), Californians (Dales, et al, 1974), and Japanese (Mimura, 1970). Thus the sensitivity of urine tests may be expected to be greater in men, and specificity less. Few data are available on the effect of other factors on renal threshold for glucose. Dales, et al (1974) found that Oriental subjects had more glycosuria than whites and blacks, at comparable blood glucose levels. Whether this difference was directly attributable to race is not known, but certainly deserves further investigation.

57

TABLE 9 Effect on Sensitivity and Specificity of Changing Diagnostic Criteria

Screening Tests	Assuming Two Hour Blood Glucose Values Greater Than 149 mg/100 ml Are Diagnostic			Assuming Two Hour Blood Glucose Values Greater Than 119 mg/100 ml Are Diagnostic		
	Sensitivity (Percent)	Specificity (Percent)	"Specificity" of Positive Tests*	Sensitivity (Percent)	Specificity (Percent)	"Specificity" of Positive Tests*
Fasting urine glucose	35.3	99.7	92.3	18.8	99.7	92.3
Urine glucose two to four hours after eating†	38.9	97.6	45.7	20.2	97.6	45.7
Urine glucose two hours after oral glucose	67.0	94.0	40.4	41.7	94.4	47.9
Fasting blood glucose (over 119 mg/100 ml)	44.0	98.0	68.8	23.4	97.8	68.8
Blood glucose two to four hours after eating† (> 129 mg/100 ml)	50.0	98.6	69.2	27.7	96.6	69.2

Source: West and Kalbfleisch (1971a).
Note: These are data on the same 1,530 subjects for whom data are presented in Table 11.
*Percentage of positive tests that were true positives.
†In a few instances (less than 10%) these specimens were drawn four to ten hours after eating.

Data of O'Sullivan, et al (1967) provide further insights concerning the relationship of postprandial blood glucose levels and results of glucose tolerance tests, as well as the factors affecting these relationships. They performed postprandial tests on 77% of the adults of Sudbury, Massachusetts. Glucose tolerance tests were also done in a representative sample. Under conditions of their study postprandial tests had only moderate sensitivity, but it was evident that this sensitivity would be greatly increased by lowering the screening level or by raising the diagnostic levels.

Other important determinants of sensitivity for all types of screening tests include the age, fatness, and other characteristics of the population tested. Table 10 shows the very considerable variation of the sensitivity and specificity of the two-hour urine glucose in ten different populations. In East Pakistan, for instance, the sensitivity of the urine glucose was high. In that circumstance a great majority of subjects had excellent glucose tolerance, but those that had diabetes were markedly hyperglycemic. In Nicaragua only 11% of those with diabetes had glycosuria. Similar interpopulation variations were seen in specificity of glycosuria. In Honduras 86% of glycosurics had diabetes; in Panama, only 22%. Thus it is a mistake to generalize too much about the sensitivity and specificity of a test. Testing methods were standardized and ages were comparable in these populations, suggesting that differences were mainly attributable to differences in the characteristics of the populations. On the other hand, even seemingly trivial differences in circumstances of testing may affect results significantly. This includes, for example, the degree of hydration of the subjects. Urine glucose tests typically measure the concentration of urine glucose, not the amount. Differences in concentration as great as threefold can be the result solely of differences in rates of urine flow that are common in daily life. When urine tests are performed after carbohydrate loads, sensitivity is often considerably enhanced by having the subject empty the bladder before or near the time of the test load. This tends to increase the concentration of glucose in the subsequent urine test.

Table 11 shows the sensitivity and specificity of five different screening tests in three populations.

Many have deprecated the fasting blood glucose as a screening test because of its purported insensitivity, but this matter appears to deserve reexamination. When traditional diagnostic criteria are employed, a substantial percentage of the older segment of well-fed populations have "diabetes", and only a small fraction of those with "abnormal" tolerance have elevated fasting levels (Hainline and Keller, 1964). But these criteria are now being challenged (Siperstein, 1974; West, 1975; Prout, et al, 1976). Data of O'Sullivan and Mahan (1968) show that persons with impaired tolerance by the traditional standards are more likely to develop florid diabetes than those with clearly normal tolerance. But only a small number of subjects were available for follow-up who initially had clearly normal fasting levels and two-hour plasma glucose values between 140 and 180 mg/100 ml. Thus the risk of diabetes in this group remains to be established. Data of Logie, et al (1974), Carlstrom, et al (1971,1972), Kobberling,

59

TABLE 10 Marked Variation in Ten Populations of Sensitivity and Specificity of Urine Glucose Two Hours After Oral Glucose

COUNTRY	TOTAL NO.	KNOWN DIABETICS URINE TEST			NO HISTORY OF DIABETES							SENSITIVITY* (PERCENT)	SPECIFICITY* (PERCENT)	"SPECIFICITY" OF POSITIVE TESTS† (PERCENT)
						DISCOVERED DIABETICS URINE TEST			NONDIABETICS URINE TEST					
		NO.	POS.	NEG	NO.	NO.	POS.	NEG.	NO.	POS.	NEG.			
Uruguay	484	17	15	2	467	16	10	6	451	37	414	63 [76]	91.4(91.8)	21(40)
Venezuela	480	7	7	0	473	28	11	17	445	7	438	39 [51]	98.4(98.4)	61(72)
Malaya	566	9	7	2	557	11	9	2	546	43	503	82 [80]	91.8(92.1)	17(27)
East Pakistan	513	0	0	0	513	9	9	0	504	29	475	100(100)	94.2(94.2)	24(24)
Costa Rica	470	4	3	1	466	23	12	11	443	22	421	52 [56]	94.8(95.0)	36(41)
El Salvador	265	2	2	0	263	7	2	5	256	7	249	29 [44]	97.3(97.3)	22(36)
Guatemala	413	6	5	1	407	12	7	5	395	7	388	58 [67]	98.0(98.2)	50(52)
Honduras	343	0	0	0	343	16	6	10	327	1	326	38 [38]	99.7(99.7)	86(86)
Nicaragua	383	5	2	3	378	18	2	16	360	8	352	11 [17]	96.9(97.7)	20(33)
Panama	345	0	0	0	345	10	4	6	335	14	321	40 [40]	95.8(95.8)	22(22)
TOTALS	4,262	50	41	9	4,212	150	72	78	4,062	175	3,887	48 [57]	95.5(95.7)	29(39)

Source: West and Kalbfleisch (1971a) where details may be found on criteria and methods.
*Numbers in parentheses are results when calculations are based on the entire population sample including known diabetics.
†Percentage of positive tests that were true positives.

et al (1975), and Jarrett and Keen (1976) show rather low rates of conversion to fasting hyperglycemia and clinical diabetes in subjects whose tolerance is slightly "abnormal" by traditional standards. There is thus still considerable uncertainty concerning the prognostic significance of slightly "abnormal" postglucose values in persons with normal fasting levels. Siperstein (1975) has also presented arguments derogating the specificity of the glucose tolerance test in persons with normal fasting values. There is some evidence that people with slightly abnormal glucose tolerance may have increased risk of vascular disease despite normal fasting glucose levels. In persons with normal fasting glucose values it is not known to what extent this relationship between vascular disease and abnormal glucose tolerance is independent of other factors with which both are associated (eg, physical indolence, obesity, hypertension). But this evidence is quite incomplete. These matters are reviewed in other sections of this book. There is little evidence that attempts to treat nonobese "diabetics" with normal fasting levels glucose have been attended by any reduction in morbidity. Obesity should be treated even if glucose tolerance is normal.

In the Pima population data are more complete in several respects than in other studies (Bennett, et al, 1976a; Dippe, et al, 1974). In general, these latter observations suggest that individuals having two-hour values high enough to be at high risk for subsequent unequivocal diabetes tend to have also an elevation of their fasting glucose concentrations. More data are needed, but it now appears that the sensitivity of the fasting blood glucose is considerably better than had been generally believed. In fact, Siperstein has suggested that the diagnosis of diabetes should probably not be made in the absence of fasting hyperglycemia. By his criteria of diabetes the sensitivity of the fasting blood glucose is 100%. Some arguments to the contrary are reviewed in the section on diagnostic tests, but these uncertainties and disagreements of interpretation deserve emphasis. Owen, et al (1970) have also emphasized the disadvantages of overdiagnosis that may attend the use of certain traditional screening and diagnostic standards, especially in their application to elderly subjects. In the United States about half of the elderly have "abnormal" glucose tolerance by some of the commonly employed criteria (Andres, 1976).

One great advantage of the fasting blood glucose as a screening instrument is its uncontested specificity. Positive screenees have diabetes unless there is a laboratory error, or unless the subject was not actually fasting. In the large group (1,057) tested by Hainline and Keller, there were 81 subjects with fasting blood glucose levels greater than 110 mg/100 ml, of whom 100% had abnormal glucose tolerance. When the fasting blood glucose is the single screening test, costs of follow-up testing are greatly reduced and overreferral avoided. In considering alternatives of screening strategy it is often overlooked that upper limits of normal for the fasting glucose are similar in subjects who have been fasting overnight and in those who have fasted for three to ten hours during the day. Overnight fasting is, therefore, not always necessary in screening for evidence of fasting hyperglycemia. The "fasting" glucose may be determined

TABLE 11 Sensitivity and Specificity of Five Screening Tests in Three Countries

	A TOTAL TESTED	B DIA-BETIC*	C NONDIA-BETIC	D POS. TESTS	E TRUE POS.	F FALSE POS.	G NEG. TESTS	H TRUE NEG.	I FALSE NEG.	SENSITIV-ITY† (PERCENT)	SPECIFIC-ITY† (PERCENT)	"SPECI-FICITY" OF POS. TEST‡ (PERCENT)
Fasting urine glucose												
Uruguay	136	11	125	7	7	0	129	125	4	63.6	100.0	100.0
Venezuela	198	20	178	5	4	1	193	177	16	20.0	99.4	80.0
Malaya	84	3	81	1	1	0	83	81	2	33.3	100.0	100.0
TOTALS	418	34	384	13	12	1	405	383	22	35.3	99.7	92.3
Average for three countries										38.9	99.8	93.3
Urine glucose two to four hours after eating												
Uruguay	348	22	326	17	9	8	331	318	13	40.9	97.5	52.9
Venezuela	282	15	267	5	3	2	277	265	12	20.0	99.3	60.0
Malaya	482	17	465	24	9	15	458	450	8	52.9	96.8	37.5
TOTALS	1,112	54	1,058	46	21	25	1,066	1,033	33	38.9	97.6	45.7
Average for three countries										37.9	97.8	50.1
Urine glucose two hours after oral glucose												
Uruguay	484	33	451	62	25	37	422	414	8	75.8	91.8	40.3
Venezuela	480	35	445	25	18	7	455	438	17	51.4	98.4	72.0
Malaya	566	20	546	59	16	43	507	503	4	80.0	92.1	27.1
TOTALS	1,530	88	1,442	146	59	87	1,384	1,355	29	67.0	94.0	40.4
Average for three countries										69.1	94.1	46.4

Fasting blood glucose (values
> 119 mg/100 ml considered
positive)

Uruguay	134	11	123	10	7	3	124	120	4	63.6	97.6	70.0
Venezuela	120	13	107	5	3	2	115	105	10	23.1	98.1	60.0
Malaya	25	1	24	1	1	0	24	4	0	100.0	100.0	100.0
TOTALS	279	25	254	16	11	5	263	249	12	44.0	98.0	68.8
Average for three countries										62.2	98.6	76.7

Blood glucose two to four
hours after eating (values >
129 mg/100 ml considered
positive)

Uruguay	341	22	319	13	10	3	328	316	12	45.5	99.1	76.9
Venezuela	150	12	138	11	7	4	139	134	5	58.3	97.1	63.6
Malaya	100	2	98	2	1	1	98	97	1	50.0	99.0	50.0
TOTALS	591	36	555	26	18	8	565	547	18	50.0	98.6	69.2
Average for three countries										51.3	98.4	63.5

Source: West and Kalbfleisch (1971a).
*Two-hour blood glucose above 149 mg/100 ml. Of 88 diabetics tested in these three countries, 55 (63%) had no previous history of the disorder. The numbers of new and previously known diabetics by country are given in Table 10.
†Sensitivity is columns E/B; specificity is H/C; and "specificity" of positive tests is D/E.
‡Percentage of positive tests that were true positives.

in late morning or late afternoon, provided that at least three hours of fasting have transpired.

Two studies have demonstrated the poor sensitivity and specificity of symptoms as screening instruments. Data of Welborn, et al (1968) have been described in Chapter 3 under current concepts. Similar results had been obtained by Jorde (1962) in his excellent and detailed studies in Bergen, Norway. He determined frequency of several symptoms in relation to age in known diabetics, in previously undiagnosed diabetics, and in the general population of adults. The most common diabetes-related symptom in occult diabetics was polyuria (17%), but this symptom was almost as common (9%) in an age-matched group from the general population. Unusual thirst was present in only 12% of undiagnosed diabetics, but the specificity of this symptom was better than for polyuria. Only 3% of the control group had this complaint. In men with undiagnosed diabetes, itching was no more common than in controls but women discovered to be diabetic by the screening program had pruritis much more commonly (10%) than controls (4%). Polyphagia (3%) and weight loss (6%) were only very slightly more common in undiagnosed diabetics than in controls (differences not statistically significant).

Sisk, et al (1970) concluded that, "Until more accurate criteria for the diagnosis of diabetes are established, the comparison of individual tests by sensitivity and specificity must remain virtually meaningless." Perhaps this view reflects an even greater degree of skepticism than is warranted, but it is useful as a reminder of the need for more critical judgments in these matters.

Follow-up, Evaluation, and Costs

The nature of the follow-up program should be strongly conditioned by the specific objectives and priorities of the screening program. As explained above, this process presents excellent opportunities for professional education and epidemiologic research as well as case detection, but the characteristics and extent of follow-up are also influenced by the resources available. Ideally, all positive screenees are followed to determine the number who do not have follow-up tests and the reasons why, as well as the results of follow-up tests. When patients are referred to their own physicians, follow-up evaluations may include ascertainment of the diagnostic methods and criteria that were applied. Finally, it is desirable, although rarely feasible, to study outcome on a long-term basis (eg, nature of treatment and response thereto). Because such data are few, there is still considerable uncertainty of the value of mass screening for diabetes.

One useful method of evaluation is to estimate in relation to cost the number of new cases discovered and/or brought under treatment. In their program Millington and Tinsman (1966) estimated a cost of $67 per new case. Details were not given and it seems likely that they did not include all indirect costs of the type discussed below. Total cost is often underestimated because a substantial portion is indirect. In Britain, Butterfield (1968) estimated the cost per new case at £5 to £30, depending on circumstances and objectives. In the massive Cleveland program the cost per new case was about $35 (Genuth, et al 1976). We carried out a screening program in which we spent less than $10 per new case. However, when we examined all the indirect costs of the whole process we found that costs per new case exceeded $150, not including the time of the screenees (West, et al, 1970). Proust and McCracken (1968) found in Australia that the cost of finding a new diabetic was $30 (about $24 US) in Goulfram, and $18 ($14 US) in Toowoomba. They indicated, however, that some substantial indirect costs were not included in their computations. Orzeck, et al, (1971) have reviewed the subject of benefits in relation to costs and have made some suggestions on how these may be estimated.

There is frequently considerable disparity between the number of diabetics identified and the number actually brought under treatment. Further, it has been argued that a substantial portion of those found to have "mild abnormalities" of glucose tolerance do not really have diabetes (Siperstein, 1974). It is also evident that only a small minority receive and follow appropriate diets (West, 1973). Finally, there is considerable uncertainty about the effectiveness of treatment even in those who follow their prescribed regimens faithfully (Butterfield, 1968). Some of these and related problems have been reviewed by Houser et al (1977). No definitive evidence is available that justifies with certainty the kinds of mass screening programs that have been traditional; nor is their decisive evidence to the contrary. Justification and priority of mass screening must therefore be based on interpretation of the incomplete evidence at hand and the application of common sense. There are several positive considerations. One is that under proper conditions the by-products of such programs as described above may be considerable. When effectively applied, early therapy of newly detected diabetics very often improves beta-cell function and reverses the severity of diabetes. Persons who know they have diabetes are very probably less likely to develop ketoacidosis and gangrene than those who are unaware of their diabetes. A substantial percentage of cases with these two complications progress to an advanced state because the patient and his physician are unaware of the diabetes. Hyperlipoproteinemia and certain types of neuropathy can often be dramatically reversed with treatment of diabetes. Present data are inconclusive but most diabetologists think that the rate of development of the vascular lesions is probably reduced by mitigation of hyperglycemia. As shown above, about one quarter of cases discovered in mass screening have unpleasant symptoms that can be relieved immediately by treatment.

Under What Conditions Is Mass Screening Justified?

There is a developing consensus, however, that mass screening should be undertaken only after careful assessment of benefits in relation to cost under the specific conditions in which the enterprise is contemplated. Malins (1974) says, "Screening of whole populations with the object of case-finding is not a rewarding exercise". Indirect as well as direct costs should be taken into

65

account. Expenses include cost of testing materials and laboratory supplies and of time of clerical and laboratory personnel. Professional time required in organizational and follow-up work is usually substantial. It has been common practice to ignore the considerable costs sustained by the screenees themselves and their families. This includes time invested in proceeding to and from the testing site. Sometimes costs sustained by positive screenees are great. These may include one or more visits to their physician for follow-up tests, charges for glucose tolerance tests, etc. Often volunteer workers contribute substantial amounts of time at no direct cost to such programs. But in deciding about cost-benefit ratios, it is usually appropriate to include all these "indirect" costs.

The recognition of costs sustained by screenees suggests the particular advantages of testing stations that are in the usual path of the screenees. This would include testing at industrial sites, homes for the aged, hospital clinics, shopping centers, etc. The benefits of combining diabetes screening with screening for other diseases is apparent and deserves emphasis. Screening for hypertension and hyperlipoproteinemia fit particularly well with screening for diabetes.

Our experience (West, et al, 1970) and appraisals of follow-up data of others (Proust and McCracken, 1968) suggest the value of on-site follow-up testing. This reduces defections by positive screenees, reduces costs of follow-up evaluation procedures, lowers costs sustained by screenees, reduces negative and positive diagnostic errors, and usually increases the percentage of the occult diabetics who are placed under treatment. The unit costs of carbohydrate-loading tests are much lower when done in large numbers at testing stations than when done one by one in the offices of individual physicians.

As they have been carried out in the past, the benefits of many mass screening programs have probably not justified their total cost. Fleeson and Wenk (1970) have described the "pitfalls of mass screening". A good argument could be made for routinely combining diabetes screening with screening for other disorders such as heart disease. Even so, there are still circumstances under which mass screening for diabetes alone is probably justified. Some of the earmarks of such conditions include:

1. A well-conceived plan for compromising the claims of economy, sensitivity, and specificity. There must be a reasonable yield of new cases per dollar spent, but overreferral should be avoided. Potentialities for cost-sharing through multipurpose screening are exploited whenever available. High-risk groups receive priority unless research objectives require more representative sampling. The three main risk factors are obesity, family history of diabetes in one or more close relatives, and age greater than thirty;

2. A program that will maximize the percentage of positive screenees who receive appropriate follow-up tests and the percentage of the new diabetics actually placed under treatment;

3. A well-designed plan for exploiting the potential by-products (public education, professional education, epidemiologic research, etc);

4. A process of systematic evaluation. This would include an estimate before and after of the total cost per new case found and per new case actually placed under appropriate treatment. Ideally, this would also include definitive tests on a sample of the negative screenees to determine the sensitivity and specificity of the screening procedures and the factors that affect them. This will also make it possible to compute prevalence rates in the screenee group and its subgroups.

DIAGNOSTIC METHODS

Designing and interpreting diagnostic tests is a function of the clinician, but an understanding of diagnostic methods and criteria is also critical in the collection and interpretation of epidemiologic data. It will therefore be appropriate to review this subject in some detail.

Many claims have been made concerning the discovery of markers other than glycemia for identifying the diabetic state. For reasons discussed in other sections of this book, none has gained acceptance as a specific sign of diabetes. The diagnosis depends on the demonstration of abnormal blood glucose levels. A variety of procedures have been developed to test the capacity of the human organism to regulate blood glucose concentration. Many problems remain in determining what tests are most appropriate, to what degree methods should be adjusted to the circumstances in which they are performed and to the characteristics of the subject tested, and what criteria of interpretation should be applied under various conditions.

Less specific tests for diabetes have been discussed in the section on screening and detection. These include symptoms and signs of diabetes, urine glucose tests, and certain kinds of procedures for measuring blood glucose.

Laboratory Tests

Measurement of Blood Glucose

Excellent reviews of this subject have been published by Cooper (1973) and by Whichelow, et al (1967). The three major variables are the laboratory procedure employed, the element analyzed (whole blood, plasma, or serum), and the source of the blood (venous or arterial).

Arterial, capillary, and venous blood
Concentration of glucose in capillary blood usually reflects the level in arterial blood (Foster, 1922; Whichelow, et al, 1967). Relative concentrations in arterial and venous blood vary with status of feeding or fasting. These A-V differences were first reported by Hagedorn in 1921. He also observed that the presence of diabetes reduced these differences, as did Rabinowitch (1927a). Results of subsequent studies on these A-V differences in normal subjects are summarized in Table 12. In the fasting state these differences are usually small or negligible. One hour after oral glucose or a meal, the differences are substantial, typically 20 to 50 mg/100 ml. At two hours differences are smaller but still

TABLE 12   Capillary-Venous Difference in Concentration of Glucose

INVESTIGATOR AND YEAR	DOSAGE OF ORAL GLUCOSE	C-V DIFFERENCE IN MG/100 ML		
		FASTING	ONE-HOUR	TWO-HOUR
Langner and Fies (1942)	50 gm	1		
Goldberg and Luft (1948)	1 gm/kg	10	26	7
Mosenthal and Barry (1950)	100 gm		37	30
Klimt (1961)	30 gm/sq m		24	13
Whichelow, et al (1967)	50 gm	6	26	−2
Joplin and Wright (1968)		3	32	
Burgi (1974)	50 gm	10	37	15
Stravljenic and Skrabablo (1975)	50 gm	16	31	14

appreciable, particularly with large glucose loads. In normal subjects these differences are well related to the prevailing levels of blood glucose and blood insulin. An interesting observation of Whichelow, et al, was that after oral glucose, blood in deep arm veins of lean subjects had lower levels of blood glucose than blood from superficial veins. Thus, A-V differences are smaller when superficial venous blood is sampled. They also found A-V differences greater in lean than in obese subjects.

All too frequently the rather substantial A-V differences that may be expected at one hour have not been taken into account in interpreting clinical or epidemiologic data. More data are needed but it would appear that cut-off points at one hour should be about 25 mg/100 ml higher for capillary levels than for venous concentration when small oral loads are employed (eg, 50 gm). With large loads (eg, 100 gm), cut-off points should be higher by about 40 mg/100 ml. With small loads, differences at two hours are usually small and in some instances negligible. After large glucose loads (eg, 100 gm), cut-off points at two hours ought to be about 25 mg/100 ml higher with capillary values than with venous values.

Plasma and whole blood

Until recent years concentration of glucose had usually been measured in whole blood. In 1965, Zalme and Knowles summarized arguments for measuring plasma levels rather than whole blood values. Their publication reflected and encouraged a trend toward use of plasma values. But it is interesting that Fredrick Allen had indicated in 1913 that determinations on serum were preferable to those on whole blood, and that the former "were likely to win general adoption". In this and other matters he was a half century ahead of the majority.

Plasma values are usually about 15% (not mg %) higher than whole blood values because the concentration is about 30% greater in plasma than in red cells. The relationship of concentration in plasma and whole blood is, however, not entirely constant. If, for example, the hematocrit is low, the difference is diminished. Nevertheless, use of a conversion factor such as 15% is in most circumstances attended by a negligible degree of error in converting actual whole blood values into estimates for the plasma levels or vice versa. This conversion figure is based on data from several laboratories. The evidence presented by MacDonald, et al (1964) and Tustison, et al (1966) is typical.

Stavljenic and Skrabalo (1975) found, surprisingly, that serum values were about 11 mg/100 ml lower than in plasma in all stages of a glucose tolerance test. The reason for this was not clear.

Our experience (West, et al, 1970) has confirmed that practicing physicians frequently fail to take into account that the normal range for plasma values extends to a substantially higher level than for whole blood values. My colleagues in the United States and abroad tell me that this problem is widespread. Physicians, who have once learned the conventional cut-off points for one-hour and two-hour whole blood values, often have difficulty in making the appropriate conversions when dealing with plasma values. Another aspect of this problem is that laboratory reports and clinical notations often fail to indicate whether the specimen analyzed was whole blood or plasma, capillary, or venous blood.

Laboratory procedures for measuring glucose

Cooper (1973) has written an outstanding review of this subject based on the observations of his own group at the Center for Disease Control of the United States Public Health Service, as well as a summary of the literature. In general, these data are very encouraging with respect to comparability of results with the methods now being widely employed. Table 13 (Cooper, 1973) shows that comparability of results is good with these six different procedures. Note that results in columns 3, 4, and 5 apply, respectively, to the traditional cut-off points for fasting values (115), for two-hour values (140), and for one-hour values (190). At each of these levels of glucose concentration, results correspond closely with the six methods.

Because it measures nonglucose-reducing substances as well as glucose, the Folin-Wu method has been almost entirely abandoned. The level of these nonglucose substances was not constant or predictable, but averaged about 20 mg/100 ml. This "conversion" figure is given because some of the older epidemiologic studies used this method.

Cooper found that the glucose oxidase method offered some slight advantages of specificity and reproducibility. For example, it was less influenced by interfering substances present in uremia than were other methods. But all the standard methods listed in the Table were highly reproducible. Coefficients of variations of clinical laboratories usually ranged between 5% and 10%. Coefficients of variation within a single run averaged 3% to 6%.

Blood glucose methods were also well summarized by the 1969 publication of the American Diabetes Association (Statistics Committee chaired by Klimt). Because fluoride prevents glycolysis for several days, it is often helpful to add this to specimens when it is necessary to delay refrigeration or the laboratory procedure. Fluoride should not be used, however, if the glucose oxidase method is employed because it interferes with that reaction. This includes the Dextrostix test.

69

TABLE 13   Comparison of Glucose Methods—Results of Selected Representative Laboratories

	Pool					
	1	2	3	4	5	6
Method	Mean (SD)	Mean (SD)	Mean (SD)	Mean (SD)	Mean (SD)	Mean (SD)
Glucose oxidase	66*	90	114	137	186	389
	(2.5)	(3.2)	(3.0)	(4.1)	(2.7)	(12.0)
Hexokinase	69	93	117	140	185	364
	(4.1)	(3.3)	(3.3)	(3.4)	(4.1)	(6.2)
o-toluidine	68	92	115	139	182	383
	(1.8)	(3.6)	(6.3)	(4.4)	(9.2)	(2.2)
Somogyi-Nelson	71	94	118	139	183	381
	(6.4)	(4.8)	(6.0)	(4.4)	(11.0)	(13.0)
AutoAnalyzer ferricyanide	71	96	119	144	188	386
	(2.3)	(2.6)	(2.6)	(3.2)	(2.4)	(2.8)
AutoAnalyzer neocuproine	72	95	120	143	189	397
	(2.9)	(1.2)	(2.0)	(2.6)	(5.2)	(14.0)
Expected values	65	90	115	140	190	390

Source: Cooper (1973).
*Measurements are in mg/100 ml.

Fasting and Random Blood Glucose Levels

These have been discussed in the section on screening and detection. Plasma glucose levels greater than 200 mg/100 ml are usually diagnostic of diabetes irrespective of time of day or status of feeding or fasting, provided they are confirmed. This confirmation is required to exclude the possibility of laboratory or clerical error, mislabeling of specimens, etc. Exceptions to the specificity of values over 200 are quite rare. They would include determinations of blood glucose during acute severe illness, after intravenous infusion of glucose, or immediately after large doses of oral sugar or injections of glucagon.

Under basal conditions fasting plasma glucose values exceeding 129 mg/100 ml are diagnostic if confirmed. Confirmation of slight elevations is particularly necessary because moderate laboratory error can be responsible for misclassification, and because false reports of fasting status are common. For example, subjects who have eaten no breakfast have sometimes consumed nutrients in drinks which they did not consider to be "food". Valleron, et al (1975) restudied 17 individuals in whom fasting hyperglycemia had been found despite normal two-hour blood glucose values. Fasting hyperglycemia was not confirmed in 9 of the 17.

Fasting venous plasma values of 115 to 129 mg/100 ml are borderline (Cooper, 1973); these subjects require further investigation. When concentration is measured in whole blood the normal range extends to about 100, and values exceeding 115 are clearly abnormal if confirmed by repeat testing. Schmidt, et al (1975) measured fasting capillary values in 500 healthy employees of a pharmaceutical company using the hexokinase method. Ages ranged from 16 to 65. The 95th percentile range extended through 99 mg/100 ml.

Values were slightly higher in men and in older subjects. The three standard-deviation range in the entire group extended to 106. The range observed in such studies would, of course, be affected by the extent and character of previous diabetes screening in the population tested.

Groups of older subjects usually have slightly higher fasting values than groups of younger subjects (Jorde, 1962; West, et al, 1964; Pozefsky, et al, 1965). Data are sparse, however. The significance of these small age-related differences is not clear; it may be attributable in part to increased rates of very mild diabetes in older subjects, or it may be partly or mainly attributable to physiologic changes in aging that bear little relationship to risk of diabetes. More data are needed.

Do persons with normal fasting values and "abnormal" tolerance have diabetes?

As pointed out in the section on screening, the sensitivity of the fasting glucose test has been widely deprecated. On the other hand, a considerable body of recent evidence suggests that the specificity is better than generally supposed. Some of these arguments have been reviewed under screening; more evidence is needed, however. The strongest current evidence is indirect. In many Western communities it has been shown that 10% to 30% of middle-aged people have, by conventional standards, "diabetic" glucose tolerance. Work of Jorde (performed in 1956 and reported in 1962) and of Unger (1957) suggest that these high rates of "abnormal" tolerance are not a particularly recent phenomenon. Yet rates of clinically significant disease in the seventh and eighth decade remain relatively modest in these same societies. In Bedford and Birmingham, England, less than 1% of adults have clinical diabetes despite the highly developed capacities in these communities for detecting such stigmata of diabetes as fasting hyperglycemia, retinopathy, glomerulosclerosis, and diabetic symptoms. It is clear that the vast majority who by traditional standards have "abnormal" tolerance are not developing in later life the morbidity that specifically attends diabetes (Jarrett and Keen, 1976). If persons who have normal fasting hyperglycemia and "abnormal" glucose tolerance were at high risk for developing fasting hyperglycemia, one would expect very high rates of fasting hyperglycemia in these same populations among those in the sixth, seventh, and eighth decade. It is clear, however, from data of the Birmingham Work Party (1963,1970) and Bedford (Butterfield, 1964) that rates of fasting hyperglycemia are low in middle-aged and elderly subjects.

Data of Dippe, et al (1974) and Bennett, et al (1976a) show that when two-hour values are high enough to be attended by high risk of morbidity, fasting levels are very likely to be elevated. In the study of the Birmingham Working Party (1970), the rate of decompensation from abnormal glucose tolerance to "florid" diabetes was 17.5% in six years, but some of these had slightly elevated fasting values initially. O'Sullivan and Mahan (1968) studied prospectively a group of 352 women with abnormal glucose tolerance but without florid diabetes. They were derived from a prenatal clinic. It was not indicated how many of these had slight elevation of fasting whole blood glucose in the range of 100 to 119 mg/100 ml. During a follow-up period of one to twelve years only 3% developed florid diabetes (postglucose values of 300 mg/100 ml, or postprandial of 180, or fasting venous whole blood values of 120 or more). The rate of development of unequivocal diabetes was 10.7% in those with abnormal tolerance, as defined by criteria similar to those of Fajans and Conn. The rate of subsequent decompensation was higher (25.9%) in those with abnormal tolerance by United States Public Health Service criteria, but this standard includes elevation of the fasting value as one of the criteria for separating normal from abnormal values. Thus, a portion of this group had abnormal fasting values initially. Data of Köbberling and Creutzfeldt (1970) suggest that a large portion of the group of subjects deemed to have abnormal glucose tolerance by USPHS criteria have abnormal fasting values.

Of 42 patients with "abnormal tolerance" followed for ten years by Walker (1975), ten had died and eight had been lost to follow-up. Retesting was performed on 24; only one of these was found to have clinical diabetes, and only this one of the 42 was known to have developed diabetes. Schliack, et al (1975) followed for five to fifteen years a group suspected of having diabetes on the basis of survey glucose tolerance tests. Twenty-five percent still had abnormal tolerance but only 5% had unequivocal clinical diabetes. According to Keen (1975) only 10% to 15% of those found to have abnormal tolerance in the Bedford survey had developed clinical diabetes in eight years, even though this group included some with two-hour values as high as 199 mg/100 ml after 50 gm of oral glucose. Carlstrom, et al (1971) followed 251 subjects with borderline tolerance for three to five years. They all had values exceeding the two standard-deviations range for their age and sex; none developed diabetes. Logie, et al (1974) followed 72 patients with abnormal tolerance and normal fasting values for a period of one to nine years. Only five developed "overt" diabetes. The results of Feldman, et al (1973) were similar.

Control data have been few in studies of this kind. Asperic, et al (1974) did measure rates of decompensation in those with normal screening values, as well as in a group with borderline tolerance. Decompensation rates in controls were almost as high as in those with borderline states. Data of Fajans, et al (1969) show that decompensation to clinical diabetes is also rare in children who have "abnormal" glucose tolerance together with normal fasting hyperglycemia. Köbberling, et al (1975) followed for five years a group of 488 close relatives of diabetics. Conversion from "abnormal" tolerance to normal tolerance was frequent. The development of "overt" diabetes was more common in those with impaired tolerance (13.6%) than in the entire group (1.3%), but only 11 of 17 found by their criteria to have "overt" diabetes were confirmed as having such by tests five years later. The data suggested that only a small fraction of those with *normal* fasting levels and abnormal tolerance would ultimately develop fasting hyperglycemia. They concluded that the glucose tolerance test had "limited prognostic value" with respect to the identification of diabetes in individual cases.

It does seem reasonable to expect that as glucose tolerance deteriorates in early diabetes, there would be a stage at which blood glucose levels would decline to normal after several hours even though definitely elevated during the first few hours. But the prevalence of this stage at any given time is probably quite low. Assume, for instance, that the rate of fasting hyperglycemia at age 80 in a certain population is 6%, and that at age 40 it is 2%. Assume further that the average duration of this interim stage (abnormal glucose tolerance with normal fasting glucose) is ten years. The number in this interim stage at any one time would be about 1%. If the interim stage lasts an average of twenty years, the prevalence of interim status would be 2%; if five years, the rate would be about 0.5%; and if one year, the rate would be 0.1%. Calculations of this kind suggest that in many populations less than 10% of those with normal fasting levels and "abnormal" tolerance will develop unequivocal fasting hyperglycemia.

For these and other reasons set forth under screening, rates of fasting hyperglycemia are probably the best indexes of disease rates. Data of O'Sullivan and Hurwitz (1966) are also consistent with this notion. It seems probable that the group of persons with normal fasting glucose values and with postglucose values in the top one to five percentiles for their age group are more likely to develop diabetes than those with lower postglucose values. But the degree of this risk is not known. Present clinical and epidemiologic evidence would not appear to warrant the widely prevalent practice of diagnosing diabetes in the absence of fasting hyperglycemia. The recent views of Siperstein (1975) to this effect were probably considered by most as quite unorthodox if not heretical. He suggested the abandonment of the glucose tolerance test as a diagnostic test for diabetes. Traditionalists will be surprised to hear that Dr. Joslin shared these reservations. In 1939 he said, "The diagnosis of diabetes with a glucose tolerance test is often difficult and most unsatisfactory, and when I say occasionally I hate to make a diagnosis of diabetes from a glucose tolerance test I am not expressing myself too strongly. The very fact in 20% of the normal group of all cases over 60 years of age there was an impairment of tolerance is disturbing". Recent epidemiologic evidence described above and below give strong support to this unorthodox conservatism concerning the glucose tolerance test.

Early diagnosis of diabetes is a decidedly useful goal. It has not been established, however, that the ratio of sensitivity to specificity is better for the glucose tolerance test than for the fasting glucose. A good argument can be made to the effect that the fasting blood glucose should be the prime diagnostic instrument. This, however, is still a minority view among diabetologists. A substantial majority of diabetologists regard as diabetic individuals who, by their particular criteria, have abnormal tolerance—even when fasting levels are normal. In sections below, the susceptibility of such individuals to vascular disease is discussed. Present data are quite incomplete. They neither exclude or confirm an *independent* effect of "abnormal tolerance" on susceptibility to vascular lesions in persons with normal fasting glucose values (Stamler, 1975; Bennett, et al, 1976a). Recent data of Jarrett and Keen (1976) and of Bennett, et al (1976a) also suggest that risk of diabetes and its microvascular lesions is very low in persons with mild "abnormalities" of glucose tolerance (of a degree usually attended with normal glucose tolerance).

73

These considerations show the need to collect and report epidemiologic data in a manner that will make clear the numbers in the samples of "diabetics" who have or do not have fasting hyperglycemia. Frequently, it will be desirable to include also in the design and analysis of such studies a subgroup with borderline fasting levels. It is not yet clear at exactly what level of fasting blood glucose increased risk begins for the development of vascular or neuropathic lesions, or for decompensation of beta-cell function. In groups with abnormal glucose tolerance followed prospectively, interpretation will be considerably facilitated by dividing the group into those with normal, borderline, and elevated fasting values. In many of the previous reports it has not been clear what percentage of the group with abnormal tolerance had slight elevation of their fasting levels. Other supplementary data will also be needed to discern the extent to which the predictive value of any given criteria are independent of known risk factors such as age and fatness.

Oral Glucose Tolerance Tests

> Presently all experts agree that a diagnosis of diabetes mellitus can be made on a completely asymptomatic patient on the basis of a carefully performed glucose tolerance test.
>
> Conn and Fajans (1961)

> I believe that the oral dextrose tolerance test as ordinarily used and interpreted is practically worthless. It is true that it will give you a diabetic type curve in a moderate-to-severe diabetic, but in those individuals a simple fasting blood sugar level will tell you just as much. In the milder diabetics the curve is so variable that it is not worth doing.
>
> Soskin (1951)

Although taken from the older literature, these views reflect well the present conflict of opinion on the utility of the oral glucose tolerance test in identifying diabetes. Conn and Fajans were in this context referring to oral glucose tolerance tests. Their views of 1961 were and are shared by most diabetologists. But Soskin's opinion no longer seems so heretical as it once did. Much recent evidence from both clinical and epidemiologic investigations suggests a need to reexamine thoroughly our traditional notions. The oral glucose tolerance test has been one of the prime instruments in epidemiologic studies of diabetes. It will be appropriate, therefore, to review in some detail the status of this and related diagnostic tests for diabetes.

History

The general use of glucose tolerance tests as clinical procedures awaited the development of methods for determining glucose concentration on small amounts of blood (Bang, 1913). But as early as 1913 Allen was able to describe a considerable research literature on glucose tolerance tests. Early pioneers in the development of these tests in man included Hofmeister (1889), Jacobsen (1913), Hopkins (1915), Hamman and Hirschman (1917), Maclean and de Wesselow (1921), Jorgensen and Plum (1923), and Malmros (1928). Two types of criteria were commonly employed in evaluating tolerance: the peak level of the blood glucose (most often measured at one hour) and the length of time required for the blood glucose to reach or approach fasting levels (most often estimated by measuring at two hours). Specific criteria of interpretation suggested initially did not differ much from those employed in recent years. These standards were usually developed by testing very small numbers of subjects, and these groups were not representative of the general populations. Goldberg and Luft (1948), Moyer and Womack (1950), and Mosenthal and Barry (1950) were among the first to test a considerable number of subjects in an attempt to develop standards of interpretation. The criteria suggested by these groups were similar, and they differed little from those later promulgated by an expert committee of the United States Public Health Service (Remein and Wilkerson, 1961). Criteria were also promulgated by Fajans and Conn (1959), and these have been widely used. These pioneering sets of criteria represented a consensus of expert opinion based on experience in testing relatively small numbers of volunteers from unrepresentative samples. More recently criteria have been proposed that take into account the gradually broadening base of evidence. These newer developments will be described below.

Tests have usually been performed in the morning after an overnight fast using as a challenge a single glucose drink. But in the 1930s and 1940s a test with a double load was widely used. In this test, designed by Exton and Rose (1934), two doses of glucose were given one hour apart; the blood glucose was then measured one hour after the second load. This test is seldom used today. Its abandonment was apparently prompted by the lack of evidence that the double load added to the sensitivity or specificity of the result. On the other hand, no evidence disproving its purported advantages has been published. There is some indirect evidence suggesting that this approach might have merit. In general, overfeeding tends to improve insulin response in normals and decrease insulin response in diabetics. Conceivably a double load might be superior to a single load in separating these two groups. Baba, et al (1970) still employ a double load.

Other developments in testing techniques and interpretation will be discussed below in the sections to which they apply. The earlier literature on glucose tolerance tests was well covered in the excellent reviews of Malmros (1928) and Jorde (1962). More recent literature is well summarized in the review of the American Diabetes Association Statistics Committee chaired by Klimt (1969), and the reviews of Lehtovirta (1973) and Duffy, et al (1975).

Amount of glucose in the load

In his excellent discussion of 1913 on glucose tolerance tests, Allen noted and deplored the absence of fixed standards of procedure. For the very reasons outlined in his review, the same divergences in practice have persisted up to the present (sixty-five years!). The considerations he so well perceived included the need to relate the challenge to body size and composition.

Attempts to further standardization of practice have had little effect. The American Diabetes Association Committee suggested a load of 40 gm/sq m; the

University Group, 30 gm/sq m; and the British Diabetes Association, 50 gm/sq m. Other dosages widely used and widely recommended include 100 gm in all subjects (Jorde, 1962); 75 gm (Kent and Leonards, 1965); 1.75 gm/kg (Polefsky, et al, 1965); 1.75 gm/kg of ideal body weight (Fajans and Conn, 1959), and 1 gm/kg (Malmros 1928; Goldberg and Luft, 1948; West and Kalbfleisch, 1966). In one large program of the United States Public Health Service a load of 50 gm was used for all subjects (Gordon, et al, 1965), while in other USPHS projects the load of 100 gm has usually been employed (O'Sullivan, et al, 1967).

For many years there was little evidence and considerable conflict of opinion about the degree to which postglucose values were affected by differences of dosage within the standard range (Maclean and de Wesselow, 1921; Hansen, 1923; Wilder, 1948). The evidence of recent years shows clearly, however, that these differences are substantial. Typical of these data are those of West, et al (1964) and of Forster, et al (1972). In some groups of young subjects with excellent glucose tolerance we found only modest differences between responses of the blood glucose after small and large dosages (eg, 50 and 100 gm). But we regularly found substantial differences in middle-aged and elderly subjects (West, et al, 1964). In several studies these dosage-related differences have been substantially greater at two hours than at one hour (Sisk, et al, 1970; Castro, et al, 1970; Forster, et al, 1972), but in some studies differences have also been great at one hour (Peterson and Reaven, 1971). In 30 patients of van't Laar (1972) with borderline tolerance, one-hour values were on the average 38 mg/100 ml higher following 100 gm than following 50 gm. He also found that such differences tended to be greater in those with mediocre tolerance than in subjects with good tolerance. The two-hour values of his patients with border-line tolerance were 60 mg/100 ml higher after 100 gm than after 50 gm. In contrast, Sisk, et al (1970) found mean differences in two-hour values of only 17 mg/100 ml when prisoners with good tolerance were tested with 50 and 100 gm, respectively. Forster (1972, 1975) also found differences in responses to these two dosages were much greater in those with "latent diabetes" than in young healthy subjects. On the basis of their data, Sisk, et al (1970) offered a formula for predicting the results with one dosage when results with the other dosage are known:

two-hour value (100 gm) = 39.4 + (0.688 × two-hour value after 50 gm)

The extent to which this conversion formula may be applicable in other populations is unknown.

Data of Castro, et al (1975) and of Forster, et al (1970) show that with glucose dosages of 100 gm, serum insulin levels are only slightly higher at one hour than those following 50 gm. At two hours the insulin levels are much higher after 100 gm. Apparently absorption of the 50-gm dose is almost complete in the first hour, while a substantial portion of the larger dose remains in the gut at one hour. Other data on this subject have been presented by Chandalia and Boshell (1970) and by Forster in a 1975 publication.

Even with the now considerable data on hand, it is difficult to create conversion factors for the comparison of results with glucose load of different sizes (de Nobel, et al, 1978). Among other problems are the effects on these differences of factors such as age, degree of tolerance, body size, and other characteristics. In middle-aged and elderly subjects one-hour values after 100 gm may be expected to be, very roughly, 25 mg/100 ml higher than after 50 gm, and about 35 mg higher at two hours.

Arguments for using a relatively large dosage include the greater challenge it provides. Forster (1975) has stressed particularly the greater duration of challenge with large loads. Hardly any direct evidence is available, however, concerning the relative sensitivity and specificity of small and large dosages in identifying diabetes. Larger dosages are more unpalatable, slightly more expensive, and more frequently produce nausea and vomiting. In testing 2,500 persons with a 50-gm load, Murray, et al (1969) observed only two instances of vomiting.

There is much to be said for relating dosage in each individual to the size of the extracellular space. Of the simple methods for doing this, the one now most frequently recommended is relating dosage to body surface area (American Diabetes Association, 1969). It would appear, theoretically, that surface area would better reflect extracellular volume than height or weight. The need for such an adjustment factor can be illustrated with examples. The women we tested in rural Pakistan (West and Kalbfleisch, 1966) weighed an average of 76 lb, less than half the weight of our Oklahoma Indian women. If both groups had been given the same dosage of glucose, the Pakistan women would have had to metabolize glucose about twice as fast to achieve comparable blood glucose levels (because their volumes of distribution of glucose are roughly half as great). Even within populations, twofold differences among subjects in sizes of extracellular spaces are not rare.

Despite its theoretical advantages, the practice of relating dosage to surface area has thus far gained little acceptance. Probably the main deterrents are the inertia of entrenched habit and the requirement for a conversion table for determining surface area from height and weight. These tables are easily obtained (American Diabetes Association, 1969), but are usually absent from testing sites unless specific efforts are made to provide continuous access to them. Furthermore, this is only a crude estimate for relating glucose dosage to body mass and extracellular space. A very muscular person and a fat person receive the same dosage if they have the same height and weight even though they differ in extracellular volume, muscularity, and adiposity. For this reason an argument can be made for relating dosage to an even simpler index such as weight. We have often used 1 gm/kg for several reasons. It is a very simple conversion to make, the size of the dosage falls in the intermediate range, and weight is easier to determine than body surface area. The American Diabetes Association Expert Group (1969) recommended the 1 gm/kg dosage as a convenient alternative to their dosage of 40 gm/sq m, pointing out that these two dosages were quite similar in most subjects.

77

Basing dosage on surface area has slight theoretical advantages. In some circumstances this may be justified, but the low rates of acceptance suggest a need to consider alternatives. Among other options we have considered cruder and simpler methods. A routine dose of 75 gm can be given to adults, with adjustment of dosage to 50 or 100 gm in persons that are quite large or quite small. An easy-to-remember formula would be 100 gm for those weighing more than 100 kg (220 lb) and 50 gm for those weighing less than 50 kg (110 lb). The standard dosage of 75 gm has received increasing acceptance in epidemiologic studies (Bennett, et al, 1976a; Kent and Leonards, 1965; Rosselin, et al, 1971; Kobberling and Creutzfeldt, 1970; West, et al, 1976). This dosage was also recommended in a recent document developed by an expert group convened by the Pan American Health Organization (1975). On the other hand, a large amount of epidemiologic data has been collected using 50 gm. This is the dosage recommended by the British Diabetes Association (Fitz-Gerald and Keen, 1964) and by the European Study Group for Diabetes Epidemiology (Gutsche and Holler, 1975). A dosage of 100 gm has also been widely used in epidemiologic studies (Jorde, 1962), particularly in the United States (Hayner, et al, 1963, 1965; O'Sullivan and Williams, 1966).

Among the small advantages of the 75 gm dosage is that it is intermediate between the other two widely employed dosages (50 and 100 gm). Two popular American loading solutions, "Glucola" and "Dexcola", are now made up in bottles containing 75 gm. In well-fed societies the average dosage with 40 gm/ sq m is similar to that when a standard dosage of 75 gm is given. A disadvantage of the standard fixed dosage is its inapplicability in children, but most epidemiologic studies in diabetes do not include children.

The following are among the considerations relevant to selection of dosage size. After a glucose load, the rates of ingress and egress of glucose from liver and muscle are the main metabolic determinants of rate of fall of blood glucose. Adipose tissue, however, has important effects of a less direct nature. Insulin levels, both fasting and postglucose, tend to correspond to the degree of adiposity, until decompensation of the beta cells occurs. On the other hand, sensitivity to insulin declines in liver and muscle with increasing adiposity. Immediately after a glucose load, fat cells receive only a small fraction of administered glucose, but with increasing fatness the size of the volume of distribution of glucose is increased. The extracellular space is not as great per gram of tissue in fat as in muscle. But data on the extracellular volume of fat tissue are incomplete and inconclusive. The extracellular volume of fat tissue, when expressed as a percentage of its weight, may vary with factors such as fat-cell size, degree of fatness, anatomic region, etc. Morse and Soeldner (1961) found the percentage of body water as high in obese subjects as in lean. Franckson, et al, (1959) found the glucose space rather well related to weight, and degree of adiposity did not seem to have much effect on the relationship of weight and volume of distribution of glucose. Data are sparse concerning the effect of fat-cell size and anatomic location of fat on extracellular volume of adipose tissues. Another problem is that the excessive weight in obese persons is usually not entirely attributable to excessive adipose tissue. Muscle mass is frequently increased also. Not much is known about the effect of body mass and composition on rates of absorption of glucose. Usually, "ideal" body weight is simply calculated from height. Height corresponds only crudely to lean body mass or muscle mass. Data are still incomplete and conflicting on the percentages of a glucose load received by muscle, fat, liver, and other tissues. There is also need for more information on how these percentages are affected by factors such as body composition and size of the glucose load.

In deciding how much glucose to administer, several alternatives exist. One can try to relate dosage to the status and characteristics of the subject (eg, size, muscularity, adiposity), or one can give a standard dosage and interpret the test in light of these characteristics (eg, sex, fatness, age). In practice a combination of these two approaches has usually been employed.

In epidemiologic work, the need for conformation to the theoretical ideal in loading dosage seems not to be as great as the need for standardization of practice, definition, and reporting. Achieving this standardization is not as easy as it might appear. A change to an international standard would make it difficult for an investigator to compare new data either to his own previous data or with results of others who had used his methods. Even if a standard fixed amount was agreed upon, difficulties would remain. For example, Oklahoma Indians weigh almost twice as much as people in most Asian populations, and body composition is very grossly different in Asians and Oklahoma Indians. The crude adjustments for weight suggested above would provide fairly satisfactory comparability while preserving simplicity. Most adult subjects would be tested with 75 gm, but very large subjects (more than 100 kg) would receive 100 gm and very small subjects (less than 50 kg) would receive 50 gm. Another of several alternatives would be a scheme for only two different dosages: 50 gm for all adults weighing up to 75 kg (165 lb), and 75 gm for those weighing more than 75 kg. The advantages of relating dosage to surface area have been discussed. On balance, however, it would appear that a scheme for standardization at a fixed dosage, with crude adjustment for weight, would be more likely to gain general acceptance. Among many considerations here is the need to simplify so that tests can be done cheaply under field conditions.

For several reasons there is need to develop epidemiologic standards that will be accepted and used by clinicians. Epidemiologic science, clinical investigation, and clinical practice have much to offer each other in this respect, provided that common methods and conventions can be achieved. This does not necessarily require unanimity of interpretation. Typical of the present difficulties is the propensity of clinicians to apply standards developed for one test inappropriately to another. Both clinicians and epidemiologists have applied the criteria of Fajans and Conn (1959) rather indiscriminately irrespective of the loading dose used. Few are even aware that the standards were based on subjects tested with 1.75 gm/kg of ideal body weight. Well-known standards for whole blood values are all too often applied to results on plasma.

Conversion from one dosage level to another would not preclude the future utility of previous data. Well-collected data on samples of these populations would permit the development of fairly satisfactory conversion factors. Admittedly, the present data for developing conversion factors (eg, to estimate what might have been expected with 75-gm tests from previous results of 50-gm tests) are not very satisfactory. This is mainly because the relationships are affected by the characteristics of the subject populations tested (age, size, etc).

Loading tests with nutrients other than glucose will be discussed below.

Absorption, concentration, temperature and rate of administration of glucose

Good reviews on glucose absorption have been published by Crane (1960) and Gerson (1971). The effects of gastrointestinal disease on the results of the oral glucose tolerance test will be discussed below. Concentration of administered glucose has an effect on rate of absorption. In some circumstances, for example, a dilute concentration is more rapidly absorbed than a highly concentrated one. Too much dilution, however, brings loading volume to a prohibitive level, particularly with glucose loads of 75 gm or more. A typical compromise is to administer the solution at a concentration of 20% to 40%. In some circumstances cold glucose is not as rapidly absorbed as glucose nearer body temperature, but in practice the drink is usually served as a cold drink, often flavored with lemon or some other flavoring agent. Standard loads may produce severe symptoms in subjects whose stomachs have been surgically removed. This is the result of the unphysiologic osmotic effect of large amounts in the upper intestine. Normal subjects may also experience nausea and other gastrointestinal symptoms. Vomiting occasionally occurs. These phenomena have not been well studied but a few observations are mentioned in the section on screening. Incidence of untoward symptoms is probably less with smaller loads and when rapid consumption of glucose is avoided.

No standardization exists with respect to rate of consumption. The Expert Group of the American Diabetes Association (1969) recommended that consumption be completed in less than five minutes. This helps to standardize the test, but requiring this of all subjects probably increases the frequency of unpleasant symptoms. Few data are available on the effects of varying the period of consumption (eg, from five to twenty minutes). Because unpleasant symptoms are rather common in some circumstances, it would probably be appropriate to limit the rate of ingestion (eg, a rate of about 5 to 10 gm/minute). This could be fixed approximately by allowing a lower and an upper time limit for consumption. The subject who drinks 75 gm would be told, for example, that the drink is to be entirely consumed before fifteen minutes, but not in less than five minutes. The test is usually timed from the beginning of consumption but there has also been some divergences of practice in that respect.

Timing of blood sampling

Many strategies of sampling have been proposed and tested. In most circumstances blood glucose begins to rise within a few minutes of ingestion of oral glucose. In normal subjects the maximum is usually reached between thirty and sixty minutes. The blood glucose then declines during the second hour, usually reaching the fasting level between ninety and one hundred fifty minutes after ingestion. Samples have been drawn most commonly at one and two hours. There is no evidence that any alternative intervals are superior in evaluating tolerance. The American Diabetes Association Expert Committee (1969) also recommended a three-hour value. This was one of the values used in the USPHS criteria (Wilkerson, et al, 1960). But these criteria were a product of authority rahter than evidence. Even so, an argument can be made that the three-hour value is useful in some respects; it often is normal in persons with "abnormal" one- and two-hour values. This sometimes prevents the inappropriate classification of these persons as diabetic (DeCoek, 1967). But use of more conservative criteria in interpreting the one- and two-hour values may overcome this problem without the necessity for a three-hour value. Extension of the test to three hours increases its cost and decreases its convenience. More data are therefore needed on the utility of this value. In clinical practice it is probably less misused than the other values. Prout, et al (1976) recommended termination of the test at two hours.

There is a general consensus, though not unanimity (Sisk, et al, 1970) to the effect that the two-hour value is the most effective single index of glucose tolerance. But direct evidence of superiority to the one- or three-hour value is scant. Rushforth et al (1975) have presented some indirect evidence suggesting that the two-hour value may be superior. Arguments of others to this effect have often been based on "circular" reasoning. The two-hour value correlates with the development of "diabetes", but diabetes has often been defined on the basis of criteria that include a particular emphasis on the two-hour level. The type of question that is most appropriate has seldom been asked. Are those with two-hour values in the top five percentiles (in the population from which they are drawn) more likely to develop unequivocal fasting hyperglycemia than those with one- or three-hour values of similar rank?

One of the reasons this needs attention is that it is often more convenient and less expensive to shorten the test to a duration of one hour. Among the theoretical advantages of the two-hour figure is that it is a reflection of both the one-hour level and of the subsequent rate of fall during the second hour. Also, it is probably less affected than the one-hour value by vagaries in rates of absorption of glucose. On the other hand, a superior sensitivity of the one-hour level could be argued on the same theoretical grounds responsible for the notion that the two-hour value is superior to the fasting value. When beta-cell decompensation is at the very earliest stage, beta cells might conceivably be able to "do the job" in two hours but not in one.

It is customary to measure the fasting blood glucose in performing a glucose tolerance test. This is probably a useful practice because of the special significance of fasting hyperglycemia. Yet an argument can be made for omitting the sample if one is prepared to make the diagnosis in the absence of fasting hyperglycemia. When the fasting value is really elevated, the postglucose values will almost always be abnormal. If the fasting value is not used either to exclude or make the diagnosis, why measure it in the diagnostic process? On the other hand, it is quite reasonable to use the fasting level if one is uncertain

81

of the significance of "impaired" tolerance in persons with normal fasting levels. Here the fasting value is used in the glucose tolerance test to distinguish diabetes from possible diabetes. There are reasonable theoretical grounds for assuming that measuring blood glucose concentration at three or four different intervals ("full" tolerance test) would provide more reliable information than is ascertained with one or two values. On the other hand, few data are available to justify the more elaborate tests. The data of O'Sullivan, et al (1966,1967) have some bearing on this issue, but much more work of this kind is needed. The most direct and relevant questions on these issues have seldom been asked. Do those whose summed values (eg, for tests at 60, 90, 120, and 180 minutes) fall in the top percentiles of all summed values have a substantially greater risk of developing fasting hyperglycemia and diabetes-related morbidity than those whose values for individual intervals (eg, two-hour) are similarly ranked? It will also be appropriate, of course, to evaluate the specificity of both the "full" glucose tolerance test and its individual elements. Condemnation of the sensitivity and specificity of lone individual values after glucose or test meals has also been based mainly on faulty circular reasoning. The sensitivity and specificity of these tests are criticized because they correspond poorly to the results of "more definitive testing". But it usually turns out that the diagnosis of diabetes is based on this same "definitive testing" rather than on fasting hyperglycemia. On the contrary, it could be argued that a single postprandial value has a specificity at least three times greater than the full glucose tolerance test because a large share who have elevated postprandial values have, or later have, unequivocal fasting hyperglycemia, while only a small fraction of these who, by conventional standards, have abnormal tolerance, actually become diabetic in this sense. This line of reasoning is also faulty because it assumes the lesser specificity is inherent in the full tolerance test. In fact, the lack of specificity is mainly the product of the method by which criteria of interpretation are derived. Roughly forty percent of elderly Americans have "abnormal" tolerance only because traditional criteria are faulty. The defective criteria do not necessarily reflect a shortcoming of the test itself. Diagnostic criteria are discussed further below in a separate section on that subject.

To summarize, the paucity of available evidence makes it difficult to formulate and justify a firm and specific recommendation on when and how many blood samples should be taken, either in epidemiologic or clinical work. Present consensus among authorities favors an oral glucose tolerance test with two to four specimens (at one and two hours; or fasting, one, two, and three hours). These conventions are based more on custom and tradition than on evidence. In the light of recent evidence some, including the author, believe the "full" glucose tolerance test (four or more specimens) to be considerably overrated as a clinical and epidemiologic instrument. When traditional criteria are applied, specificity of the glucose tolerance test in predicting risk of diabetes is poor in those with clearly normal fasting values, even when four or more specimens are included. When criteria are raised sufficiently to achieve reasonable specificity, fasting hyperglycemia is usually present (Dippe, et al,

1974; Bennett, et al, 1976a). Prevalence of diabetes and risk of morbidity are probably best judged by determining prevalence of fasting hyperglycemia. But most diabetologists have much more confidence in glucose tolerance tests than the author. Only more evidence can resolve this disagreement and uncertainty.

Effect of previous diet and time of day

Previous diet   It was well known in the 19th century that severe starvation impaired glucose tolerance (Allen, 1913). Among other designations this was called "vagabond diabetes" and "cachetic diabetes". Scientists contributing observations on this phenomenon included particularly Claude Bernard and Hofmeister. Kaguera demonstrated impairment of tolerance with low-carbohydrate diets in 1922. In 1927 Shirley Sweeney performed systematic studies of the effect of antecedent diet on the glucose tolerance test. Tolerance was impaired substantially after two days of high-fat, low-carbohydrate diet. It was also much worse after two days of total starvation. Tolerance was also impaired, but to a lesser degree, after a high-protein, low-carbohydrate diet. Malmros (1928) confirmed these observations. Several papers of Himsworth (cited elsewhere in this book) also showed the deleterious effect of carbohydrate deprivation on glucose tolerance in normal subjects.

In 1940 Conn reported on abnormal glucose tolerance secondary to severe carbohydrate deprivation and suggested that a special preparation diet be administered routinely prior to glucose tolerance tests to preclude false-positive results. This diet provides 300 gm of carbohydrate daily for three days. It is little known that Ross had suggested this specific diet in 1938 as a means for evaluating the significance of equivocal results of glucose tolerance tests. Use of this "preparation" diet has been fairly extensive, although many have challenged its necessity as a routine procedure (Irving and Wang, 1954; Wilkerson, et al, 1960; Nillsson, 1962; Hughes, 1975; Anderson and Herman, 1972, 1975). Data of Himsworth (1935) suggested that an intake of about 125 gm of carbohydrate daily was adequate to prevent deterioration of tolerance. This was later confirmed by Irving and Wang (1954) and by Wilkerson, et al (1960).

More recent studies confirm that severe carbohydrate deprivation, even without reduction in calories, will impair glucose tolerance—at least in short-term conditions. Muller, et al (1971) showed that ratios of insulin to glucagon were substantially reduced in such circumstances. But in their studies, levels of carbohydrate were extremely low (19 gm daily) and fat consumption was high (154 gm daily). In the studies of Persson, et al (1967) showing impairment of tolerance in children on low-carbohydrate diets, only 5% of calories were from carbohydrate.

Many of the studies addressed to this issue have been difficult to interpret because other changes have attended reduction of dietary carbohydrate (eg, reductions in calories or substantial increases in fat). Data of Anderson and Herman (1975) suggest that in some circumstances impairment of tolerance on low-carbohydrate, high-fat diets may be attributable more to the excess of fat than the paucity of carbohydrate. They also showed that high-protein diets did

83

not impair glucose tolerance when levels of fat were controlled. Evidence will be cited below that effects of short-term carbohydrate deprivation may differ from those of long-term low-carbohydrate diet.

An important related question is whether in persons consuming ordinary amounts of carbohydrate, glucose tolerance is improved by increasing dietary carbohydrate for a few days, with or without adding calories. Available evidence is to some degree inconsistent in this respect. Goldberg and Luft (1948) found no effect when they increased dietary carbohydrate substantially. On the other hand, Tolstoi (1929) described a few data of John to the opposite effect.

A positive argument for increasing consumption of carbohydrate and calories prior to testing is that it might increase the sensitivity of the test. Normal subjects tend to develop higher insulin levels with short-term overfeeding, while those with early diabetes tend to develop beta-cell decompensation. This would be more properly referred to as dietary "challenge" rather than dietary "preparation". Further studies would be of interest. Such studies should be controlled to determine whether observed effects, if any, are attributable to changes in carbohydrate, starch, sugar, fat, or calories.

Although the general purpose of the "preparation" diet is well understood, there are many problems in its execution. Should persons who require 4,000 kcal/day (eg, manual laborers or athletes) be given the same amount of carbohydrate as those who require 1,500 to 2,000 (eg, small old women)? Should carbohydrate be reduced in those who habitually eat more than 300 gm daily? Most of the people in the world eat more carbohydrate than this. Should one assume that the effects of sugar and starch are the same? Should those who usually eat substantially more, or much less, than 300 gm of carbohydrate daily be instructed to raise or reduce their other nutrients to keep the diet isocaloric? Which nutrients? Should standardization be based on percentage of calories as carbohydrate rather than the absolute amount of carbohydrate? Goschke (1977) found that in obese subjects glucose tolerance remained unchanged despite starvation for 6 days.

In the aggregate, present evidence suggests that a preparation diet is unnecessary, and perhaps undesirable, except for individuals who have been losing weight or in those who have recently restricted carbohydrate to less than 125 gm daily. Even in those on long-term low-carbohydrate diets the effects of carbohydrate restriction have not been well defined in those consuming sufficient calories to maintain weight. Certain Eskimo groups have shown excellent glucose tolerance despite very low levels of carbohydrate intake (Heinbecker, 1928; Mouratoff, et al, 1967; West, 1974). Asians and Africans typically consume 300 to 500 gm of carbohydrate daily. In the Occident levels of 200 to 400 gm daily are typical, but levels of consumption as low as 150 gm are not rare in small elderly people whose weights are stable. Unger (1957) found no evidence that carbohydrate tolerance was more likely to be impaired in normal persons who gave a dietary history of low levels of carbohydrate consumption.

Although diets moderately low in carbohydrate are probably not a cause of abnormal tests in persons consuming sufficient calories to maintain weight, it may be that postglucose values are slightly lower in groups prepared routinely with diets higher in carbohydrate than their usual diets. Effects may depend on whether calories are kept constant or allowed to rise. It is not yet known whether standards of interpretation should be the same in subjects on their ordinary isocaloric low-carbohydrate diets (eg, 150 to 250 gm daily) and in those who have observed Conn's preparation diet (300 gm). Studies of Wilkerson, et al (1960) and other suggest that the effects of the preparation diet are slight in those who eat as much as 125 gm of carbohydrate, but these data are not sufficient to exclude a small effect of the preparation diet in certain elements of populations in whom carbohydrate consumption is low. Seltzer (1970) reported some data consistent with this possibility, but numbers tested were not sufficient to be decisive. Keen, et al (1975) found glucose tolerance somewhat better in Englishmen consuming high carbohydrate diets. We (West, et al, 1976) found no relationship of glucose tolerance to sugar consumption in Oklahoma Indians, even though differences in sugar intake of two- to fourfold were common.

Another argument for a routine preparation diet is that those who order the test may be ignorant of the need to evaluate the diet by history, or they may forget to do so, or they may not know how. Fortunately, those needing preparation are few, and they can usually be identified by very simple screening questions: Have you been on a diet lately? Have you lost any weight recently? Have you cut down lately on starches or sugars? One screening method deserving more evaluation is the urine ketone test. Those in need of special preparation probably have ketonuria. The delay in testing necessary with a preparation diet often adds expenses for the patient. The diet counseling also adds a bit to cost. Preparation diets also increase the costs of epidemiologic studies.

One approach in epidemiologic studies is to perform glucose tolerance tests after screening questions on diet but without dietary preparation. One could then retest, after dietary perparation, the small portion who demonstrate both impairment of tolerance and a history of dietary restriction. This would probably require retesting only a very small fraction. There would be additional advantages in retesting these persons anyway. It would also be of interest to retest a control group after similar dietary instruction. In some circumstances other approaches would be preferable.

Another relevant consideration is that the number of middle-aged and elderly subjects with "abnormal" results is greatly diminished by employment of the newer more conservative criteria. This substantially reduces the number in whom the issue of previous diet is likely to arise.

In a study Gerard et al (1977) there was an inverse relationship of previous alcohol consumption and glucose tolerance, except that persons who consumed more than eight drinks daily had *better* glucose tolerance.

Another factor that influences glucose tolerance is the temporal relationship of the test to the most recent meal. Traditionally tests have been performed after an overnight fast. But frequently this is an inconvenient requirement in both

85

epidemiologic and clinical work. For this reason glucose tolerance has with increasing frequency been assessed after shorter periods of fasting. Several recent studies have been designed to evaluate the effects of varying this interval. A major problem has been that results may be affected by both interval of fasting and the time of day. It has, therefore, often been difficult to determine which of these factors is responsible for a given result.

The data of Hayner, et al (1965) showed a dramatic effect of interval of fasting on glucose tolerance. When tests with 100 gm of glucose were done within four hours after a meal, one-hour blood glucose levels were about 25 mg/100 ml lower than in individuals tested after longer fasts. Even after a fast of only five hours, mean values were 19 mg/100 ml higher than when the period of fasting had been four hours or less. In these studies no effect of time of day of testing was observed. On the other hand, under the conditions of our studies (West and Kalbfleisch, 1971), we observed no effect of interval of fasting on results. One probable reason for this was that few tests were done within two hours of the last meal. Our unpublished data and observations of others suggest that the priming effect of "prefeeding" is strong when tests are performed two hours after a feeding. Gordon, et al (1964) found that after 50 gm of glucose one-hour values were somewhat lower when the load was administered one to two hours after breakfast than when it was given three to four hours after breakfast. This difference was not observed, however, after lunch or supper. Afternoon values one hour after glucose were not higher than morning values except when glucose was administered one to two hours after lunch (as compared to tests performed one to two hours after breakfast). In a study in prisoners using loads of 50 gm, Hayner, et al (1963) observed little influence of interval of fasting on response to glucose. Using a dosage of 75 gm, Gough, et al (1970) found "no constant effect" of fasting interval on results.

Walsh, et al (1976) obtained rather different results under other conditions. They gave a load of 50 gm in the morning on three occasions to each of 33 subjects. Period of fasting was twelve hours on one occasion, eight on another, and four on another. Postglucose values were slightly but significantly *higher* with the test performed after the four-hour fast than that after the twelve-hour fast. When the test was done after an eight-hour fast the results were intermediate. Interval of fasting had little effect on results of tests in young adults, but tests of subjects over forty years of age were affected substantially. Duffy, et al (1973) found that the blood glucose levels of their fasting subjects given a 75-gm load were quite similar to those loaded one to four hours after eating. But values were higher in subjects who had fasted four to six hours than in those who had fasted overnight. This difference was not the result of diurnal phenomena.

Thus the effects of interval of fasting appear to differ considerably depending on several variables.

Effect of time of day　The recent interest in diurnal variations in response to glucose dates from the observations of Roberts (1964) and Bowen and Reeves (1967). Diurnal variations had, however, been reported sporadically in previous generations. In 1923 Brill observed that blood glucose was "apt to rise higher" after lunch than after breakfast even when the test meal was constant. Brill also thought the reproducibility of morning tests better than that of afternoon tests.

Roberts (1964) and Bowen and Reeves (1967) found responses to oral glucose substantially higher in the afternoon than in the morning. This was confirmed by others including Jarrett and Keen (1969,1970). Jarrett and Keen found that diurnal differences were smaller in obese persons and in those whose morning values were high. Carroll, et al (1973) performed tests at 7 AM and 7 PM. They found insulin response to oral glucose tolerance better in the morning. No diurnal variation was seen in response to intravenous insulin. Injections of tolbutamide also produced a greater insulin response in the morning. Carroll, et al (1973) reviewed much of the previous literature on this subject (58 references). Melani, et al (1976) also found insulin response to glucose greater at 8 AM than at 6 PM, even though a ten-hour fast preceded both the morning and afternoon test. Capani and Sensi (1976) found blood glucose responsiveness to insulin greater in the morning than in the late afternoon except in obese subjects. Beck-Nielson (1976) observed that insulin binding to monocytes was greater in the morning than at certain other periods of the day.

Figure 2 summarizes data of Mayer et al (1976). These results show clearly that both period of fasting and time of day have a considerable effect. These and other data of Mayer showed that these two effects were independent.

Several uncertainties remain concerning the diurnal variation. When oral glucose tolerance is tested in the afternoon it is difficult to know what correction factor should be applied in interpreting results. The degree of diurnal differences appears to differ with several factors, including adiposity, status of feeding or fasting, and degree of tolerance. It is clear, however, that epidemiologic and clinical studies should take this phenomenon into account in their design and interpretation. In a group tested by Jarrett and Keen (1970), one-hour blood glucose levels were 30 mg/100 ml higher in the afternoon; and two-hour values were higher by 35 mg/100 ml. Because of their large numbers of data of Mayer, et al (Figure 2) are probably the best available as a basis for extrapolating results from one time of day to those that might be expected at another time of day. But these results might not be applicable to all circumstances. For example, diurnal differences with 50-gm loads are probably not quite the same as those with 100-gm loads. It is not known whether the sensitivity or specificity of the afternoon test is worse or better than that of the morning test. The morning test is now preferable, but only because more data are available as a basis for defining its limits of normal. It should be emphasized that the higher afternoon values have not been observed under all conditions (Duffy, et al, 1973; Gordon, et al, 1964; Gough, et al, 1970; Hayner, et al, 1963).

Factors affecting glucose tolerance that have little relation to risk of diabetes
There are hundreds of factors that may influence glucose tolerance. Some of these are important causes of diabetes (eg, acromegaly, obesity). Many of these factors, however, have little etiologic significance although they may signifi-

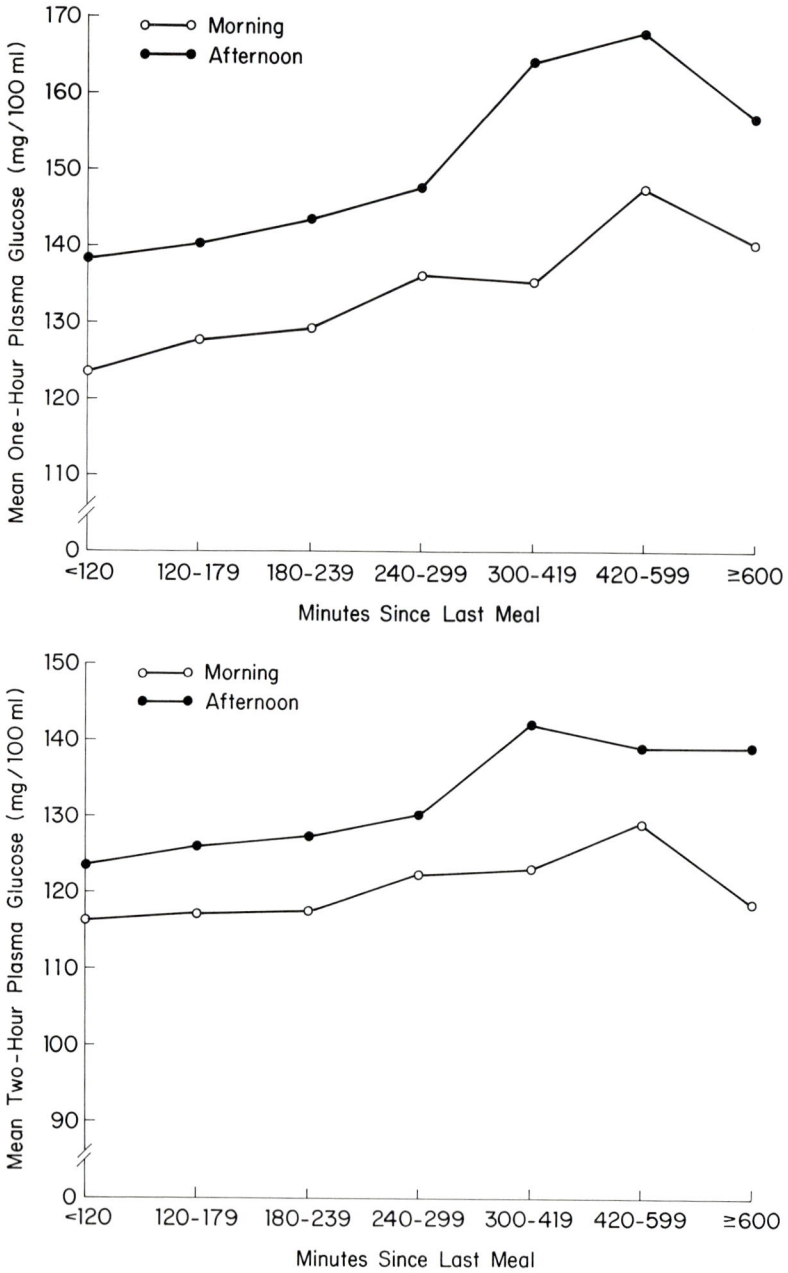

FIGURE 2.   Relationship of time of day and time since last meal to one-hour (upper graph) and two-hour (lower graph) postload (100 gm) plasma glucose (Mayer, et al, 1976).

cantly influence glucose tolerance. Under some conditions such effects may lead to an erroneous diagnosis of diabetes. Some of these factors are listed below. The effects of dietary restrictions have been discussed above.

Factors that may produce falsely positive glucose tolerance tests

1. *Medications:* Contraceptive steroids, ACTH, glucocorticoids, high dosages of certain thiazides and other diuretics, diphenylhydantoin (Dilantin), nicotinic acid, colchoicine, L-asparaginase, lithium carbonate, caffeine, sympathomimetics, nalidixic acid, mannoheptulose, marijuana, indomethacin; also nicotine and phenothiazines may have a weak effect

2. *Marked reduction in exercise*

3. *Acute or severe illness* (eg, myocardial infarction, stroke, infection, azotemia)

4. *Recent trauma, surgery, or severe stress*

5. *Severe depletion:* of potassium, chromium, pyridoxine, calories, or carbohydrates

6. *Gastrectomy* (particularly if peak blood glucose volume substantially influences diagnostic interpretation)

7. *Other diabetogenic factors:* as listed in Table 4. These latter agents include those that are significant causes of clinical diabetes such as pheochromocytoma (epinephrine), acromegaly (growth hormone), Cushing's syndrome, thyrotoxicosis, hyperaldosteronism, and hepatic cirrhosis. Many other drugs not listed above will impair tolerance in toxic doses (eg, alloxan, streptozotocin, thyroid).

Some factors affecting disposition of an oral glucose load

1. Capacity of beta cells to secrete insulin

2. Rate of absorption of glucose
   a. Integrity of intestinal epithelium and its circulation
   b. Intestinal motility
   c. Rate of stomach emptying (anatomic, physiologic, and biochemical determinants that include status of pylorus, nausea, etc)
   d. Temperature and concentration of glucose
   e. Presence of other nutrients in the load

3. Hormonal responses of gut

4. Size of glucose space

5. Body composition (muscularity, adiposity, etc)

6. Integrity, functional capacity, and blood supply of liver

7. Other hormonal factors such as changes in levels of glucagon and growth hormones in response to glucose

8. Other factors determining tissue sensitivity or resistance to insulin and glucose (age, previous diet, adiposity, status of insulin receptors, enzyme systems, serum potassium, etc)

9. Renal threshold for glucose

The traditional admonition that glucose tolerance tests should be performed only in the "basal" state was promulgated in an attempt to avoid overdiagnosis resulting from the factors listed above. But in a segment of the population over fifty years of age a very large proportion are for various reasons not in a truly basal state, free of all conditions that might influence glucose tolerance. Often it will be appropriate to perform the test in the circumstances that prevail, even though conditions are not entirely "basal", keeping in mind these circumstances in interpreting the test. When tolerance is found to be abnormal this knowledge may have some clinical utility. It may, for example, show the need to consider discontinuing a certain medication.

In epidemiologic work it is often desirable to record systematically information concerning the factors that most frequently produce falsely positive results. These include any acute or severe illness, marked reduction in exercise, contraceptive steroids, strenuous dieting, and glucocorticosteroids. The effects of restricting exercise on glucose tolerance are discussed in a section on exercise in Chapter 7. General screening questions are sometimes appropriate: Have you been sick lately? Have you lost weight recently? Are you taking birth control pills? Are you taking any drugs or medicine regularly? The priority and extent of such screening may be considerably reduced if criteria of diagnosis are conservative (eg, when only decidedly elevated values are considered diagnostic).

Effects of gastrointestinal factors on glucose tolerance have been reviewed by Mehnert and Forster (1968). Gastrointestinal disease may affect tolerance substantially through its influence on rate of absorption (Soskin, 1951). Persons whose stomachs have been surgically removed tend to have early high peaks in their blood glucose levels. Usually these blood glucose levels are restored to normal at the second hour if glucose tolerance is normal. When absorption is poor, mild abnormalities of glucose tolerance may be missed. This can occur with delayed gastric emptying or with generalized disease of the small bowel. But most "flat" glucose tolerance curves are not attributable to poor absorption of glucose or gastrointestinal disease. This phenomenon (flat curve) is common in healthy subjects (Gupta and Whitehouse, 1971; Nolan, et al, 1972). Rate of absorption is significantly affected by gastrointestinal motility, and also by posture (Nisell, 1957; Lewis and Said, 1961; Desai and Antia, 1966). But effects do not appear to be sufficiently large to warrant special requirements of posture or special criteria of interpretation in subjects who are tested in various conventional postures (eg, sitting or standing). Nisell (1957) thought it better for subjects being tested to avoid the supine position because of the possibility of significant slowing of absorption. In most reports upon which criteria of diagnosis have been based, no information was provided on the postures of the subjects tested. Severe exercise before or during the test may increase assimilation of glucose, but effects of minimal exercise do not require its complete proscription during the course of the test. Effects of contraceptive steroids on glucose tolerance have been well summarized by Winegerd and Duffy (1977).

Under some conditions smoking decreases tolerance, and it is traditionally prohibited during the test. Evidence of the need to prohibit smoking and the drinking of black coffee before and during testing is not wholly convincing. It has long been known that nicotine may stimulate release of epinephrine, but it is not yet clear whether the effect on glucose tolerance in chronic smokers is sufficient to warrant prohibition of smoking during the test. Conceivably, withdrawal itself might have an effect in a chronic smoker. The literature on this subject was well summarized by Goldman and Schecter in 1967. This literature includes both positive and negative evidence. Recent studies of Winegerd and Duffy (1977) and of Walsh, et al (1977) were impressively negative. Feinberg, et al (1968) reviewed previous publications on the effects on glucose tolerance of caffeine and coffee. Under conditions of their studies coffee *improved* glucose tolerance slightly but significantly. Conceivably, the effects of both serving and withdrawing coffee might be different in those who drink coffee habitually and in those who do not. Under some conditions caffeine and coffee have appeared to have an unfavorable effect on glucose tolerance, but it isn't yet certain whether proscription of coffee before or during the test is necessary. In some of the studies it was not possible to tell whether observed effects were caffeine-related or whether they were secondary to effects on gastrointestinal motility, absorption, or on release of enteric hormones.

Reproducibility

In 1927 Lennox showed that intraindividual variation of results is considerable with oral glucose tolerance tests. This has been confirmed by many.* We (West, et al, 1964) analyzed our own results and those of seven other investigators. Coefficients of correlation ranged from 0.36 to 0.82 when results of duplicate tests were compared. Values of about 0.6 were most common. In our groups intraindividual variability was similar for the one- and two-hour values. Variability was also similar with glucose loads of three different sizes. In a small group of 47 subjects, intraindividual variation of response was less with a breakfast of standard size than with glucose. This, among other possibilities, suggested that vagaries of absorption might be less with a more palatable and physiologic load. But Kosaka, et al (1966) found intraindividual variation of comparable degree with rice and with glucose loads.

Data of Olefsky and Reaven (1974) suggest that a part of the variation in response is attributable to a considerable variation in levels of insulin secretion

---

*References: (Freeman, et al, 1941; Goto, 1955; Hayner, et al, 1963; West, et al, 1964; Unger, 1957; MacDonald, et al, 1965; Kosaka, et al, 1966; Johnson, et al, 1968; Olefsky and Reaven, 1974; Troxler, et al, 1975).

when duplicate tests are performed. R. A. Jackson, et al (1970) observed substantial intraindividual variation in assimilation of glucose when the metabolism of forearm tissue was studied.

In persons with normal fasting glucose levels, we (West, et al, 1964) observed as much intraindividual variation in response to glucose in those with good tolerance as in those with relatively high postglucose values. These data and those of others indicate that intraindividual differences of 20 mg/100 ml or more occur in about one half of the test pairs at both one and two hours. Variations as great as 40 mg/100 ml are not at all rare, indicating the need for a broad range of normal values. It also suggests the appropriateness of a fairly broad range for those considered as borderline.

Intraindividual variations of considerable degree have also been observed over time (O'Sullivan and Hurwitz, 1966; Kahn, et al, 1969; Carlstrom, et al, 1971; Kobberling, et al, 1975; Aspevik, et al, 1974).

In 1959 J. A. Wulf and the author did continuous analyses of blood glucose levels in several normal subjects. We found that waves of considerable amplitude interrupted the general ascent and decline of the blood glucose during the course of carbohydrate tolerance tests. These data were not published because we could not be certain that these waves were not attributable in part to technical defects in the system of flow of blood into the analyzer. Subsequently, however, Burns, et al (1965) and others using more advanced technical methods confirmed the presence of these "waves". Their amplitude and frequency of occurrence indicate clearly that the usual results, with traditional intermittent sampling at thirty- to sixty-minute intervals, are often a poor reflection of the actual curves. When tests were repeated in the same individual we found, moreover, that the positions of the waves were not predictable. Peak values occurred as early as thirty minutes and as late as sixty minutes with considerable interindividual and intraindividual difference in time of occurrence.

O'Sullivan and Mahan (1966) studied the degree of variation, intraindividually and interindividually, both of individual values and of the sums of blood glucose values. Intraindividual variation was less for summed values than for individual postglucose values. The design of their observations permitted them to determine how much of the interindividual variation of postglucose values was attributable to the day-to-day inconsistencies in results of the tests when duplicate tests were performed in the same individual. About half of the variation observed among individuals was attributable to this factor. They also examined the correlation among postglucose values obtained during a single test at one, two, and three hours. Correlation coefficients were modest (r values from 0.4 to 0.7 in various groups).

Results of Sisk, et al (1970) were different in some respects. They found that the reproducibility of the summed values was not significantly better than that for individual values. It is possible, however, that with larger numbers a small but significant "superiority" might have been demonstrable for the summed values. The same correlation coefficient for repeat tests was slightly better (0.72) for four summed values than for single postglucose value (0.60 for one-, 0.58 for two-, and 0.61 for three-hour values).

Diagnostic criteria

Table 14 summarizes some of the criteria most commonly employed. As pointed out above, the standards promulgated before 1965 are based more on tradition than on evidence and have been challenged with increasing frequency.* The history of the development of traditional criteria was well summarized by Glodberg and Luft (1948). Table 14 shows the wide divergence of opinion that currently exists concerning diagnostic standards.

Figure 3 also illustrates the extent of this uncertainty and disagreement. Twenty leading authorities in diabetes were asked for their criteria in interpreting the glucose tolerance test of an asymptomatic middle-aged subject to whom a glucose load of 75 gm (1 gm/kg) had been given. Details were described in the original report (West, 1975). Several of these respondents were also well known for their work in the epidemiology of diabetes. A substantial divergence of criteria was evident among both clinicians and epidemiologists. These widely-differing criteria were applied to data from several populations to estimate the effects of such differences on the portion of the middle-aged population judged to be "diabetic". In some populations in which borderline glucose tolerance was not common, effects of these differences in criteria were modest. But in populations of Europe or North America such differences in criteria would have resulted in markedly different rates of prevalence. Typically, one criterion would classify as "diabetic" less than 5% of middle-aged subjects, while another would classify more than one third as diabetic!

Nadon, et al (1964) performed both oral and intravenous tests in a group of 81 subjects, interpreting results by standard criteria. Disparate results with the two tests were common. These investigators concluded that neither test was an accurate instrument for identifying early diabetes.

The data of Gordon (1964) on a representative sample of the United States population were among the first upon which such standards might have been based. These results are summarized in Chapter 5 on prevalence. Unfortunately, tradition overcame common sense, and the old standards based on the much weaker evidence were used by most to interpret the new data, rather than the reverse. We Americans were joined in this folly by the British, most of whom interpreted their excellent data from Birmingham and Bedford in the light of their traditional criteria, rather than the reverse. Jarrett and Keen (1976) have, however, proposed a new look, and a revision of these conventional standards.

As pointed out above, many investigations have shown that the range of normal response in subjects over forty years of age extends well above the ranges suggested by the early studies in small groups of young volunteers. Among these newer and more relevant data are those of Stamler, et al, cited by Cooper (1973). They determined one-hour plasma glucose levels in 1,916 male employees of a Chicago gas company to whom glucose (50 gm) was given

---

*References: (Unger, 1957; Nadon, et al, 1964; Hayner, et al, 1965; West, 1966; Andres, 1971; Duffy, et al, 1973; Prout, 1975; Jarrett and Keen, 1976; Siperstein, 1975; West, 1975).

TABLE 14 Proposed Criteria for Interpreting Oral Glucose Tolerance Tests in Adults

PROPOSERS	GLUCOSE LOAD	CUT-OFF POINTS		COMMENT
		ONE-HOUR GLUCOSE*	TWO-HOUR GLUCOSE*	
USPHS (Wilkerson, et al, 1960)	100 gm	195	140	Diagnosis made by point system, 2 pts diagnostic. Abnormality of fasting level (130) is 1 pt; of three-hour (130) is 1 pt; of one-hour is ½ pt; and two-hour is ½ pt.
Fajans and Conn (1959)	1.75 gm/kg ideal weight	185	140	Original criteria also required that a ninety minute value be 160 or greater. ADA (1974) modification raises cut-off pts. 10 mg/100 ml per decade beginning with sixth decade.
British Diabetes Association (FitzGerald and Keen, 1964)	50 gm	180	130	Converted from whole blood values of 160 and 110
College of General Practitioners, Birmingham Working Party (1970)	50 gm		135 (capillary)	
WHO (1965)	50 to 100 gm		140 (capillary)	
Hayner (1965)	100 gm	180–270 (age-dependent)		Values 120–129 considered borderline Allowed for wide range of "indeterminate" status. In middle-age diagnosis would be made when one-hour levels were about 240.
Japan Diabetes Society (1970)	50 gm	180	140	Both one- and two-hour values must be elevated
	100 gm	180	160	

European Diabetes Epidemiology Study Group (1970)	50 gm	220 (capillary)	150 (capillary)	One-hour values of 160–220 considered borderline, as are two-hour levels of 120–150
Mimura (1970) (Japan) Andres (1971)	100 gm 1.75 gm/kg	200 (capillary) (age-dependent)	150 (capillary) 170–260 (age-dependent)	In middle-age diagnosis would require two-hour values of about 210
American Diabetes Association (Meinert, et al, 1972)	40 gm/sq m body surface			When one-, two-, and 3-hour values are summed, values of 600 or more are diagnostic
University Group Diabetes Program, Klimt, et al (1967)	30 gm/sq m body surface			When four plasma values are summed (fasting, one-, two-, and 3-hour), values of 575 or more are diagnostic
Danowski, et al (1973)	1.75 gm/kg			When four values are summed (as above), values over 800 indicate diabetes, of 650–759 suggest probable diabetes, while of 500–649 are considered borderline
Cooper, USPHS Center for Disease Control (1973)	Not stated	195	140	
Kobberling and Creutzfeldt (1970)	75 gm			Abnormal if one-hour plus two-hour is 300 or more
Siperstein (1975)				Suggested that diagnosis be limited to those with fasting hyperglycemia
Bennett, et al (1976a)	75gm		204–245 (age-dependent)	

*Venous plasma values in mg/100 ml unless otherwise specified.

Two-Hour
Glucose
(mg / 100 ml)

200
190
180
170
160
150
140
130
120
110
100

| Mean | 160 | 140 | 161 | 132 |

| Lowest Value Considered Clearly Abnormal | Highest Value Considered Clearly Normal | Lowest Value Considered Clearly Abnormal | Highest Value Considered Clearly Normal |

Responses of American Group

Responses of International Group

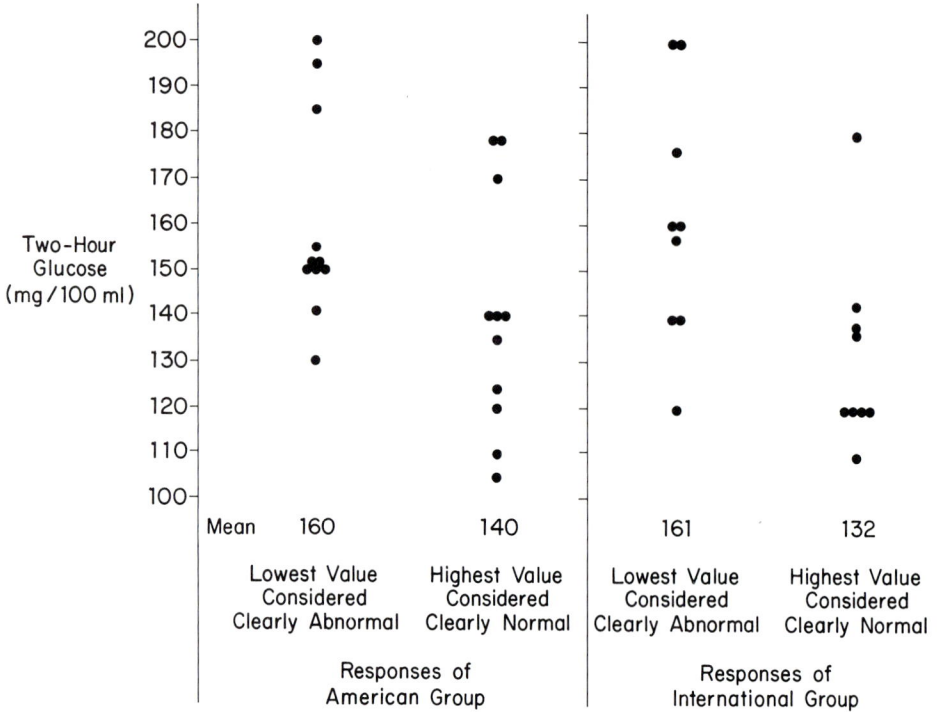

FIGURE 3. Two-hour levels of plasma glucose in a middle-aged subject considered normal or abnormal by each of 20 prominent diabetologists. Details are provided in the original report (West, 1975).

orally. In subjects 40 to 59 years of age the two standard-deviation range extended to 240 mg/100 ml. This wide range of normal responses is not peculiar to the United States. The range is also broad in other affluent societies where samples from the general population have been studied. These include groups in Norway (Jorde, 1962), Britain (Keen and Jarrett, 1975), and Australia (Welborn, et al, 1968; Boyer, et al, 1974). The data of Jarrett and Keen on a representative sample in Bedford, England, are shown in Table 15. Mayer, et al (1976) tested a group from 30 to 64 years of age in Chicago. In the course of a multiphasic screening program 1,673 subjects without known diabetes were given 100 gm of oral glucose after an overnight fast. The two standard-deviation range for the two-hour plasma glucose level on venous blood extended to 252 mg/100 ml. The mean value was 125.1 with a standard deviation of 63.4. By traditional standards about one third had "abnormal" two-hour values.

As shown by O'Sullivan and his colleagues (1966,1970), the poor specificity of traditional cut-off points for individual values can be greatly mitigated by requiring for diagnosis that values be elevated at each of two or three cut-off points. Even when this is done, rates of abnormal tolerance with conventional criteria are much higher than the number who can be expected to become diabetic, particularly in older subjects. Data of Jarrett and Keen (Table 15) also show the profound effect of modest changes in diagnostic criteria.

Fortunately, useful comparisons can be made in epidemiologic studies without achieving agreement concerning diagnostic criteria. For example, it may be of interest to know what percentage of a certain age group in populations A and B have values exceeding the Fajans-Conn cut-off points, irrespective of one's beliefs about their specificity in the diagnosis of "diabetes".

Some of the principles to be used in developing such standards will be discussed. Common sense requires that the rate of abnormality with a test should not greatly exceed the number who may be expected to develop the disease. One of the main problems here is that, in most circumstances, large-vessel disease rates are excessive in those with borderline or slightly impaired tolerance (Ostrander, et al, 1975). This suggests the possibility that mild glucose intolerance causes atherosclerosis, and that persons with these slight "abnormalities" of glucose tolerance should be regarded as diabetic. But the extent to which this association of atherosclerosis and mild glucose intolerance is causal or coincidental is not known (Stamler, 1975). For this reason, and because atherosclerotic lesions are not specific for diabetes, it is appropriate to define diabetes by criteria relevant to the aberrations specific to diabetes. These include risk of subsequent fasting hyperglycemia and microvascular disease. Rates of glomerulosclerosis and clinically significant retinopathy are trivial or nil in persons without fasting hyperglycemia (Jarrett and Keen, 1976). Not one in 10,000 autopsies on such persons shows unequivocal evidence of glomerulosclerosis together with a history of impaired renal function. Some disagreement exists about the frequency of significant diabetic retinopathy in persons with normal fasting values, but the frequency of impaired vision from diabetic retinopathy is virtually nil in persons who have never had fasting hyperglycemia. Putting it another way, there are probably at least a thousand cases of impaired vision from diabetic retinopathy in those with fasting hyperglycemia

TABLE 15 Effect of Varying Criteria upon Prevalence of "Diabetes" in Random Sample of Bedford Population Undergoing Standard 50-gm Oral Glucose Tolerance Tests

AGE	PERCENT WITH "DIABETES" WHEN BLOOD GLUCOSE (MG/100 ML) IS:			
	120+ AT Two Hours	140+ AT Two Hours	180+ Peak	PEAK 180+ AND 120+ Two Hours
20–	7.3	2.1	11.5	2.1
30–	6.4	1.1	14.9	1.1
40–	9.7	4.3	29.0	6.5
50–	15.4	6.6	48.4	14.3
60–	18.4	5.7	51.7	11.5
70–	40.2	22.0	61.0	34.1
TOTAL	15.7	6.6	35.2	11.1

Source: Jarrett and Keen (1976).

for every one in persons who have never had fasting hyperglycemia. Neuropathy sometimes occurs before the discovery of fasting hyperglycemia, but evidence that diabetic neuropathy ever exists before hyperglycemia is not conclusive.

From this line of reasoning it is evident that the number at risk for development of morbidity secondary to diabetes corresponds very closely to the number who will develop fasting hyperglycemia. This number is not known precisely for any population. It is doubtful that the risk of unequivocal fasting hyperglycemia during a lifetime exceeds 7% in any large country. In certain special small populations that are very fat, risk is considerably higher (eg, Pima Indians). Arguments set forth in the section above on the specificity of the fasting blood glucose suggest that the portion who at any one time have normal fasting levels together with truly abnormal glucose tolerance is quite small, probably less than 3%, even in populations in which diabetes is common.

Table 14 provides a list of the various criteria that have been proposed for interpreting oral glucose tolerance tests. As evidence has accumulated, the range of normal has been expanded, particularly for older subjects. The need for age-dependent criteria is now rather generally accepted, although some uncertainty and disagreement remains concerning the appropriate degree of adjustment and the age at which it should begin. The age-dependent criteria of Andres (1967) would classify as diabetic about 7% of those over 70 years of age in his population (Maryland). This was based on a cut-off point of about 236 mg/100 ml for the two-hour plasma glucose value. This rate of 7% did not include known diabetics. His criteria classified about 8% more of this age group as "probably diabetic" (two-hour plasma values about 215). In addition to this 15% (7% diabetic and 8% possibly diabetic), about 7% of Americans of this age have clinically diagnosed diabetes (Bennett, et al, 1976). Some of the latter group have levels of glucose tolerance that Andres would classify as normal. These considerations suggest that even by these conservative criteria, at age 70, about 12% of Americans would be classified as "diabetic". If those with "probable diabetes" are included, the portion considered diabetic would include about one fifth of this age group. With the traditional two-hour cut-off point of 140, about two thirds of these values in old people would be classified as "diabetic". The recent brochure of the American Diabetes Association (1974) suggests a cut-off point of 160 at this age. Data of Andres suggest that about one third of elderly Americans fall into the "diabetic" range by these criteria of ADA.

These criteria of Andres are based on results with a large glucose load of 1.75 mg/kg. In persons 70 years of age, I would guess that two-hour values would be roughly 20 mg/100 ml lower with dosages of 75 to 100 gm, and 35 mg/100 ml lower with loads of 50 gm. Subjects of Andres weighing 70 kg (154.3 lb) received a dosage of 123 gm. Even after these corrections for glucose dosage are applied, about one third of persons over 59 years of age from the population of Andres have abnormal values when traditional criteria are used in interpreting the two-hour value (eg, cut-off point of 140 for the two-hour plasma values on venous blood). Rates of abnormality may be appreciably lower in less indolent leaner populations, but in affluent populations of North America and Europe abnormal tolerance is extremely common in older subjects when conventional criteria are employed. The effect of aging on glucose tolerance is discussed in detail in a separate section of this chapter.

Few data are available to support the cut-off points traditionally recommended. Most of the studies in representative samples of general populations were limited to a single value at one or two hours. Frequency distribution data for summed values have seldom been presented in the general populations in which multiple glucose values have been obtained. Particularly sparse are data on summed values for the older segment of the population. Some theoretical advantages of the summation method have been discussed under timing of sampling. In general, the criteria suggested for interpreting summed values have better specificity than those conventionally employed in interpreting individual values. But this advantage is mainly attributable to a more reasonable placement of the cut-off point suggested for the summed values. These were assigned after it had become apparent that the range of normal responses was broader than was appreciated initially.

In most populations of adults frequency distribution of results of glucose loading tests are distributed unimodally with a slight but definite skew to the right (West, 1966; American Diabetes Association, 1969; Keen and Jarrett, 1969). This unimodality obtains no matter how results are expressed (eg, height of curve, width of curve, area under curve, sum of values). Lack of bimodality makes it impossible to separate clearly normal from abnormal values by any statistical procedures or criteria relating to frequency distribution. Nor is this problem overcome with any of the other diagnostic tests for diabetes (eg, steroid-modified tests, intravenous glucose tests, tolbutamide tests). Bimodality was, however, observed in the Pima population where rates of diabetes are exceedingly high (Figure 6). Separation of the two modes was not complete but was impressive. It is not yet clear whether this bimodality of distribution of two-hour values in Pima is peculiar to a few populations, or whether it is mainly or wholly attributable to the high disease rate. An important related observation was that analysis of the bimodality suggested a level of separation of modes that was much higher than that prescribed by tradition (Rushforth, et al, 1971; Bennett, et al, 1976a). These levels of separation are summarized in Figure 6. They are age-dependent ranging from 204 to 245 mg/ 100 ml (two-hour plasma values). Another pertinent related observation was that subjects with two-hour levels exceeding these cut-off points usually have some elevation of their fasting values (Dippe, et al, 1974). The criteria of diagnosis suggested by the frequency distribution data also fit well with observations in this population on susceptibility to the microvascular lesions of diabetes (Bennett, et al, 1976a). Recently, bimodality was observed in another population in which diabetes rates are very high. In Polynesians of Nauru Zimmet and Whitehouse (1977) found that the division of modes was at approximately the same level as that observed in the Pimas. These results

99

suggest that the dividing line between normal and abnormal values may be substantially higher than the one traditionally employed.

More evidence is needed but it appears that when interpreted by traditional standards the one- and two-hour values have poor specificity. The specificity of the USPHS criteria are better than most of the other older criteria, for reasons that are seldom appreciated. Although one- and two-hour cut-off points are quite low, and although these results are considered in the point score, the score cannot reach a diagnostic value unless the fasting or the three-hour value is elevated. Even if both the one- and two-hour values are 100 mg/100 ml above the USPHS cut-off points, they are not in themselves diagnostic. When the USPHS criteria are used in patients without fasting hyperglycemia, results of the one- and two-hour values are almost inconsequential to classification. Inspection of the data of Köbberling and Creutzfeldt (1970) illustrates this. In 95 patients tested positive by these USPHS criteria there were 27 who did not have elevated three-hour levels. All but one of these had abnormal fasting values. Of 181 in this group with negative results by USPHS criteria, only six (3%) had three-hour levels (venous whole blood) above 109 mg/100 ml. Of these six, only two had values greater than 138 mg/100 ml. Both of these also had two-hour values well above the cut-off point (172 and 152 mg/100 ml). They were classified by these criteria as nondiabetic because all other values were normal.

Köbberling and Creutzfeldt compared several different standards after performing oral glucose tolerance tests (75-gm) in 746 adults who were close relatives of diabetics. Disparities of classification were great. They described new simplified criteria from which the results with other standards diverged only to a modest degree. By their formula the results were considered positive when the sum of the one- and two-hour values exceeded 299 mg/100 ml (venous whole blood). These investigators stressed that their new criteria were not based on any direct evidence of sensitivity and specificity. They were promulgated only on the bases of their simplicity and their applicability as a "consensus" of the divergent results of other traditional criteria. These various criteria did not include any of the newer criteria that employ much higher cut-off points such as those of Andres (1971). Valleron, et al (1976) also found very poor agreement when results of a group of tests were classified using each of six of the most widely-used criteria.

I suspect that in some circumstances a common reason for diagnosis with the USPHS criteria is a slight elevation of the "fasting" level in persons who are thought to be fasting and are not. When this event is combined with slight "elevations" of the one- and two-hour values, a diagnosis may be made despite a normal three-hour value. Data of Valleron, et al (1975) are consistent with this possibility. Under circumstances of their study, slight elevations of the fasting level were often not confirmed with repeat tests.

It is common practice to base ranges of normal (mindlessly) on a two standard-deviation range. This has also been done in setting limits of certain indexes of glucose tolerance. Fortunately, in many adult populations rates of occult diabetes are not very different from the percentages that have values above this range. Unfortunately, groups tested to derive this range have often been quite unrepresentative. As pointed out by Andres (1971), when representative groups have been tested the results have typically been considered inconveniently high and quite out of keeping with traditional notions. For this reason, the two standard-deviation range has usually been abandoned as inapplicable. In the discussion above on sensitivity of the fasting blood glucose, these matters have been considered in some detail. Let it suffice to say here that the ideal percentile range for normal values is unknown for any population, and this optimum would vary considerably depending on the characteristics of the population under consideration (eg, age distribution, fatness, rate of prevalence of diabetes). For reasons set forth in that previous section, the percentage classified as diabetic in any age group should seldom, if ever, exceed 5% of those who are without fasting hyperglycemia. Because of the poor reproducibility of glucose tolerance tests, an argument can be made for creating a "suspect" or "borderline" range as broad as ten percentiles, but in most populations the very high-risk group probably includes less than two percentiles, after those with fasting hyperglycemia are removed. Data of Bennett, et al (1976a) suggest, for example, that a substantial portion of those who will develop diabetes are drawn from those who had clearly normal tolerance a few years before. In Birmingham, England (Birmingham Diabetes Survey Working Party, 1976), a cohort with varying degrees of glucose tolerance was followed for ten years. Persons with borderline tolerance developed diabetes much more frequently than did those with clearly normal tolerance, but a substantial portion of those who had borderline results initially, had clearly normal results ten years later. It was not clear to what extent the predictive value of status of glucose tolerance in those with normal fasting levels was independent of known predictors such as age and fatness.

It is now rather generally agreed that criteria of interpretation of glucose tolerance tests should be adjusted for age. Less certain is the degree to which criteria should be related to other characteristics such as sex, fatness, race, muscularity, activity levels, diet, etc. In interpreting a specific result it is desirable to know the frequency distribution of blood glucose values in the general population from which that individual is drawn. This is, however, only one of several indexes to be used in interpretation. It is of further help to know the frequency distribution in persons with matching characteristics of age, fatness, etc.

There are three important trends in recent years in interpreting glucose tolerance tests. One is to adjust interpretation for age; another is to extend the limits of normal range. It may be noted, for example, that in Table 14, cut-off points proposed in recent years have been substantially higher than those proposed earlier. The third trend is an increasing acceptance of a broad range for borderline values. This reflects both a knowledge of the limited reproducibility of such tests and an appreciation of the paucity of information on the significance of values in the upper percentiles in subjects with normal fasting

101

levels. Data of several kinds are needed, including long-term prospective studies of the relationship of glucose tolerance to risk of future fasting hyperglycemia and morbidity. Pioneer small-scale efforts to this end have been described, but these should be expanded and intensified.

Diagnostic criteria in children have been discussed by Danowski (1957), Nilsson (1962), Drash (1975), and by several authors in the volumes edited by Laron (1972) and by Rosenbloom, et al (1973). Suggested criteria have been quite similar to those promulgated for young adults. Few data are available in groups of children that could be considered representative of the general population of children, and not much is known about the effects of geographic, ethnic, and environmental differences on glucose tolerance in children, or the significance of such differences. Lestradet, et al (1976) studied the relationship of age to response in 70 healthy children. When oral glucose loads of 30 gm/sq m of body surface were administered, glucose levels in children less than 6 years of age were somewhat lower than in older children, despite higher levels of insulin secretion in older children. Florey, et al (1976) found insulin levels somewhat higher in girls than in boys when oral glucose was administered to children from 9 to 12 years of age. The greater adiposity of the girls did not appear to explain these differences.

Discussions elsewhere in this volume call attention to the very incomplete evidence concerning the significance, in children with normal fasting levels, of postglucose values that are borderline or slightly "elevated" by traditional standards (eg, in the section on juvenile diabetes in Chapter 8).

Conclusion A majority of scholars in this field still believe that the oral glucose tolerance test is a useful and appropriate diagnostic instrument, even in persons with clearly normal fasting blood glucose levels. There is a general trend, however, to employ more conservative criteria that provide wider ranges for normal and borderline values, particularly in older subjects. There is a very wide disparity of opinion about the limits of the normal ranges in the various age groups. Part of the problem is the lack of data concerning risk of unequivocal diabetes for the various levels of glucose tolerance in persons with normal fasting blood glucose levels. Indeed, it is not established that the oral glucose tolerance test is capable of identifying diabetes with acceptable specificity in persons with normal fasting values.

Pregnancy

There is an extensive body of literature on glucose tolerance in pregnancy. A long and well-selected bibliography is appended to the excellent publication of Pehrson (1974). The very considerable contributions of O'Sullivan and his colleagues are described in other sections of this book (eg, in the reviews of pregnancy as an etiologic factor in Chapter 8 and in Chapter 9 on prediabetes). O'Sullivan and Mahan (1964) have published data on the range of responses to oral glucose in pregnancy. On the basis of these results with 100-gm tests they suggested cut-off points for the one-hour values (venous whole blood) of 165 mg/100 ml, and 140 for the two-hour value. Thus, two-hour plasma values up to about 160 mg/100 ml would be regarded as normal. O'Sullivan, et al (1976) pointed out that these criteria were not necessarily applicable in all populations of pregnant women.

Arguments have been made for and against the use of intravenous tests in pregnancy. Silverstone, et al (1963) recommended intravenous testing. There appears to be some reduction in rate of intestinal absorption of glucose in pregnancy. Montgomery, et al (1970) compared an oral glucose test in pregnancy with a cortisone-glucose test and an intravenous procedure. Their results did not provide any basis for a "clear preference" among these tests, nor do data of other investigators. In the studies of Hohe (1971) the blood glucose level two hours after oral glucose was found to reflect very well the results by more complex indexes.

Results have been conflicting with respect to the effects of the various stages of pregnancy on oral and intravenous tolerance. This rather extensive literature has been summarized by Pehrson (1974). Most, but not all, workers have found slight diminution of oral glucose tolerance as pregnancy progresses. Welsh (1960) and others have found a poor correlation in pregnancy between results of intravenous and oral tests. Most studies have shown no decrease in intravenous tolerance with pregnancy. Both Silverstone, et al (1963) and Picard, et al (1963) found intravenous tolerance increased in the first trimester. O'Sullivan, et al (1976) have shown that, in part, the apparent conflicts with results in intravenous testing are the result of technical problems. O'Sullivan found a slight decline of intravenous tolerance in the course of pregnancy when he corrected certain of these technical difficulties. He pointed out that some of the disparities between results have been secondary to inadequate matching of methods by which criteria of interpretation were developed. I have considered the possibility that changes with pregnancy in volume of distribution of glucose might account for some of the problem of interpretation of the decline in blood glucose levels after intravenous glucose.

Steroid-modified tests have been used frequently in pregnancy, but there is little evidence of their utility (Pehrson, 1974). They are discussed in detail below.

Calderon, et al (1966) evaluated intravenous glucose tolerance in pregnant women living at altitudes in Peru. Blood glucose levels were lower than in pregnant women living at sea level, but the slope of the descent of the blood glucose was similar in the two groups. Perhaps the lower glucose values were the result of a larger volume of distribution in the women who lived at altitude. The hypoxic condition was not the only environmental factor that differed in these two groups.

Effect of age

There is a vast literature showing the effects of age on glucose tolerance. The National Library of Medicine prepared a bibliography on this subject published as Literature Search 19-68. Although it covered only four and one-half years (January 1964 to July 1968) and concerned only studies in man, there were 123 citations. Some of the earliest observations in this field were reviewed by Allen in 1913. Other pioneer observations included those of Spence (1921), Malmros (1928), Deren (1936), and Chessrow and Bleyer (1955). Among the modern reviews are those of Andres (1967,1971,1976) and O'Sullivan (1974). Recent data of interest include observations of West, et al (1964), Gordon, et al (1964), Hayner, et al (1965), Andres (1967), Chlouverakis, et al (1967), O'Sullivan, et al (1971a), Nolan, et al (1973), and Duffy, et al (1973). The profound effects of age on glucose tolerance are well illustrated by the data from Busselton, Australia (Bowyer, et al, 1974). In this population the decline is progressive beginning with the fourth decade.

Data are in some respects conflicting. It is not clear, for example, the extent to which reduction in tolerance is attributable to poor beta-cell function or to insulin resistance. There is rather general agreement that, in most populations, a substantial decline occurs with age and that this is usually greater than can be accounted for by age-related increases in the incidence of diabetes. For this reason most scholars in this field recommend that diagnostic criteria be adjusted substantially for age. There is disagreement about the age level at which this adjustment should begin and its degree. Jarrett, et al (1970) showed that some of the conflict may be ascribed to differences of method. When they used only 50 gm in Bedford, no significant effect of age on two-hour values could be detected until the seventh decade. However, well-marked changes could be seen much earlier on values in the earlier part of the test.

The effect in various circumstances of aging on incidence of diabetes will be discussed below in greater detail in the section on etiologic factors in Chapter 7. It has also been reviewed above in the section on incidence in Chapter 5. Let it suffice here to say that relationships of age to incidence of diabetes differ considerably by population. In most Western populations incidence rises sharply from the third to the sixth decade. But it is not yet clear, for reasons explained in the other sections, whether incidence increases, decreases, or plateaus in the seventh, eighth, and ninth decades. On the other hand, postglucose values in these populations continue to rise in the seventh, eighth, and ninth decades.

Mean glucose values have risen with age to variable degrees in the different studies. Results of Andres (1971) are typical. In adults not previously known to have diabetes the mean one-hour and two-hour values both increased about 6 mg/100 ml in each decade. In some studies even larger age-related increments have been found (Hayner, et al 1965; Duffy, et al, 1973). In the study of Lauvaux and Staquet (1969) there was little change with age in the level of the fifth percentile. This suggested to them the possibility that the higher values in the older subjects might be mainly secondary to a greater frequency of diabetes in the elderly. But in several populations it has been shown that about half of elderly subjects have "abnormal" tolerance by certain traditional standards. These include the general population of the United States (Gordon, et al, 1964).

It is now clear that the increases with age are, in most circumstances, attributable to an increasing incidence of diabetes and also to factors unrelated to risk of diabetes. Most observers believe that the increase in incidence of diabetes is, although significant, of lesser importance in accounting for these age-related rises (Andres, et al, 1976). Among age-related factors that may contribute include lower exercise levels, increasing degree and duration of adiposity, decreasing muscularity, increasing insulin resistance (many causes), and less effetive beta-cell function.

Andres (1967) also gathered age-related data on responses to the steroid-glucose tolerance test and the tolbutamide response test, with very similar results. Andres has published a convenient nomogram that permits an easy determination of approximate percentile rank by age for any given two-hour blood glucose value (see Figure 4). This nomogram is not necessarily applicable to other populations, but probably is applicable to the general population of the United States and roughly applicable, with the reservations cited below, to most other Western societies.

In interpreting the excellent data of Andres and the diagnostic criteria developed from them, several considerations should be kept in mind. In selecting the subjects an attempt was made to recruit a representative group of volunteers, but the responses of this group may not reflect precisely those of the general population from which they were drawn. The number tested was substantial (600), but the years of age ranged from 17 to 103 so that the average number per decade was modest. They received large dosages of glucose 1.75 gm/Kg. By this formula most subjects receive more than twice as much glucose as those in other studies in which loads of 50 gm were employed. By this formula a 70-kg subject receives 123 gm. Finally, the results of Andres were expressed as whole blood values. Plasma values would have been about 15% higher.

There is considerable uncertainty concerning which methods and criteria are best for appraising glucose tolerance in children. Several papers were addressed to these issues in a special issue of *Metabolism* (Rosenbloom, et al, 1973), and in the volume edited by Laron and Carp (1972). A popular oral loading dose has been 1.75 gm/kg. Several investigators have published mean and standard deviation ranges for blood glucose values at various intervals after such tests (Drash, 1975). These ranges are similar to those found in young adults. Both capillary and venous blood have been used, more commonly capillary specimens. When glucose dosage is based on weight, responses seem to vary little by age in children. However, data are rather limited on glucose tolerance in children and many factors may affect it. Very few data are available on the sensitivity and specificity of values at the upper end of the scale.

There are two general possibilities with respect to the prognostic significance of postglucose values above the two standard-deviation range in children with normal fasting values. One is that a substantial portion may be individuals with "chemical diabetes" or "maturity-onset diabetes of youth". Another possibility is that a substantial majority of these are normal. Present evidence, although not decisive, gives more support to the latter view, although it is probably less popular. This evidence is reviewed in some detail in other parts

Age

Two-Hour
Blood Glucose
(mg / 100 ml)

Percentile
Rank

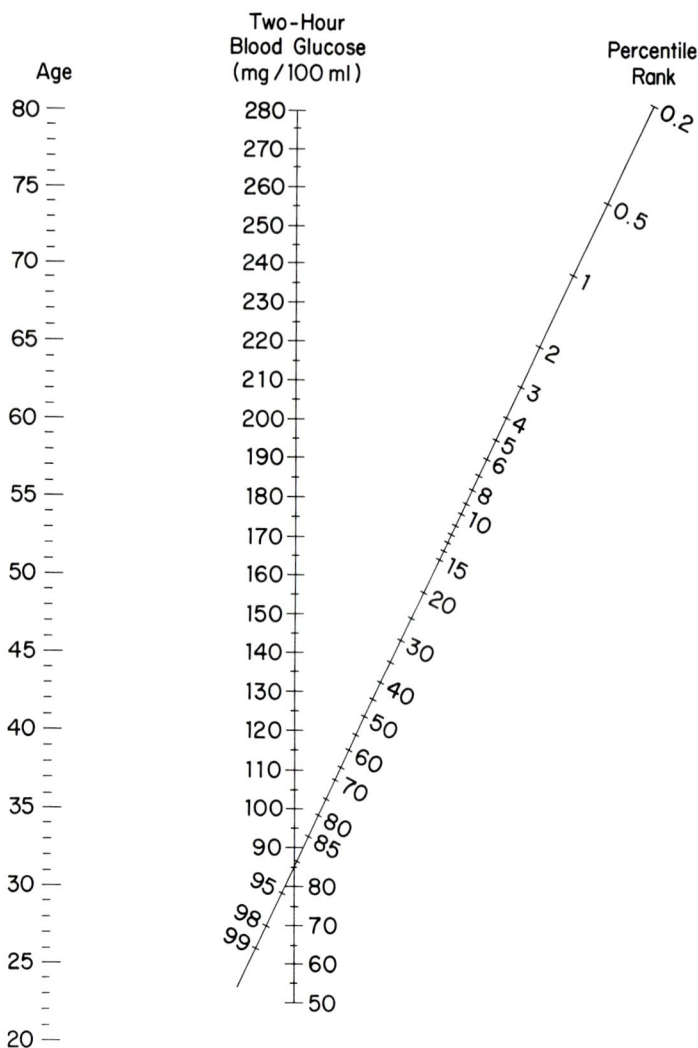

FIGURE 4. Nomogram of Andres (1971), based on data from a general population in Maryland. When age and two-hour glucose (whole venous blood) are known the approximate percentile rank of the value within the population may be computed. These data are based on results with a large glucose load (1.75 gm per kg).

of this book, including the section on mild diabetes of youth. This negative evidence includes the low rate of decompensation to unequivocal diabetes in these children. Another consideration is that the prevalence of unequivocal diabetes is very low even in the oldest children, far lower than the 2% that were above the two standard-deviation range five or ten years before. Conceivably children with normal fasting values and poor glucose tolerance may be more likely to develop diabetes as adults, but there is little evidence for or against that possibility. It is quite possible that a substantial majority of new youth-onset diabetics come from the group which had clearly normal tolerance five years before.

The reproducibility of results of oral glucose tolerance tests has not been so extensively investigated in children as in adults. The rather considerable intraindividual variability in adults gives reason for interpreting borderline results conservatively. In neither children or adults is the future risk of diabetes known in persons considered to have abnormal tolerance and *normal* fasting glucose values. Indeed, it has not been proved that glucose tolerance tests have any clinical utility in children, although there is some evidence in support of that possibility (Rosenbloom, et al, 1973).

Pioneering observations on glucose tolerance in children were made by Ross (1938), who also provided an excellent review of the early history of the development of glucose tolerance tests.

LOADING TESTS WITH NUTRIENTS OTHER THAN GLUCOSE

There are theoretical and practical advantages and disadvantages in using glucose as a challenge. More data are available with glucose loading tests than with any other agent. This is sometimes an advantage in interpreting results in either individuals or groups. Glucose is relatively cheap and produces no permanently harmful effects under ordinary circumstances. Interpretations of responses are in some respects simplified by the absence of the somewhat more complex effects that follow the administration of other loads such as mixed meals.

On the other hand, administration of glucose is in a sense unphysiologic. Glucose is present in the diet in only very small amounts. Persons with moderate or severe diabetes do not require glucose tolerance tests. Those who require such tests are those with mild diabetes. These persons did not become diabetic because they could not tolerate oral glucose; they became hyperglycemic because they could not tolerate their normal diets. An argument could therefore be made that the best test is one that simulates the loads ordinarily sustained by the subject to be tested. Another disadvantage of glucose is that it is unpalatable in concentrated amounts. In dosages ordinarily employed it produces unpleasant gastrointestinal symptoms fairly frequently, and vomiting occasionally. These considerations have led to the evaluation and use of other loads.

Test meals

The alternative most frequently employed is the test meal. Three general approaches have been used: constituents of the meal may be specifically prescribed, all specifications may be omitted, or less specific prescriptions may be employed (eg, "large meal", "meal containing at least three pieces of bread"). Sakaguchi introduced a rice test meal in 1926.

107

Until rather recently it was thought that the carbohydrate content of the meal was the dominant determinant of respose, and that responses expected after glucose were quite similar to those after meals containing equal amounts of rapidly digestible carbohydrate (CHO). Even in the excellent Joslin textbook (Marble, 1971, p 202), it is indicated that " . . . for sake of simplicity we use the same criteria for both food and glucose tolerance tests". Recently, however, it has become evident that responses to mixed meals and to glucose differ more than had been commonly supposed. The main factor accounting for this difference is probably the substantial effect of protein and fat in stimulating beta-cell secretion when these other nutrients are administered through the gut along with carbohydrate (Kipnis, 1972). In most circumstances intravenous fat has little direct or immediate effect on insulin secretion, but when administered orally with carbohydrate it may greatly enhance insulin response (Dobbs, et al, 1975). In some circumstances oral fat may inhibit immediate glycemic response to a test meal by delaying the rate at which the stomach empties.

The higher insulin levels achieved after mixed meals may sometimes have a considerable effect on glucose values. We (West, et al, 1964) found in 46 subjects that two-hour values were, on the average, 21 mg/100 ml higher after 75 gm of oral glucose than after breakfasts containing 75 gm of carbohydrate (plus the usual protein and fat in a typical breakfast). These data are shown in Figure 5. Mean one-hour values ere 49 mg/100 ml higher with oral glucose (23 paired tests).

Data of O'Sullivan, et al (1967) also suggest strongly that postglucose values are much higher after glucose loads of standard size than after ordinary meals. In Sudbury these investigators tested 1,991 adult subjects from the general population one to two hours after an unmeasured meal. Only 2% of the two-hour venous blood glucose values exceeded 138 mg/100 ml. Other data of these investigators indicate that after 100 gm of oral glucose, two-hour values above this level are much more common (by sevenfold). In Bedford (Keen, 1964) glycosuria was more than seven times as frequent after 50 gm of oral glucose than postprandially. The much greater tolerance for meals probably explains most of the huge discrepancy between the purported prevalence rates (very low) in Oxford, Massachusetts, and the very high rates in American groups in which glucose tolerance tests were performed in all subjects (O'Sullivan and Williams, 1966). In Oxford only those with "high" postprandial values were retested after oral glucose.

Kosaka, et al (1966) studied the effects of a rice meal (270 gm cooked rice, two eggs, and small amounts of vegetables) compared to those of a glucose load containing about the same amount of carbohydrate (100 gm). Mean blood glucose values were only slightly higher after glucose (by 6 mg/100 ml at one hour) in a group of mild diabetics but the standard deviation was greater with glucose at both one hour and two hours. At two hours it was 37 mg/100 ml with rice and 58 with glucose. Crapo, et al (1976) found in 19 subjects that two-hour plasma glucose values were similar after cooked rice and cooked potato, but one-hour levels were higher after potato, though not quite as high as after an

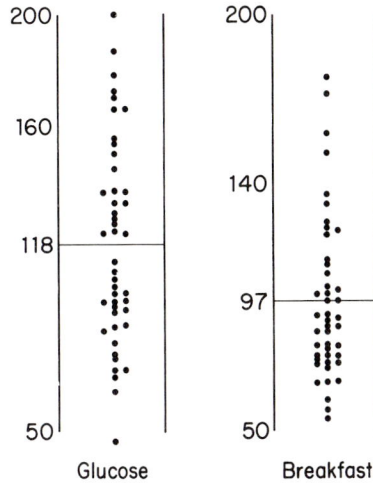

FIGURE 5. Two-hour blood glucose values (in mg/100 ml) for 46 subjects after 75 gm oral glucose and after 75 gm carbohydrate given as part of a mixed meal. Mean responses were 21 mg/100 ml higher after glucose than after the mixed meal ($p < .001$). From West, et al, 1964.

equal amount of carbohydrate (50 gm) in the form of glucose. Lenner (1976) found blood glucose levels higher after bread starch than after equal amounts of carbohydrate in the form of disaccharides (lactose, fructose, or sucrose). Ziegler, et al (1973) compared the effects of feedings containing different nutrients but the same amounts of carbohydrate, protein, fat, and calories. Blood glucose levels and insulin levels were higher when the carbohydrate (50 gm) was mainly glucose than when it was mainly starch (whole-wheat flakes).

It was believed formerly that blood glucose levels were higher after oral glucose than after test meals because of the much greater rapidity of absorption of glucose. But to a considerable degree, the difference is attributable to the greater insulin response to mixed meals. It is true that absorption of certain kinds of complex carbohydrates is much slower, as shown, for example, by Campbell (1970a). But many of the dietary starches are quite rapidly absorbed. When Swan, et al (1966) administered bread starch, levels of plasma glucose and insulin were only slightly lower at one hour than with oral glucose. One-hour levels of insulin and glucose were very slightly higher with starch than with sucrose. These latter differences were probably insignificant. At two hours plasma glucose levels were virtually identical with the three nutrients. Plasma insulin levels were slightly higher with starch and glucose than with sucrose.

On the basis of a rather small amount of data, Kjer (1925) had concluded that the effects on blood glucose of glucose and potato were similar, whereas rises of blood glucose after bread and oatmeal were somewhat less abrupt. Cooking of starches frequently accelerates very considerably the rate at which starchy foods are absorbed. If absorption of carbohydrate in mixed meals were decidedly slower, one would expect higher two-hour values than with oral glucose, but this is not the case, as indicated above. Much is left to be learned. It is clear the responses vary substantially depending on both the characteristics and sizes of the meals. Comparisons are needed with larger numbers.

Although blood glucose values are generally lower after mixed meals than after glucose, it does not necessarily follow that tests with meals are less sensitive. Indeed, such tests might be more sensitive since they may under some conditions stimulate beta cells to a greater degree than does glucose. Almost no direct evidence is available evaluating these two methods directly by appropriate means. It is generally believed that glucose tests are much more sensitive as indexes of diabetes, but this is not based on any conclusive evidence. In the past the question has usually been asked in the wrong way: Does the universe of those with two-hour plasma values above 140 mg/100 ml after oral glucose contain more diabetics than those that have such values after a meal? A more appropriate question is one of this type: In persons with normal fasting glucose values, do those with glycemic responses at the 95th percentile after oral glucose have greater risk of developing diabetes than those with responses at the 95th percentile after a standardized meal?

Turner et al (1977) observed subjects with normal responses to breakfast in whom glucose tolerance was "abnormal" by traditional standards. They thought this reflected a greater sensitivity of the glucose tolerance test. An alternate explation is that the glucose test is less specific when interpreted using traditional standards.

An additional advantage of test meals is their palatability, and the lack of unpleasant symptoms that often attend the administration of oral glucose. Another theoretical asset is that, without producing these gastrointestinal symptoms, a greater insulinogenic challenge can be delivered.

More data are needed on the frequency distribution of responses to test meals and how it is affected by the characteristics of the subjects tested (eg, age, adiposity). Most of the present data in population studies were obtained in circumstances of rather limited standardization. Often the interval between the meal and testing has not been precisely standardized, and characteristics and quantities of these meals has seldom been controlled. Data of both types are useful (standardized and unstandardized conditions), but there is a particular need for more information in circumstances where meal characteristics are known and standardized, and where interval between eating and testing is known and standardized.

It would usually be desirable that these meals conform in characteristics to the typical diet of the population tested. An example of this is the rice tolerance test that has been used in Japan (Sakaguchi, 1926). A simple test meal for Western subjects consists of: three bread exchanges (45 gm CHO); two fruit exchanges as fruit or fruit juices (20 gm CHO); 10 gm sugar as jam, small dessert, or sugar added to tea or coffee; 3 oz of meat (about 21 gm protein and 15 gm fat); and two fat exchanges (10 gm fat). This meal contains approximately 75 gm carbohydrate, 27 gm protein, and 25 gm fat. It can be served as a breakfast or lunch. Where fruit is not easily accessible, 200 ml of a soft drink may be substituted for the two fruit exchanges (20 gm of simple CHO). The well-known exchange lists (American and British Diabetes Associations, etc) provide many options with respect to partial or complete substitutions for the prescribed bread (crackers, starchy vegetables, etc) or meat (cheese, eggs, etc).

There is some theoretical advantage in giving a meal of greater size. On the other hand, to the extent that it is made larger, the number who cannot eat it all increases. Thus, standardization is lost. One of the several options would be to relate test meal size to weight. This could be done crudely with some very simple formulas. One might, for example, give the test meal described above (75 gm CHO) to all subjects except those weighing more than 75 kg. These might be given 90 gm (one more bread exchange).

In population testing, when meal size is not standardized, one of the many variables that may affect results is the behavior of those who know they are to be tested for diabetes. Some may change to some degree the size or character of their meal. An approach that is often appropriate in screening surveys is the simple request that subjects eat a large meal. In screening surveys or studies in which meal characteristics are not prescribed, it is desirable to define the term "meal". We have sometimes coded along these lines: Subjects who have consumed no nutrients in the previous three hours are considered "fasting". A "meal" is defined as a feeding containing more than 30 gm of carbohydrate. Lesser feedings are classified separately as "snacks". Sometimes it is appropriate to consider very small amounts of carbohydrate as negligible (eg, less than 10 gm, as in 1 tsp of sugar in a cup of coffee). For certain purposes of analyses, results from two of these three categories can be lumped. It is often difficult to interpret tests performed immediately after meals. In screening it is usually better to delay testing until at least forty-five minutes after the ingestion of food.

Other forms of sugar

Allan and Georgson (1960) described a candy tolerance test. A modification of this was used quite effectively by MacDonald, et al (1963) in a mass screening program. Jelly sandwiches have been used. Most commercial soft drinks (sweet drinks) have a sugar concentration of only about 10% to 12%. This makes it difficult for many subjects to consume as much as 50 gm of sugar in this form (about 450 to 500 ml). But it is sometimes feasible to use popular sweet drinks or modifications thereof as part or all of a test load in screening programs.

Leonards, et al (1965) developed a loading solution later called "Glucola" (Ames Company), which has had wide use in the United States. This is a partial hydrolysate of cornstarch flavored as a "cola" and carbonated. It contains 30% glucose, 18% maltose, 13% maltotriose, and 39% higher saccharides. Average molecular weight is almost three times that of glucose. Most subjects find

Glucola decidedly more palatable than glucose, even when the latter has been flavored with lemon or other flavors. In North America, Glucola is available in 7-oz bottles containing 75 gm of carbohydrate. In other geographic areas, including Latin America, a dry powder called "Dexpack" containing similar constituents is marketed, from which a loading solution can be made. Glucola is not as sweet as glucose and the osmotic effect is considerably less than with glucose.

Kent and Leonards (1965) administered 75-gm dosages of Glucola to 50,000 persons. They reported an incidence of nausea of less than 0.1%, and vomiting was not observed. We have observed vomiting occasionally with 75-gm dosages of this solution, but only four cases of vomiting and nausea can be recalled, all women. The author is not aware of any controlled studies comparing gastrointestinal symptoms after Glucola with those after glucose or sweet drinks without carbohydrate (eg, cyclamate).

Several investigators have found that levels of glycemia and insulin secretion are very similar after glucose and Glucola (eg, Genuth, 1969).

INTRAVENOUS TESTS

Intravenous tests offer both theoretical and practical advantages, but also disadvantages. They are uninfluenced by the vagaries of gastrointestinal absorption that sometimes make oral tests difficult to interpret. In general, results are less subject to intraindividual variation than with oral tests. They usually require less time to complete than oral tests. Disadvantages include the need to give an intravenous injection. Usually this is well-tolerated, but concentrated glucose is quite irritating to tissues if any of the material is inadvertently injected outside the vein, or if it escapes from the vein in substantial amounts. Most of the intravenous tests prescribe several samples of blood, which requires repeated punctures or placing a catheter in a vein. In some respects intravenous tests represent an unphysiologic challenge. Glucose does not enter through the portal system (the normal route). In most of the standard tests a rapid bolus is given that has little correspondence to the challenges sustained in daily life. The typical intravenous challenge is much more abrupt and intense, but much smaller than ingestion of an ordinary meal. The total amount of carbohydrate given (eg, 25 gm) is usually less than that in one sandwich or in 300 ml of a typical soft drink.

It is now clear that gastrointestinal factors play an important role in determining beta-cell responses to meals (Scow and Cornfeld, 1954; Dupre and Chisholm, 1971; Kipnis, 1972; Dobbs, et al, 1975). Intravenous tests do not measure the integrity of this element of the system for regulating carbohydrate metabolism. Another problem is that only a small minority of physicians understand the meaning of the usual expressions of results of intravenous tests. If, for example, the medical record or letter of referral says the K value is 1.03, only a small percentage of physicians are able readily to interpret such a report.

There is a large body of literature on comparisons of oral and intravenous tests, but there is little direct evidence on their comparative sensitivity and specificity as diagnostic instruments. In some circumstances results of the two types of test correspond rather closely, and in other conditions the correlation has been poor (Nadon, et al, 1964; Welsh, 1960; Olefsky, et al, 1973). Age seems to affect glucose tolerance to about the same degree whether it is determined orally or intravenously (Schneeberg and Finestone, 1952; Silverstone, et al, 1957; West, et al, 1964). Use of intravenous tests in pregnancy has been discussed in the section on pregnancy earlier in this chapter.

The modern history of the development of these tests was reviewed by West and Wood (1959). Many workers made early contributions to the development of these tests.* Several others contributed subsequently.† Intravenous tests had been employed rather frequently prior to 1913 (Allen, 1913). Butterfield, et al (1971) and Pehrson (1974) have published more recent reviews. Ross (1938) credited F. J. von Becker with having crudely evaluated intravenous tolerance in 1854. Urine glucose tests were performed in rabbits after intravenous glucose.

The procedure employed most commonly in recent years is the rapid injection of concentrated glucose (typically 50%). The dosage most commonly employed in adults has been 25 gm. After a postinjection period of extracellular equilibration (about ten to twenty minutes), blood glucose levels are measured serially for periods of thirty to sixty minutes at intervals of about five minutes. When values are plotted on semilog paper (time on horizontal axis and glucose level on the vertical by log value), the descent usually forms a straight line (Hamilton and Stein, 1942). From these data the rate of decline of the blood glucose can be determined. Usually this rate is expressed as a K value that indicates the percentage decline per minute. Some investigators have based calculations on the increment values. These are computed by subtracting the fasting value from each of the postinjection blood glucose values. Under certain conditions the serial plots of the logs of these incremental values also form a straight line. Greville (1943), Amutuzio, et al (1953), and Duncan (1956a) presented evidence in support of using increment blood values rather than absolute values. On the other hand, West and Wood (1959) presented contrary arguments, as did Franckson, et al (1962) and Butterfield, et al (1967a). This technical point is not a crucial one. Both methods measure fairly satisfactorily the rates at which glucose disappears. When absolute blood glucose values are used to calculate the K values ("total index"), figures of 0.9 to 1.2 are borderline, values greater than 1.2 are normal and values below 0.9 are probably diabetic except in old age. Results of Lundbaeck (1962) are typical. In his healthy subjects mean K was 1.72 with a standard deviation of 0.53. In

---

*References: (Thannhauser and Pfitzer, 1913; Jorgensen and Plum, 1923; Ross, 1938; Tunbridge and Allibone, 1940; Lozner, et al, 1941; Hamilton and Stein, 1942; Greville, 1943; Goldberg and Luft, 1948).

†References: (Conard, Franckson, Bastenie, et al, 1953; Amutuzio, et al, 1953; L. J. P. Duncan, 1956; Ikkos and Luft, 1957; West and Wood, 1959; Hlad and Elrick, 1959; Lundbaeck, 1962; Nilsson, 1962; Lunell, 1966).

diabetics, mean K was 0.63 ($\pm$0.18). But these ranges in groups of controls and diabetics are influenced by many factors, such as definition of "diabetic" and "healthy", age (Silverstone, et al, 1957; West, et al, 1964), and physical conditioning. Standards for interpretation are even less well established for intravenous tests than for oral tests.

West and Wood (1959) have shown that under certain circumstances single forty-minute values in such tests reflect rather well the K values as determined by more elaborate methods (correlation coefficient of minus 0.91 between the simple test and the elaborate test). Amutuzio, et al (1956) observed that the sixty-eight-minute increment value corresponded very well (negatively) with the K value when a load of 25 gm was given. Theoretically, correspondence would be better if the initial peak values were similar interindividually. Standardization of peaks can be achieved by relating loading dosage to the volume of distribution of glucose. This volume may be crudely estimated on the basis of weight (Franckson, et al, 1959). Our simplified test (West and Wood, 1959) provided for a glucose load of 0.1 gm/lb. Glycosuria is negligible with this dosage, but appreciable with large dosages in the first ten to twenty minutes of the test (West and Wood, 1959). On the other hand, Nilsson (1962) thought that the glucose space was probably related better to fat-free weight than weight. This deserves further study. Since extracellular volume of adipose tissue is somewhat less than in muscle but appreciable, the appropriate index is probably intermediate between weight and fat-free weight. This would be fairly well reflected by surface area.

Verdy, et al (1971) evaluated glucose tolerance when intravenous tests were repeated after one hundred fifty minutes. In normal young lean subjects glucose tolerance was usually not quite as good with the second test, although still normal. In older heavier subjects with poor glucose tolerance, K values were somewhat better with the second tests. Insulin levels were also higher immediately after the second glucose injection. In contrast, those who initially had normal tolerance had lower insulin levels immediately after their second injections than after their first. In some respects the results of Metz and Friedenberg (1970) were the same. They performed consecutive tests in triplicate, one hour apart. Tolerance subsequently improved in individuals whose tolerance was poor initially. This improvement was associated with improved insulin secretion in response to the later challenges. Tolerance also improved in those whose first tests had been normal, but this improvement was not associated with a change in insulin response. When Holten, et al (1957) performed duplicate intravenous tests two hours apart in patients without known diabetes, they noted no significant change in response to the second test.

For reasons outlined above, intravenous tests have not usually been employed in epidemiologic or clinical work except under special conditions. In some special circumstances, they are preferable to the oral methods. When one attempts to measure changes in tolerance over time in small groups of subjects, the intravenous method may be preferable because intraindividual variations of response are usually less than with oral tests. There are other circumstances in which it is particularly desirable to eliminate the influence of gastrointestinal factors. Intravenous tests have been widely used in epidemiologic studies relating to pregnancy (O'Sullivan, et al, 1970a; Pehrson, 1974). Some of this work is discussed above under criteria for interpreting oral glucose tolerance tests in pregnancy. Not many data are available on intravenous tolerance in children. Among the few such studies performed were those of von Euler and Larsson (1962). They found K values quite similar to those previously reported for adults, as did Robert Jackson, et al (1973). Steroid-modified intravenous tests will be discussed below.

Steroid-Modified Tests

Glucocorticoids related to hydrocortisone, when administered in supraphysiologic doses, impair glucose tolerance. Indeed, persons who receive long-term therapy with large dosages of these compounds frequently develop diabetes. So do persons with excessive endogenous secretion of these steroids. This led Berger to propose in 1952 a challenge test with corticotrophin (ACTH) as a means for identifying latent diabetes. On the basis of rather limited data, Berger concluded that the sensitivity of the glucose tolerance test was increased by the ACTH. He found positive tests more commonly in nondiabetic siblings of diabetics than in a group without a family history of diabetes. Fajans and Conn (1954) found these data of Berger "uninterpretable". One of the problems was that evidence of matching of the characteristics of the two groups (eg, baseline glucose tolerance) was lacking.

The major factor in the popularization of steroid-modified tests was the report of Fajans and Conn in 1954 and a follow-up report in 1961 (Conn and Fajans). They designed a standardized test in which a dose of 50 mg hydrocortisone (62.5 mg for those over 160 lb—about 73 kg) was administered by mouth eight and one-half hours, and again two hours, before an oral glucose tolerance test (1.75 gm/kg of ideal body weight). They then determined the range of responses to cortisone and glucose of a small "control" group (37) of young adults with normal glucose tolerance. These responses were compared to those in 75 persons with a normal glucose tolerance and a strong family history of diabetes (parent, sibling, or offspring of a diabetic). It was found that, after cortisone and glucose, two-hour values of 140 mg/100 ml or more were much more common (24%) in subjects with strong family history of diabetes than in controls (3%). Moreover, rates of development of diabetes (26%) and "probable diabetes" (9%) were much higher during a follow-up period of seven years in the group with "positive" cortisone tests than in those with "negative" cortisone tests (only 3% developed "diabetes", none developed "probable diabetes"). For these reasons a provisional criterion provided that tests would be regarded as positive if the two-hour glucose level was 140 mg/100 ml or greater (venous whole blood). The most encouraging finding of Fajans and Conn was that *differences* between blood glucose values after cortisone and glucose, as compared to those after glucose alone, were greater in persons with a family

115

history of diabetes than in controls. Not unjustifiably, these investigators concluded that this priming with cortisone might increase the sensitivity of the glucose tolerance test.

The very considerable amount of negative evidence that has subsequently accumulated suggest a need to reexamine the circumstances of the original studies of Fajans and Conn. Indeed this was done by Fajans and Conn themselves (1961) with a conclusion that their test should be regarded only as a research procedure requiring further investigation. Thus, the widespread misuse of this and related tests as diagnostic instruments is not based on advocacy of its creators.

In interpreting the results of Fajans and Conn the following considerations apply. This was intended as a preliminary report containing promising, but not definitive results. The control group was small (37) and somewhat younger than the group with a family history of diabetes. Subsequently, it was found that response to steroids is influenced by age (West, 1960; Sanders, 1961; Pozefsky, et al, 1965). The groups with and without family history of diabetes were not from the same universe and may have differed in other significant respects also. All subjects in both groups had clearly normal glucose tolerance, but tolerance was slightly better in the control group. So far as can be ascertained, the frequency and number of follow-up tests were not systematically matched in the two groups in these exploratory studies of Fajans and Conn. It is now much more evident than before that the frequency with which abnormalities of glucose tolerance tests are demonstrated is strongly related to the number of times tests are repeated (Kahn, et al, 1969). For example, subjects who have three follow-up tests during a given interval are more likely to exhibit abnormal tolerance than those who have two follow-up tests during the same period. Older subjects with a strong family history of diabetes are usually tested more frequently for diabetes than younger subjects with no family history. Since ages of those with a family history of diabetes were greater than those of the "controls", the rate of new diabetes would be expected to be lower in the "controls". This is because incidence of diabetes rises very rapidly with age in the age range of these subjects. In a group studied by Hayward and Lucena (1965), incidence of diabetes in the fifth decade (age 40–49) was more than twice that in the fourth decade (age 30–39). Data of Falconer, et al (1971) in Edinburgh showed that at age 55, incidence of diabetes was about four times greater than at age 35.

Fajans and Conn also demonstrated positive cortisone tests in obese subjects in whom previously abnormal glucose tolerance had been reversed by weight loss. It was not indicated whether any of these subjects had achieved an ideal weight. Data of German (1958) and Kahn, et al (1969) suggest the possibility that this positivity to the steroid test after weight reduction may have been partially or entirely secondary to factors other than hyperresponse to cortisone. These possibilities include ages greater than controls, high-normal glucose tolerance levels, and intraindividual variability of tests. Rates of positivity were decidedly age-related (Conn and Fajans, 1961). This and other evidence led

Conn and Fajans (1961) to conclude that the cortisone test was not a specific marker for genetic diabetes. Rather, certain of their data were consistent with the possibility that steroid tests might reveal diabetes at an earlier time, perhaps by a decade. This seemed to be a reasonable hypothesis, but acceptance of this possibility creates other problems in interpreting their data and that of others. Twenty-six percent of those with normal glucose tolerance and a family history of diabetes had abnormal cortisone tests, and another 19% had abnormal tolerance with glucose alone (Conn and Fajans, 1961). An additional percentage of those with a strong family history of diabetes have clinical diabetes. Thus, the total percentage who had positive cortisone tests was more than 45%. If, after each new decade, an additional increment of positive tests is expected, the percentage expected to develop positive tests would approach 100% in a very few decades. Actual risk of diabetes over a lifetime in those with a family history of this degree is very roughly 20%, a figure that cannot be reconciled with these latter extrapolations. There are several alternative explanations for the very high rate of positives on follow-up testing. One is that the cortisone identifies virtually all with a genetic diathesis for diabetes. But this possibility has been excluded, as Conn and Fajans (1961) subsequently observed. A remaining alternative is that the specificity of the test is very poor. Another possibility is that a portion of those judged to be diabetic on this basis of follow-up glucose tolerance tests may not be diabetic. The number with fasting hyperglycemia was not given. Conn and Fajans (1961) indicated that some of these difficulties might relate only to the criteria of interpretation employed in judging results of the cortisone tests. The criterion now so widely employed was offered only provisionally by these investigators (Conn and Fajans, 1961). They also pointed out that the dosage regimens of cortisone were proposed only on a trial basis. Despite these modest claims and the problems cited above, the cortisone glucose tolerance has been widely accepted as a standard test for identifying diabetes at an early stage and as the most sensitive test for diabetes.

The rate of positivity with the cortisone test to be expected in persons over 40 could not be discerned from the data of Fajans and Conn (37 controls, average age 28). In their follow-up report Conn and Fajans (1961) mention a larger group of 105 controls. Their mean age was 27 years. Present data are not sufficient to establish with precision the frequency distribution of responses to the Fajans-Conn test in subjects over 40 years of age. Many who subsequently reported results with steroid tests did not follow the protocol of Fajans and Conn closely enough to permit conclusions applicable to the test of Fajans and Conn. Data of Pozefsky et al (1965) suggest that "positive" cortisone-modified tests can be expected in about one third of middle-aged subjects and about half of elderly subjects in populations with characteristics similar to those of Americans. Even in subjects with normal glucose tolerance, positive steroid tests are extremely frequent in subjects over 45 (Pozefsky, et al, 1965).

Many others subsequently confirmed certain of the observations of Fajans and Conn. For example, it has been found repeatedly that persons with a strong family history of diabetes are more likely to have positive steroid-modified tests than those with no such history. But only in a few studies was the effect of the steroid examined independently of the effect of glucose to evaluate whether sensitivity to the steroid was a significant determinant of these differences (eg, Goto, et al, 1960; Medley, 1965). Well-controlled studies, including both those with negative and those with positive results, have been rare. In general, groups with and without family history of diabetes were not well matched for other characteristics. In studying a small group whose parents were both diabetic, I found greater responses to certain steroid-modified tests than in groups with no family history of diabetes (West, 1957). Subsequent reexamination of these data revealed that for the most part this was attributable to the greater number of high-normal values when glucose alone was administered in these "prediabetics".

Several other studies yielded negative results. Some of these workers used the methods of Fajans and Conn and some employed other kinds of steroid-modified tests. German (1958) and West (1960) showed that the apparent response to cortisone (difference between the two-hour value when both glucose and cortisone are administered and the two-hour value after glucose alone) was highly variable from day to day in the same subject. In 44 subjects with no family history of diabetes, these responses ranged from -23 to $+121$ (West, 1960). The reproducibility of the cortisone-modified test leaves much to be desired. The range of intraindividual differences in 44 subjects tested in duplicate was 1 to 50 mg/100 ml with an average day-to-day variation of 18 mg/100 ml (West, 1960). Most of this variability is probably attributable to the well-known variation in response to the oral glucose element of the test, but these results indicate the difficulty in using this means for identifying interindividual differences in response to cortisone.

German (1958) also found that responses to cortisone were no greater in his obese subjects than in his lean subjects. Because risk of diabetes is substantially higher in those with two diabetic parents than in the group studied by Fajans and Conn, I examined responses to cortisone and other steroids in this group (West, 1960). In 26 such subjects with normal glucose tolerance, responses to cortisone were not significantly different than those of a control group of 44. Mean age was 37 in the "prediabetics" and 32 in the controls. Our control group was well matched for adiposity with the "prediabetic" group, but exhibited one of the same shortcomings of the Fajans-Conn controls. In neither study were controls drawn from the same element of the population as the "prediabetics". This may not be critical if age, adiposity, and glucose tolerance are matched, but probably a better control group would be a group such as the spouses or friends of the "prediabetics".

Positive steroid-glucose tolerance tests were, indeed, much more common in our "prediabetics" than in controls, but it could not be demonstrated that any of these differences were attributable to cortisone priming itself. In 26 other subjects with slight impairment of glucose tolerance, responses to cortisone did not exceed those of a control group. No evidence of bimodality was observed in this or any other study with respect to response to cortisone or other steroids (West, 1960; Klimt, 1961).

In contrast to these negative results, Goto, et al (1960) observed greater responses to prednisone in subjects with poorer glucose tolerance, but their subgroups differed substantially in other characteristics such as age, origin, and adiposity. The numbers in the subgroups of Goto, et al were quite small (eg, 10 normals). Although far from decisive these data were consistent with the possibility that certain elements of the population with borderline tolerance may in some circumstances be more sensitive to steroids than age-matched subjects with better glucose tolerance. This author found that healthy young men adjusted well to steroid therapy after a few days of mild hyperglycemia. After a week, glucose tolerance was normal (West, 1960). In contrast, the older subjects (patients) of Bastenie, et al (1954) did not tolerate the hyperglycemic effects of these dosage regimens as well. Engel had observed the same contrast. This was reported by Engel in the discussion of the initial report of Fajans and Conn (1954). Among the possibilities for these differences are the better glucose tolerance of younger healthy subjects. But when age groups were matched we found no difference in response to the Fajans-Conn dosages of cortisone in those with normal and those with slightly impaired tolerance. This issue should be evaluated further with greater numbers in subgroups drawn from a single population. This question is not as important, however, as whether prediabetics with clearly normal tolerance have increased responses to steroids.

Medley (1965) found that a small group of 19 nonobese mothers of large babies (10 with a family history of diabetes) had responses to prednisone much greater than those of a control group. When intravenous tolerance was measured with and without prednisone, 17 of the 19 "prediabetics" had a greater decrease in tolerance than any observed in a "control" group of 30. Responses in obese subjects without a family history of diabetes were only slightly greater than controls. These subgroups were not drawn from the same population, so differences might be attributable to factors other than prediabetes status. It seems very unlikely that the rate of subsequent diabetes in these lean mothers will approach the very high rate of positivity to the steroid test (17 of 19). Another consideration is that recent studies, described in Chapter 9, suggest that a history of large babies is not an independent marker of prediabetes. Rather, the association is entirely or almost entirely secondary to the occult hyperglycemia and/or obesity that are so frequently present in mothers of large babies (Pehrson, 1974). The "prediabetic" subjects of Medley were neither obese nor hyperglycemic. Ten of 19 did have a family history of diabetes. Medley correctly observed that the lesser intraindividual variations of intravenous tests would be an advantage in estimating the hyperglycemic effects of a steroid. This had been suggested originally by Duncan (1956). One possible interpretation of Medley's results are that his test identified persons with a genetic diathesis for diabetes. But Goto, et al (1960) found responses to prednisone were slightly greater in patients with pancreatic disease than in subjects

119

with a family history of diabetes. Moreover, the considerations discussed above and below appear to exclude the possibility that responses to such brief steroid challenges are genetic markers for diabetes. This view is shared by Conn and Fajans (1961).

When Nilsson (1962) tested relatives of young diabetics and controls he found a significant effect of prednisone on intravenous tolerance in both groups, but no difference was observed in the effects of prednisone or hydro-cortisone in those with and without diabetic heredity.

Lambert, et al (1961) found positive tests common in his control group in whom an oral cortisone-glucose test was evaluated. They observed little difference between responses of those with and without a family history of diabetes. Kahn, et al (1969) studied 155 subjects with two diabetic parents. This evidence in a very large group was very damaging to any remaining hope that the cortisone test might have practical utility. It was found, for example, that the oral glucose tolerance test was positive in 33%, while the cortisone-glucose test was positive in only 13%. No evidence of hyperresponse to cortisone itself was observed in these subjects. The steroid-modified test was less capable of distinguishing the control group from the prediabetic group than the standard oral glucose tolerance test. The evidence presented suggested that the slightly higher rates of response to the cortisone-glucose test in prediabetics as compared to controls was probably related to their higher responses to glucose and their greater fatness.

Jackson, et al (1972) evaluated a triamcinolone test using dosages of 8 mg. This dosage has a hyperglycemic potency comparable to that of the 50-mg dosages of cortisone employed by Fajans and Conn. Offspring of two diabetic parents had positive tests more frequently than controls, but no evidence was found that the test was more sensitive or discriminating than a standard glucose tolerance test. Upon reviewing these and other results of their own and those of other investigators, they concluded that the triamcinolone test was of no value, and that the utility of other steroid tests was not established. Montgomery, et al (1970) studied cortisone-glucose tolerance in pregnancy. They found no evidence that it was a more sensitive method than conventional tests for diabetes.

A review of certain theoretical considerations provides ground for further pessimism about the potentialities of such tests. Results of oral steroid-modified tests are not distributed bimodally. Intraindividual variation of response is great. Even if there was a difference in sensitivity to cortisone between true prediabetic and normals, beginning a decade prior to the development of abnormal glucose tolerance, it would be difficult to identify this by the Fajans-Conn test. The incidence of diabetes in adults with a family history of diabetes is only about 2% per decade. For these reasons the frequency distribution of values at any given time would be expected to be very similar in those with and without a family history of diabetes (parent, sibling, or child with diabetes). Separation would be somewhat greater in those with two diabetic parents because of the higher incidence of diabetes. But separation would only be substantial if the test were a specific marker for the development of diabetes at least two or three decades in the future. Data of Kahn, et al (1969) and of West (1960) indicate that this is not the case.

The intravenous tests may deserve more study. Direct evidence on their utility is scant. The evidence of Duncan (1956) and Medley (1965) was encouraging but not conclusive for reasons cited above. In North America and Europe about 80% of diabetics are, or have been, obese. Several studies have shown that obese subjects more frequently have positive tests than nonobese subjects, but no evidence is available to show that obese subjects are more responsive to the steroid itself (after control for level of glucose tolerance and age). In the study addressed most directly to this issue (German, 1958), results were negative.

Taton, et al (1964) performed the Fajans-Conn test in 38 "prediabetics" (offspring of two diabetic parents or identical twins of diabetics). There were 10 abnormal responses, but other clinical diagnostic tests were positive in six. There were four with positive cortisone tests in whom results of other tests were normal, but there were three others with normal cortisone tests and abnormal oral glucose tolerance tests. There was no evidence that one test was more sensitive than the other. Kaplan (1961) also cited four cases in which oral glucose tolerance was abnormal and the cortisone test normal.

Twenty-five years have elapsed since steroid tests were introduced. The initial reports were in some respects promising, but subsequent experience has been quite disappointing. As pointed out by Conn and Fajans (1961) it is possible that other strategies of this kind might prove useful even if the pioneering methods proved to be unsatisfactory. These newer regimens should be tried in circumstances more conducive to definitive results than those prevailing in the studies of the previous quarter century. Elements of such strategies include testing of groups at very high risk (eg, both parents diabetic), whose characteristics really match those of controls. Preferably this should be achieved by drawing the control and test groups from the same elements of the population with matching for age, adiposity, and baseline glucose tolerance.

Although some favor further evaluation of the present types of steroid tests, this author does not because the negative evidence appears so impressive. One of several possibilities for revision of technique would be to test the fasting blood glucose after a greater dosage or a regimen of longer duration. Therapy of longer than one or two days would probably be impractical and perhaps inadvisable. One of the advantages of using the fasting blood glucose is its great stability and reproducibility. Single doses of glucocorticoids in the usual pharmacologic range regularly elevate the fasting blood glucose. Degree of response is well related to dosage (West, 1959). Perhaps other steroid-challenge tests will be more effective instruments, but present evidence does not provide a basis for optimism.

The main point of this discussion is to show that the wide acceptance of the steroid-modified tests as an especially sensitive instrument for detecting early diabetes is not justified, either by the available evidence or by the conclusions of those who introduced these procedures. Pyke (1968) observed that cortisone-augmented tests, " . . . are no more likely than other tests to differentiate reliability between diabetes and abnormality". Malins (1968) suggests that the cortisone test, " . . . has no place in the general clinical practice of medicine". Most authorities, however, have endorsed these tests as "research tools". But after a quarter century of rather unproductive application in investigative studies one may also doubt the continuing utility of these tests in research, at least in their present form. Another purpose of this discussion is to raise this latter issue. Certainly those who subsequently use these tests as clinical, epidemiologic, or research instruments should be more aware of the large body of evidence suggesting they are probably worthless.

Tolbutamide-Response Tests

The tolbutamide-response test has been proposed as a diagnostic test for diabetes (Unger and Madison, 1958). This test does offer some practical and theoretical advantages. In normal subjects sulfonylureas induce prompt release of insulin from beta cells. The amount released is, in general, proportional to the functional capacity of these cells. Severe diabetics do not respond at all; in mild diabetics there is a response, but this is usually less than in normals. Tolbutamide is an especially suitable sulfonylurea for this purpose because of its short biologic half-life and its low toxicity. This test is probably less affected by factors unrelated to beta-cell integrity than are glucose tolerance tests. As ordinarily performed it is quite simple and convenient, requiring only twenty to thirty minutes. Results are reproducible (Kaplan, 1961), although present data do not establish precisely the degree of intraindividual variation. Conn and Fajans, on the basis of a small number of observations, concluded that change of status from positive to negative, or the reverse, was not uncommon. Some other disadvantages will be described below.

The test described by Unger and Madison (1958) provides for the intravenous administration of 1 gm of tolbutamide over a two-minute period. After an overnight fast a sample of venous blood is first drawn for determination of a baseline blood glucose value. The test is timed from the midpoint of the injection. Additional specimens are drawn at twenty and thirty minutes to measure the decline in blood glucose induced by tolbutamide. A sugar-containing drink such as orange juice is provided immediately following the last sample to prevent symptoms of hypoglycemia. Breakfast should follow promptly.

Results are classified according to the extent of decline of the blood glucose. According to Unger and Madison (1964) normal subjects regularly exhibit blood glucose levels at twenty minutes that are less than 76% of their baseline values, while diabetics usually have twenty-minute values that are greater than 84% of their fasting levels. Persons whose thirty-minute values have not declined below 76% are considered diabetic. Kaplan (1961) has presented additional data, making possible better understanding of the normal range of responses with this test, including the effects of age, liver disease, pregnancy, and other factors.

Discriminating powers of this test probably could be improved slightly by relating dosage to the volume of distribution of tolbutamide. This would further standardize the concentration of tolbutamide "seen" by the beta cells. Mainly because of binding of tolbutamide to albumin (Johnson, et al, 1960), this space is not easy to compute with precision, but Johnson, et al have found that it is fairly well related to weight. We have, therefore, used tests in which challenge dosage was related to weight (eg, 15 mg/kg). Dosage with this latter formula corresponds closely with the standard 1-gm dosage, except in subjects who are quite large or small.

The disadvantages of this test are several. Deprivation of carbohydrate, and probably of calories, may produce false-positive results. Idiosyncrasy or allergy to the drug is very rare but not unknown. Hypoglycemia is usually mild and trivial, but occasionally more substantial and of longer duration. Small laboratory errors may have a decisive effect because the changes being measured are small. For this reason Unger and Madison recommend duplicate laboratory determinations. The base of data for establishing diagnostic criteria is much smaller than for glucose tolerance tests. The effects of factors such as age, race, body composition, physical activity, and diet have not been studied extensively. The best data available are those of Kaplan (1961).

It has been claimed that results of this test are more specific than with oral glucose tolerance tests. This is so if certain traditional criteria are used for interpreting oral glucose tolerance tests. This hypersensitivity of oral glucose tests is, however, probably mainly attributable to the inappropriate manner in which these standards were arrived at. Very few data are available using appropriate indexes for comparing tolbutamide tests to other tests. On the basis of their data, Conn and Fajans (1961) thought that oral glucose tolerance tests were better than tolbutamide tests for distinguishing between those with and without early diabetes. But when comparing the sensitivity and specificity of these tests in identifying diabetes, they apparently used impairment of oral glucose tolerance as one of the indexes of "diabetes". Kaplan measured cortisone-glucose responses in persons with a family history of diabetes and normal oral glucose tolerance tests. He found that 12 (28%) had positive cortisone-modified tests. All 12 had normal tolbutamide tests.

Kaplan showed that correspondence between results with tolbutamide tests and those with oral glucose tests was strongly related to degree of intolerance. In persons with slight impairment of glucose tolerance, tolbutamide tests were usually normal. These data and those of Conn and Fajans (1961) comparing the two tests could mean either that the tolbutamide test is less sensitive, that the glucose tolerance test is highly unspecific when older traditional criteria are used, or both. For reasons discussed elsewhere in this chapter, a major reason for this lack of correspondence may be that the conventional criteria for interpreting oral tests are faulty. Correspondence of results of glucose tolerance tests and tolbutamide tests was good in subjects of Kaplan with two-hour blood glucose values greater than 170 mg/100 ml. On the other hand, Conn and Fajans found normal tolbutamide responses in four of 14 subjects who had fasting values less than 110 and two-hour levels after oral glucose greater than 180 mg/100 ml. Kahn, et al (1969) tested a group, each of whom had two diabetic parents, using both of these tests. Divergence between responses of the normals and the "prediabetes" group was somewhat greater with the oral glucose test, but incomplete matching of methods and subjects made these data difficult to interpret in some respects. Not all those tested for oral glucose tolerance were tested with tolbutamide. Rates of positive tolbutamide tests were zero in 30 lean "prediabetics" less than 41 years of age, 24% (3 of 17) in older lean subjects, 78% (7 of 9) in obese subjects of all ages, and 20% for the entire group (11 of 56). Rates of positivity with oral glucose tolerance tests were 25% (38 of 152) in lean young "prediabetics", 37% (25 of 67) in older (above 40) subjects, 48% (29 of 61) in obese of all ages, and 32% (92 of 280) in the total group of "prediabetics".

Results of Kaplan suggested the possibility that the responses to tolbutamide may be affected somewhat less by age and by liver disease than is glucose tolerance. On the other hand, tolbutamide response is strongly affected by pregnancy (Kaplan, 1961). Response declines progressively during the course of pregnancy. About half of women have abnormal tests in the ninth month. Reactivity returns promptly to normal after delivery. In a small group of obese patients Kaplan found positive responses to oral glucose tolerance tests commonly, while results of intravenous glucose tolerance tests and tolbutamide tests were usually normal in these same subjects. But on the whole, obese subjects were less responsive to tolbutamide than lean normals.

There apparently are no prospective studies in progress designed to compare the sensitivity and specificity of the intravenous tolbutamide test with the glucose tolerance test (oral or intravenous).

The ordinary therapeutic tablets of tolbutamide are absorbed very gradually, but the sodium salt of tolbutamide is absorbed quite rapidly (West and Johnson, 1960). This makes possible the testing of response to oral tolbutamide as an index of beta-cell capacity. This method has been described by Boshell, et al (1963) and by Vechio (1964). In general, results correspond well with those obtained when other diagnostic methods are employed. Despite the rapid absorption of tolbutamide it does not seem likely that this test will prove generally useful. The main problem is that in normal subjects counterregulatory responses are rapidly induced when hypoglycemia occurs. When response of the blood glucose at thirty minutes is suboptimal, it is difficult to exclude the possibility that this is attributable to slow absorption of the drug. At one hour, lack of hypoglycemia may be due to a counterregulatory response to earlier hypoglycemia. These problems can be greatly mitigated by frequent sampling to insure that a nadir will not be missed. But this makes the test more complex.

OTHER TESTS

Other agents used to measure beta-cell response include glucagon. Castells, et al (1976) employed a "maximum" challenge that included a combination of glucagon, glucose, and tolbutamide. A modest amount of data exists concerning the normal range of beta-cell response to other nutrients such as amino acids, yet these data are not yet adequate to develop and evaluate standardized tests as diagnostic instruments for diabetes.

It has been repeatedly claimed that qualitative or quantitative peculiarities of insulin secretion in response to glucose are helpful in separating normals from prediabetics or from "diabetics" with normal fasting blood glucose values. None of these views has gained general acceptance. Some of these claims deserve further investigation, but at present measurements of insulin response to glucose are not accepted as diagnostic instruments in persons with normal fasting blood glucose levels. Kosaka et al (1977) reported that in persons with impairment of glucose tolerance those with delayed early insulin responses were especially likely to develop unequivocal diabetes subsequently. Savage, et al (1975) found insulin-secretion patterns normal in a group who later developed maturity-onset diabetes. Glucagon levels are usually elevated in established diabetes, but they are probably normal in very early diabetes and prediabetes.

Summary on Diagnostic Methods

There is much uncertainty and disagreement concerning diagnostic criteria. It is appropriate, therefore, to point out that there is agreement concerning several aspects of the diagnostic process. Persons who have fasting venous plasma glucose concentrations that persistently exceed 130 mg/100 ml are diabetic. Adults with normal gastrointestinal function may be considered to be free of diabetes if, with oral glucose loads of 50 gm or greater, the one-hour venous plasma glucose value is below 180 mg/100 ml and the two-hour value below 140. There is much evidence to suggest that values considerably higher than this may also be normal, particularly in older subjects, but evidence is still inadequate to determine precisely either diagnostic criteria or degree of risk of diabetes by level of response.

Interpretation of oral glucose tolerance tests should take into account that results are not highly reproducible. Intraindividual variations in the one-hour and two-hour values as great as 40 mg/100 ml are not rare, and variations greater than 20 mg/100 ml are quite common. In many affluent populations about one quarter of middle-aged subjects and about half of the elderly have "abnormal" glucose tolerance by older traditional standards. There has been a general trend in recent years to broaden the ranges of values considered normal or borderline. Indeed, it is not yet established that glucose tolerance tests are capable of identifying persons at risk of developing diabetes with acceptable specificity when fasting glucose values are clearly normal.

Many different diagnostic methods have been introduced as possible alternatives for the standard oral glucose tolerance tests. These include tolbutamide-response tests, intravenous glucose tolerance tests, and steroid-modified glucose tolerance tests. None of these alternatives has gained general acceptance as a prime instrument of diagnosis.

125

Glucose tolerance tests are not necessary or desirable as diagnostic instruments when fasting hyperglycemia is present. When oral glucose tolerance tests are performed, blood glucose levels are usually measured at one hour or at two hours, or both. Some authorities recommend additional determinations (eg, at ninety minutes, at three hours, or both).

Standardization of method has not been achieved in the performance of oral glucose tolerance tests, and no immediate prospect is in sight for uniformity of practice or interpretation. The variables to be taken into account in interpreting or comparing data include the size of the load, its relationship to the characteristics of the subjects tested (eg, weight, surface area, extracellular fluid volume), sources of blood (eg, capillary, venous), element of blood analyzed (plasma, serum, or whole blood), time of day, duration of fasting, intervals and time of sampling, technique of measuring concentration of glucose, and methods of expressing the results (eg, area under a curve, summed values). Although not ideal, there are now some data that make possible comparisons of data when different methods have been used. For example, plasma glucose values appear to be in most circumstances about 15% (not mg %) higher than whole blood levels. At one hour, capillary values are usually 20 to 40 mg/100 ml higher than venous values, while at two hours these differences usually range from 0 to 20 mg/100 ml. Degree of hyperglycemia is usually greater when oral glucose tolerance tests are performed in the afternoon, and less when performed from one to four hours after a meal. When small glucose loads are administered (eg, 50 gm), two-hour values are substantially lower than when large loads (eg, 100 gm) are administered. Differences in one-hour values tend to be less but are also significant. The degree of these differences varies with factors such as the level of glucose tolerance, but in some circumstances mean glucose levels at two hours may be as much as 30 mg/100 ml higher with large loads. Data of Cooper (1973) provide a fairly satisfactory basis for comparing results from several of the different methods for measuring glucose concentration. In general these latter differences are quite small.

There is no direct evidence that response to oral glucose is any more sensitive and specific as a diagnostic instrument than response to a typical meal of mixed nutrients. But the body of data available for evaluating the glucose tolerance test is far greater. Because of the unpalatability of glucose and its propensity to produce unpleasant gastrointestinal symptoms, there is a trend toward the employment and evaluation of other nutrients. These include sugars that challenge beta-cell function while producing a lesser osmotic effect in the small intestine.

There is an urgent need to evaluate further the sensitivity and specificity of glucose tolerance tests and other diagnostic procedures in persons with normal fasting values, and to relate such results to variables such as age and adiposity.

5
CHAPTER

Prevalence and Incidence

METHODS

Methods for ascertainment and counting of known cases and for diagnosis have been discussed above in the chapters on epidemiologic methods (3) and on screening and diagnosis (4). The sensitivity and specificity of some of these methods will be discussed further below in the section on prevalence in the United States and its subpopulations. These methods of estimating prevalence include examinations of medical records, estimating total drug consumption, and interviewing or testing of population samples. Another method is to count cases to whom antidiabetic drugs or diets are dispensed (Lancaster, 1951; Harris, 1971). Occasionally, counts of cases have been made in the practices of a sample of physicians (Adelstein, 1975; Dunstone, 1976).

In many populations, rates of diabetes have been underestimated considerably. Reasons for this include difficulties in identifying all known cases, and use of insensitive testing methods. A common mistake has been to assume that negative screenees do not have diabetes. Several factors, other than actual prevalence, profoundly affect apparent or stated rates. Except possibly in the elderly, overdiagnosis has not been perceived as a major problem. But in some populations it has been estimated that as many as 10% of diagnosed diabetics do not have the disease (Silwer, 1958). Because of the increasing numbers of glucose tolerance tests, overdiagnosis is becoming a significant problem. In the past the main difficulty in estimating prevalence has been underascertainment, the degree of which is typically unknown. Based on his experience in Mecklenberg, East Germany, Schliak (cited by Silwer, 1958) estimated that the ratio of undiagnosed to diagnosed cases was about 5 to 1. Rates of "abnormal" glucose tolerance in adults of Bedford, England were about 20 times as high as rates of diagnosed diabetes (Jarrett and Keen, 1975).

One crude index of prevalence is diabetes mortality rate. This relationship is discussed in detail in Chapter 6 on mortality.

In a few populations, rates of diabetes have been estimated using sensitive methods. These results will be summarized in a separate section below. Since the sensitivity and specificity of the *same* screening tests are highly variable among different populations (West and Kalbfleisch, 1971a), reliable interpopulation comparisons of prevalence are not possible on the basis of screening data even when methods are standardized, unless diagnostic tests are performed on representative samples of negative screenees. Even when prevalence rates are based on glucose-loading tests performed on all subjects, there may be problems in making interpopulation comparisons. Among the factors incompletely standardized have been the sizes of glucose loads, criteria of diagnosis, laboratory methods for measuring blood glucose, time of day of tests, status of feeding and fasting, type of specimen (capillary or venous blood, plasma, or whole blood), age distribution of subjects, inclusion or exclusion of known diabetics, and methods of ascertainment of known diabetes. When complete data have been presented concerning these variables, fairly reliable extrapolations have usually been possible, but direct and precise comparisons have rarely been possible. Our studies (West and Kalbfleisch, 1966–1971) in ten countries were highly standardized, but even these were not ideal. For example, sampling was only crudely representative, and sample sizes were quite small (only about 500 subjects per country).

Agreement on diagnostic criteria is not a requisite for making comparisons of disease rates among populations and subpopulations. If data are presented by frequency distribution, comparisons can be made using any diagnostic criterion of glucose level. Fairly satisfactory data are available for matching of results obtained by different standard laboratory methods for measuring blood glucose (Cooper, 1973). The other methodologic differences pose more formidable problems. In the United States the most popular dosage of oral glucose has been 100 gm. Recently loads of 75 gm have also been widely used. The National Health Survey (Gordon, 1964) used 50 gm. A dosage of 1.75 gm/kg of ideal weight has been used frequently in clinical studies. In Britain 50 gm has been standard. In Scandinavia 1 gm/kg has been widely employed. The University Group Diabetes Program used 30 gm/sq m of body surface; and 40 gm/sq m was recommended by an Expert Committee of the American Diabetes Association (1969). In our international studies we expected to encounter very wide variations of body size. We therefore selected a simple method for relating dosage crudely to extracellular space (1 gm/kg of body weight). In Chapter 4 on diagnostic methods the differences in response with varying dosages of glucose are described. Comparisons are possible even when populations have been tested with different dosages of glucose, but the required extrapolations are imprecise.

As indicated in Chapter 4 on diagnostic methods, there is no decisive evidence on whether the smaller or larger glucose loads are best. In the field, it is often difficult to prepare and administer dosages related to the specific characteristics of each subject. In these circumstances a fixed dosage has advantages, but not infrequently subjects are encountered whose sizes vary as much as twofold. In East Pakistan, for example, the average weight of our women was 76 lb (34.5 kg); in Plains Indian women, 162 lb (73.5 kg). One possible compromise would be a standard dosage of 75 gm, with an alteration to 50 gm in those weighing less than 50 kg and to 100 gm in those weighing more than 100 kg. An expert committee of the Pan American Health Organization has described the advantages of the standard 75-gm dosage (PAHO, 1975). A load of 75 gm is being used in the NIH studies of Pimas. It was used also in Cleveland by Kent and Leonards (1967). We are now using this dosage in our studies of Oklahoma Indians (West, et al, 1974,1976).

Surprisingly few data exist on the fasting blood glucose values of populations. One problem here is that results are considerably distorted if even a very small percentage of those purporting to be in the fasting state have actually eaten. One way to control for this would be to repeat all positive tests or a representative sample thereof. As indicated in Chapter 4, a good argument can be made for use of fasting hyperglycemia as the index of the frequency of diabetes. Data of Dippe, et al (1974) show, for example, that subjects with two-hour values sufficiently high to be at substantial risk of developing clinical stigmata of diabetes usually have a concomitant elevation of the fasting blood glucose. Observations of Jarrett and Keen (1976) also lend support to the notion that rates of clinically significant diabetes are probably best reflected by the prevalence of fasting hyperglycemia. The prevalence of fasting hyperglycemia is not known for any country!

Studies of the type performed by O'Sullivan and Mahan in Sudbury, Massachusetts (1968) have the potential for determining the level of fasting blood glucose that is diagnostic of diabetes. But as yet data are not adequate to make this determination. One difficulty here is that a very large number of subjects is required in order to yield a cohort of adequate size with borderline values. It would be desirable to study prospectively at least 500 adults with fasting plasma glucose values in the borderline range (100 to 130 mg/100 ml), and to compare subsequent fasting values for at least a few years to those of individuals whose initial fasting levels were in the clearly normal range. In order to derive a borderline group of this size, a universe of about 10,000 would be necessary. Assuming that 500 (5%) of the 10,000 would develop unequivocal fasting hyperglycemia in a period of thirty years, the number of new cases per year would be small (about 17 per year or 166 per decade) in the total group. Even if it were possible to follow a 10% sample (1,000) of this group, only about

17 new cases per decade would be expected. Rates of decompensation would probably be higher in the subgroup of 500 with borderline values, but even if they were excessive by a factor of four, only about four new cases would be expected annually in this subgroup. If prospective "short-term" (five to ten years) studies of this type are to yield meaningful results, the initial study group will have to be quite large. The same may be said of prospective studies of the predictive value of varying degrees of glucose intolerance.

Estimation of Incidence

Falconer, et al (1971) discussed in some detail the several problems involved in determining incidence. Incidence may be very crudely estimated by examining data on prevalence and purported duration of diabetes. Such estimates must be corrected for the effect of mortality, which is higher in diabetics than in the general population. Anderson (1966) has performed calculations designed to estimate crudely the average duration of diabetes before its discovery (roughly a decade). This interval would of course be influenced by many variables, including age distribution, frequency of testing in the population, diagnostic criteria, and fatness of the population. Even when data are available on the number of new cases reported in a given year, there are usually problems in converting this to a figure for annual incidence. Reporting is seldom complete. In many populations intensity of screening varies from year to year. Not only will apparent incidence rise during years of mass screening projects, rates in immediately subsequent years may fall as a result of the previous identification of a substantial portion of those with occult diabetes. Interpopulation comparisons of incidence have seldom been possible because of lack of standardization and the paucity of data.

The incidence of childhood diabetes has been measured in a few populations (eg, by the Registry for Britain and Ireland). These findings are reviewed in the section on juvenile diabetes. A rare study of incidence is being performed in the Pima population. Incidence of diabetes and its stigmata are being related to factors such as fatness and status of glucose tolerance (Hamman and Miller, 1975; Bennett, et al, 1976a). Results of these studies are reviewed elsewhere in this book, including the section on incidence below.

PREVALENCE AS MEASURED BY LESS SENSITIVE METHODS

These less sensitive methods are not necessarily to be deprecated. In fact, the prevalence of moderate or gross hyperglycemia is in some respects a better index of the importance of the disease than a rate that includes those who have slight or equivocal hyperglycemia by conventional standards. On the other hand, lack of standardization also makes it difficult to compare estimates of prevalence of moderate and severe hyperglycemia. Rates of known cases are often related more to methods of ascertainment and the frequency with which they are applied than to the frequency of the disease. Even so, the interpopulation comparisons of the frequency of known clinical disease are sometimes better indexes for comparison than rates based on mass screening enterprises. This is because of the vast differences in the sensitivity of the various screening strategies and methods.

Measurements of prevalence of fasting hyperglycemia would be of considerable interest, but as indicated above, data are very, very few.

Counts of known cases have been made in many populations and some have been related sytematically to the characteristics of those populations, such as age, sex, and weight. Table 16 provides a list of such surveys and their results. Older studies on prevalence are summarized in the excellent publication of Silwer (1958). Silwer also reported the results of a classic comprehensive study of diabetes prevalence in a whole community (Kristianstad, Sweden). The number of known diabetics identified was 1,326 (0.51% of the total population). Silwer concluded that the actual rate of diagnosed diabetes was a bit higher because his counts were not quite complete. Nevertheless, this is one of the most complete surveys of diagnosed cases yet made. Details were given relating prevalence to age and sex; and distribution of type of treatment was well studied. Some of these details are reviewed in other sections of this volume to which they relate. Silwer's review of the older data on prevalence indicated that the relatively low prevalence rates of the past were often the result of low rates of ascertainment.

Among the best of the community studies on prevalence was that of Grönberg, et al (1967) in Sweden. On the basis of their data they estimated the aggregate risk of developing clinically-identified diabetes up to age 50 as 2.1% for males and 1.9% for females. Aggregate risk at 70 was estimated at 4.7% in males and 9.0% in females; at age 90, 6.5% in males and 13% in females. By a life-table expectancy method they estimated the lifetime risk of developing clinical diabetes at 4.8% for males and 10.3% for females. The approximate rate of diabetes in the 1965 Swedish population was judged to be 2.05%. For age 15 and over the approximate rate was 2.6%.

These rates of known diabetes in Sweden are about three times the rates of known cases reported in Birmingham, England (0.64%) by Malins (1974b); in Edinburgh (0.62%) by Falconer, et al (1971); and in Bergen, Norway (0.7%) by Jorde (1962). Rates in Sweden were slightly higher than rates in Busselton, Australia (Welborn, et al, 1968) and in Sudbury, Massachusetts (O'Sullivan, et al, 1967). The rates of known diabetes in Sweden are about the same as reported by the United States National Health Survey of 1973 (2.0%). Rates in Sweden were very similar to those in Rochester, Minnesota, where the frequency of known cases was 4.3% in males and 3.8% in females in the segment of the population over 40 years of age (Palumbo, et al, 1976). It seems likely that the higher rates in Sweden and the United States reflect a truly greater disease frequency as compared to that in Britain, but it is difficult to exclude the possibility that a substantial part of these differences are apparent only. Among

TABLE 16   Prevalence of Clinically-Diagnosed Diabetes as Estimated in General Populations

RATE IN PERCENT	LOCALITY	DESCRIPTION (AGE GROUP)	INVESTIGATOR AND YEAR OF PUBLICATION
2.0	USA	Representative sample, 1973	National Diabetes Commission, 1976 (Questionnaire survey of Natl. Center for Health Statistics
	Massachusetts		
1.1	Oxford	Adults	Wilkerson and Krall (1947)
1.1	Sudbury	Adults	O'Sullivan, et al (1967)
	Minnesota		
1.6	Rochester	All ages	Palumbo, et al (1976)
4.1	Rochester	Over forty years	Palumbo, et al (1976)
0.8	*Porcupine and Hawksbury, Ontario, Canada*	Over six years	Kenny and Chute (1953)
	England		
0.6	Cornwall	All ages	Andrews (1957)
0.5	Newcastle	Over thirty years	Redhead (1960)
0.8	Ibstock	Over five years	Walker (1959)
0.6	Halstead	All ages	Harkness (1962)
0.6	Birmingham	All ages	College of Practitioners Birmingham Working Party (1963)
	Scotland		
0.6	Edinburgh	All ages	Falconer, et al (1971)
0.5	Forfar	All ages	Stewart and Robertson (1963)
	Germany		
1.3	East Berlin	All ages	Schliack (1969)
0.7	Herrenberg	All ages	Glogner and Durr (1964)
2.0	Munich	All ages	Mehnert, et al (1967)
	Finland		
1.5	Entire country	Over fourteen years	Reunanen, et al (1976)
1.1	Nokia	All ages	Pessi (1964)
0.4	*Denmark*	All ages	Lindhardt (1954)
	Sweden		
2.0	Entire country	All ages	Grönberg, et al (1967)
2.7	Kristianstad	Adults	Nilsson, et al (1964)
1.0	Malmohus Lan	Over 15 years	Brandt, et al (1964)
0.9	Ølekinge	All ages	Munke (1964)
0.7	*Bergen, Norway*	All ages	Jorde (1962)
0.3	*Iceland*	All ages	Albertson, (1953)
1.3	*Valencia, Spain*	All ages, small sample (2,193)	Varo-Uranga, et al (1969)
2.5	*Naples, Italy*	All ages	Licenziati (1968)
1.1	*Zagreb, Yugoslavia*	Over fifteen years	Jaksic and Skrabalo (1969)
1.8	*Czechoslovakia (Bohemia and Moravia)*	All ages	Czechoslovak Group (1975)
2.4	*Malta*	All ages	Maempel (1965)

Rate in Percent	Locality	Description (Age Group)	Investigator and Year of Publication
1.1	*Roumania*	All ages	Mincu, et al (1972)
	Australia		
0.9	Busselton	Adults	Welborn, et al (1968)
1.3	Cunderdin	Adults	Welborn, et al (1968)
0.3	Goulburn	Over nineteen years	Smithurst, et al (1968)
0.6	Toowomba	Over nineteen years	Smithurst, et al (1968)
	New Zealand		
0.6	Entire country	All ages	Beaven, et al (1974)
1.6	Rangiora	Over twenty years	Murray, et al (1969)
	Rhodesia		
0	Blacks, rural	All ages, small sample (999)	Wicks, et al (1973)
0.3	Blacks, urban	All ages, small sample (1,078)	Wicks, et al (1973)
	South Africa		
0.7	Bantus	Over ten years	Marine, et al (1970)
1.8	Indians	Over ten years	Marine, et al (1970)
1.4	Malays	Over fifteen years	Marine, et al (1970)
0.8	Whites	Over sixteen years	Jackson (1970)
1.8	Natal Indians	Over ten years	Goldberg, et al (1970)
0.7	British Guiana, rural (East Indians and blacks)		Weinstein (1962)
	Argentina		
2.9	Rosario	Adults	Cardonnet and Nusimovich (1968)
2.0	Santa Fe	Adults	Cardonnet and Nusimovich (1968)
	Cuba		
0.7	Artemisia	Adults	Mateo DeAcosta, et al (1973)
1.6	Havana	Adults	Mateo DeAcosta, et al (1973)
0.2	Rural Areas	Adults	Mateo DeAcosta, et al (1973)
0.7	*Semerang, Indonesia*	Over thirteen years (11 of 1,571)	Djokomoeljanto (1975)
	Japan		
0.43	Kumamoto	All ages	Mimura (1970)
1.3	Yao, rural	Over thirty-nine years	Sasaki, et al (1964)
1.6	Yao, semiurban	Over thirty-nine years	Sasaki, et al (1964)
	India		
0.8	Chandigarh	All ages	Berry, et al (1966)
0.03	Cuttack	Over nine years (before screening)	Tripathy, et al (1970)
0.09	Rural	Over fifteen years	Gupta, et al (1975)
1.4	Urban	Over fifteen years	Gupta, et al (1975)
1.0	*Jerusalem area*	Over two years	Cohen (1961)
0.2	*Okinawa*		Sakumoto (1970)

TABLE 16   (Continued)

Rate in Percent	Locality	Description (Age Group)	Investigator and Year of Publication
	SOME OTHER PRIMITIVE AND ABORIGINAL POPULATIONS		
	Greenland		
0.03	Eskimos	Over thirteen years	Sagild, et al (1966)
	Alaska		
0.02	Athabascan Indians	All ages	Mouratoff (1969)
0.03	Eskimos	All ages	Mouratoff, et al (1967)
10	Cherokee Indians, North Carolina	All ages	Stein, et al (1965)
14	Seneca Indians, New York	Adults	Frohman, et al (1969)
10	Alabama-Coush-atta Indians, Texas	All ages	Johnson and McNutt (1964)
2.9	Sioux and Assini-boine Indians, Montana	All ages	Petersen (1969)
	Arizona		
5.3	Papago Indians	All ages	Reinhard and Greenwalt (1975)
6	Pima Indians	Over four years	Bennett, et al (1971)
40	Pima Indians	Over thirty years based on glucose tolerance testing	Bennett, et al (1971)
	Oklahoma		
5	Indians (Multitribal)	All ages	West (1974)
10	Indians (Multitribal)	Adults	West (1974)
30	Indians (Multitribal)	Over thirty years based on glucose tolerance testing	West (1976)
8	Urbanized Abo-rigines, Australia	Over twenty years	Wise, et al (1970)
0	Papua, rural	None among 2,182 adults	Hingston and Price (1964)
34	Nauru	Over fourteen years (based on glucose tolerance data)	Zimmet, et al (1976)

Note: Unless specified otherwise, these data do not reflect results of intensive screening with sensitive methods, in which circumstances rates are often much higher. Comparison among these populations should be made with great caution, particularly because of marked variability in the ratios of known to undiagnosed cases. For example, in the study of Tripathy, et al cited above, a screening survey increased the number of known cases by more than tenfold.

countries there are differences in "popularity" of the diagnosis, frequency of testing, diagnostic criteria, sensitivity of testing procedures, and other factors relating to rates of ascertainment.

The Edinburgh study of Falconer, et al (1971) will be discussed further under incidence. In some respects it was a model study. Rate of ascertainment of diagnosed cases was estimated to be in the range of 90% to 95% for the whole community. The characteristics of 2,932 diabetics were studied; prevalence of known diabetes was 0.6%.

Adelstein (1975) reported on results of a British survey of a sample of 100 practices of individual physicians in general practice. In the year 1971–1972, 45 cases were identified per 100,000 patients. The sensitivity of this method is unknown, but the rate of diabetes reported was somewhat less than these in Britain when other methods were used. On the basis of data on the dispensing of antidiabetic drugs, Harris (1971) estimated that about 300,000 diabetics were receiving these drugs in England, Scotland, and Wales. This represented about 0.6% of the population.

Table 16 shows that rates of known diabetes in whole populations (all ages) have ranged from less than 0.1% to more than 4%. In European populations, rates of about 1% are now typical. In most primitive societies, rates are far lower; and in several special circumstances rates are much higher (eg, certain American Indian tribes). Although the age ranges are given for the populations listed in Table 16, the data are not corrected for the considerable differences in age distribution. These latter differences also tend generally to increase the disparity between poor and rich societies in rates of clinical cases. But data presented elsewhere in this book show that these differences are to a considerable extent real. In the primitive Eskimo groups, for example, extreme paucity has been confirmed by surveys employing sensitive methods (Sagild, et al, 1966; Scott and Mouratoff, 1970).

In a cooperative autopsy study of WHO, methods were well standardized and whole populations were studied (Kagan, et al, 1977). Moreover, from 60% to 80% of decedents over 10 years of age were autopsied. Rates of diagnosed diabetes in decedents were determined for each of five populations. Prevalence in Prague was 8.6%, Malmo 8.6%, Yalta 3.3%, Tullin (USSR) 3.4%, and in Ryazan (USSR) 2.1% (Zdanov and Vihert, 1977).

Many of the previous estimates of total prevalence in the various populations as determined by screening surveys, are more misleading than informative. This is mainly because they so frequently assume that rates are zero among negative screenees. Prevalence rates for two different populations may be stated as the same when in fact they differ fourfold. Or they may be stated to differ fourfold when they are in fact quite similar. In its *Source Book on Diabetes* (1969) the United States Public Health Service estimated that 5% of middle-aged Americans had diagnosed diabetes and 2% had undiagnosed diabetes. But another element of the Public Health Service (Gordon, 1964) found that impaired glucose tolerance (by traditional criteria) was present in about 20% of middle-aged Americans. Even as measured by conservative criteria, the actual rate of occult diabetes is at least three times the rate originally estimated in the *Source Book*. The main reason for this huge discrepancy was the unfortunate tradition of assuming that negative screenees had a zero rate of diabetes. In the sections on screening sensitivity and specificity (Chapter 4), some of the other factors are discussed that make it extremely difficult to compare rates of prevalence among populations when these rates

135

have been based on typical screening surveys. This is why no attempt is made here to show by population, in tabular form, rates of total prevalence (rate of diagnosed diabetes plus rate of undiagnosed diabetes). However, figures are given in the text below for several populations in which more precise data are available.

PREVALENCE AND INCIDENCE IN THE UNITED STATES AND ITS SUBPOPULATIONS

Two sources have provided the most useful information on prevalence in the United States population. Both consist of data gathered by the surveys of the National Center for Health Statistics on samples of the entire population. Except that persons in institutions are excluded, the samples are representative. Although neither the interview method nor the examination method has been ideal, these data are better in most respects than those available for other countries. Moreover, these methods are being improved and prospects are good for even more informative results in surveys that are underway (eg, glucose tolerance tests in a representative sample).

Interview Methods

One method used by the National Center for Health Statistics is a questionnaire administered in a group of representative households (Bauer, 1967). The interview data, for 1973, were summarized in the report of the National Diabetes Commission by its work group on epidemiology (Bennett, et al, 1976). In this 1973 survey a representative sample of households was selected. About 200,000 people (including children) residing in the households were the subjects of a questionnaire that included questions on diabetes; 4,190 (2.0%) were reported to have diabetes. The design of these studies is such that the questions are often answered by a member of the household other than the subjects about whom questions are being asked. It seems likely that diabetes rates would be a bit higher if each subject was an interviewee.

Table 17 summarizes these data by age, color, sex, economic status, educational level of head of household, urban-rural status, and geographic region. These differences (eg, by sex, age, income) are discussed in detail in the various sections of this book to which they relate.

By a very similar method the rates of known diabetes were also determined in a survey of 1964–1965 (Bauer, et al, 1967). In those reported to be diabetic, information was obtained on type of treatment. Twenty-five percent were taking "insulin only", 55% were receiving "oral drugs only" and 23% were receiving "no antidiabetic drugs".

The limitations of this method of estimating prevalence are considerable, as discussed above. The data should be interpreted with these reservations in mind.

Prevalence Rates Based on Results of Glucose Loading Tests

Table 18 summarizes data obtained by the National Center for Health Statistics by measuring *whole blood* glucose values on venous blood one hour after an oral glucose load of 50 gm in a representative sample of the US population (Gordon, et al, 1964). The tests were not performed in the fasting state routinely, and some were not performed in the morning. Details concerning circumstances of testing and their effects on results were included in the aforementioned publication. Persons with known diabetes were not included. The Table shows the results by sex and age. In intepreting these results it is important to keep in mind that values would have been about 30 to 50 mg/100 ml greater with measurement of *plasma* values and larger doses of glucose (eg, 100 gm). Thus, one-hour values of 150 with this test are roughly equivalent to one-hour plasma values of 190 with a larger load. In the total group (ages 18 to 79), 7.6% had one-hour whole blood values greater than 149 mg/100 ml and 3.6% had levels exceeding 189. Data discussed elsewhere suggest that roughly 3% of American adults have diabetes that has been discovered. These and other data cited elsewhere in this volume indicate clearly that when traditional standards are employed in interpreting glucose loading tests, rates of occult "diabetes" are much higher than rates of known diabetes.

PREVALENCE STUDIES IN AMERICAN COMMUNITIES

Results in individual American communities of studies employing glucose loading tests confirm the findings in the National Survey. These local studies include surveys in Cleveland (Kent and Leonards, 1968), Dallas (Unger, 1957), California (Searcy and Low, 1967), and in Sudbury, Massachusetts (O'Sullivan, et al, 1967). It is still not clear, however, whether substantial intercommunity differences exist in the United States with respect to rates of diabetes after correction for race and social status. This is because of the lack of standardization of obtaining, interpreting, and expressing results. Modest differences by state in diabetes mortality rates are discussed in the section on mortality. Except for the low mortality rates in Alaska, reflecting mainly the low rates in Eskimos and Indians, these differences are rather small. They may be mainly the result of differences in the ratios of diagnosed to undiagnosed cases. Very little difference was found by region in blood glucose levels by the National Health Survey of 1960–1962 (Gordon, et al, 1964).

In Tecumseh, Michigan, detailed results were given for those with no apparent diabetes on blood glucose values in persons over 15 years of age who received 100 gm of oral glucose within four hours after a meal (Hayner, et al, 1965). These results are summarized in Table 19. In persons to whom glucose loads were administered in the fasting state, values averaged 25 mg/100 ml higher. When traditional standards are applied to the results in Table 19, the proportion with "abnormal tolerance" is about one quarter in middle-age and one half in old age. Glucose tolerance is probably somewhat better in Sudbury

TABLE 17 Prevalence of Diabetes Reported in Health Interviews by Age and Selected Characteristics: United States, 1973

CHARACTERISTICS	NUMBER OF DIABETICS					DIABETICS				
	ALL AGES	UNDER 17 YR	17–44 YR	45–64 YR	65 YR & OVER	ALL AGES	UNDER 17 YR	17–44 YR	45–64 YR	65 YR & OVER
TOTAL	4,191	86	704	1,813	1,589	20.4	1.3	8.9	42.6	78.5
Sex										
Male	1,620	35	261	819	506	16.3	1.1	6.9	40.6	60.3
Female	2,571	51	443	993	1,083	24.1	1.6	10.8	44.4	91.3
Color										
White	3,570	74	576	1,518	1,402	19.9	1.4	8.3	39.6	75.9
All other	622	*	128	294	187	23.9	*	12.8	70.0	104.5
Family income										
Less than $3,000	737	*	50	234	445	45.0	*	9.8	81.4	89.0
$3,000–$4,999	666	*	70	236	350	35.9	*	12.9	68.0	74.8
$5,000–$6,999	512	*	67	202	236	23.8	*	8.5	48.5	77.7
$7,000–$9,999	519	*	117	238	153	17.3	*	9.5	40.4	74.1
$10,000–$14,999	733	*	181	372	151	14.4	*	8.4	37.8	81.1
$15,000 or more	693	*	178	387	110	12.9	*	8.0	30.5	62.7
Education of head of family										
Less than 9 yr	1,665	*	149	667	833	38.0	*	13.7	56.6	84.3
9–11 yr	805	*	122	387	271	22.5	*	9.6	48.5	86.9
12 yr	935	*	220	438	253	13.9	*	7.7	34.5	68.8
13 yr	723	*	204	298	204	12.8	*	7.8	31.2	63.6

Usual activity status										
School age (6–16 yr)	76	76				1.7	1.7			
Usually working (17 yr & over)†	1,393		410	856	128	18.0		8.6	31.5	48.8
Usually keeping house (females 17 yr & over)	1,754		219	666	869	44.1		12.3	55.1	88.4
Retired (45 yr & over)	669			201	468	74.6			97.6	67.8
Place of residence										
All SMSA†	2,863	64	520	1,249	1,030	20.2	1.5	9.3	42.6	79.3
Central city	1,431	*	261	598	548	23.0	*	10.7	46.3	84.5
Not central city	1,431	40	259	651	482	18.0	1.6	8.2	39.7	74.1
Outside SMSA										
Nonfarm	1,178	*	165	500	492	20.8	*	7.9	44.8	76.9
Farm	150	*	*	64	68	20.4	*	*	31.0	78.3
Geographic region										
Northeast	984	*	154	425	384	20.2	*	8.4	39.6	74.9
North Central	1,187	*	199	505	456	21.1	*	9.3	43.5	79.9
South	1,355	*	199	617	521	20.8	*	7.9	47.2	83.5
West	665	*	151	266	228	18.7	*	10.6	37.4	71.8

Source: National Center for Health Statistics.
Note: Total includes unknown income and education.
*Figure does not meet standards of reliability or precision.
†Urban and suburban.

TABLE 18   Percent of Adults according to Blood Glucose Level after Challenge,* by Age and Sex: United States, 1960–1962

BLOOD GLUCOSE LEVEL* (IN MG/100 ML)	TOTAL 18–79 YR	18–24 YR	25–34 YR	35–44 YR	45–54 YR	55–64 YR	65–74 YR	75–79 YR
				PERCENT OF ADULTS				
Both sexes								
150 or more	20.9	5.8	9.7	15.9	22.6	35.7	42.9	49.3
160 or more	15.5	3.4	6.2	11.0	16.5	26.4	36.0	41.5
170 or more	11.6	2.1	4.2	8.0	12.0	20.9	27.2	34.6
180 or more	8.4	1.1	2.9	5.2	8.2	15.0	21.8	29.5
190 or more	6.0	0.6	1.9	3.1	5.7	11.8	15.2	22.4
200 or more	3.9	0.5	1.1	1.9	3.7	7.3	9.3	19.9
210 or more	2.7	0.3	0.7	1.2	2.2	5.6	7.5	13.9
220 or more	1.9	0.2	0.4	0.6	1.5	4.2	6.1	9.0
230 or more	1.6	0.1	0.4	0.4	1.3	3.3	4.8	8.0
Men								
150 or more	16.3	2.7	7.6	14.9	17.1	27.1	33.5	35.9
160 or more	11.8	1.3	5.0	11.0	13.2	17.7	27.4	24.7
170 or more	8.9	0.4	3.8	7.7	9.8	13.6	22.1	21.9
180 or more	6.4	0.4	2.8	5.8	5.7	10.4	15.1	19.5
190 or more	4.4	0.4	1.7	3.2	3.1	8.3	10.9	17.3
200 or more	2.9	0.2	1.4	1.7	1.9	5.5	6.9	16.2
210 or more	2.0	0.2	0.7	1.1	1.2	3.9	5.2	10.9
220 or more	1.4	0.2	0.4	0.6	0.6	3.1	4.5	7.6
230 or more	1.2	—	0.4	0.4	0.5	2.6	4.3	7.0
Women								
150 or more	25.1	8.4	11.6	16.9	27.9	43.7	50.5	62.5
160 or more	18.8	5.1	7.3	11.0	19.6	34.5	43.0	58.2
170 or more	14.0	3.6	4.6	8.3	14.1	27.7	31.3	47.1
180 or more	10.3	1.7	3.0	4.7	10.7	19.3	27.2	39.3
190 or more	7.4	0.8	2.1	3.1	8.1	15.0	18.7	27.4
200 or more	4.7	0.7	1.0	2.0	5.4	9.0	11.2	23.6
210 or more	3.4	0.3	0.6	1.3	3.1	7.1	9.4	16.8
220 or more	2.4	0.2	0.5	0.5	2.3	5.3	7.3	10.3
230 or more	1.9	0.2	0.5	0.4	2.1	4.0	5.2	9.1

Source: Gordon (1964).
Note: Excludes known diabetics—definite or questionable.
*On venous whole blood after 50 gm oral glucose.

(O'Sullivan, et al, 1967), but direct comparisons are not possible because of methodologic differences. O'Sullivan (1967) has discussed some of these problems. He points out, for example, that even when the same load and cut-off points are used, apparent interpopulation differences in prevalence may not be real. In each of two hypothetical surveys, for instance, a two-hour plasma value greater than 150 mg/100 ml is a diagnostic criterion. In one of the surveys, however, this is the sole "criterion", while the other requires as a condition of diagnosis that the one-hour value also be elevated. Data of O'Sullivan and

Williams (1966) show that factors of this kind can affect substantially the purported rate of prevalence.

Results in Cleveland (Kent and Leonards, 1968) suggest that the prevalence of diabetes is similar to that observed in Tecumseh and in the sample tested in the National Survey. This detection project in Cleveland was not designed as an instrument for measuring prevalence. It is possible that the recruitment of high-risk subjects substantially influenced the frequency distribution of blood glucose values, but the data suggest strongly that impairment of tolerance is very common in adults of Cleveland when conventional criteria are used. In Oklahoma City we (West, et al, 1970) found the rate of positive screening tests was greater in those with a strong family history of diabetes (diabetes in a sibling, parent, or child). But there was no increase in rates of positivity in those with a family history of lesser degree (diabetes in grandparents, uncles, aunts, cousins, grandchildren).

Samples in Dallas (Unger, 1957) and Southern California (Searcy and Low, 1967) were not necessarily representative of these populations, but in these groups distribution of results of glucose loading tests were similar to those in Tecumseh and in the National Survey. In the Southern California survey of 456 apparently healthy adults, 32% of men and 36% of women had two-hour plasma glucose values greater than 140 mg/100 ml after 100 gm of oral glucose. Glucose tolerance was much better in the younger subjects of this group, and worse in the elderly. In a subsample of 88 adults (all ages), only four had fasting plasma glucose levels greater than 119, mg/100 ml, and only two had fasting levels greater than 125. Rates of known diabetes were not studied in this population.

Studies of O'Sullivan, et al in Sudbury, Massachusetts, are in some respects the most informative of the population surveys. Postprandial blood glucose tests were performed in 4,626 (77% of the eligible adults), and full oral glucose tolerance tests were done on a 5% sample (O'Sullivan and Williams, 1966). It

TABLE 19 Twentieth, fiftieth, and eightieth percentiles of one-hour blood glucose in mg/100 ml for persons challenged within four hours of eating, by sex and age (Tecumseh, Michigan)

		MALES				FEMALES		
AGE	N	20TH	50TH	80TH	N	20TH	50TH	80TH
16–19	120	77	94	122	109	89	106	137
20–29	253	86	107	137	281	88	111	145
30–39	373	98	125	158	368	94	123	161
40–49	257	103	136	176	242	104	131	174
50–59	161	112	147	185	143	125	156	200
60–69	74	119	155	198	79	121	158	196
70–79	36	135	172	226	27	114	182	224
TOTAL	1,274				1,249			

Source: Hayner, et al (1965).

Note: N—number of persons tested. Specimens were whole venous blood. Results are for general population of Tecumseh, Michigan, after 100 gm oral glucose.

was shown that rate of prevalence of occult diabetes could have been stated to be as low as 0.8% or as high as 13.4%, depending on diagnostic criteria and methods of calculation. After appropriate extrapolations necessitated by differences in methods and criteria, it appeared that rates of abnormal glucose tolerance in Sudbury were roughly similar to those in Bedford (Butterfield, et al, 1964) and in the United States general population (Gordon, et al, 1964).

Elsewhere in this volume, data are reviewed on prevalence of diabetes in various US Indian tribes. The Pima tribe is the only one for which rates are known precisely (Table 20, Figure 6). Unfortunately, no equally satisfactory data are available in US whites for comparison. Probably the best data available are those of Hayner in Tecumseh and O'Sullivan in Sudbury. Very crude extrapolations suggest that Pimas have rates of diabetes about four times that of the US white population. Rates are also two to four times higher in other American tribes than in US whites (West, 1974,1977).

Prevalence Based on Screening Surveys and Other Methods

Crude studies of prevalence have been made in many other US communities using a variety of methods. Typically, these have been based on results of screening programs that did not include study of rates of occult diabetes in negative screenees. Results of this kind are difficult to evaluate, but they may be useful in suggesting that the rate of diabetes is above a certain level (at least 1%, at least 2%, etc). Lack of information on age distribution often adds to the difficulty of interpretation. Another frequent problem is that population samples tested are unrepresentative. They may, for example, include a disproportional number from high-risk groups.

In the United States few attempts have been made to count known cases in individual communities. Centralized medical record systems are rare except in special groups such as rural Indian tribes. A rare study of this kind has, however, been performed by Palumbo, et al (1976) in Rochester, Minnesota. In this community 1.6% had diabetes that had been diagnosed. In those over 40 years of age the rate was 4.3% for males and 3.9% for females, as summarized below. In Framingham 3% of adults over 34 years of age had diagnosed diabetes (Garcia, 1974).

Another crude indicator of prevalence is mortality rate. This is covered in Chapter 6 on mortality. Rates of diabetes in the employees of *certain* types of large companies probably reflect fairly well the rate of adult-onset diabetes in the general population. Pell and D'Alonzo have published some carefully collected data on diabetes in employees of the DuPont Company. Among young employees diabetes rates were probably considerably less than in the general population because several factors relating to youth-onset diabetes reduce the frequency of their employment. In employees over forty, however, there was in this circumstance little evidence of discrimination or other bias. Rates of diabetes were slightly less than those found in the National Health Interview Survey. In men, for example, diabetes was known to be present in

TABLE 20 Two-Hour Postload Glucose Levels and Prevalence of Diabetes in Half-to Full-Blooded Pima Indians

Age Group (Yr)	Number Examined	Two-Hour Venous Plasma Glucose (mg/100 ml) After 75 gm Oral Glucose							With Diabetes			
		0–99	100–139	140–159	160–199	200–299	300–399	400 and Over	Previously Recognized		>160 mg/ 100 ml*	
									No	%	No	%
Males												
5–14	547	280	249	16	2				0	0.0	2	0.4
15–24	239	121	95	15	3	2	1		1	0.4	8	3.4
25–34	135	39	58(1)	8	8	8	3	2	8	5.9	30	22.2
35–44	142	39(1)	44(1)	8	6	8	15	10	26	18.3	51	35.9
45–54	94	12	35	8	7	8	12	20	21	22.3	39	41.5
55–64	84	16	25	8(1)	4(1)	7	11	12	23	27.4	35	41.7
65–74	76	9(1)	20(1)	11	9	7	7	11	21	27.6	36	47.4
75+	41	4	13	6	5(1)	6	3	3	7	17.1	18	43.9
TOTAL	1,358								107	7.9	219	16.1
35 and over	437								98	22.4	179	41.0
Females												
5–14	604	272	293	24	13	2			0	0.0	15	2.5
15–24	307	131	143	18	9	2	1	3	3	1.0	15	4.9
25–34	187	39	87	20	15	12	5	9	11	5.9	41	21.9
35–44	178	11	64(1)	14	26(3)	17	21	21	41	23.0	89	50.0
45–54	107	9	26	5(2)	12(2)	17	8	26	40	37.4	67	62.6
55–64	102	4	16(1)	12(1)	4(4)	15	18	27	54	52.9	70	68.6
65–74	59	1	15	8	6	13	9	7	21	35.6	35	59.3
75+	15	2	6	8		5	2	7	2	13.3	7	46.7
TOTAL	1,559								172	11.0	339	21.7
35 and over	461								158	34.3	268	58.1
Both sexes												
TOTALS	2,917								279	9.6	558	19.1
35 and over	898								256	28.5	447	49.8

Source: Bennett. et al (1976a).

*Includes subjects. shown in columns 3–6 in parentheses. who had diabetes clearly confirmed by medical record review and were mostly taking hypoglycemic agents. but in whom the two-hour plasma level was lower than 160 mg/100 ml.

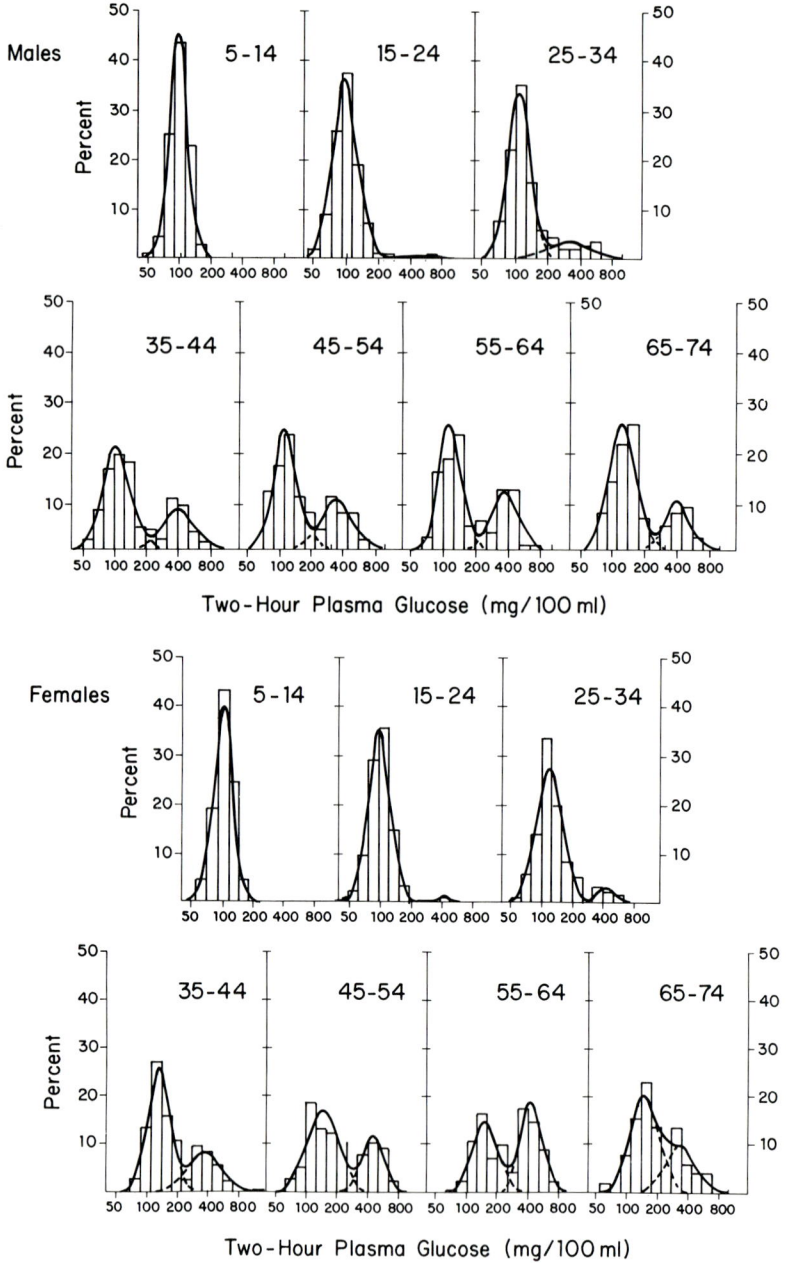

FIGURE 6.   Frequency distribution of two-hour plasma glucose levels after 75 gm oral glucose in Pima Indians (Bennett, et al, 1976a).

144

2.4% of those 55–59 years of age (142 diabetics) and 3.5% in those 60–64 (111 diabetics).

The *incidence* of diabetes in the United States is discussed below in the section following prevalence.

Is Prevalence Really Rising?

It is widely believed that rates of diabetes have increased substantially in recent years. But there is surprisingly little evidence to support this opinion. The number of diabetics identified in the 1973 United States National Health Survey did substantially exceed the number counted in the National Survey of 1965. This must be interpreted, however, in the light of two considerations. The manner of questioning about diabetes was more thorough in 1973 than in 1965. During this eight-year interval there was also a great increase in the number of blood glucose tests. This was mainly due to the introduction of automated systems that measure the concentrations of as many as 12 or more blood elements simultaneously, of which one is usually glucose. Formerly, blood glucose determinations were usually performed selectively; they are now very often done on all patients seen in hospitals and clinics. It is therefore difficult to know whether the rise in diabetes rates is real or apparent. Americans are probably fatter than heretofore, but evidence to this effect is not wholly convincing. This is discussed in detail in the section on obesity in Chapter 7.

As shown in Chapter 6, data on mortality show little change in the past twenty-five years. Data prior to 1949 on mortality are not comparable to subsequent figures because revision of guidelines in that year reduced substantially the sensitivity of this index. Between 1920 and 1950, age-adjusted mortality observed by the Metropolitan Insurance Company remained quite constant, rising only from 15 per 100,000 in 1920 to 17 in 1950 (Joslin, et al, 1959).

No data are available on glucose loading tests in the general population previous to the present generation. Data of Unger in Dallas food-handlers, reported in 1957, suggest that levels of glucose tolerance were similar to those found in more recent studies. Review of data in selected groups tested between 1920 and 1950 revealed low rates of impaired tolerance in some and high rates in others. The numbers were small in all groups in which tolerance was superior to that observed subsequently in larger groups. It does seem likely that the continuing decline in exercise requirements would have a deleterious effect. Palumbo, et al (1976) found little evidence of change in the incidence of diabetes in Rochester, Minnesota between the years 1945 and 1970. There was a small temporary increase coinciding with the introduction of automated methods for measuring blood glucose. Kahn and Hiller (1974) found no evidence of any recent increase in diabetes-related blindness, except in nonwhite women. Evidence discussed elsewhere in this book clearly establishes recent sharp increases in diabetes in certain special groups, such as Indians and blacks, but it is not clear whether age-adjusted rates are any higher in whites than in 1920. Changes in rates of juvenile diabetes are discussed in the section on that subject in Chapter 8.

In Europe, diabetes mortality rates have risen sharply in several countries since 1950. Probably prevalence of diabetes did increase in these countries during the decade after World War II, but subsequent increases in prevalence may only be apparent. The numbers of blood glucose determinations increased substantially in Europe during the past two decades.

PREVALENCE IN OTHER COUNTRIES
AS ASCERTAINED BY GLUCOSE LOADING TESTS

Prevalence by country receives detailed discussion in other sections including those on mortality (Chapter 6) and geography (Chapter 7). Also, data on prevalence as determined by less sensitive methods are summarized above in Table 16. The discussion below reviews results from studies in which prevalence has been determined by performing glucose loading tests in whole populations or representative samples thereof.

Bergen, Norway

One of the first such studies was that of Jorde in Bergen, Norway, in 1956 (Jorde, 1962). In this classic investigation he tested 2,273 men and 3,657 women from the Nygard district. This represented 53% of the population of the eligible age group. The characteristics of the sample tested were systematically compared to those of the general populations of Nygard district and of Bergen. In general, the frequency distribution of these characteristics (eg, age, weight, socioeconomic status) seemed quite similar in the three groups. The youngest age included was 14. The number of known diabetics was counted (22 men and 24 women). This represented a rate of 0.6% in the adult population. A screening random blood glucose was performed, and a specimen of urine was tested that had previously been collected by the subject, usually one to two hours after a meal containing bread. On the basis of follow-up studies of positive screenees the rate of occult diabetes in this age group was estimated to be about 1.2% and the total rate (known plus occult) about 1.8%. Jorde noted that this rate was quite similar to the rate reported in Oxford, Massachusetts, in which similar methods had been used. But Jorde's survey was unusual in that a sample of 194 "normal" subjects from this population was tested after a glucose load. In 102 subjects from thirty to fifty-nine years of age, the mean two-hour capillary glucose after 100 gm of glucose orally was 128 mg/100 ml with a standard deviation of 20. In 53 normal subjects over 60 years of age, the mean two-hour value was 138 with a standard deviation of 26. Rates of "chemical diabetes" in the group over 30 years of age may be stated to be as high as 40% or as low as

2%, depending on the criteria employed, but when traditional criteria were employed (eg, two-hour value above 140 classified as abnormal), rates of occult diabetes were more than ten times the rate of known diabetes in this adult population. Details were not given for the frequency distribution of fasting blood glucose values, but fasting hyperglycemia was not common. Even in the subjects over 60 years of age the two standard-deviation range extended only to 119 mg/100 ml. In the total group (194), the two standard-deviation range extended to 116. In all screenees who said that they had not eaten for more than three hours (1,693), the mean blood glucose was 99 with a standard deviation of 17.

Jorde also gathered some excellent data on the relationship of blood glucose levels to several other factors. These included urine glucose, duration of fasting, weight for height, age, and sex. This study is too little known. In several respects it was a model survey. This publication also included an excellent review of the older literature on several aspects of the epidemiology of diabetes.

Sweden

The excellent study of Nillson, et al (1964) was not intended as a study of prevalence but did yield some information in that respect. In a random sample of the adult population of Kristianstad, 8 of 301 (2.7%) had known diabetes. These diabetics and ten others with "disabling" diseases were excluded from a testing program that included oral and intravenous glucose tolerance tests. Attrition of recruitment further reduced the sample to 207. The oral glucose load was 30 gm/sq m of body surface. Blood glucose was determined on capillary blood. Details given include the mean and standard deviation for one- and two-hour blood glucose values after oral glucose, by age and sex. Glucose tolerance in these Swedes was similar to that in Bergen and Sudbury; and, as shown below, also similar to tolerance in Bedford and Birmingham, England. For example, in subjects of Kristianstad 40–59 years of age the one standard-deviation range for two-hour values extended to about 111 mg/100 ml. In older subjects aged 60 to 79, it extended to 138.

There have been many other studies of diabetes prevalence in Scandinavia, but the studies in Bergen and Kristianstad were unusual in that glucose tolerance tests were performed in samples from the general population. Many of these other studies are mentioned elsewhere in this volume because of their epidemiologic significance in other respects.

Finland

Heinsalmi and Hiononen (1967) reported the results of a survey of four areas of East Finland in which plasma glucose levels were measured one hour after an oral glucose load of 40 gm/sq m of body surface. This test was performed in

5,636 persons (78.5% of whom were over 14 years of age). Persons with equivocal or slightly elevated levels were tested again with full glucose tolerance tests. From these data it was estimated that 16.7% of this population (over 14 years) had "abnormal" glucose tolerance.

Birmingham, England

In 1963 the College of General Practitioners published the first of a series of reports on their survey of 1960–1961. The "Working Party" included Dr. John Malins whose publications have subsequently drawn on the results of this excellent project. A population of 19,412 served by ten general practitioners was the subject of this detection project and study. Postprandial urine glucose determinations were performed in 95.5% of the eligible population. Glucose tolerance tests were performed in a representative sample (343) who were negative screenees, and also in all available positive screenees. Publications also reported on subsequent morbidity and on the course of glucose tolerance in those with varying degrees of impairment or with normal tolerance (Birmingham Working Party, 1970,1976).

Known diabetics were not tested but were counted (119). They constituted 0.6% of this population. Glycosuria was found in 493 subjects (2.7%). Of the 493 glycosurics, 464 were tested after 50 gm of oral glucose. In these glycosurics the rate of "florid" diabetes (fasting capillary blood glucose above 130 mg/ 100 ml) was modest, 55 of 464 (12%). These glycosurics with "florid diabetes" represented only 0.3% of the total populaton. In the representative sample of 343 negative screenees who had glucose tolerance tests, there was only one florid diabetic (0.3% of negative screenees). Thus, the rate of undiagnosed "florid" diabetes in this population was about 0.3%.

When traditional criteria were employed, details of which are given by Malins (1974b), 28 of 343 negative screenees (8.2%) had "diabetic" glucose tolerance curves. This includes the one with "florid" diabetes. In the 464 positive screenees, 47 (10%) had impaired tolerance without florid diabetes. Thus the total with "abnormal" tolerance in this subgroup was 47 plus 55 with florid diabetes, or 104 (22% of all positive screenees tested). In addition to these "abnormal" glucose tolerance tests, there were a large number with equivocal results (eg, lag storage curves, elevated two-hour values with normal one-hour values). Of all positive (630) and negative (464) screenees available for retesting in 1966–1967, only 200 had had glucose tolerance tests deemed to be "normal" in every respect (Birmingham Working Party, 1970).

These highly informative data bring out well the many problems involved in estimating and comparing rates of prevalence. The rate of known diabetes was 0.6%. When rates are based on the rather complete follow-up of the almost comprehensive screening survey, the apparent frequency increases to about 1.2%. When calculations are based on those data plus results of glucose tolerance tests in a representative sample, the rate of "diabetes", by traditional

148

criteria, is much higher (about 9%). Moreover, this rate could be expressed as 1% or 20% depending on criteria for defining "diabetes"!

Bedford, England

The design and results of the excellent studies in Bedford were similar in some respects to those in Birmingham. The Bedford data receive considerable attention in several other sections of this book. This work was started in 1962 as a cooperative enterprise of local and national elements of the Ministry of Health and expert consultants, including the scientists from Guy's Hospital, London (Sharp, 1964). Two thirds (25,700 of 38,400) of those on the Bedford electoral role submitted urine samples that they had been asked to collect postprandially. About 4% of these adults had glycosuria (Keen, 1964). When oral glucose tolerance tests were performed on glycosurics, about one third of these glycosurics had two-hour capillary blood glucose levels of 120 mg/100 ml or more after 50 gm of oral glucose. Glucose tolerance tests were also performed in a sample (543) of negative screenees (Butterfield, 1964). In this group the rate of elevated two-hour values was 14% (76 of 543). In a sample (570) from the entire population that included both negative and positive screenees, 90 (18%) had impaired glucose tolerance by the standards employed. Based on these latter data, Butterfield (1964) estimated that the rate of abnormal tolerance in the general population was about 12% to 14% when traditional criteria were employed for interpreting results of glucose tolerance tests.

Under conditions of the Bedford study (Keen, 1964), glycosuria after 50 gm of glucose was observed more than seven times as frequently as after a meal (30% and 4%). In 245 subjects with two-hour glucose levels below 120 mg/100 ml, the rate of glycosuria was 3% after a meal and 26% after glucose. In those with higher two-hour values, glycosuria was observed in 4% after a meal and in 30% after glucose. On the other hand, 9 of 10 persons whose two-hour values exceeded 159 had glycosuria after oral glucose.

The Bedford investigators (Butterfield, 1964) have presented data on the frequency distribution of two-hour blood glucose values. Rates of prevalence can, therefore, be estimated using any of the several diagnostic criteria that have been advocated. Again, rates of "diabetes" in this population of adults would vary greatly depending on diagnostic criteria employed. Rates are higher in this adult population than in the Birmingham study (all ages), but these differences in rates are probably attributable wholly or mainly to the age differences. Table 15 summarizes some of these data from Bedford by age.

These rates of "abnormal" glucose tolerance in England seem to be roughly comparable to those in Sudbury, Massachusetts (O'Sullivan and Williams, 1966) and somewhat lower than those in Tecumseh, Michigan, but differences in methods and criteria exclude the possibility of precise comparisons in which one can place confidence. Glucose tolerance in England was also roughly the same as in Bergen, Norway and Kristianstad, Sweden.

149

Arbroath, Scotland

Mitchell and Strauss (1964) performed postprandial and glucose loading tests (50 gm) on glycosuric and aglycosuric subjects from the general population of those over 5 years of age. By traditional standards it was estimated that 12% had impaired tolerance.

Australia

There have been some surveys in Australia in which glucose loading tests have been used in examining whole communities or samples thereof. These were performed at Busselton (Welborn, et al, 1968; Bowyer, et al, 1974), at Toowomba (Smithhurst, 1969), and at Cunderdin (Welborn, et al, 1968). The Busselton surveys were exemplary in several respects. In a total adult (over 20 years of age) population, 89% were examined (3,331 of 3,741), with a group of tests that included a determination of glucose on venous blood about one hour after 50 gm of oral glucose (Welborn, et al, 1968). This test was performed at varying times of the day. Known diabetics were excluded. The frequency distribution of results was presented by age and sex. Only 59 (1.8%) had one-hour values over 199 mg/100 ml. Fifty-six of these (95%) were retested with a full glucose tolerance test. In this group, 29 (52%) had diabetes by conventional criteria, 10 (18%) had clearly normal tolerance, and 17 (30%) had equivocal results.

On the basis of these results it was estimated that the rate of occult diabetes in women was 1.0% and in men 0.7%. The rate of previously known diabetes was 1.2% in women and 1.6% in men. The estimated rates of diabetes were, therefore, 2.3% in women and 2.4% in men. Negative screenees were not tested with glucose tolerance tests. One should keep in mind that even if the rates of "abnormal" tolerance in negative screenees were as low as 5%, the rate of "diabetes" (abnormal glucose tolerance) would be increased about threefold by taking this into account in estimating the rate of prevalence for this community.

In Busselton glucose tolerance was related to several other factors including age, weight for height, symptoms of diabetes, obstretric history, and stigmata of cardiovascular disease. Results were quite similar in a subsequent Busselton survey reported by Bowyer, et al (1974). The latter data were well presented by frequency distribution in relation to age and sex. These results are discussed elsewhere in this book in the sections to which they apply.

It does seem that glucose tolerance in Busselton is better than in Tecumseh, Michigan, but difference in methods prevent precise comparisons.

In Cunerdin, Australia, rates were similar to those found in Busselton (Welborn, et al, 1968).

Rangiora, New Zealand

In Rangiora, Murray, et al (1969) measured glucose levels on *whole* venous blood two hours after 50 gm of oral glucose in 2,486 adults of Rangiora (93% of

TABLE 21   Two-Hour Blood Sugar Results (mg/100 ml) in a New Zealand Town

Age (yr)	Number	Mean	SD	X ± 2 SD	95th Percentile	50th Percentile
Males						
21–29	206	78.5	14.0	51–107	47–108	78
30–39	208	80.7	15.5	50–111	45–113	80
40–49	211	79.7	28.4	23–136	43–109	76
50–59	214	82.4	27.9	27–138	40–116	79
60–69	182	92.0	43.9	42–180	36–132	84
70+	124	95.4	43.3	21–180	45–133	88
Females						
21–29	193	80.2	14.1	52–108	52–106	79
30–39	204	79.5	14.1	51–108	51–105	78
40–49	210	83.4	28.1	27–140	42–117	80
50–59	249	88.0	39.2	10–166	43–120	82
60–69	220	91.6	29.3	28–145	50–123	87
70+	174	106.3	50.1	26–206	42–143	95

Source: Murray, et al (1969).
Note: Subjects comprised 93.1% of a 2,500 New Zealand European urban population (see text).

the population). Tests were performed between 8:00 AM and 1:00 PM in the fasting state. The frequency distribution of blood glucose results by age and sex are shown in Table 21. Follow-up glucose tolerance tests were performed on all available subjects in the group with screening two-hour values greater than 129 mg/100 ml. On the basis of these studies it was concluded that about 9.6% of the adult population had diabetes. This included 1.7% with previously diagnosed diabetes. Although not completely matched, methods were similar to those employed in Bedford and Birmingham. It seems that glucose tolerance was somewhat better in Rangiora than in Bedford or Birmingham, but it is difficult to be certain.

South Africa

Extensive and informative studies have been performed in various ethnic groups of South Africa by Jackson and his colleagues who have included Goldberg, et al (1969), Marine, et al (1969), and G. D. Campbell (1970). These were well summarized by Jackson (1972,1977) and Marine, et al (1969). Although methods were not completely standardized, the degree of standardization was considerable, making possible some unusual opportunities for comparisons of prevalence. Data on age and other characteristics were well collected. Population sampling techniques were far from ideal in some instances, but on the whole, these samples were more representative than those usually available. In Tongaat, a community of Indians near Durban, 2,427 were tested. This represented 90% of the eligible population.

In the various South African groups, after 50 gm of oral glucose was administered, venous plasma glucose was measured at one hour, and in some groups a two-hour value was also obtained. Among the various ethnic groups, comparative prevalence varied substantially by age. In Capetown Indians, for example, diabetes was uncommon in subjects 15–34 years of age but very frequent in those over 55; in blacks, however, diabetes was moderately common in those 35 to 54 but rare in those over 55. In general, age-related rates of diabetes were about the same in Capetown blacks and whites. Rates were roughly twice as great in Indians, Malays, and in the group of "colored" persons (mixed racial origins). The frequency distribution of two-hour glucose values was very similar in Tongaat Indians (near Durban) to that in Transvaal Bantus (Goldberg, et al, 1969).

Examination of distribution of blood glucose values by age for the Capetown groups suggested that glucose tolerance was somewhat better in Capetown whites than in Bedford, England (Butterfield, 1964) or in the United States (Gordon, 1964). By traditional criteria, "abnormal" glucose tolerance is very frequent in urban Indians of South Africa; it is not yet clear whether this rate is any higher than for whites in certain United States communities (Hayner, 1965; Searcy and Low, 1967).

These data from South Africa are of special interest in several respects and receive attention in other sections of this book, including those on race, geography, nutrition, vascular disease, and genetics. Many other studies have been performed in Africa on prevalence in which loading tests were not used as the first-stage procedure. These have been reviewed by Tulloch (1962,1966), Campbell (1970), and Jackson (1970,1977).

Asia and Latin America

Many population surveys have been performed in Asia and Latin America, particularly in India, Japan, and Argentina. But only a few have included glucose loading tests on all subjects or a representative sample thereof. In rural Jamaica, Florey, et al (1972) studied blood glucose values after subjects ingested 75 gm of Glucola in a sample of 696 persons 25–64 years of age. The mean one-hour values on whole blood were 126 ± 36 mg/100 ml in men, and 138 ± 43 in women. In India a cooperative study is now underway that will ascertain the frequency distribution of blood glucose values in several communities (Ahuja, 1976).

Figure 9 in Chapter 7 summarizes rates of prevalence in ten populations of Asia and Latin America (West, 1972). For comparison, approximate rates are also given for Cherokee Indians and for the general population of the United States. In all populations only persons over 29 years of age are included, and average age in all groups was approximately 50. Details of the methods have been published (West and Kalbfleisch, 1966,1970). These rates are based on dividing normals from diabetics at a two-hour blood glucose value of 150 mg/100 ml (venous whole blood after 1 gm/kg of oral glucose). But data have been presented by frequency distribution (West and Kalbfleisch, 1966,1970), so that rates can be compared using either higher or lower values as diagnostic criteria. In Bangor, Pennsylvania, 17% of whites in this age group had diabetes by this criterion when these methods were used (West and Kalbfleisch, 1970). In all these populations the rates presented *include* known diabetics.

These methods overcame or mitigated many of the usual problems in estimating and comparing rates of diabetes. Conditions were, however, not ideal. The samples were more representative than those usually available but were by no means optimal. The samples were small, averaging only about 500 per country. For these reasons, small differences (eg, between 4% and 6%) may not reflect a truly significant difference. But note that many of the differences are very great (range from 2% to 25%) despite the standardization of methods, criteria, and age distribution. These data provide strong evidence that real interpopulation differences as great as fivefold are common, and are not the result of incomplete ascertainment or differences of methods and criteria.

Primitive Populations

Glucose tolerance tests have been performed in samples of a few primitive populations. These have included studies of Mouratoff, et al (1967) in Eskimos and in Athabascan Indians (1969). In these groups diabetes was exceedingly rare and glucose tolerance excellent. Similarly, the Broayas of the Sahara had very low blood glucose values and no diabetes (DeHertogh, et al, 1975). In Micronesians and Polynesians studied by Reed, et al (1973) and by Prior (1966,1971), levels of glucose tolerance ranged from very good in primitive people to mediocre or poor in some groups living under "modernized" conditions. West (1974) reviewed rates of prevalence in more than 80 populations of the New World. Irrespective of race (Indian, Eskimo, Micronesian, or Polynesian), rates have been low in primitive groups and moderate or high (Zimmet and Whitehouse, 1977) in those subjected to acculturation. Interpopulation differences as great as tenfold in rates of diabetes were common in these aboriginal groups. This same spectrum has been observed in different groups of Melanesians (Campbell, 1963; Winterbotham, 1960) and Australian aborigines (Wise, et al, 1976; Finlay-Jones and McComish, 1972).

INCIDENCE

Data on incidence are few and rather difficult to interpret. Using household interview data of the National Center for Health Statistics, the epidemiology workgroup of the National Diabetes Commission (Bennett, et al, 1976) estimated crudely the annual incidence of diabetes in the United States. This estimate was 612,000 cases annually or 300 cases per 100,000 population (0.3%). In children (less than 17 years of age) the rate was roughly 30 per 100,000 (0.03%). The highest rate was in females over 64 in whom annual incidence was 1,100 per 100,000 (1.1%).

These very crude extrapolations also suggested to Bennett et al that the probability of developing diabetes upon surviving to age 85 was about 23% in males and 35% in females. In Rochester, Minnesota the annual incidence rate was 133 cases per 100,000 (Palumbo, et al, 1976). Some of the problems involved in such estimates will be discussed below.

In certain respects the best data on incidence in a population are from the intensive studies in the Pima Indians, where glucose tolerance tests are performed periodically in the entire population of adults. Hamman and Miller (1975) reported on incidence in Indians over 14 years of age. Because length of follow-up varied they used a life table method to compute incidence in an eight-year period. The rate was 19.6% or about 2.5% per year (2,500 per 100,000). The very high rate is probably attributable to two factors: the peculiarly high rate of diabetes in this population and the very sensitive method of ascertainment. Related studies of these investigators are discussed further below and in other sections of this book, concerning the effects of fatness and of blood glucose level on incidence rates.

In Canberra, Australia circumstances were such as to permit a crude estimate of incidence (Proust and Smithurst, 1968). Based on a three-year experience, the incidence was approximately 61 per 100,000 per annum. In those less than 20 years of age the age-specific incidence rate was 3 per 100,000 at risk; in persons 20 to 39 the rate was 32 per 100,000; in those 40 to 59 the frequency was 118 per 100,000. In those over 59 the age-specific rate was 300. These rates are much lower than rates reported above for the United States and about the same as those reported below for populations in Europe. It is not clear to what extent the much higher rates in the United States are real or apparent. A review of all the circumstances suggest that differences of circumstance and methodology are partly responsible, but very probably incidence rates are really higher in the United States.

In Odense, Denmark incidence rates were estimated by Horstmann (1972). In 1961 the frequency was 86 per 100,000, very similar to the rate of 61 in Canberra. For the Danes over 39 years of age incidence was 183 in men and 225 in women. Maximum incidence was at age 70, with lower rates in older and younger Danes. On the basis of these data, Horstmann showed that death certificate information greatly underestimated prevalence.

In Israeli men more than 39 years of age, annual incidence was 775 per 100,000 (Herman, et al, 1970). To a substantial degree, the high rate was the result of the circumstances of the study, in which regular testing was performed in cohorts under intensive study. Incidence rates were higher in men from the Middle East (1,015) than in men from Eastern Europe (425).

Studies by Joslin, et al (1936) were probably the first in which data on incidence by age were properly corrected for age distribution of the population at risk. This method, which related incidence by age of Joslin clinic patients to the age distribution of the population of New England, was far from ideal, particularly because the age distribution of these patients probably reflected imperfectly the age distribution of all diabetics in the general population. The results are of interest, even though they should be interpreted with caution. In both sexes incidence peaked in the sixth decade before declining moderately in the seventh and eighth decades. More recent studies of age-incidence patterns in Joslin Clinic patients were performed by Hirohata (1969). The distribution of age of onset had shifted somewhat to the right (toward older ages). In the period 1950–1956 the peak incidence occurred during the first part of the seventh decade before declining slightly. Among several possible explanations of this shift is the increasing use of blood glucose testing that would tend to identify a greater portion of the particularly mild cases of hyperglycemia seen in old age. In some societies old people have more medical attention, and for this reason, diabetes is more likely to be discovered than in younger age groups.

Falconer, et al (1971) pointed out several problems in calculating age-specific incidence from the kinds of data usually available. These include excessive death rates in diabetics and differences over time in the ratio of diagnosed to undiagnosed diabetes. Even when age and age of onset of diabetes are known and properly related to the age distribution of the general population from which they are drawn, it is difficult to calculate incidence retrospectively. Mortality rates in both the numerator (diabetics) and denominator (general population) vary greatly by age, and mortality rates in diabetics vary by duration of diabetes. Some of these difficulties can be avoided by basing calculations on a short interval of time, but this requires study of a very large representative population. It is clear from these discussions on prevalence and on diagnosis that incidence rates and their relation to age are profoundly affected by frequency and sensitivity of testing and by diagnostic criteria, particularly in the older age groups.

Excellent data on age of onset were collected by Malins et al. (1972) in Birmingham, England, and by Gamble and Taylor (1969) in London. These are discussed in other sections of this book. The data of Gamble and Taylor only crudely reflected incidence by age because they were not related to the number at risk in each of the age groups. The data in Birmingham were related to the number in each age group at risk by Hayward and Lucena (1965). They are, therefore, among the most informative available. These investigators point out that conditions were not ideal for establishing age-specific incidence rates, but circumstances suggest that their figures are at least crudely representative, particularly for adults under 70 years of age. In the 1950s incidence per annum was about 0.006% per year in the third decade, 0.009% in the fourth decade, 0.018% in the fifth, 0.05% in the sixth and 0.06% in the seventh. In the eighth decade incidence declined in men and increased in women, but the authors pointed out that these data in the elderly were less representative and more subject to error. In the ninth decade incidence declined substantially in both sexes, but as pointed out by these authors and by Falconer, et al (1971), this apparent decline may not have been real. In Birmingham, there was little difference between the sexes in incidence up to age 70. Prevalence of diabetes in this population was about 0.6%. My calculations from the data of Hayward and Lucena for the 1950s yielded an overall incidence rate of about 0.04% per year or 0.4% per decade. Other crude calculations suggested that about 3% of those that survived to age 80 could be diagnosed as diabetic if the incidence rates of the 1950s continued to prevail. It seems likely, however, that incidence rates will be increased by an increasing sensitivity and frequency of testing. This prediction is based mainly on the expected effects of the development of cheap automated methods for determining blood glucose levels. Another study in this population (Birmingham Working Party, 1970) has shown that "abnormal" glucose tolerance is exceedingly common when traditional criteria of interpretation are used.

The earlier plateau or decline of incidence in men than in women is interesting. This fits well with the observation (West, 1973) that in well-fed societies women continue to gain weight into the seventh decade, while in men mean weight tends to plateau in the fifth decade and decline in the seventh. Part of this decline is probably due to the higher death rate in fat men, but part is apparently secondary to weight loss with old age that begins about a decade earlier in men.

Probably the most informative publication on incidence is that of Falconer, Duncan, and Smith (1971). This outstanding paper is too little known. Its special merit is attributable both to the unique excellence of the design of the studies and the highly perceptive review and analysis of the many problems in determining incidence. These investigators performed a comprehensive study of diabetes in Edinburgh, Scotland. The study group probably included more than 90% of all diagnosed diabetics in this population. Age and age of onset were determined for each of 2,932 diabetics in the study, and the data were related to the distribution by age of the general population of Edinburgh. They found that incidence rose only slightly between ages 15 and 30 before rising sharply until a plateau was reached in the seventh decade. These data are summarized in Figure 7. In young adults annual rates were about 200 per 100,000, in middle age about 800, and in old age about 2,000 (2% per year). A similar relationship of age to incidence was observed in Rochester, Minnesota (Palumbo, et al, 1976), but incidence continued to rise slightly even in the eighth decade.

Falconer, et al also calculated potential lifetime risk of diabetes in this population (about 8% in those surviving to age 80). This figure is considerably lower than such estimates for the United States (Bennett, et al, 1976). In part, the higher rates of lifetime risk in the United States appear to be a result of differences in methods of calculation, but are also attributable to higher incidence. Prevalence of diagnosed diabetes in Edinburgh was about 0.7%; in the United States it is about 2%. Methods of ascertainment were not matched, but it does seem that actual rates are higher in the United States. In Rochester, Minnesota the prevalence of diabetes was found to be 1.6% by methods similar to those employed in Edinburgh, where prevalence was 0.6%.

The data of Bennett, et al (1976a) on Pima Indians are of particular interest for several reasons. A complete population is being followed with periodic

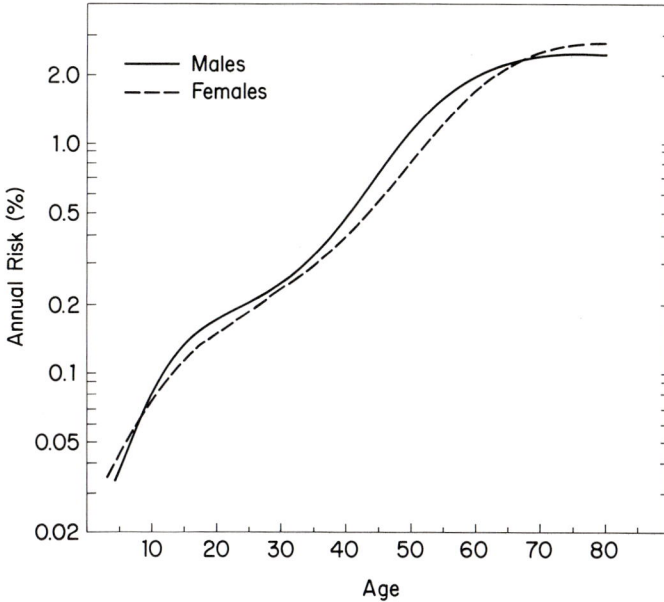

FIGURE 7. Incidence of diabetes by age in Edinburgh (Falconer, et al. 1971).

glucose tolerance tests. In these circumstances results have been quite different with respect to the relationship of incidence to age. Here, incidence peaked at age 30 in males and at age 40 in females before declining steadily and markedly. One possible explanation is that criteria of diagnosis were more conservative than those usually employed. This eliminates a large number of elderly persons from the "diabetic" group. A second factor is that ascertainment occurs earlier under these circumstances, where frequent glucose loading tests are performed in the entire population. Finally, it seems quite possible that the elderly Pimas were never as fat as their offspring. These data do fit with the possibility that the high incidence of diabetes in the elderly may be to a considerable degree spurious, because of greater frequency of testing in older people, inappropriate diagnostic standards, and delay in diagnosis because of infrequent testing in adults under 40 years of age.

SOME SUGGESTIONS FOR FUTURE STUDIES

It would be of considerable interest to have more and better data on incidence of diabetes and the factors that affect it. Previous experience suggests that such data are often very difficult to interpret. Probably the greatest problem is that huge effects in apparent incidence are produced by variations in frequency and sensitivity of testing and in criteria of diagnosis. In many

157

populations it has been shown that by certain commonly employed standards, frequency of abnormal tolerance is as much as ten times more common than the frequency of known clinical cases. This is discussed in detail in other sections. Meaningful interpretations and comparisons will therefore require greater standardization of methods and conventions.

The most workable criterion of "diabetes" for purposes of comparison would probably be the frequency of fasting hyperglycemia. Among those with normal fasting glucose levels, risk of diabetes is quite likely higher than in persons who have poorer glucose tolerance, but the degree of this increased risk is unknown. Moreover, to the degree that this increased risk was really appreciable it would soon be reflected in a higher subsequent incidence of fasting hyperglycemia. Results of glucose tolerance tests are difficult to compare unless conditions, methods, and criteria are fully standardized. There is no immediate prospect of such standardization.

For these and other reasons it is suggested that fasting hyperglycemia be the main index of comparison. In all age groups venous plasma values greater than 129 mg/100 ml could be regarded as abnormal. In some instances it might be useful to create also a borderline subgroup having values of about 115 to 129 mg/100 ml. Conventions might require that all values of 130 to 149 be confirmed at least once. Adequate data are now available (eg, Cooper, 1973) for converting blood glucose values determined by other methods to these standards. This would include capillary specimens, whole blood specimens, and results with the various laboratory procedures used for determining blood glucose. Corrections for the varying ratios of diagnosed to undiagnosed cases could be made by testing a sample of modest size with no apparent diabetes in each of the various age groups. In some circumstances it would also be necessary to test elements of the group with diagnosed diabetes to estimate the number who have never had abnormal fasting levels.

6
CHAPTER

Mortality

Two of the better general reviews on the subject of mortality are the chapter by Marks and Krall in Joslin's book (Marble, et al, 1971) and the report of the workgroup on mortality of the National Diabetes Commission of the United States (Tokuhata, et al, 1976). Several aspects are well reviewed in the publication of Grönberg, et al (1967).

To what extent does diabetes shorten life? Intraindividual variation is very great. Death may occur as early as a few weeks after onset when, for example, ketoacidosis is the first detected manifestation. I recently saw a patient in whom onset of diabetes had occurred at age 51. At age 97, she had survived for 46 years, about twice as long as a 51 year old nondiabetic would have been expected to survive. Generalizations therefore have limited application. Nevertheless, well-collected data on mortality have considerable potential for promoting a better understanding of the nature of diabetes and the factors that increase or decrease prevalence, morbidity, and survival.

HISTORY AND METHODS OF STUDY

One of the best sources of information on mortality in diabetes is the data assembled by E. P. Joslin and his associates, which have been set forth in eleven editions of Joslin's book. The first edition appeared in 1916 and the most recent in 1971 (Marble, et al). The physicians at the Joslin Clinic have for many years received substantial assistance in their mortality studies through collaborations with the statistical and medical departments of the Metropolitan Insurance Company. These collaborators have included Dublin, Marks, and Entmacher. Joslin also undertook pioneering cooperative projects with Lombard of the Massachusetts Department of Public Health. Their publication of 1926 was one of the first to use the term epidemiology in reference to diabetes-related studies. In a subsequent publication (Lombard and Joslin, 1947) they showed that the average age at death of Massachusetts diabetics had increased from 52 years in 1900 to 67 years in 1945. They also added to knowledge of the sensitivity and specificity of death certificates as an instrument for quantitative and qualitative studies of diabetes mortality. They found, for example, that very commonly the death certificates of diabetics did not mention diabetes.

Systematic collection of death registration data on diabetes began in the 19th century, and in some localities statistics were gathered as early as 1850. By 1901 a considerable degree of international standardization had developed with respect to methods of death registration. Some of the early data on diabetes were summarized in the book of Lepine (1909). They included early observations in France of Bertillon whose publication of 1912 is cited below. In their landmark paper of 1924 Emerson and Larimore drew heavily on mortality data by locality and in localities over time. These included observations in Berlin, Paris, and New York City. Williamson (1909) was one of the first to use mortality data in studying the geographic and environmental determinants of diabetes prevalence. He and Saundby (1908) evaluated and compared data in Britain and many other parts of the world. Other important publications on mortality by country or locality included those of Hoffman (1922), Gore (1927), and Mills (1930). In 1948 Moriyama reviewed some of the problems that had arisen in collecting and interpreting data from registration of deaths. These problems will be discussed below.

In 1958, Hargreaves published a paper on the "Epidemiology of Diabetes Mellitus", in which he cited differences in diabetes mortality rates among countries and among regions of Britain as possible clues to the etiology of diabetes. The further standardization of methods in death registration under sponsorship of the World Health Organization was an important development of more recent years. Recent worldwide statistics gathered by WHO will be presented below. Moriyama, Langberg (1971), and others at the US National Center for Health Statistics have contributed substantially in this field.

The development of modern epidemiologic methods has made it possible to evaluate the death registration procedures and to measure diabetes mortality rates and causes by other means. These have included population-based studies of the kind performed in Scandinavia by Grönberg, et al (1967) and Westlund (1969), and follow-up studies of the type carried out by Goodkin (1975) in insurance applicants. Important studies on causes of mortality include population-based studies of Keen and Jarrett (1975) in Bedford, by Bennett, et al (1976a) in Pima Indians, and by the investigators studying the population of Framingham, Massachusetts (Garcia, et al, 1974).

Among the methods used to study causes of death are data from hospital records and from reports of autopsies. Because of the special character of the population of diabetics dying in hospitals, these data should be interpreted with some caution, but on the whole they have been informative. The results of Bell (1952) in a very large autopsy series, and those from other autopsy studies are discussed elsewhere in this volume, particularly in the section on large-vessel disease. Mimura (1970) and others (Tsuji and Wada, 1970; Baba, et al, 1975) have called attention to the profound geographic differences in the results of such autopsy studies. Among the more informative reviews of the now considerable literature on autopsy studies are Joslin's book (Marble, et al, 1971) and the publications of Mimura (1970) and Kurihara, et al (1970).

Causes of death in diabetes differ substantially with environment. For this reason it will be quite important to gather more and better mortality data in diverse populations. This was well demonstrated in the volumes on diabetes in Asia edited by Tsuji and Wada (1970) and Baba, et al (1975).

The Death Registration Process

One of the main instruments for appraising the quantitative and qualitative aspects of diabetes mortality is the registration of deaths. Certification is to a considerable degree standardized by international conventions under the coordinating sponsorship of the World Health Organization. But it is important to keep in mind that these conventions have changed over time. Prior to the sixth revision of the international system of classification (1948), diabetes was assigned as the "underlying" cause of death in most deaths of diabetics. In a study by Altshuler in 1940, for example, it was found that 65% of deaths of diabetics in Detroit were assigned to diabetes. In this same group only 39% of these same deaths were assigned to diabetes by the physicians who completed the medical records of these diabetics. The more recent conventions of classification have resulted in a considerable increase in the portion of deaths of diabetics that are assigned to other causes (eg, ischemic heart disease, stroke). In Britain a change of conventions introduced in 1938 and implemented in 1939 and 1940 resulted in a substantial reduction (about one third) in the portion of deaths of diabetics that were assigned to diabetes itself. Changes of this type make it difficult to evaluate trends over time. Applications of conversion factors make possible very crude comparisons, but the effects of changes in conventions are not the same in different populations and different circumstances. In some populations the changes produced by the criteria introduced in 1949 were relatively modest. In others a very great effect was evident. In New York City diabetes mortality rates fell to about 45% of the previous level with the sixth revision of the international standards (Erchardt and Weiner, 1950). On a national basis it was found that in 1950 about 44% of deaths that would formerly have been assigned to diabetes were being assigned to other causes (Joslin, et al, 1959).

It has also become apparent that substantial differences exist among physicians and groups of physicians in criteria of assignment of underlying and contributing causes, and in the frequency with which known diabetes is mentioned on the death certificates. A physician's handbook on medical certification (US National Center for Health Statistics, 1970) is available, but not much used. A similar guide has been published by WHO (1952). In most statistical reports only cases in which diabetes is assigned as the underlying cause of death have been counted. In recent years diabetes has been assigned as a cause of death in roughly one third of those cases in which it has been mentioned on the death certificate, but this proportion varies considerably by locality as indicated below.

In the well-known studies on the Joslin Clinic patients, the specific cause of death has been cited, and "diabetes" is not used as one of these specific designations. Often data of these kinds have been inappropriately compared with death registration data that have included a substantial portion in which death was attributed to "diabetes". Despite these problems, death registration data have been a highly useful source of information. But these vagaries of practice require attention and caution in interpreting such data. These problems are discussed in detail below, in a section on death registration data.

LONGEVITY AND RISK OF MORTALITY

In Joslin Clinic patients Hirohata, et al (1967) found that mortality was quite uncommon in the first fifteen years of juvenile diabetes. Between the 15th and 25th year, mortality rates were very high; even so, 82% of these Joslin Clinic patients with juvenile-onset diabetes survived for at least twenty-five years. Degree of excessive mortality in adult-onset cases was also strongly related to duration of known diabetes, but in this latter group the sharp rise began after five years rather than fifteen years. Among the factors that may account for this difference is that, on the average, onset of diabetes probably exceeds discovery of diabetes by about a decade in maturity-onset cases, while duration of occult diabetes is much shorter in those with onset in childhood. Another factor is that susceptibility to atherosclerosis is much greater in older persons. Survival was somewhat better for cases first seen in 1944 than for those first seen in 1939, but no significant further improvement in longevity was seen in those with discovery of diabetes in 1959.

In interpreting these and other studies on Joslin Clinic patients, these special circumstances should be kept in mind. Numbers are usually large and data are well collected. On the other hand, these patients are not a representative sample of the diabetics in the populations from which they are drawn. Comparisons with results of other investigators suggest that the effects of these sources of bias are modest, but they should be kept in mind. Patients followed from the beginning by the Joslin Clinic are particularly advantaged, while patients referred to the Joslin Clinic for complications, difficulties in control, etc, may be disadvantaged with respect to longevity because of these problems. In

general, the more famous and prestigious the clinic, the more there are potentialities for bias relating to selection.

Nevertheless, these studies of the Joslin group and their collaborators have
provided many useful insights. Results of Kessler (1971) are illustrative. He
studied mortality in 21,447 Joslin Clinic patients followed from four to thirty
years. During this period 10,066 deaths were recorded. Increased risk of mortality (as compared to age-matched elements of the general population) was
greatest in the fourth decade. Probably this was mainly because the disparity
between diabetics and nondiabetics in rates of coronary disease is maximal at
this age, and because death from glomerulosclerosis is also common at this age
in long-duration juvenile diabetics. In males (all ages), observed rates of death
exceeded by 66% those expected for age-matched males of the general population (standardized mortality ratio of 1.66). In females the standardized mortality ratio was 2.18. But these ratios varied greatly depending on age, age of onset
of diabetes, and duration of diabetes. In elderly males this ratio was only
slightly in excess of unity, while in young diabetics of long duration it reached
levels as high as 20 in some cohorts. In general, results of Kessler were similar
to those of Hirohata, et al, but there were some differences even though both
studied Joslin Clinic patients. For example, in maturity-onset patients studied
by Kessler, little effect of duration of diabetes was observed. Kessler appropriately attributed these to differences in the methods employed. In his study, all
Joslin Clinic patients from Massachusetts were included, while in studies of
Hirohata cases were excluded that had not been studied from the beginning of
their illness. One of several possibilities is that subjects later referred to Joslin
Clinic contained a high proportion of short-duration diabetes with complications increasing risk of death. There are advantages in both of these
approaches, but in some respects bias is less in the group followed from the
onset of disease.

Further details on mortality and longevity in the Joslin Clinic patients are
presented in the informative publication of Marks (1965) and in the excellent
chapter of Marks and Krall (1971) in the Joslin textbook.

When expressed in years, survival is longer in diabetics with early onset.
When longevity is expressed as percentage of normal life expectancy it has
usually been found to be greater in patients with older onset (Bale and Entmacher, 1977). When mortality is expressed as a rate at a certain age compared
to rates of age-matched elements of the general populations, these standardized
mortality ratios are typically in the range of 2 or 3 in patients with maturity-
onset diabetes and 5 to 10 in childhood-onset cases. When mortality is
expressed as rate per year, such rates are much higher in maturity-onset
diabetes because they are older and risk of death from factors other than
diabetes is so strongly related to age. Marks (1965) reported that in diabetics
annual mortality per 1,000 rose from less than 1 in the first decade of life to
greater than 80 in persons 65 to 74 years of age. Of diabetics in whom the
disease begins before age 30, about 90% survive more than ten years. When
onset occurs between 60 and 74 years of age, less than 40% survive ten years.

Even so, mortality risks in relation to those in age-matched nondiabetics are much higher in the younger diabetics.

Two highly informative studies on mortality have been performed in Scandinavia by Grönberg, et al (1967) in Sweden and by Westlund (1966,1969) in Oslo. As compared to the Joslin Clinic patients, the group of maturity-onset diabetics studied by Grönberg was in some respects more representative of the general population of diabetics in the localities from which they were drawn. These Swedish investigators explain, however, that the samples are by no means perfect representations. Patients (3,759) were from four county hospitals. The organization of health services in these districts and the circumstances of the study were such that a high percentage of all known adult diabetics residing in these districts were identified. Children were also included in the study, but this sample was small and much less representative. Mortality was studied in a group in which 398 deaths were observed during 16,440 observation years. Incidence of death was increased about sixfold in childhood-onset cases, but only about 30% (standardized mortality ratio of 1.3) in diabetics with onset after the fourth decade. These investigators also studied for all of Sweden data from death certificates for the period of 1961 through 1963. They concluded that the excess mortality from diabetes did not exceed 15%, but pointed out that excess was much higher in the group with youth-onset diabetes.

The effect of diabetes was also relatively benign in Denmark in studies of Dryer and Hey (1953,1954). They found a standardized mortality ratio of 1.8 in males and 1.7 in females. In comparing and evaluating such data from different populations one needs to take into account several factors: the distribution of age and duration of diabetes, the method of ascertainment of cases, and other aspects of methods, definitions, and criteria. Some factors affecting results when death registration data are employed will be discussed below.

Bale and Entmacher (1977) estimated life expectancy of diabetics in Iowa using death certificate data. Average life expectancy for diabetic females was judged to be about 6.7 years shorter than in all females. In diabetic males average life expectancy was reduced by about 9.1 years. The degree of these differences inversely relates to age of onset of diabetes. Results in Pennsylvania were similar when analyzed by these authors.

Westlund (1966,1969) studied mortality in 3,832 diabetic residents of Oslo who had been discharged for the first time with a diagnosis of diabetes from thirteen hospital departments. Follow-up periods ranged from six to thirty-six years. In this group the effect of diabetes was less benign than in the studies of Grönberg, and of Dreyer and Hey. During the period 1956–1961 the standardized mortality ratios of these Oslo diabetics (based on data from age-matched elements of the general population of Oslo) were 2.9 for males and 2.6 for females. These ratios were very high in diabetics from 5–39 years of age, 10.0 in males and 7.5 in females. But even in diabetics over 70 years of age, ratios considerably exceeded the standard of unity (2.3 in both sexes). In the age range 40-69, ratios were 3.9 for men and 4.4 for women. The circumstances of these observations suggest that although the study group consisted of patients discharged from hospitals, it was probably a fairly satisfactory representation of the universe of known diabetics in Oslo. It does seem likely, however, that risk of death is lower in the small minority of diabetics who have not been in a hospital since diagnosis nor at the time of diagnosis.

Diabetes mortality in Birmingham, England was studied by Hayward and Lucena (1965). This excellent publication is too little known. They followed 5,545 diabetics for periods up to fifteen years. The number lost to follow-up was quite small. There were 1,325 known deaths and 32,816 exposure years. A small minority of diabetics who had care outside the National Insurance System were not included. The authors were aware that this probably influenced certain aspects of their results. Degree of increased risk of mortality was strongly related (inversely) to age and several other factors. On the whole, increased risk of mortality was only moderate in diabetics over 49 years of age. In these older diabetics the risk of death was only increased about one third. Indeed, it could not be demonstrated with certainty by these data that mortality risk was elevated in elderly diabetics. These investigators pointed out that the group of fee-paying diabetics excluded from these studies probably included a disproportionately higher number of severely ill patients. The inclusion of this latter group would probably have raised the mortality rates somewhat.

The number of cases under 40 was small and this sample of young patients may have been less representative than the sample of older patients. But the data for younger diabetics showed the same trend as in other studies. Risk of death was increased several fold in youth-onset diabetics as compared to age-matched elements of the general population. Several other aspects of the results of Haywood and Lucena will be discussed below, including data on causes of death, and effects of personal characteristics and of types of therapy.

Insurance Company Statistics

Some of the most informative data on diabetes mortality have been gathered by the insurance industry. In addition to the aforementioned data of the Metropolitan Company and of Hayward and Lucena, other important results include those of George Goodkin (Goodkin and Wolloch, 1968; Goodkin, 1971; Goodkin, et al, 1975) at the Equitable Life Insurance Society. These investigators (Goodkin, et al, 1975) studied 10,538 diabetic applicants for life insurance including *both* accepted and rejected applicants. There were 83,687 exposure years and 1,478 deaths. Follow-up ranged from one to twenty years and averaged 7.9 years. Only 5.9% of applicants were excluded from the study because they could not be traced to death or completion of the study. Eighty-nine percent were males. Average age at entry was 42, with a range of 15 to 60.

Standardized mortality ratio for the diabetics was 3.35. The degree of increased risk was strongly related (inversely) to age at application. The standardized mortality ratio was 11.08 for those who entered the study in their third decade, and it declined progressively with age, reaching 2.64 in the sixth decade. In the group of 7,638 rejected applicants (all ages), the mortality ratio was more than twice as high (3.95) as that in accepted applicants (1.67). This difference of substantial degree between these two groups prevailed at every age level. Criteria for acceptance, discussed further below, included judgments about status of control and presence of complications. In all age groups mortality was strongly related to duration of diabetes, but the strength of effect of duration was greatest in young diabetics. At all ages studied, standardized mortality risk imcreased in the first fifteen to twenty years of diabetes, after which it plateaued. Tables 22–24 show some of these data.

Entmacher (1972) reviewed results of his own studies at the Metropolitan Life Insurance company and those of Barch at the Lincoln National Company, and found them quite similar to those of Goodkin. However, the effect of duration of diabetes was not so impressive: in the group of Barch a peaking of mortality risk was observed after seven to twelve years of diabetes. Results in the studies of Entmacher were similar in this respect. Several factors might account for the less apparent effects of duration in the latter studies, as compared to those of Goodkin. Goodkin's numbers were larger, particularly with respect to the subgroup with long duration. Age distributions were different in these studies, and Goodkin's group was probably more representative because he followed a large segment of the universe of rejected applicants. Study of all these and other data suggest the possibility that standardized mortality ratios plateau in juvenile-onset cases at about twenty years; and in maturity-onset cases a peak occurs at about ten years. It should be kept in mind that these ratios are strongly affected by mortality rates in the denominator of the ratio (age-matched elements of control populations). The lessening ratios with age and duration are in part the result of sharp age-related rises in the mortality rates of the control groups. When known duration of adult-onset diabetes is ten years, actual duration is typically about twenty years. Table 22 shows data of Goodkin, et al (1975), relating mortality risk to age of onset corrected for duration and vice versa. Here the mortality ratio is expressed as a percentage of the standard (eg, a twofold excess is 200%).

In studies of smaller North American groups of insured diabetics, results were similar to those of Goodkin (Cochran and Buck, 1961; Briehaupt, 1961; Pollock, et al, 1967). The Metropolitan Life Insurance Company summarized in its May 1973 *Statistical Bulletin* some of its mortality statistics, covering the same group described by Entmacher (1972). In all these studies of insured diabetics, numbers of women have been small.

Other Studies

Pell and D'Alonzo (1970) studied mortality in diabetic employees of the DuPont Company. During a ten-year period 25.4% of diabetics died, while only 9.7% of a matched group of nondiabetic employees died. As in the Insurance studies, increased risk of mortality (as compared to age-matched controls) was much greater in the younger diabetics and in persons requiring insulin.

In his publication of 1971 Knowles reported his experience on longevity in a group of childhood-onset diabetics treated in Cincinnati, Ohio. He also summarized studies of other investigators on this subject, including the experience of Larsson and Sterky (1962) in Sweden and that of Hirohata, et al (1967) in the Joslin Clinic patients. Patterns of longevity were quite similar in all three groups. About 80% survived twenty years, but only about half survived more than three decades, and only about half reached their 40th birthdays.

Factors Influencing Mortality

Oakley, et al (1974) and Ryan, et al (1970) studied large groups of diabetics who had survived for very long periods. In both groups the propensity to leanness was striking. The patients of Oakley, et al (1974) who had survived more than forty years of diabetes had particularly low blood pressures.

Nondiabetic females enjoy a high degree of immunity to coronary disease prior to the sixth decade and a lesser degree in the sixth and seventh decades. In diabetic women this immunity is completely or almost completely lost. In diabetics risk of death from coronary disease is high and approximately equal in the sexes, even in young adults. Data on risk of death from all causes are not ideal, but it appears to be still somewhat higher in men. The higher death rates for diabetes observed in women in many countries seem to be mainly the result of a higher prevalence of diabetes in women. In Oslo, however, the rates of mortality were studied using as a denominator the number of diabetics at risk, rather than the traditional method of confining the analysis to number of deaths per 100,000 of the general population. Rates of death were increased more in females by diabetes, but rates of death were still somewhat higher in the diabetic males than in the diabetic females. In the Joslin Clinic diabetics, survival was very slightly better in males but mortality rates (as percentage of the number of diabetics at risk) were quite similar for the two sexes (Hirohata, et al, 1967).

The extent to which observed racial differences in mortality rates of diabetics are genetic or environmental is not yet clear. Rates of fatal vascular disease are much higher in Indian than in black diabetics of South Africa (Jackson, et al, 1970). Probably this is mainly the result of nongenetic factors such as diet and exercise levels, but significant racial factors cannot be excluded. American black diabetics have rates of vascular disease similar to those of US white diabetics. Japanese diabetics appear to lose their immunity to coronary diseases when they take on Western ways. Diabetic Pima Indians have less coronary disease than American diabetic whites (Ingelfinger, et al, 1976). These racial and geographic factors are discussed elsewhere in this volume.

The influence of age of onset and duration of diabetes have been discussed above. Further data of Marks and Krall (1971) are presented in Table 23. It is not entirely clear why the rate of death is especially high in youth-onset diabetes. Some of the factors involved are discussed in greater detail in other sections of this book. The greater hyperglycemia in youth-onset cases is probably an

TABLE 22   Diabetic Mortality Study of Goodkin 1951–1970: Relationship of Risk to Age and Duration of Diabetes

DURATION OF DIABETES AT TIME OF APPLICATION (YR)	ENTRANTS	EXPOSURE YEARS	ACTUAL DEATHS	EXPECTED DEATHS	A/E RATIO*
Ages 1–19					
0–5	200	1,662.32	7	1.49	470%
6–10	101	816.16	1	.69	144%
11–14	48	457.00	4	.42	968%
15–19	11	87.00	0	.08	
20 & over	0				
ALL	360	3,022.48	12	2.68	448%
Ages 20–29					
0–5	657	5,713.96	35	5.86	598%
6–10	451	3,983.54	39	3.95	988%
11–14	280	2,524.01	46	2.60	1,766%
15–19	208	1,722.73	28	1.76	1,585%
20 & over	110	1,046.25	18	1.10	1,636%
ALL	1,705	14,990.49	166	15.27	1,087%
Ages 30–39					
0–5	1,078	9,615.59	65	20.79	313%
6–10	425	4,113.23	35	9.41	372%
11–14	235	2,412.70	44	5.38	818%
15–19	251	2,326.25	46	5.08	905%
20 & over	268	2,463.17	61	5.38	1,134%
ALL	2,257	20,930.94	251	46.04	542%
Ages 40–49					
0–5	1,695	12,826.38	193	65.90	293%
6–10	559	4,730.91	85	25.17	337%
11–14	212	1,883.53	34	10.08	337%
15–19	182	1,644.59	36	9.04	398%
20 & over	233	1,830.01	39	9.38	434%
ALL	2,881	22,915.42	387	119.57	324%
Ages 50–59					
0–5	1,477	10,323.43	225	106.84	211%
6–10	445	3,087.11	106	33.16	320%
11–14	164	1,183.33	46	11.36	405%
15–19	119	887.58	40	9.44	424%
20 & over	110	704.00	28	6.70	337%
ALL	2,315	16,185.45	445	167.50	266%

168

Duration of Diabetes at Time of Application (Yr)	Entrants	Exposure Years	Actual Deaths	Expected Deaths	A/E Ratio*
Ages 60 and over					
0–5	478	2,768.57	103	48.67	212%
6–10	165	1,030.41	46	19.78	233%
11–14	52	253.91	16	4.86	329%
15–19	52	316.00	24	6.08	395%
20 & over	52	242.91	10	3.87	226%
ALL	799	4,611.80	199	83.26	239%
All ages—Duration unknown					
	220	1,031.14	18	6.32	285%

Source: Goodkin, et al (1975).
Note: These follow-up data on life insurance applicnts include both accepted and rejected applicants.
*A/E—Ratio of actual to expected deaths.

important contributing factor, but the available evidence in this respect leaves much to be desired.

Degree of Hyperglycemia

Much of the evidence linking level of glycemia and risk of mortality is indirect. The insurance company studies show that those who require insulin seem to have higher mortality rates even after correction for age and duration of diabetes (Goodkin, et al, 1975; Cochran and Buck, 1961). This was confirmed in a large industrial population studied by Pell and D'Alonzo (1970). Age-corrected data from Birmingham, England (Malins, 1966) and from Framingham, Massachusetts (Garcia, et al, 1974) also show this. In general, blood glucose levels are higher in patients in whom insulin is required. There is little reason to believe that insulin itself increases risk of mortality in childhood-onset cases. In the study of Goodkin, et al (1975) mortality was not related to dosage of insulin in youth-onset cases. Table 24 shows the strong relationship of mortality risk to type of treatment. In animals, effects of degree of hyperglycemia have been variable depending on species and conditions, but there is some evidence that both large- and small-vessel disease is proportional to degree of hyperglycemia (eg, Kalant, et al, 1964; Bloodworth, et al, 1973; Mauer, et al, 1975; Cahill, et al, 1976; Lundbaek, 1974; Engerman et al, 1977).

Data of Goodkin, et al (1975) are especially persuasive with respect to the relationship of blood glucose levels to risk of mortality. *At the time of entry* into the study, level of control of glycemia was judged by a series of specific criteria. Those judged initially to have poor control had death rates more than twice as high as the other cases. Study of the other characteristics of these two

169

TABLE 23 Principal Causes of Death among Diabetic Patients by Age at Onset of Diabetes and Duration of Disease

PERCENT IN SPECIFIED CATEGORY

CAUSE OF DEATH	UNDER AGE 20 AT ONSET				AGES 20–39 AT ONSET				AGES 40–59 AT ONSET				AGES 60 AND OVER AT ONSET			
	DURATION OF DIABETES (YEARS)															
	<10	10–19	20–29	30+	<10	10–19	20–29	30+	<10	10–19	20–29	30+	<10	10–19	20–29	30+
All Causes	100	100	100	100	100	100	100	100	100	100	100	100	100	100	100	100
Cardiovascular-renal	21	78	84	81	38	77	82	80	66	79	80	75	72	78	77	100
Large vessels	13	16	29	56	30	51	66	74	62	73	75	73	69	75	74	75
Cardiac	3	15	23	46	23	44	58	61	52	58	57	49	51	52	46	75
Cerebral	10	2	5	9	2	5	7	9	8	12	15	19	14	18	17	
Other*			1	1	5	2	1	3	2	3	3	5	4	5	11	
Small vessels	8	61	55	25	8	26	16	6	4	6	5	3	3	2	4	25
Nephropathy	5	55	46	22	3	17	10	4	1	3	2		1	1	1	
Other renal	3	6	9	2	5	9	6	2	3	2	3	3	2	2	2	25
Diabetic coma	28	4	1	2	3	2		2		1	1	1		1		
Cancer	15		1	5	13	6	8	7	19	11	9	8	17	10	6	
Infections	8	10	5	6	20	8	3	6	4	4	5	7	5	7	9	
Violence	10	3	3	3	8	1	2	3	3	1	2	3	1	2	5	
Other and unknown	18	5	6	3	17	6	5	2	8	4	3	5	4	3	3	
Number of deaths	39	179	285	179	60	379	467	354	842	2,193	1,287	306	1,406	1,053	171	4

Source: Marks and Krall (1971).
Note: Experience of Joslin Clinic, Boston, Mass., 1956–1968. Includes all deaths reported up to December 31, 1968.
*Chiefly arteriosclerosis without additional details and diabetic gangrene.

TABLE 24 Diabetic Mortality Study of Goodkin 1951–1970: Relationship of Mortality to Type of Treatment

Type of Treatment	Entrants	Exposure Years	Expected Deaths	Actual Deaths	A/E Ratio* (%)
Diet only, no medication	1,659	13,374.75	212	95.52	222
Oral medication	2,582	13,759.05	210	87.45	240
Insulin	4,976	46,392.37	872	194.77	447
Insulin & oral medication	102	665.82	6	2.48	242
Unknown	1,219	9,495.73	178	60.42	295
ALL	10,538	83,687.72	1,478	440.64	335

Source: Goodkin, et al (1975).
*A/E—ratio of actual to expected deaths.

TABLE 25 Diabetic Mortality Study of Goodkin 1951–1970: Relationship of Control of Diabetes at Entry to Mortality Risk

Type of Control	Entrants	Controlled* Exposure Years	Actual Deaths	Expected Deaths	A/E Ratio (%)
Insulin, < 50 units	875	8,874.57	82	40.41	203
50-74 units	326	3,039.60	28	8.48	330
≥ 75 units	65	681.34	5	2.36	212
Amount unknown	3	22.00	0	0.09	
All with insulin	1,269	12,617.51	115	51.34	224
Unknown	145	1,265.22	7	6.87	102
Insulin & oral medication	31	216.00	1	0.99	101
Oral medication only	830	4,571.83	37	24.21	153
Diet only	625	5,178.93	31	31.15	100
ALL	2,900	23,849.49	191	114.56	167
		Poor Control†			
Insulin, < 50 units	523	4,917.12	76	17.84	426
50-74 units	299	2,621.14	36	5.83	614
≥ 75 units	106	990.58	15	3.08	487
Amount unknown	18	107.82	1	.25	400
All with insulin	946	8,636.66	128	27.00	474
Unknown	86	843.42	16	5.02	319
Insulin & oral medication	21	129.00	0	0.38	
Oral medication only	118	764.51	9	4.14	217
Diet only	90	905.49	25	7.03	356
ALL	1,261	11,279.08	178	43.57	409

Source: Goodkin, et al, 1975.
Note: See text for further explanation.
*Issued cases.
†Cases declined for the following reasons: (1) excessive glycosuria or poor blood sugar test on examination only; (2) history of recent high blood sugar; (3) history of coma or insulin shock only.

groups (eg, age, age of onset, type of therapy, duration of disease) failed to account for more than a small part of the excessive mortality in patients with poor control. These results are not decisive, but suggest strongly that degree of glycemia is an independent risk factor for mortality. Table 25 summarizes data of Goodkin (1971) on the relationship of control to mortality in those matched for type of treatment.

Many researchers have attempted to study the effects of degree of control of hyperglycemia on outcome, including mortality. Conflicting results have been obtained. None has been decisive, but a majority suggest that risk of morbidity and mortality is related to degree of glycemia.

Gottlieb (1974) studied longevity in Joslin Clinic patients, and its relationship to several factors. She found that persons who reported hypoglycemic episodes (reactions to insulin) had a significantly increased longevity. Ryan, et al (1970), Rogers and Holcomb (1960), and Deckert, et al (1975) thought their patients with great longevity had had on the whole exceptionally good control of hyperglycemia. Oakley, et al (1974) were not certain whether this was the case in their long survivors.

Kaplan and Feinstein (1973,1974) have identified and analyzed many of the problems in designing and interpreting studies of outcome in diabetes and the factors to which it relates. The importance of matching for factors such as co-morbidity was emphasized. Most studies attempting to relate degree of gly-cemia and outcome have been difficult to interpret because of defects of design of the types described by Kaplan and Feinstein.

Major Causes of Death

Although death from ketosis is more common in youth-onset cases, in most affluent societies this factor is no longer a leading cause of death. In the Joslin Clinic patients, it accounted for only 4% of deaths in patients with onset before 20 years (Marks and Krall, 1971). The studies of insurance companies cited above also confirm that diabetic coma is a significant but not major cause of death in childhood-onset cases. The US National Commission Study (Ganda and Marble, 1976) found that about 10% of deaths (all ages) were from ketosis in the group in which diabetes was assigned as the underlying cause. Since diabetes is now assigned as a cause of death in less than one third of deaths of known diabetics, ketoacidosis probably accounts for only about 3% of deaths of North American diabetics. In a youth-onset group ketosis probably accounts for 4% to 8% of deaths, although this portion is much higher in those who die in childhood. In some societies a very considerable portion of insulin-dependent diabetics die of diabetic coma. In a group of Bantu diabetics studied at autopsy in South Africa, about one third died of coma (Bhoola, 1976).

In affluent Western societies the main cause of death in diabetics is ischemic (coronary) heart disease. Details will be given in a special section on that subject. As early as 1944 Beardwood had shown that arteriosclerotic heart disease was a very common cause of death in diabetes. Several autopsy studies before and after that time showed the high level of coronary artery disease in diabetics. Data of Kessler (1971) suggest that most of the excess mortality of American diabetics is attributable to this factor alone. Death from coronary disease was increased by a factor of 1.66 in men and 2.18 in women. Studies in Framingham yielded similar results (Garcia, et al, 1974). In Oslo, Westlund (1969) also found that this factor accounted for most of the excess in mortality with diabetes. In diabetic men under 70 years of age, fatal coronary heart disease was 4.3 times more common than in controls. The rate was increased by a factor of 8.6 in women! In the insured populations of America rates of coronary-related fatalities have also been high in diabetics, but generally these excesses were more modest in degree except for the very excessive rates in the fourth and fifth decades (Goodkin, et al, 1975). However, it seems very likely that some of the mortality attributable to coronary disease in these data is hidden among deaths assigned to "diabetes". Data from the National Center for Health Statistics (Langberg, 1971) support this contention. On death certificates of persons 45 to 64 years of age in whom the underlying cause of death assigned was "diabetes", arteriosclerotic heart disease was mentioned 12 times more frequently as a contributing cause than on certificates on which diabetes was not assigned as the underlying cause of death. The relationship was confirmed by examining it in the reverse manner for this same age group (45–64). When arteriosclerotic heart disease was the underlying cause of death, diabetes was mentioned 2.1 times more frequently as a contributing cause than in certificates listing other underlying causes of death.

Moriyama, et al (1966) found in a study of death certificates and from supplementary clinical data that about 14% of Americans dying of heart disease had diabetes. But this latter group represents only a modest portion of all those who have heart disease and diabetes at death. In 1968, heart disease was cited as a contributing factor on 57% of those death certificates citing diabetes as the underlying cause. Additional certificates (unknown number) doubtless cited both diabetes and heart disease as contributing factors. Moreover, it is well known that a substantial percentage of patients with ischemic heart disease have undiagnosed diabetes; and often the death certificates of previously diagnosed diabetics do not make any mention of diabetes.

High rates of mortality from coronary disease in diabetics is mainly attributable to the high prevalence of coronary atherosclerosis, but there are other contributing factors. For example, most studies have shown that diabetics with myocardial infarction are more likely to die during such episodes than are nondiabetics. This is discussed further in Chapter 10 under heart disease. Even those diabetics with little coronary disease have congestive failure more commonly than nondiabetics (Hamby, et al, 1974).

Diet appears to play a major role in determining risk of fatal large-vessel disease. This is reviewed in detail in the section on vascular disease. Probably the high-salt diet observed in many parts of Japan contributes to the high rate of stroke in the diabetics of some localities of that country. Rates of fatal coronary disease seem to be high in groups of diabetics that consume high levels of

173

saturated fat, and low in localities where intake of saturated fat is low. Many other factors, such as exercise and smoking, may influence risk of fatal large-vessel disease in diabetics. The possible role of hyperglycemia itself in accelerating atherosclerosis will be discussed in other sections including that on atherosclerosis in Chapter 10. Present evidence is not entirely decisive but does suggest that the degree of hyperglycemia probably affects the rate of atherogenesis, at least under some conditions.

In diabetics of some other societies the excess of deaths from ischemic heart disease has not been great. In Sweden, Grönberg, et al (1967) found the rate of death from coronary disease only slightly excessive in diabetics. In Birmingham, England diabetics the mortality rate from "diseases of the circulatory system" was about 80% above controls in women and about 60% greater in men (Hayward and Lucena, 1965). In these two studies some additional diabetics dying from coronary disease may have been hidden in the group in which death was ascribed to "diabetes".

Interpretation of data on death from coronary disease is complicated by incomplete standardization among physicians and groups of physicians with respect to nomenclature, conventions, and concepts. In identical cases of coronary disease some physicians would assign ischemic heart disease as the underlying cause of death, while others would cite "diabetes" as the underlying cause. Another problem is that idiopathic congestive heart failure is common in diabetics, sometimes secondary to coronary disease and sometimes not. This is discussed in detail in Chapter 10 in the section on heart disease. These cases of idiopathic congestive heart failure have usually been called ischemic heart disease unless an autopsy has revealed unobstructed coronary arteries. But most such cases are not autopsied, and death certificates are sometimes completed before autopsy. There are also differences in the priority assigned to hypertension as an underlying cause of death in diabetics with hypertension and ischemic heart disease. Very commonly diabetics have a terminal illness that includes severe renal failure and either severe heart disease or stroke. In these cases, it is often difficult to select which cause should be underlying and which contributing. Doubtless there are differences among physicians and groups of physicians in how they code such events. These differences are mitigated to some extent by international standards of practice by coders who convert the physician's conclusion to the statistical data. But this standardization does not fully erase or correct the effect of poor standardization of data supplied by the physicians. Among physicians, knowledge is quite variable concerning the standard guidelines for completing death certificates. In some countries a substantial share of deaths are not certified by a physician. These considerations should be kept in mind in interpreting mortality data. Some investigators (eg, Kessler) have analyzed the deaths assigned to "diabetes" and reallocated them to more specific causes such as ketoacidosis or glomerulosclerosis, while others have not done so. On the other hand, Gillum, et al (1976) found death certificates to be a fairly reliable source of information on heart disease, in a circumstance (Framingham, Massachusetts) where it was possible to compare the death certificate with information from other sources.

In North America and at least several countries of Western Europe, heart disease accounts for about half of deaths of diabetics. Marks and Krall (1971) report that in their Joslin Clinic diabetics, cardiac disease was assigned as the underlying cause of death in 54.6%. In 43.9% the underlying cause assigned was coronary disease. In their patients with onset of diabetes between 40 and 59 years of age the underlying cause of death was "cardiac" in 56%. Entmacher (1973) found in an insured population of diabetics that 55.4% who died had heart disease as the underlying cause. Tokuhata, et al (1976) has recently summarized mortality data from the US National Center for Health Statistics for 1968. Heart disease was assigned as the underlying cause of death in 40.1% of death certificates on which diabetes was also mentioned. "Diabetes" was assigned as the underlying cause of death in 29.9% of all certificates mentioning diabetes. Probably coronary disease was the actual underlying cause of some of this latter group. In this group in which diabetes was assigned as the underlying cause of death, heart disease was mentioned as a contributing factor in 57%; and in an additional 22.4% arteriosclerosis (anatomic location unspecified) was mentioned.

In Oslo (Westlund, 1969) only about one quarter of diabetics died of "coronary disease" but coronary disease was by far the leading cause of death in diabetics, and the rate of coronary mortality in diabetics was more than three times that in the Oslo general population.

In Britain coronary disease is also the leading cause of death in diabetics, but rates are not as high as in the United States (Hayward and Lucena, 1965). In a hospital study in Australia of a small series of deaths there was little difference in rates of death from coronary disease between diabetics and nondiabetics, but death occurred at an earlier age in the diabetics with coronary disease (Seymour and Phear, 1963).

In most countries of Asia (Tsuji and Wada, 1970) and Africa (Seftel, 1964; Tulloch, 1964) coronary disease is much less prevalent in diabetics than in US diabetics. This reflects the low rates of mortality from coronary disease in these areas. In special populations of Asians, such as Indians of South Africa, coronary disease is common (Jackson, 1972). These environmental differences are discussed more fully in the section on coronary disease.

Data from Israel (Najenson, et al, 1970,1973; Lavy, 1973) suggest that stroke mortality is considerably higher in diabetics than in nondiabetic Israelis. In certain parts of Japan, stroke is a somewhat more common cause of death in diabetics than coronary disease (Mimura, 1970; Goto and Fukuhara, 1968). Also, it appears that cerebral thrombosis is more common in Japanese diabetics than in nondiabetics, but more data are needed. Kuzuya and Kosaka (1970) found cerebral infarction more frequently in diabetics than nondiabetics in a small autopsy series. In most Western societies stroke is also a more common cause of death in diabetics than in nondiabetics. In the Oslo studies of Westlund (1969) death from "apoplexy" was about four times as common in diabetics under 70 as in controls. In contrast, Kessler's report on mortality in Joslin Clinic patients showed rates for cerebrovascular diseases that were only slightly higher in diabetics than controls. In diabetics of the West it is probable

175

that rates of mortality from stroke are diminished by high rates of mortality from coronary disease.

Other observations on stroke and diabetes, including accounts of autopsy studies, are summarized in the section on cerebrovascular disease in Chapter 10. In diabetics the degree of excess of stroke and death from stroke has been highly variable among populations. More data are needed, but it appears that in general the effect of diabetes on the cerebrovascular system is not so deleterious as its effect on the coronary vasculature.

Gangrene is seldom the main and direct cause of death in diabetes, but is often a contributory cause. Langberg (1971) reported that gangrene was mentioned on the death certificate 20 times more frequently when diabetes was the underlying cause of death.

Glomerulosclerosis as a cause of death is discussed in detail in the section of Chapter 10 on that subject. About half of childhood-onset cases die from nephropathy. In societies such as Japan where coronary disease is uncommon, the portion of childhood-onset cases dying of glomerulosclerosis may be even greater. Moreover, glomerulosclerosis is a more important cause of death in adult-onset diabetes in populations where coronary disease is uncommon (Tsuji and Wada, 1973; Baba, et al, 1975). In societies where medical care is poor the proportion of childhood-onset cases that die from ketoacidosis may be substantial, and consequently the fraction dying from kidney disease may be less. In Western affluent societies the fraction of deaths caused by glomerulosclerosis in cases with onset of diabetes after age 40 is typically less than 10%. In childhood-onset cases as indicated by data of Marks and Krall (1971), glomerulosclerosis accounts for most of the deaths that occur in the second and third decades of diabetes. Glomerulosclerosis is also a common cause of death in childhood-onset cases that survive for more than three decades, but in this subgroup death from macrovascular disease is somewhat more common. Table 23 shows the relationship of cause of death to age of onset of diabetes (Marks and Krall, 1971).

Severe macrovascular disease and severe nephropathy often contribute jointly to death, making it difficult to assign a single underlying cause. Pyelonephritis and other kidney disease often contribute substantially to fatal renal failure in diabetics, but most of these renal deaths are primarily attributable to glomerulosclerosis.

Other diseases found by Westlund (1969) to be especially common as a cause of death in diabetics included tuberculosis (increased by a factor of five) and cirrhosis of the liver (increased threefold). Kessler (1971) found little relationship of mortality from diabetes and cirrhosis. He did find a higher rate of tuberculosis-related deaths in diabetics (increased by a factor of 1.5). The strength of this latter relationship seems to be proportional to the rate of tuberculosis in the population. In some populations where tuberculosis is rife, it is a leading cause of death in diabetics, and rates of tuberculosis are far higher in diabetics than in nondiabetics. The relationships of diabetes to tuberculosis and liver diseases are discussed in detail in Chapter 7.

Are Death Rates from Some Causes Particularly Low in Diabetics?

There have been some reports of decreased death rates for certain diseases in which diabetes is cited on the death certificate. In the study of Kessler of deaths of Joslin Clinic patients, fatal cancer of the lung was less common in diabetics than in controls. It is not clear why rates observed in male diabetics were only 59% of those observed in male controls. One possibility is less smoking in the diabetics. No significant difference in rates of cancer of the lung were found by Westlund in Oslo. Smoking was slightly less in diabetics, but this difference was not statistically significant for diabetics and controls. In the studies of Kessler rates of mortality from peptic ulcer were slightly less in diabetics, but this difference was not statistically significant. Data of Westlund showed a trend in this respect, but differences were not great and may or may not have been significant. The relationship of diabetes to cancer and peptic ulcer are discussed further in Chapter 7.

DEATH REGISTRATION DATA

Sensitivity and Specificity

The general nature of the death registration process has been described above, including some considerations that require caution in the use of rates of registered deaths as indexes of prevalence of diabetes. Although few data are available on specificity of the citation of diabetes on death certificates, it does seem likely that, in most circumstances, only a very small portion of citations of diabetes are incorrect ("false positives"). Emerson and Larimore (1924) cited some older investigations of Cabot, who concluded that such false citations were then rare. With the recent advent of blood glucose testing on a massive scale, false or questionable citations are probably becoming more frequent, but this does not appear to have been a major problem in the past. Rather, the main problems have been undercitation, and variations in the degree of this under-reporting with time, place, and physician.

The problem is nicely illustrated by the recent study of Tokuhata, et al (1975). They found that in Pennsylvania 2.2% of deaths were attributed to diabetes (underlying cause), but diabetes was mentioned in 8.6% (2.2% under-lying, 6.4% contributing). Diabetes was cited as the underlying cause of death on only 26% of certificates on which it was mentioned. Moreover, many death certificates of diabetics did not mention diabetes at all. In a small sample of 311 patients whose death certificates did not cite diabetes, 8% were found to have had diagnosed diabetes. On the basis of these figures for 1968–1969 it was estimated that about 16.9% of all decedents were known diabetics. Diabetes was cited as the underlying cause of death in only about one eighth of diagnosed diabetics. It is not yet clear to what extent Pennsylvania results are typical of other states or nations. It seems likely that the same general situation prevails elsewhere. In Rochester, Minnesota, diabetes was mentioned on the death certificates of only 32% of previously diagnosed diabetics (Palumbo, et al, 1976). Diabetes was assigned as the underlying cause of death in only 7% of all deaths of these diabetics!

Langberg (1971) estimated that in 1967 diabetes was mentioned on about 86,000 American certificates of which 35,049 (41%) cited diabetes as the underlying cause. In earlier years, before changes in classification criteria, a greater percentage of diabetics were identified by counts confined to deaths in which diabetes was assigned as the underlying cause. In Britain, Stocks (1944) estimated that about 60% of death certificates of diabetics attributed death to diabetes. In Birmingham, England, Hayward and Lucena (1965) found more recently that diabetes was assigned as the underlying cause of death in only about 10% of diabetic deaths. In Sweden diabetes is cited as the underlying cause in about 31% (Grönberg, et al, 1967) of those certificates that mentioned diabetes. Entmacher and Marks (1965) cited reports suggesting that in France diabetes was assigned as the underlying cause of death in about two thirds of the certificates that mentioned diabetes, while in England and Wales the figure was about one third. In the Netherlands 46% were assigned to diabetes. In Osaka, Japan, diabetes was assigned as the underlying cause in 56% (Sasaki, et al, 1976), in Israel only 10% (*Israel Journal of Medical Sciences*, 1971). In Australia, Lancaster and Maddox (1958) found that about one third of deaths of diabetics were attributed to diabetes. It is not known precisely in any country with what frequency death certificates of diagnosed diabetics fail to mention diabetes at all (either as an underlying or as a contributing cause); nor is it known what percentage have occult diabetes at time of death.

In studying deaths from vascular disease on a sample of US deaths, Moriyama, et al (1966) found that in only 25% of diabetics was diabetes mentioned anywhere on the death certificate. Grönberg, et al (1967) estimated that diabetes was mentioned on the death certificate of about half of diabetic women in Sweden, and on about two thirds of the certificates of diabetic males. In Ceylon, Weerasinghe followed a group of diabetics, for whom diabetes was cited on the death certificate of 59%, and listed as the underlying cause of death in 27.5%. In some circumstances diabetes mortality rates may reflect as few as one fifth of deaths of diabetics when counts are limited to those in which diabetes is cited as the underlying cause of death.

Entmacher and Marks (1965) called attention to the very strong inverse relationship between age of death and proportion of deaths of diabetics attributed to diabetes as the underlying cause. Data of Grönberg, et al (1967) also showed this in Sweden.

Below are summarized some of the many factors that influence the sensitivity and specificity of death registration data as indexes of diabetes prevalence:

Sensitivity

1. Frequency with which existing diabetes is diagnosed
   Frequency of testing, sensitivity of tests, diagnostic criteria, "popularity" of the diagnosis

178

2. When diabetes is known to be present
   Frequency with which it is cited
   Frequency with which it is cited as underlying cause (statistical analyses have only rarely included data on contributing causes)

   Criteria employed by physicians in assigning underlying cause
   Characteristics of diabetes in the population (eg, frequency of ketosis)
   Characteristics of the diabetics (age, age of onset, sex, adiposity, etc); some past data have been age-specific or age-adjusted, but often details not available
   Characteristics of environment (diet, exercise, etc)
   Effectiveness of therapy, or preventive measures (eg, rate of ketosis, coronary disease)
   Criteria and procedures of statisticians (individually or collectively) in assigning underlying cause

Specificity

1. Frequency of false-positive diagnosis
   Faulty diagnostic criteria
   Frequency and type of testing

Death registration has many uses in assessing the diabetes problem, of which crude estimation of prevalence is only one. Even with all its shortcomings as an instrument for measuring prevalence, mortality rate has been the method most widely used in comparing prevalence in populations. One reason for this is that, although standardization is quite incomplete, procedure and practice are somewhat standardized. Until very recently standardization was even worse for other methods. When, for example prevalence data are based on screening and follow-up, sensitivity of such methods varies as much as fivefold depending on screening procedures used, diagnostic criteria, methods of calculations, and other factors.

It seems likely that the introduction of inexpensive blood glucose determinations with automated procedures will lower the prevalence of undiagnosed diabetes, particularly in the older segment of the population. This may be expected to raise the frequency with which diabetes is cited on the death certificate, but probably will not increase substantially the frequency with which diabetes is assigned as the underlying cause of death unless present criteria and practices are changed.

Grönberg, et al (1967) have considered in detail the practical and theoretical problems of estimating rates of prevalence of diabetes from death certificate data. It is clear from their observations as well as those cited above that extrapolations are very hazardous when the only data available are those on cases in which diabetes is assigned as the underlying cause of death. In the past, regular and complete reports have seldom been available by country or locality on death certificate information other than underlying cause of death.

179

In the United States, for example, analyses of data on contributing causes have been performed and published only for data of 1950 and 1967 (Langberg, et al, 1971). Among the information that would be useful would be computation on a regular basis of the distribution of contributing causes of death on diabetic decedents, both when diabetes is the underlying cause and when it is a contributing cause, and an appraisal of the relationship of these distributions to age, sex, race, etc. There is also need for more studies on the sensitivity, specificity, and reliability of death certificate data and the factors affecting them. The potentialities for linking death registration data to other data sources (eg, hospital records) deserve further study.

It has been little recognized that the character of manifestations of diabetes may greatly affect the sensitivity of death registration data as indexes of prevalence. If, for example, macrovascular disease is rife, as in the United States, most deaths of diabetics are attributed to this cause, while only one third or less are attributed to diabetes. In contrast, a very substantial percentage of deaths in diabetics are attributed to diabetes in societies where macrovascular disease is uncommon. Present evidence is incomplete, but probably the portion attributed to diabetes is about twice as high in Japan as in the United States. Thus, if diabetes death rates are about twice as high in the United States, the prevalence of diabetes is probably about four times as high as in Japan.

Mortality by Country and Locality

Some details have been given above for studies in Sweden (Grönberg, et al, 1967), Oslo, Norway (Westlund, 1969), Birmingham, England (Hayward and Lucena, 1965), and Japan (Kurihara, et al, 1970). Data over time are also available for several other countries and cities. Many of these have been presented in the 11 editions of Joslin's book (1916 to 1971). Some older data for countries and a few major cities were reviewed by Williamson (1909), Lepine (1909), Emerson and Larimore (1924), and Mills (1930).

Since its foundation shortly after World War II, the World Health Organization has coordinated the collection and publication of national figures. In recent years more detailed collections and presentations have been possible for some of the countries, such as age-specific data. Some of these were presented for selected countries by Entmacher and Marks (1965), by Kurihara, et al (1970), and by Marks and Krall (1971).

The traditional method for expressing mortality rates has been number of deaths per year per 100,000 population. Most of the poor countries with high birth rates have not collected and submitted complete information on diabetes rates. Thus, age distributions among countries submitting data were not so different as they might have been. Even so, rather substantial age differences have existed among some of the countries submitting data (eg, Britain and Thailand), making corrections for age highly desirable. In Sweden diabetes death rates were, for example, more than 40 times higher in the eighth decade than in the second decade (Gronberg, et al, 1967). The same problem applies when diabetes death rates are expressed as a percentage of all deaths. Another consideration is that the distributions of incidence and prevalence of diabetes by age are greatly different among societies. In North America and Europe prevalence of diabetes is many times higher in the seventh decade than in the third, but this is not the case in very lean societies. These considerations make it difficult to develop simple methods for comparing data by country. Among the better procedures for this purpose is presenting figures as age-specific rates. In this instance the number of deaths in an age range (eg, 5 to 20 years) is related to the estimated number of persons in that age range in the population at risk. This approach can also be used to show diabetes-related deaths as a percentage of all deaths in each specific age group.

Because of the many problems explained above it is usually not certain whether interpopulation differences of moderate degree in diabetes mortality reflect real differences in incidence or prevalence. It is also possible that actual intercountry differences in prevalence as great as two- to threefold could be hidden by under-reporting in the country with the higher rate. It does seem likely that age-specific interpopulation differences as great as two- or threefold reflect real differences in prevalence when there are not gross interpopulation differences in the frequency and sensitivity of screening tests. The number of diabetes-related deaths is of course affected to some extent by the quality of treatment available. But it does not seem likely that differences among populations in diabetes death rates are affected to any substantial degree by this factor. A more significant problem in using diabetes death rates as an index of prevalence is the considerable difference among populations in the portion of diabetics that are undiagnosed.

Despite all these difficulties of interpretation it was mainly interpopulation difference in diabetes mortality rates that suggested the strength and importance of the environmental determinants of risk of diabetes. The future utility of such data will be substantially increased by systematic determination of their sensitivity in each of the populations in which they are collected. This can be done with intensive investigation of samples in the manner of Tokuhata, et al (1975) and of Moriyama, et al (1966), but these representative samples of death certificates need to be somewhat larger than those studied heretofore. The samples should include groups of certificates in which diabetes is mentioned and groups in which diabetes is not mentioned. There is also need for integration of studies on mortality with studies in living populations. For example, in interpreting mortality data on diabetics and nondiabetics who die in the sixth decade, it would be useful to know the rate of known and occult diabetes in that population for those who are in the sixth decade.

Table 26 shows by country the most recent data available from the World Health Organization. These and other intercountry comparisons are discussed in other parts of this book (eg, in sections of Chapter 7 on geographic and etiologic factors). Table 27 shows age-adjusted data for selected countries. Table 28 gives for selected countries some age-specific data for the group 45–64 years of age.

TABLE 26   Diabetes Mortality Rates by Country

COUNTRY	RATE PER 100,000		
	1970	1971	1972
Africa			
Egypt		6.0	
Mauritius			12.9
America			
Canada			14.3
Chile	8.9		
Costa Rica		8.8	
Dominican Republic		4.8	
El Salvador		3.9	
Mexico			15.8
Panama, excluding tribal Indians			9.0
United States			18.8
Uruguay		23.8	
Venezuela, excluding tribal Indians		8.9	
Asia			
Hong Kong			4.4
Israel, Jewish population		7.2	
Japan			7.4
Singapore			9.6
Thailand		2.1	
Europe			
Austria			17.4
Belgium	36.7		
Bulgaria			7.5
Czechoslovakia		18.0	
Denmark		13.9	
Finland		14.1	
France			15.7
German Democratic Republic		19.4	
Germany, Federal Republic of		30.1	
Greece		22.7	
Hungary			8.1
Iceland			3.3
Ireland		10.4	
Italy		22.8	
Luxembourg			58.3
Malta			76.3
Netherlands			11.5
Norway		7.6	
Poland			8.5
Portugal			10.2
Romania			3.7
Spain		16.6	
Sweden		11.9	
Switzerland		25.6	

Country	Rate per 100,000		
	1970	1971	1972
United Kingdom:			
England and Wales			10.8
Northern Ireland			11.8
Scotland			13.6
Yugoslavia		7.5	
Oceania			
Australia			14.2
New Zealand		13.0	

Note: Data from WHO (1974) for 1972 or most recent year available. These data are not adjusted for age.

TABLE 27   Age-Adjusted Mortality from Diabetes (United States, Canada, and Selected European Countries, 1967–1968)

Country	Average Annual Death Rate* per 100,000	
	Male	Female
United States		
White	13.1	13.6
Nonwhite	19.9	31.6
Total	13.5	14.9
Canada	11.6	12.6
Denmark	8.4	8.5
Norway	4.5	4.4
Sweden	10.5	10.9
Netherlands	9.1	15.1
United Kingdom		
England and Wales	5.0	5.6
Northern Ireland	5.0	6.8
Scotland	7.2	9.0
Ireland	5.9	6.9
Belgium	13.9	23.4
France	9.8	10.0
Germany, Federal Republic of	9.0	11.6
Switzerland	12.0	14.1
Italy	11.4	15.6
Spain	7.7	10.2
Portugal	7.6	8.0

Source: Metropolitan Life Insurance Company Statistical Bulletin, 1972.
*Adjusted on the basis of age distribution of the United States total population, 1940. Basic data from reports of Division of Vital Statistics, National Center for Health Statistics; World Health Statistics Annuals, World Health Organization; and Demographic Yearbook, Statistical Office of the United Nations.

183

TABLE 28   Age-Specific Diabetes Mortality by Country (mean annual death rate from diabetes mellitus per 100,000 in persons from 45 to 64 years of age, 1966–1967)

COUNTRY	MALES	FEMALES
Norway	5.9	5.3
Northern Ireland	6.0	7.9
Israel	6.5	8.2
England and Wales	6.8	7.3
Philippines	8.3	8.4
China (Taiwan)	8.4	11.9
Republic of Ireland	9.3	10.1
Yugoslavia	9.9	10.8
Hungary	10.2	14.4
Poland	10.3	13.5
Bulgaria	10.4	13.9
Finland	10.8	12.3
Netherlands	10.9	15.5
Denmark	11.5	10.6
Scotland	11.6	15.3
Japan	11.9	10.3
Sweden	12.9	10.5
Portugal	14.3	11.9
Federal Republic of Germany	14.6	15.6
New Zealand	14.8	12.7
Australia	15.2	14.3
Canada	15.8	15.0
Switzerland	16.9	19.1
Austria	17.0	15.7
Greece	17.6	23.9
France	17.7	15.6
Chile	18.7	18.1
Belgium	18.9	32.5
Czechoslovakia	20.2	25.7
United States	21.6	23.5
Venezuela	26.5	28.6
Trinidad and Tobago	81.5	99.2

Source: *Israel Journal of Medical Sciences* (1971).
Note: Includes all countries for which age- and sex-specific rates for 1966–1967 were provided by WHO. The countries are ranked according to the rates for males in 1966–1967.

Kawate, et al (1975) have compared diabetes mortality rates of Japanese in Japan and Hawaii with those in whites of Hawaii. In recent years rates in Japanese in Hawaii have been very similar to those of whites. Both of these rates are roughly four times as high as in Hiroshima. These comparisons are necessarily crude, however, because of incomplete standardization of methods.

Data of the US National Center for Health Statistics show differences in diabetes mortality rates by state that are in a few instances as much as twofold (Tokuhata, et al, 1976). To a considerable degree these differences are probably attributable to regional differences in frequency and character of screening and diagnostic procedures. Such differences by region were not observed when population samples were actually tested in various regions (Gordon, 1964). In the period from 1968 to 1971 the US age-adjusted diabetes mortality rate was 14.1 per 100,000. Only two states had rates that differed substantially from the mean. Rates were highest in Delaware (22.0) and lowest in Alaska (6.7). Rates are very low in the Eskimos and Indians of Alaska, as shown elsewhere in this volume. These natives make up a substantial portion of the Alaskan population. Similar regional variations of modest degree have been observed in Sweden (Grönberg, et al, 1967) and Japan (Kurihara, et al, 1970). The extent to which these apparent differences are real is not clear.

Variations of Mortality with Time

Variations over time in methods and criteria employed in certification of causes of death make it very difficult to interpret the meaning of changes in diabetes mortality rates. The available data suggest that the prevalence of diabetes was increasing in most, if not all, Western countries during the period between 1850 and 1914. But it is certain that much of the increase in diabetes death rates was secondary to improved ascertainment. Emerson and Larimore (1924) published interesting figures for the pre-insulin era in New York City. Although there are many problems in interpreting these data, they are, in some respects, the best American data for examining mortality rates over time during that period. Between 1866 and 1900 there was little change in the diabetes mortality rate for persons less than 20 years of age, while rates rose tenfold in those more than 44 years of age. Between 1900 and 1920 the mortality rate rose from 1.0 to 2.5 per 100,000 in this younger age group, and from 50.3 to 81.7 in persons over 44 years of age. Much of the tenfold increase observed for the older subjects during the period of 1866 to 1900 was probably the result of great increases in the frequency of testing. Since juvenile diabetics are usually symptomatic, it is not surprising that rates of increase during the same period were far less. On the other hand, it is quite possible that much of the dramatic increase in the rate of increase in diabetes mortality in older subjects reflected a substantial increase in actual incidence of the disease. The discovery of insulin (1921) and its wide application in 1923 had a dramatically favorable influence on diabetes mortality rates in children, but the effect on overall diabetes mortality rate was small because only a small segment of the total US population of diabetics required insulin for survival. In the years just before the use of insulin, mortality rates (all ages) in Britain were typically about 11 per 100,000. In Germany, France, Italy, and the United States these rates were about 15 to 20. But in Boston they were 29, and in New York 25. Dramatic declines occurred in Germany and France with World War I, and a modest decrease occurred in Britain. In these three European countries peaks in mortality rates for the period before the discovery of insulin were reached at the onset of the war (Joslin, 1923).

Gore (1927) examined changes in diabetes mortality over time for 14 countries for the period 1901 to 1925. Most of the increases ranged from 33% to 100%. Doubtless much of this was attributable to improvements on methods of ascertainment of diabetes.

It is generally believed that the prevalence of diabetes has increased substantially in the last half-century. In certain elements of society (eg, American blacks and Indians, Africans who migrated to cities, Indians who migrated to South Africa) diabetes rates have certainly increased dramatically. Evidence that rates have increased substantially in Western urban societies is less convincing. Age-corrected mortality rates are in many localities about the same in 1974 as in 1914, in some cases substantially less. Because of differences of reporting methods, modern rates of 10 per 100,000 are probably equivalent to rates of about 20 per 100,000 in 1914. On the other hand, the sensitivity of diagnostic methods and the frequency with which they are applied are now very much greater than heretofore. It is probable that diagnosed diabetes is more common even after age correction, but the actual incidence of diabetes may not be much different in urban Europe and urban America than immediately prior to World War I. Between 1920 and 1949 no significant change in the diabetes mortality rate was recorded either by the US Public Health Service or by the Metropolitan Life Insurance Company (Joslin, et al, 1959). This lack of change does not seem to be the result of a substantial effect of insulin therapy. A slight fall in mortality did occur in 1923 and 1924, coinciding with the introduction of insulin, but rates in 1949 were only slightly higher than those in 1925, at a time when insulin had become widely available. Perhaps the worldwide economic depression of the 1930s had a favorable effect on diabetes mortality. In 1950 mortality rates of diabetic policyholders of the Metropolitan Life Insurance Company declined from 17 to 9.6 per 100,000. This reflected only a change in international conventions promulgated by the Sixth Revision of the Classification of Deaths. Between 1969 and 1973 there was a slight decline of 5% in diabetes mortality among an insured population of Americans (Metropolitan Life Insurance Company, 1975).

During the period 1950–1967 there were no major changes in the system of classification and no change was observed in age-adjusted diabetes mortality rates for the United States (Langberg, 1971). Mortality rates declined slightly in women and rose slightly in men. A very large rise occurred in the nonwhite population (mainly blacks), but the size of this minority population was not sufficiently large to raise the rate for the total population. These results compiled by Langberg and his colleagues at the National Center for Health Statistics are summarized in Figure 8. Data of this type were among the first clues to the epidemics that occurred in American blacks and Indians. Data from the Center also showed that rates in American Chinese and American Japanese were similar to those in US whites, and much higher than rates in Taiwan or Japan (Entmacher and Marks, 1965). In 1952 diabetes mortality in Hawaii was twice as high in whites as in Japanese; by 1968 the rates were equal (Kawate, et al, 1975).

Data are quite incomplete on death rates over time in youth-onset diabetes. In

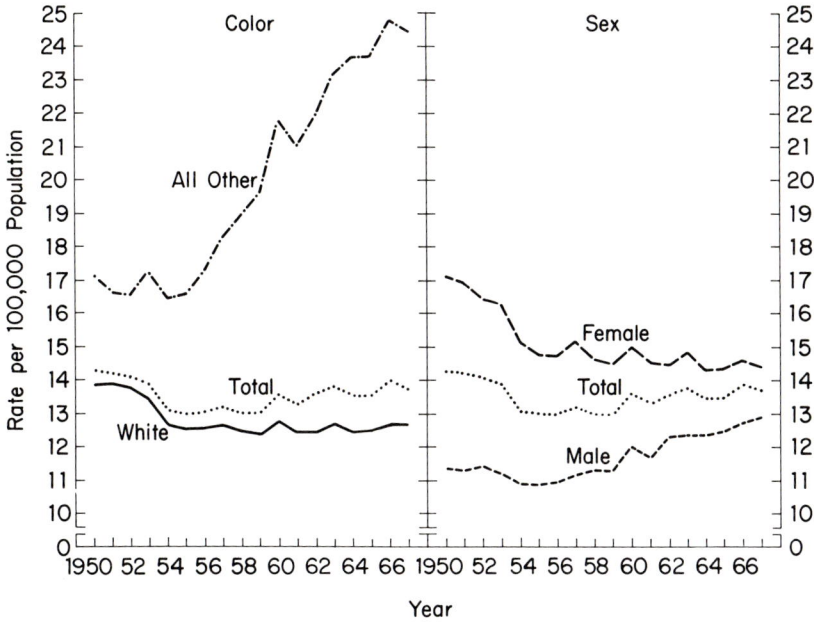

FIGURE 8. Age-adjusted diabetes mortality rates for the United States by sex and color over time. Data of the US National Center for Health Statistics (Langberg, et al, 1971).

Norway (Westland, 1966) and Britain (Smith and Hudson, 1976), there is little evidence of any recent change in frequency.

In most European countries diabetes mortality rates rose sharply between 1950 and 1967 (*Israeli Journal of the Medical Sciences*, 1971). It is probable that the considerable increase in affluence following World War II was responsible for these increases in diabetes mortality. But changes of methods of classification and more intensive screening make it difficult to determine the extent to which rates have really increased during the past several decades in Europe or elsewhere. In some countries (eg, Britain) "uncorrected" mortality rates were only about half as great in 1967–1968 as in 1915. In 1914 the diabetes mortality rate had already reached 23 per 100,000 in Berlin (Joslin, 1923). In Asia (eg, Japan) the very great increase in diabetes mortality rates probably reflect a real and substantial increase in prevalence as well as increased ascertainment.

Table 29 shows age-specific rates of diabetes mortality for the period 1950–1973 in the United States.

Seasonal Variations

Several observers have noted a seasonal variation in death rates from diabetes, with higher death rates in winter and early spring. Brigham commented on

TABLE 29   Age-Specific Death Rates per 100,000 Population for Diabetes Mellitus (United States, 1950–1973)

Year	Total	0–1	1–4	5–14	15–24	25–34	35–44	45–54	55–64	65–74	75–84	85+
1973	18.2	0.5	0.1	0.2	0.6	2.0	4.6	11.8	34.1	85.4	179.7	245.9
1972	18.6	0.5	0.2	0.2	0.6	2.4	4.9	12.3	33.8	89.7	181.5	255.3
1971	18.6	0.6	0.1	0.2	0.6	2.3	5.1	12.4	35.2	89.5	182.4	248.0
1970	18.9	0.3	0.2	0.3	0.7	2.2	5.3	12.8	36.7	92.1	186.8	230.2
1969	19.1	0.3	0.1	0.2	0.7	2.5	5.4	13.1	37.1	96.7	185.9	262.0
1968	19.2	0.5	0.1	0.2	0.7	2.6	5.3	13.0	39.2	99.5	183.3	258.3
1967	17.7	0.4	0.1	0.2	0.7	2.5	4.8	12.3	36.2	94.2	169.4	234.8
1966	17.7	0.5	0.2	0.3	0.7	2.6	5.0	12.1	35.7	95.7	171.5	234.4
1965	17.1	0.5	0.2	0.3	0.7	2.6	4.7	11.9	36.1	92.6	166.4	220.0
1964	16.9	0.6	0.2	0.3	0.8	2.6	4.8	12.0	37.3	91.4	161.6	204.9
1963	17.2	0.4	0.2	0.3	0.9	2.6	5.0	12.1	37.5	95.1	165.9	206.6
1962	16.8	0.6	0.2	0.3	0.8	2.5	4.6	11.7	36.9	94.0	160.2	206.7
1961	16.4	0.3	0.2	0.3	0.7	2.7	4.7	11.3	35.9	91.4	162.9	184.2
1960	16.7	0.4	0.3	0.4	0.9	2.3	4.5	12.1	37.9	93.4	163.7	181.7
1959	15.9	0.3	0.2	0.4	0.9	2.6	3.8	11.4	37.5	89.9	154.5	158.8
1958	15.9	0.3	0.3	0.3	0.9	2.5	4.1	11.2	37.0	91.6	151.7	169.9
1957	16.0	0.3	0.3	0.4	1.2	2.6	4.5	11.2	38.0	92.5	149.8	158.1
1956	15.7	0.5	0.2	0.3	1.0	2.4	3.8	11.0	37.5	92.1	151.7	162.6
1955	15.5	0.6	0.3	0.4	1.0	2.4	3.9	10.9	37.3	91.7	150.6	163.1
1954	15.6	0.5	0.3	0.4	1.0	2.2	3.9	11.3	38.3	92.3	153.9	155.3
1953	16.3	0.5	0.3	0.4	1.2	2.4	4.1	11.7	41.7	96.2	161.7	156.4
1952	16.4	0.8	0.5	0.6	1.3	2.3	4.0	12.3	40.8	99.7	161.5	152.8
1951	16.3	0.4	0.4	0.5	1.2	2.2	3.9	12.4	42.7	99.8	161.2	151.1
1950	16.2	0.7	0.3	0.6	1.1	2.2	4.2	12.4	42.1	101.2	166.7	150.3

Source: US National Center for Health Statistics.

this in 1868. Emerson and Larimore (1924) presented detailed evidence of this variation in diabetics of New York City. It seems likely that this has been secondary to the effects of the seasonal incidence of respiratory infection, a common terminal event in the elderly and in persons with severe heart disease. Although few data are available, it seems likely that the seasonal variation in diabetes-related mortality has diminished since the availability of antibiotics.

Other Uses of Death Registration Data

Death registration data have provided many other useful clues in the study of diabetes. These receive discussion in several other sections of this volume including those on sex, geography, race, and morbid effects.

Grönberg, et al (1967) have estimated from mortality data the risk of becoming diabetic during a lifetime or before any certain age. They recognized clearly the several problems in such extrapolations. According to their estimates, lifetime risk of developing diabetes in Sweden was about 4.8% for males and 10.3 for females. At age 50 risk was about 2.0% in males and 1.9% in females; at age 70, about 4.7% in males and 9.0% in females. These investigators also estimated prevalence from mortality data. Their estimate in Sweden was that "clinically manifest" diabetes was present in about 1.5% of all males and 2.6% of all females.

Seltzer and Jablon (1977) computed standardized mortality ratios for diabetes in veterans of the U.S. Army. Diabetes was less common as an underlying cause of death than in other American men. In privates the SMR was 0.658, in noncommissioned officers 0.500, but in commissioned officers only 0.175!

7
CHAPTER

FACTORS ASSOCIATED
WITH OCCURRENCE OF DIABETES

HEREDITY

A full discussion of the genetics of diabetes is beyond the scope of this book. The book of Rimoin and Schimke (1971) contains a good review with more than 300 references. The volume edited by Creutzfeld, et al (1976) is an excellent and detailed account of the subject. Although there is considerable confusion, controversy and uncertainty in the field, it is clear that genetic factors are quite important in the etiology of diabetes. Rosenthal, et al (1976) concluded that "diabetes mellitus in man, regardless of age of onset, is primarily genetic in origin, with environmental factors apparently influencing only the time of appearance of the disease." A considerable amount of evidence contradictory to the latter conclusion is outlined below, but these contrasting views illustrate nicely the need for better and more complete information concerning the genetics of diabetes.

Falconer (1967) estimated that the "hereditability" of diabetes was approximately 35%, with a higher degree of "hereditability" of youth-onset diabetes and a somewhat lower degree in maturity-onset diabetes. Simpson's conclusions (1969) were similar in this respect. She estimated "hereditability" at 50%,

---

Some additional etiologic factors relating to insulin-dependent diabetes and other special types of diabetes are discussed in Chapter 8.

with a greater degree in youth-onset diabetes and a lesser degree in maturity-onset cases. The conclusions of Goodman and Chung (1974) were also similar. Simpson's data (1968) were especially enlightening in some respects: numbers were large and there were control families. She found that when diabetes was discovered after age 40 in the proband, risk for siblings and children was increased by a factor of only 2 to 3. But, when diabetes was discovered before age 20, risk was increased about 12-fold in siblings, and more than 30-fold in offspring of the proband. On the other hand, both Gottlieb, et al (1974) and Tattersall and Pyke (1972) found a lesser degree of concordance for diabetes in identical twins with youth-onset diabetes (about half) than in those pairs in whom diabetes in the index case had developed after age 40. In these older pairs concordance for diabetes exceeded 90%. But in both these studies ages were much less in twins of early-onset cases. Data on previous and present fatness were not reported for either diabetic or nondiabetic subjects. It is possible that to some degree the high concordance for diabetes in the older pairs were attributable to concordance for fatness. Rosenthal, et al (1976) thought that the relatively modest rates of concordance of insulin-dependent diabetes in the identical twins studied by Tattersall and Pyke (1972) would become substantially greater with longer follow-up, but this prediction cannot be supported or refuted on the basis of present evidence.

It should be emphasized that estimates of "hereditability" of diabetes have sometimes been based on incomplete data and a considerable degree of extrapolation. Moreover, results of this kind are not necessarily applicable to populations other than those from which the data are derived. Simpson's data (mentioned above) and those of Goodman were from Canada (Prince Edward Island), and Falconer's were from Scotland.

Opinions have differed widely concerning the genetic mechanisms responsible for diabetes. Several factors account for the highly contradictory conclusions that have been offered with respect to the degree and character of genetic influences.

1. Many have failed to take into account sufficiently the differences between familiality and heredity. In most circumstances, relatives of nondiabetics are less likely to be tested for diabetes than relatives of diabetics. When diabetes is present in relatives, diabetics are more likely to know about it or remember it than are nondiabetics. For both genetic and nongenetic reasons, relatives of obese diabetics are more likely to be obese than relatives of age-matched nondiabetics from the general population.

2. Genetic studies have often failed to take into account the importance of descriptive data on the probands. This includes age, age of onset of diabetes, severity and character of the diabetes, type of treatment, adiposity (past and present). Only in a very few studies has an attempt been made to measure maximum degree of adiposity and duration of obesity. Often a specific definition of "diabetes" is not provided. This is crucial because in certain age groups of some populations, diabetes rates may

vary as much as several fold, depending upon criteria of diagnosis and methods used.

3. Nomenclature, criteria, and definitions are poorly standardized (Baum-slag, et al, 1970).

4. Information has often been scant on the family members, as pointed out by Keen and Track (1968). Useful data that are sometimes missing include sex, age, age at onset of diabetes, type of diabetes, and status of glucose tolerance. Only rarely has information been gathered on extent and duration of adiposity in the family members. Methods of ascertainment of the presence of diabetes have often been poorly matched in groups and subgroups. In general, data from these genetic studies have been overanalyzed, overinterpreted, undergathered, and underdefined. Sometimes uncertain or erroneous conclusions have been the result of inadequate numbers of diabetics, families, or family members, but more often the main problem has been inadequacy of description and definition.

5. Control data have often been absent or unsatisfactory. As pointed out previously, by certain criteria the rate of abnormal glucose tolerance in those over 40 years of age is as high as one third in some societies. This often necessitates careful matching of methods and definitions in relatives of diabetics with those in control families.

6. Until quite recently, the design of most studies failed to take adequately into account the possibility: (a) that environmental factors have a potent effect; (b) that multiple genetic factors may contribute to the genesis of diabetes in a single individual; and (c) that different types of diabetes sometimes have distinctive genetic mechanisms.

7. An important consideration usually ignored in interpreting and describing genetic studies in diabetes is that obesity itself has a strong genetic background (Seltzer, 1969).

Rimoin (1971) has reviewed the evidence for and against the various genetic mechanisms by which susceptibility to diabetes might be transmitted. Several recent reports have shown relationships of mild to moderate degree between susceptibility to insulin-dependent diabetes and presence of certain genetically-transmitted histocompatibility antigens. It has now become clear from experience in both man and animals (Dickie, 1970; Renold, et al, 1971) that many different genetic mechanisms play a role in causing diabetes, acting separately or together. Most recent data suggest that the principal mechanisms are to a substantial degree separate for juvenile- and maturity-onset diabetes (Simpson, 1968; Lestradet, et al, 1974; MacDonald, 1974; Barta, et al, 1976; Köbberling, 1971). Among 210 parents of Israeli juvenile diabetics (Cohen, 1970) only five had known diabetes. Tattersall and Fajans (1975) showed that only 2% of the offspring of two maturity-onset diabetics developed juvenile diabetes. As pointed out by the authors, rates might have been affected by the method of ascertainment of these diabetic couples. Thirteen couples were identified through diabetic offspring, but it was not clear how many of these 26 were juvenile diabetics. Studies of Tattersall and his associates suggest that there probably is a distinctive mechanism for the genetic transmission of a mild type of diabetes with onset in youth (Tattersall, 1974; Tattersall and Fajans, 1975). Rimoin (1976) listed 35 different genetic disorders in man associated with increased rates of impaired glucose tolerance or diabetes! It is still conceivable that a single genetic mechanism accounts for most cases of insulin-dependent diabetes, but present data do not establish this. Data in twins do, however, confirm the very strong hereditary features in both insulin-dependent and typical maturity-onset cases.

The possibility has been considered repeatedly that inbreeding might account for high rates observed in some populations. Present evidence cannot prove or entirely refute this possibility. There are, however, some reasons to be skeptical about this notion. All of many subpopulations of North American Indians have high rates of diabetes when they become fat, irrespective of present or past degree of isolation (West, 1974). All lean American Indian subpopulations have low rates. All isolated subpopulations of other races that have been studied have low rates of diabetes if they are lean. High rates of diabetes observed in presently or previously isolated populations might be attributable to environmental factors. A relatively isolated small population on Mabuiag Island, North of Australia, has high rates of diabetes; but they are fat. It is, however, possible that inbreeding or natural selection would lead to a greater frequency of genes enhancing risk of adiposity. Jackson, et al (1974) found high rates of diabetes in an isolated Tamil population in South Africa. Although they were fat (Fredman, 1972), rates of diabetes seemed to be even higher than one would expect with the degree of adiposity observed. Inbreeding is a possible explanation for the high rates of diabetes, but many other populations of less isolated Indians have also developed high rates of diabetes with changing social and dietary circumstances, increasing indolence, etc. In the Capetown Tamils there was little apparent difference between rates of diabetes in the general population and rates in those whose parents were both diabetic. In Israelis and Israeli immigrants (Cohen, 1970), cousin marriages were common, but such matings were not especially common in parents of juvenile diabetics. In dogs, Gepts and Toussant (1967) found diabetes more common in mongrels than in pure breeds.

Neel (1962) suggested that, through natural selection in time of relative famine, the frequency of a certain genetic trait or traits might be increased. These advantageous "thrifty" genes might later be disadvantageous in circumstances of relative abundance. Neel offered this as a working hypothesis and not as a conclusion. It fits in some respects the circumstances of the Pima Indians. On the other hand, all other races probably lived for millions of years under conditions of intermittent famine, and many other populations lived for long periods in desert environments similar to that of the Pimas. Cherokees who have lived in the temperate woodlands now have rates of diabetes that are roughly comparable to those in Pimas. It is true, however, that very high rates of obesity and maturity-onset diabetes have often been observed in populations that have moved rapidly from primitive to modern conditions. The extent to which genetic and environmental circumstances are responsible for this remains to be determined. Opperman, et al (1975) observed that fasting produced a smaller decline of blood glucose in nondiabetic KK mice than in another strain less susceptible to diabetes.

Environmental conditions may increase or reduce rates of maturity-onset diabetes several fold. This does not indicate that heredity is unimportant, but it shows closely the great discrepancy that may prevail in some circumstances between rates of genetic susceptibility and rates of diabetes, even when subjects are followed over a lifetime. This discrepancy probably has two aspects. Studies in identical twins of maturity-onset diabetics suggest that a substantial majority of genetically susceptible individuals who live in affluent societies will ultimately develop maturity-onset diabetes. The very low rates in lean societies suggest that a substantial majority of genetically susceptible persons will never develop maturity-onset diabetes if they remain very lean. The other aspect is that persons who remain very fat over long periods probably do not require any other special genetic potential to develop diabetes. Present data are inadequate, but it appears that a substantial majority of those who remain quite fat for more than thirty years will develop diabetes (see below). Köbberling (1971) found the rate of impaired glucose tolerance to be much lower in close relatives of fat maturity-onset diabetics who did not require insulin than in age-matched relatives of leaner maturity-onset diabetics who did not require insulin. Indeed, rates of diabetes in the nonobese close relatives of those in whom diabetes followed gross obesity of long duration appeared to be little, if any, higher than in the general population of the nonobese.

Since adiposity in diabetics may decline with age, or with uncontrolled or diet-treated diabetes, epidemiologic and genetic studies should take into account that present weight is often an imperfect index of weight prior to discovery of diabetes. Detailed documentation of this contention is given in the section below on obesity. The very high rate of concordance found in identical twins, when onset in the index twin develops after 40, attests to the strong effect of heredity in maturity-onset diabetes. It should be kept in mind, however, that environmental factors tend to be very similar in twins. Furthermore, obesity is strongly genetic (Seltzer, 1968). Since few data are available on adiposity in twin studies, the extent to which concordance of maturity-onset diabetes is attributable to concordance of adiposity is not yet clear. Finally, from evidence to be reviewed below, it seems likely that duration of obesity is important in the induction of beta-cell failure. But duration of obesity has seldom been measured in genetic or epidemiologic studies in either probands or their relatives.

Not all studies show high degree of familiality. In Colombia there was little relationship between glucose tolerance and family history of diabetes (Sanchez Medina, et al, 1970). In Tamils of Capetown glucose tolerance in offspring of two diabetic parents was similar to that of the general population of Tamils

195

(Jackson, et al, 1974). The relatives of fat diabetics of Köbberling (1971) had little more diabetes than those of nondiabetics. Wicks and Jones (1974) studied 107 African diabetics in Rhodesia, only five of whom had a family history of diabetes. Only 2% of Zulu diabetics had a family history (Campbell, 1963a). Tulloch (1962) listed four other studies in tropical populations in which the hereditary aspects of diabetes were judged to be "not important". In Nagasaki, Japan, there was little evidence of familiality of diabetes (Freedman, et al, 1965). In our preliminary studies in Plains Indians we have found little evidence of familiality of diabetes that is independent of obesity and its familiality (West and Mako, 1976). Low rates of family history of diabetes have often been reported in populations in which obesity is rare. This fits the possibility that much of the familiality of maturity-onset diabetes in the West is secondary to the familiality of obesity. In follow-up studies of O'Sullivan and Mahan (1968) in a group with equivocal or slightly abnormal glucose tolerance, rates of decompensation were strongly related to obesity, but not related to family history of diabetes.

In view of the problems discussed above, it is not surprising that relative importance of the different genetic mechanisms remains uncertain. There is, however, a developing consensus on several points:

1. Many different genetic mechanisms may increase risk of diabetes.
2. Environmental factors exert powerful influences in both maturity-onset and youth-onset diabetes.
3. The various genetic mechanisms differ not only in their capacity for inducing diabetes, they also differ sometimes in the type of diabetes they induce.

Rimoin (1971) has summarized evidence suggesting that some of the differences among societies in the manifestations of diabetes may also have a genetic basis. Certain data of Pyke (1973) indicate that this may be true for retinopathy.

The specific mechanisms by which genetic defects induce beta-cell failure are not clear. There are several possibilities, including peripheral antagonism to insulin, excessive secretion of growth hormone or glucagon, and qualitative or quantitative aberrations of beta-cell secretion. Data and conclusions on insulin secretion patterns of prediabetics have been quite conflicting (Johansen, et al, 1974). Recently Savage, et al (1975) reported unique data from adult Pima Indians. They had collected data on insulin secretion on 14 "true" prediabetics. These were persons with clearly normal glucose tolerance who later developed unequivocal diabetes. Prior to diabetes their insulin secretion patterns had been quite normal during the course of an oral glucose tolerance test.

It is clear that a substantial portion of diabetes is neither purely genetic or entirely environmental. Rather, individual cases of diabetes are very frequently the result of an interaction between multiple environmental factors and one or more genetic factors. Future epidemiologic and genetic studies need to take this into account to a much greater degree than has previously been done.

Studies designed to determine *the* genetic mechanism for diabetes or *the* genetic marker for diabetes will continue to meet with failure. That such naiveté is still widely prevalent may be illustrated by an example. A recent inquiry addressed to the American Medical Association for information on diabetes yielded a brief informative document. Although it listed some predisposing factors, the document indicated that "*the* cause of diabetes is unknown" (italics added).

Most of the variables that require better documentation and definition in the epidemiologic aspects of genetic studies have been mentioned above. It is also suggested that both cases and family members be divided between those with and without fasting hyperglycemia. One way to do this would be to set an arbitrary definition (eg, in the absence of antidiabetic therapy, a plasma glucose level above 130 mg/190 ml). Whenever possible, data should be collected and presented by frequency distribution. This would include, for example, data on weight in relation to height (and, whenever feasible, lifetime maximum weight) in both probands and family members.

More studies are needed to examine the relationship between the genetics of insulin-dependent diabetes with onset in youth and in adult life. More information is needed on the genetics of mild maturity-onset diabetes in persons who have never been fat, and the genetic relationship of this disorder to the several other types of diabetes.

Genetic factors in some of the special types of diabetes receive discussion in Chapter 8. This includes the section on typical juvenile-onset diabetes. Nelson and Pyke (1976) have shown recently that youth-onset cases with mild hyperglycemia of the kind described by Tattersall are different from the more typical cases of juvenile diabetes in that they do not exhibit excessive rates of diabetes-related histocompatibility antigens.

RACE AND ETHNIC GROUP

This section will review racial variations in the occurrence of diabetes. Interracial differences in the *manifestations* of diabetes are discussed in Chapter 10. Other observations on interracial differences will be cited in the following section on geography and in Chapter 8 on special types of diabetes.

Early Observations

It is possible that the frequency and character of certain diabetogenic genes differ among the races and ethnic subgroups. Differences in rates of diabetes among ethnic groups had been cited as early as 1885 by Hirsch and in 1891 by Saundby. In 1909, Williamson noted differences in prevalence among races, but he was aware that environmental circumstances might account for a substantial part of the differences. Montel (1924) observed in Indochina that diabetes was rare in natives but common in local Hindus (Indians).

197

Jews

It has been widely held that Jews are especially susceptible to diabetes. In both Europe and America at the turn of the century diabetes was often referred to as "judenkrankheit". According to Emerson and Larimore (1924), Billings had gathered data reported in the 1890 Bulletin of the United States Census Bureau to the effect that diabetes rates were excessive by a factor of sevenfold in Jewish men and 16-fold in Jewish women! Wallach reported in 1893 that death rates from diabetes in Jews of Frankfurt, Germany were about six times as great as in the general population. Morrison (1916) described observations made by Stern and by Judisch and Aronson in the latter part of the 19th century. They reported high rates of diabetes in Jews of New York City. In 1920, diabetes death rates in New York City were more than ten times as high in Germans and Poles (mostly Jews) than in either Greeks or Norwegians (Emerson and Larimore, 1924).

Early in this century diabetes was especially common in Jews of Budapest (Auerbach, 1908), Bengal (Chakravarti, 1907), and Boston (Morrison, 1916), but less well known was its rarity in Cairo Jews (Sandwith, 1907). The same disparities persist in more recent times. Rates were high in Sephardic Jews of Rhodesia (Krikler, 1969), and extremely low in both Yemenite and Kurdish Jews upon their arrival in Israel (Cohen, 1961). Blotner and Hyde (1943) studied rates of diabetes in 45,650 draftees and volunteers of World War II at a Boston induction station. Prevalence was high in Jews. Hargreaves (1958) noted that mortality rates from diabetes were high in a Jewish community in England. He also noted, however, that diabetes mortality was very low in Israel. Dr. Joslin studied the subject of diabetes in Jews over a lifetime. He held the view that the high rates seen in some Jewish groups was just a reflection of too little exercise and too much food (1923). In the Joslin Clinic patients, the proportion of Jews is much lower among juvenile cases than among adult-onset cases (Graham and White, 1971). Diabetes rates are high in Jews of modern Turkey (Ipbuker, et al, 1970).

The important studies in Israel on rates of diabetes and its various subpopulations are reviewed in detail in other sections of this book, including those sections on sugar consumption, geographic factors, and juvenile diabetes. By standards of North America and Western Europe, rates of diabetes appear to be low in Israel.

Chinese

Early reports on diabetes in China and Chinese are cited in the section immediately below on geography. Havelock Charles commented in 1907 on the rarity of diabetes in China, but noted that it was common in Chinese of Calcutta. Saundby in a publication of 1908 related a survey by Burge conducted in about 1888 among the members of the Shanghai Medical Society. None of these physicians had ever seen a case of diabetes in a Chinese patient! But

Saundby was aware that this immunity might have strong environmental aspects. He mentioned cases in Chinese of Singapore which he attributed to their "European" ways. After an excellent survey Reed (1915) reported on the rarity of diabetes in China, but he did not conclude that Chinese were less susceptible. Rather, he thought that the very low rates might be attributable to factors other than race. Reed warned of the dangers of anecdotal evidence. Physicians in North China told him that diabetes was more common in the South, while southern doctors told him that diabetes was more common in the North! Chun (1923–1924) summarized data from seven hospitals in various parts of China for the period 1914–1922. Rates of diabetes in outpatient and inpatients ranged from 0 to a "high" of 0.2% of patients!

Diabetes is still somewhat uncommon in modern China. A survey reported by the Endocrinology and Metabolism Division of Peking Hospital in 1959 summarized "recent" data from 11 Chinese hospitals of Peking, Shanghai, Nanking, Tientsin, Chengtu, Changsha, and Hangchow. Only 0.45% of all patients were diabetic. It was interesting, however, that a range of tenfold was observed among rates for the 11 hospitals (0.12% to 1.18%). Chung reported in 1962 that only 1.2% of patients were diabetic in the First Teaching Hospital of Shanghai.

In Americans who are Chinese, diabetes mortality rates are somewhat higher than in the general US population (Entmacher and Marks, 1965). In the study of Dales, et al (1974) "orientals" of northern California had blood glucose levels about the same as those of whites. At comparable blood glucose levels they had more glycosuria.

American Indians

This subject has recently been reviewed in detail (West, 1974,1977). In most tribes of North American Indians, rates of maturity-onset diabetes are much higher than in white North Americans, but there are many social, cultural, and environmental differences in the two races that could account for part or all of these differences. Widely different rates have been observed in fat and lean genetically-related tribes living in different circumstances (West, 1974). Juvenile diabetes is uncommon. In some tribes incidence rates suggest that a majority may be expected to become diabetic before reaching old age. The following listing gives information on prevalence of diabetes by tribes of aboriginals of the New World. (Indians, Polynesians, Micronesians and Melanesians.

High rates

Cherokees (North Carolina)
Alabama-Coushattas (Texas)
Choctaws (Mississippi)
Choctaws (Oklahoma)
Kiowas (Oklahoma)

Comanches (Oklahoma)
Pimas (Arizona)
Papagos (Arizona)
Yumas (Arizona)
Hualapis (Arizona)

199

Havasupis (Arizona)
Cocopahs (Arizona)
Chemehuevis (California)
Pawnees (Oklahoma)
Seminoles (Oklahoma)
Seminoles (Florida)
Washoes (Nevada and California)
Paiutes (Nevada and California)
Caddos (Oklahoma)
Senecas (New York)
Winnebagos (Nebraska)
Maricopas (Arizona)
Omahas (Nebraska)
Mojaves (California)
Sioux (Montana and Dakotas)
Assiniboines (Montana)

Passamaquoddy (Maine)
Cherokees (Oklahoma)
Creeks (Oklahoma)
Chickasaws (Oklahoma)
Cheyenne-Arapahos (Oklahoma)
Osages (Oklahoma)
Sauk-Foxes (Oklahoma)
Kickapoos (Oklahoma)
Shawnees (Oklahoma)
Polynesians
  Hawaiians
  Maoris (New Zealand)
  Rarotongans
Micronesians
  Chamorro females (Guam)
  Chamorro females (California)

Rates probably high
Poncas (Oklahoma)
Otoes (Oklahoma)
Potawatomies (Oklahoma)
Ft. Sill Apaches (Oklahoma)
Delawares (Oklahoma)

Wichitas (Oklahoma)
Kiowa-Apaches (Oklahoma)
Umatillos (Oregon)
Zunis (New Mexico)

Low rates
Eskimos
  Eastern and Western Greenland
  Eastern, Central, and Western
    Canada
  Alaska
Navajos (Arizona)
Hopis (Arizona)
Apaches (Arizona)
Western Shoshones of Nevada (1954
  report only)
Athabascan Indians
  Canada
  Alaska
Micronesians
  Truk and Marshall Islands
  Gilbert Islands

Paluans of Peleiu and
  Ngerchelong
  (Western Caroline Islands)
Chamorro males of Rota
  (Marianas)
Polynesians
  Pukapukans
  Western Samoans
  Tongatapuns
Melanesians
  Fijis
  Natives of New Hebrides
  New Caledonia and the
    Solomon Islands
Central American Indians
  Guatemala
  El Salvador

The preceding listing is taken from West (1974). Sources are cited in the original publication. In some of these populations where rates were formerly low, more recent studies have shown moderate or high rates (eg, in the Navajos).

Although diabetes was rife in Cherokees of North Carolina, it may not be any more frequent than in those whites of Bangor, Pennsylvania who are equally fat (West and Kalbfleisch, 1970). It does seem likely that there are genetically determined racial factors that influence susceptibility to obesity. The high rates of obesity in American Indians and in black women of certain societies may be in part the result of such factors. My colleagues who have studied the Pima Indians believe that diabetes is probably more common in Pima adults than in US whites even after corrections for adiposity (Bennett, et al, 1976a). It seems likely, however, that the high rates of diabetes in some tribes are mainly or entirely the result of their adiposity. I will describe below some evidence from our studies in Oklahoma Indians suggesting that the high rates of diabetes are largely, if not wholly, attributable to the obesity of these people.

Data are few on South American Indians, but Filho (1977) has recently reported on blood glucose levels in Caripuna and Palikur Indians of Brazil. Diabetes is no longer rare in these Indians. Rates also appear to be increasing in aboriginals of Guyana, Surinam and Chile.

In some tribes elevated levels of insulin have been reported (West, 1974). Rimoin (1969) observed high levels in lean Navajos. High levels of insulin were found by Bennett, et al (1976a), and by Frohman, et al (1969) in Senecas. In neither instance was it thought the high levels were explained entirely by the corpulence of these tribes. In contrast, the high insulin values in Oklahoma Plains Indians seem to be entirely attributable to the degree of fatness observed (West and Mako, 1976).

Peculiarities of the manifestations of diabetes in American Indians are discussed in Chapter X. The studies of Bennett and of Miller, et al, in the Pimas are among the most informative of all epidemiologic investigations. They are also reviewed in some detail in several of the sections below. Results of other studies in American Indian populations of Oklahoma and elsewhere are also discussed in several other parts of this book.

Asian Indians

Early observations on high rates of diabetes in India and South Africa are reviewed below in the section on geography of diabetes. High rates of diabetes have been described in several widely separated groups of Indians whose ancestors lived on the Indian subcontinent of Asia. These have been summarized by Ahuja (1976). Rates of diabetes are, for example, much higher in certain Indians of South Africa than in whites and blacks of the same communities (Cosnett, 1959; Jackson, 1970). Walker (1966) reported a range of prevalence of diabetes in South Africa from a low of 1% in certain rural blacks to as high as 32% in a group of urban Indians. It should be pointed out, however, that interpopulation differences of the same magnitude have been observed among groups of the same race (eg, in Jews by Cohen in 1961, and in American Indians by West in 1974).

Seftel (1964) has reviewed evidence concerning the difference among populations of Indians of India and South Africa in the prevalence and in the manifestations of diabetes. Differences of substantial degree have been reported among various ethnic and social groups in India, but with few exceptions their degree has not been measured with precision; nor is it clear to what extent the differences are determined by genetic or environmental factors (Ahuja, 1976). A cooperative study is underway in which rates of diabetes are being compared in several subpopulations of India using standardized methods (Gupta, et al, 1975; Ahuja, et al, 1976).

Rates of diabetes in Fiji are about nine times greater in Indians than in the Fiji natives (Cassidy, 1967); and in Singapore rates are much higher in Indians than in Chinese or Malays (Cheah, et al, 1975). But even in the same localities the way of life of these different races is still quite dissimilar in many ways. Differences include quantity and character of diet, levels of exercise, occupations, income levels, etc. In general, high rates of diabetes in such Indians have been associated with a very sedentary life and considerable adiposity (Campbell, 1964; Cassidy, 1967; Jackson, et al, 1970). Moreover, rates of impaired glucose tolerance in most of these subpopulations of East Indians in South Africa are probably not greater than in whites of Tecumseh, Michigan (Hayner, et al, 1965), Bangor, Pennsylvania (West and Kalbfleisch, 1971), Cleveland, Ohio (Kent and Leonards, 1968), or in the US general population (Gordon, et al, 1964). In general, however, rates of diabetes in Indians of South Africa are higher than those of local whites. In British Guiana (Weinstein, 1962) and in Trinidad (Wright and Taylor, 1958) rates in Indians were about the same as in local blacks. We found low rates in diabetes in the lean Indians of Malaya; rates were quite similar to those in local Chinese and Malays (West and Kalbfleisch, 1966). All three races were very lean. Rates of diabetes were also modest in Indians of Trinidad studied by Poon-King, et al (1968).

In Bengal diabetes was much more common in Hindus than in Mohammedans (Sen, 1893; Williamson, 1909), but we found little difference in Malaya between these two ethnic groups where environmental circumstances and diets were less disparate (West and Kalbfleisch, 1966).

Additional research in various Indian populations of the past and present are discussed in several other sections of this book including those on atherosclerosis (Chapter 10) and on geography (immediately below).

African Blacks

Jackson and his associates (1968) studied in South Africa a group of black women in whom rates of diabetes were low despite considerable weight. One of several possibilities is that these Bantu women have a lesser frequency of diabetic genes. Other possibilities include greater muscularity or more physical exercise than whites of equal weight; or a shorter duration of adiposity.

In other sections of this book many examples are cited of low rates of diabetes in black populations past and present. In 1944, for example, Dubois had observed that diabetes was very rare in the Congo. Saundby reported in 1908 that his colleague Dr. Tyson had never observed a case of diabetes in a Negro in the course of his extensive experience in Philadelphia. Data of Emerson and Larimore (1924) showed that in the early part of this century diabetes mortality rates were much lower in blacks than whites of rural America, but in cities differences were much less. The degree of difference in rural areas was probably attributable in part to the lesser frequency of testing for diabetes in blacks. Mills (1930a) cited evidence that diabetes was probably quite rare in certain parts of Nigeria in the 1920s.

It now appears, however, that these low rates in blacks were mainly the result of environmental rather than racial factors. By 1958 diabetes had become fairly common in certain urban areas of Africa (Dodu, 1958; Tulloch, 1962). In US black women rates of diabetes are now much higher than in white women. There is no evidence, however, that black women have special susceptibility to maturity-onset diabetes after corrections have been made for the greater adiposity of the black women. Dales, et al (1974) found glucose tolerance decidedly better in black than in white or oriental participants of a Northern California Health Plan of the Kaiser Corporation. These differences were not explained by differences in level of education or adiposity. Stamler, et al (1973) found that black employees of a Chicago industry had better glucose tolerance than white employees. Data of the National Center for Health Statistics (Gordon, 1964) show poorer tolerance in black women than white, but at comparable levels of education the glucose tolerance of black women was at least as good. Glucose levels were quite similar in black men and white men.

It should be recognized, of course, that there are considerable differences among various populations with black skin in respect to physical attributes, genetic makeup, etc. Other data from studies in black populations are reviewed in several other sections of this book, including Chapter 5 on prevalence and the section immediately below on geography.

Japanese

Diabetes is considerably less common in Japan than in the United States, but Japanese of Oahu, Hawaii, have at least as much diabetes as their white countrymen (Bennett, et al, 1963). Age-adjusted death rates from diabetes in Americans who are Japanese (9.7 per 100,000) are only slightly lower than in whites (12.6). The latter are data of the National Center for Health Statistics for 1959–1961 cited by Marks and Entmacher (1965). Kagan, et al (1974) found that lean Japanese men in Japan had much better glucose tolerance than fatter Japanese men in Hawaii or California. Gordon (1967) reported age-specific death rates from diabetes of Japanese-Americans for the years 1959 through 1961. These data were compared by me with data from other sources on Japanese of Japan and white Americans. Rates of death from diabetes in the Japanese-Americans were intermediate, but more similar to the higher rates in white Americans. Diabetes appears to be more common in Hiroshima than in Nagasaki (Freedman, et al, 1965). The reason for this is not clear. Many other data from Japan receive attention elsewhere in this book.

203

Other Races

In Wales, Ashley (1967) found diabetes to be somewhat more common in persons with Welsh names than in those whose names were not typically Welsh.

Eskimos have, in general, low rates of diabetes, but their immunity tends to disappear when they are removed from their primitive conditions (West, 1974; Mouratoff and Scott, 1976). Both low and relatively high rates of maturity-onset diabetes have been reported in each of many races, including Chinese, Japanese, Indians, American Indians, Jews, blacks, Australian Aborigines, Polynesians, and Micronesians (see specific citations above and below). Recent epidemics of diabetes have been reported in several Polynesian populations (West, 1974; Zimmet, 1976). This was first noted in Maoris (New Zealand Department of Health, 1960; Prior, 1962) and in Hawaiians (Sloan, 1963).

Other differences among ethnic groups are reviewed below under geography.

Special Types of Diabetes

It is possible that susceptibility to certain of the less common types of diabetes differs among the races. Among populations there are profound differences, as shown below, in the frequency distribution of types of diabetes. A major part of this is attributable to the low rates of obesity-related maturity-onset diabetes in some populations. Although the relative frequency of youth-onset diabetes is great in some poor populations, the absolute frequency in this age group is regularly low when the number of children at risk is taken into account. Indeed, in most disadvantaged populations the rate of youth-onset diabetes seems to be substantially less than in the United States or Western Europe. Although this apparent paucity may be, in part, the result of incomplete counting, it is probably real. It seems very likely, for example, that juvenile diabetes is less common in India than in the United States. Racial factors in typical juvenile diabetes are discussed in detail in the section on juvenile diabetes (Chapter 8).

Certain other special types of diabetes will be discussed below, including racial, genetic, and environmental aspects. This will include the insulin-dependent diabetes of youth, that associated with pancreatic calcification, and the ketosis-resistant type of insulin-dependent diabetes.

Insulin Secretion Patterns

Differences among populations in insulin secretion patterns have been described by Rimoin (1971), Aronoff et al (1977), and in Africa by Rubenstein, et al (1969), Joffe, et al (1971), Wapnick, et al (1972), Asmal and Leary (1975), Walker, et al (1972), Wise, et al (1976), as well as in Pygmies by Merimee, et al (1972). The extent to which these differences are racial or environmental remains to be determined. Because of profound differences in diet, exercise, and fatness, it seems likely that environmental factors contribute substantially to these differences. After correcting for adiposity and blood glucose levels we found no differences in the insulin secretion patterns of Plains Indians and Ohio whites (West and Mako, 1976).

Strong Contribution of Environmental Factors to Racial Differences

In India, Cheevers (1886) and Sen (1893) were among the first to note profound differences in prevalence of diabetes in different elements of the same race in whom there were differences in diet, social customs, and way of life. Most of recent evidence also suggests that environmental and social circumstances are more important than race in determining susceptibility to typical adult-onset diabetes. But the strong interracial differences deserve further investigation. It appears, for example, that American Indians may be especially susceptible to diabetes under certain circumstances.

In the section on geography I will describe our worldwide studies on prevalence of maturity-onset diabetes using standardized methods in 13 societies. These studies included whites, blacks, Indians, Malays, Chinese, Pakistanis of Bangladesh, and aboriginal Indians of Central and North America. After corrections for adiposity very little difference could be found in rates of maturity-onset diabetes even though rates varied as much as tenfold among these societies.

GEOGRAPHY

Geographic variations in the *manifestations* of diabetes will be discussed elsewhere in this volume. This section will summarize some of the major geographic differences in prevalence. The significance and interpretation of some geographic differences in frequency are also discussed in other sections (eg, the section above on race and Chapter VI on mortality). Other geographic variations have been discussed in Chapter V on prevalence, particularly those demonstrated by the testing of representative samples with more sensitive methods. But many interesting and important differences have been identified using less optimum methods. A full appreciation of the degree and significance of these geographic variations must await the application of more thorough and sophisticated methods. Nevertheless, the present less complete evidence is worthy of review because it provides some useful clues.

History

Rollo (1798) found diabetes rare in the West Indies and America during a lengthy tenure of practice ending in 1796 before his return to Scotland. In 1811 Thomas Christie described his experience with diabetes in Ceylon where he found the condition common. He called attention in the West to the description of diabetes by ancient Indian physicians. In most of the authoritative works on diabetes of the 19th century there were little or no epidemiologic data. Austin Flint (1867) deplored the remarkable paucity of "well-ascertained" facts. Possibly the most informative review of the time was written by a Harvard medical student who received a special prize for his essay (Brigham, 1868). Brigham quoted Harley to the effect that diabetes was considered to be much more common in Britain than on the Continent.

August Hirsch (1885) cited several examples of apparent geographic differences in rates of diabetes. He also noted the difficulties in determining the extent to which these apparent differences were real. He cited evidence that diabetes was fairly common in some of the major European cities, but apparently rare in St. Petersburg. He reviewed reports indicating that diabetes was common in Vera Cruz, Ceylon, Bengal, and on the Coromandel coast of India, but rare in Bombay. Diabetes was said to be rare or absent in the West Indies, Peru, China, Japan, Australia, Guiana, certain parts of West Africa, and in the Pacific Islands. In 1886 Norman Cheevers reported in his book on the diseases of India that diabetes was very common in affluent men in Bengal. He cited an editorial in the Indian Medical Gazette of 1871 that had described an extraordinary instance of familial diabetes. In three generations of first-degree relatives there were nine known diabetics! These observations were later extended by Sen (1893) and Bose (1895) who cited examples of very high and very low rates of diabetes in different parts of India, but these important facts were little appreciated at the time.

Saundby mentioned in 1891 that diabetes rates were much higher in Malta than in England. Osler reviewed evidence in 1894 that lead him to conclude that diabetes was uncommon in America by European standards. In 1901 Cook reported that in comparison to his native Britain, diabetes was "rather uncommon" in Uganda. Martin observed in 1906 that diabetes was rare in the natives of West Africa.

A splendid account of geographical differences was published in 1907 by the *British Medical Journal.* This symposium on diabetes in the tropics was chaired by Havelock Charles. Although the available evidence left much to be desired, it was already clear that diabetes was much more common in Bengal than in upper India, and much less common in the Sudan (Christopherson, 1907) and the Cameroons (Ziemann, 1907) than in Europe. Reviews on diabetes of Futcher (1907), Saundby (1908), and Lepine (1909) were the best of the period and gave some attention to geographic differences, including an apparent rarity of diabetes in Japan and China. Saundby (1908) reviewed impressive evidence of differences by locality in Europe. For example, he noted a mortality rate of 14 per 100,000 in Paris, 7 in London, and 1.5 in Italy. Both Saundby and Futcher thought that previous reports of low rates in America might be attributable, at least in part, to incomplete reporting.

Except for the pioneering brief report of Hirsch (1885), the first systematic review of the epidemiology of diabetes was published by R. T. Williamson in 1909. This outstanding publication cited many geographic differences, some of which will be related below.

Lambert reported in 1908 that diabetes was exceedingly rare in Chinese of Nanking. The report of Reed (1915) on the rarity of diabetes in China has been mentioned previously. Reed told of a report from a colleague of VanBuskirk that he had never seen a case of diabetes in Seoul, Korea during thirty years of practice. In Allen's book of 1913 many examples are given of geographic differences in prevalence. Magnus-Levy cited some differences in rates by city in 1913. Morrison, in 1916, reported that rates of diabetes were high in the Irish of Boston, and Mills (1930) subsequently pointed out that rates were considerably lower in Ireland. Hoffman (1922) published data on mortality rates for 15 countries or regions *in persons over 20 years of age*. Rates ranged from 67.8 per 100,000 in Malta to 8.6 in Italy, at a time when the United States rate was 16.4. Williamson (1909) had cited the high rates in Malta in 1909, as well as low rates in Cyprus, Hong Kong, Malaya, Aden, Sierra Leone, British Honduras, Cuba, Labrador Eskimos, Fiji, and in certain populations of Indians and Chinese! Williamson also summarized available evidence on rates by time and place in many European populations. In the report of Hoffman (1922) diabetes mortality rates (all ages) ranged from 38.4 in Malta to 1.1 in Venezuela. Statistics were also given for 26 cities. Berlin had a rate of 17.9 (highest), London 10.3, Toronto 11.1, and Tokyo 4.1. None of these latter data were age-adjusted. Similar data were published in the many editions of the books of Joslin beginning in 1916, and in a series of papers of Joslin, Dublin, and Marks (1933–1936).

Among the early systematic studies of prevalence in Europe were those of Gottstein and Umber in Germany (1916) and by Hunziker in Switzerland (1919). Emerson and Larimore gave extensive data by geography in 1924 based mainly on mortality statistics. In 1927 Gore published on the geography of diabetes, citing its rarity in the tropics. C. A. Mills in 1930 and Harold Himsworth in 1935–1936 published landmark papers on differences by country, climate, and nutrition, showing the very great geographic differences in reported rates of diabetes. Mills cited evidence on the rarity of diabetes in China, Japan, and Venezuela. In the 1930s reports were published on the very low rates in certain Eskimos and American Indians (West, 1974). Diabetes was apparently rare in Iceland prior to 1940 (Albertson, 1952). Other pioneer studies of prevalence in various European populations (1916–1952) have been well summarized by Silwer (1958).

Modern Observations

In 1954 S. M. Cohen published a landmark paper citing marked differences among American Indian tribes in rates of diabetes. In 1957 Cosnett described very high rates of diabetes in Indians in South Africa that were estimated to be about 30 to 40 times as frequent as in local blacks! Cosnett published details in 1959. Observations on other groups of Indian migrants have been reviewed in the section on race. In 1961 A. M. Cohen demonstrated a very dramatic difference in rates of diabetes between long-term residents of Israel who were

Yemenites and new arrivals who were Yemenites and Kurds. The outstanding work of Tulloch (1962) added greatly to our knowledge and understanding of these geographic variations. The following listing, taken from Tulloch's book (1962), summarizes his conclusions as to the countries in which diabetes was to be considered common or uncommon. Insufficient information was available at that time to classify the countries in the "indefinite" list; however, diabetes has recently become common in some of these populations, as we have indicated. For example, diabetes is now common in Cuba and Tahiti, and very common in Mexico and the Ellice Islands (Zimmet, et al, 1976).

Common

Antigua

St. Kitts

Trinidad

Jamaica

British Guiana

Curaçao

Bermuda

Fiji

Nauru

Tonga (moderately)

Hawaii

Singapore

Mabuiag Island

Ceylon

Bengal

Tanganyika (Asians)

Natal

Ghana

Congo (moderately)

Senegal

Indefinite

St. Lucia

Puerto Rico

Cuba

Tahiti

Indonesia

Malaya

The Yemen

India

Nyasaland

Cameroun

Nigeria

Mexico

Uncommon

Grenada

British Honduras

Bahamas

Honduras

El Salvador

Costa Rica

Colombia

British Solomon Islands

New Hebrides

New Caledonia

US Trust Territories of the Pacific Islands

Cook Islands

Gilbert and Ellice Island Colony (but now common)

Western Samoa

Netherlands New Guinea

Papua and New Guinea

Sarawak

Brunei

Phillipines

Thailand

Vietnam

Hong Kong

Seychelles

Muscat

Queensland and the Northern Terri-   Somaliland Protectorate
   tories of Australia (aborigines)   Southern Rhodesia
Ethiopia   Bechuanaland Protectorate
Kenya   Sierra Leone
Uganda   Gambia
Portuguese East Africa   St. Helena

Tulloch's methods included death certificate data, rates in outpatient and inpatient groups, results of systematic surveys, and clinical impressions of colleagues throughout the world. The limitations of some of these methods were well recognized by Tulloch. In his book, the conclusions provided in this listing are supported by descriptions of the evidence on which the conclusions were based. It ranged from rather scant to considerable. In a publication of 1966 Tulloch lists rates of diabetes in several populations of outpatients and inpatients.

In the section above on American Indians are listed many aboriginal populations of the New World in which rates of diabetes have appeared to be either low or high in relation to the rates that prevail generally in North America and Europe. The specific sources upon which this list is based are given in the original publication (West, 1974). Rates of diabetes in populations may change dramatically over time. In several groups, rates are now much higher than those reflected in my listing and that of Tulloch. Extreme variations of prevalence have been observed in various groups of Polynesians and Micronesians (Sloan, 1963; Bassett, et al, 1966; Reed, et al, 1970,1973; Prior, 1971; West, 1974; Zimmet, et al, 1976).

Table 26 in the chapter on mortality gives most recent data of the World Health Organization on death rates from diabetes by country. With some reason, it was widely believed that to a very considerable degree these geographic differences in rates of diabetes might be more apparent than real. It was clear, for instance, that the frequency of testing was usually much lower in the group of societies in which diabetes rates were purportedly low. Disadvantaged populations also have a proportionately smaller number of older adults in relation to their total populations. Generally, testing methods used in poor countries are less sensitive. Another problem is the variation in frequency with which death is attributed to diabetes itself in diabetics who die. This has been discussed above under mortality. It is very probable that the degree of this latter disparity varies by geography, and over time in the same region. Thus, data on mortality rates must be interpreted with caution. One cannot be certain, for example, that apparent variations of moderate degree are significant. But it does seem likely that differences of as much as threefold are usually attributable to real differences in prevalence rates, particularly if they are at least crudely adjusted for age.

For these reasons a large group of collaborators undertook in 1961, under sponsorship of the US Interdepartmental Committee on Nutrition, a series of

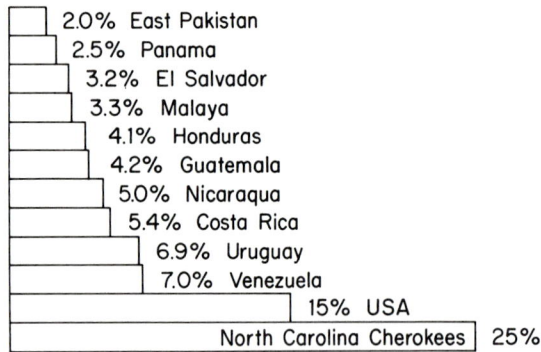

FIGURE 9. Prevalence of abnormal glucose tolerance (2-hr glucose concentration more than 149 mg/100 ml on venous whole blood after 75 gm oral glucose) in subjects over 29 years of age. In all population samples mean age was near 50 years. From West (1972).

direct investigations on prevalence of diabetes using standardized methods and criteria together with matching for age. Figure 9 summarizes results in 12 societies concerning rates of diabetes in persons over 29 years of age. Details of procedures and criteria have been published (West and Kalbfleisch, 1966-1970). Small but crudely representative samples averaging about 500 per country were tested. *All* subjects had a blood glucose determination two hours after one gm/kg of oral glucose.

These and other data established clearly that the purported differences among societies were to a very considerable degree quite real. It is now evident that environmental differences frequently account for interpopulation variations as great as tenfold in rates of diabetes. Indeed, these differences may be as great as 50-fold in some instances. In some societies such as primitive Eskimos or Broayans of the Sahara, rates of impaired tolerance in adults may be as low as 1%, while almost half of adult Pima Indians have impaired tolerance. Although rates by country relate rather well to levels of social and economic development, exceptions are not rare. In Malta mortality rates from diabetes are now more than three times greater than those in the United States. Rates for Belgian women are about five times greater than in Norwegian women, despite very similar levels of social and economic attainment.

Appendix 7A, which follows this chapter, lists population groups in which rates of diabetes have been reported to be high or low. It refers to but does not duplicate the 1962 listing of Tulloch (above), except when subsequent studies have provided additional information. Appendix 7A also refers to but does not include the large number of populations of American Indians, Eskimos, Polynesians, and Micronesians listed in the American Indian section above.

Mimura (1970) summarized diabetes mortality rates by age for five Asian countries from data provided by WHO. He also showed these by age in Australia, New Zealand, and the United States. When all ages are included, rates ranged from 1.5 per 100,000 population in Thailand to 17.7 in the United States. In interpreting these data it should be noted that diabetes mortality rates have usually been related to total population with no adjustment for the differences of age distribution of the various populations. Death rates relating to diabetes are typically 3 to 12 times higher in the United States than in Asian countries. After appropriate adjustments for the age distributions of these populations, these differences would be greater in young segments and less in older segments. Typically, the net effect of adjusting for age is to narrow the gap between diabetes death rates in rich and poor countries by about half. Thus, age-adjusted death rates are typically about two to six times greater in the United States than in Asian countries. Some of this difference is of course only a reflection of the greater frequency of testing for diabetes in the United States than in Asia.

It has often been mistakenly concluded that diabetes in certain Asian communities is as frequent as in the United States. This has sometimes been the result of assuming that rates of diabetes in the United States are those based on the Oxford Studies published in 1947. It should be kept in mind that these excellent studies used the relatively insensitive methods of the time. Rates of diabetes were not determined in negative screenees by examining a representative sample. It is now clear from subsequent studies that rates of diabetes in Americans over 40 range from 7% to 30% depending on diagnostic criteria (Gordon, et al, 1964; Hayner, et al, 1965; O'Sullivan, 1967; Kent and Leonards, 1968; West, 1966; Prout, et al, 1976).

In both Britain (Hargreaves, 1958) and the United States (Tokuhata, et al, 1976) there are modest differences by region in diabetes mortality rates. The extent to which these represent real differences in incidence is not clear. In the United States hospitalization for diabetes is somewhat less common in the West than in other regions (Ranofsky, 1977). But at least part of this paucity may be attributable to the relative youth of Westerners.

In the sections that follow the significance of these geographic differences will be discussed in detail, particularly in the sections on nutritional factors.

BLOOD GROUPS

Several investigators have examined the frequencies of blood types in diabetics and controls. These studies have included those of McConnell, et al (1956), Anderson and Lauritzen (1960), and Jolly, et al (1969). Jolly, et al (1969) reviewed the results of 12 such studies, pointing out the lack of any consistent relationships between diabetes and either ABO or Rh type. Vague et al (1977) observed that 31% of 137 diabetics were Lewis negative. This rate of negativity was approximately three times higher than in the general population from which these diabetics were drawn (Marseille, France).

211

The histocompatibility antigens and their geographic distribution are discussed in the section on juvenile diabetes (Chapter 8).

AGING

Figure 10 shows the age of discovery of diabetes in a large group of diabetics of London cared for at King's College Hospital. Circumstances there are such that this sample probably reflects rather well the frequency distribution by age of onset in all London diabetics. This distribution is very similar to that found by Malins (1972) in a large portion of all diabetics in Birmingham, England, and by Vinke, et al (1958) in the Netherlands. Data from the US National Health Surveys exhibited a similar frequency distribution of age of diagnosis. The curves in Figure 10 reflect the distribution observed in many affluent societies for both insulin-independent and insulin-dependent diabetes. It should be noted that these data are not adjusted to reflect rates for each age group in

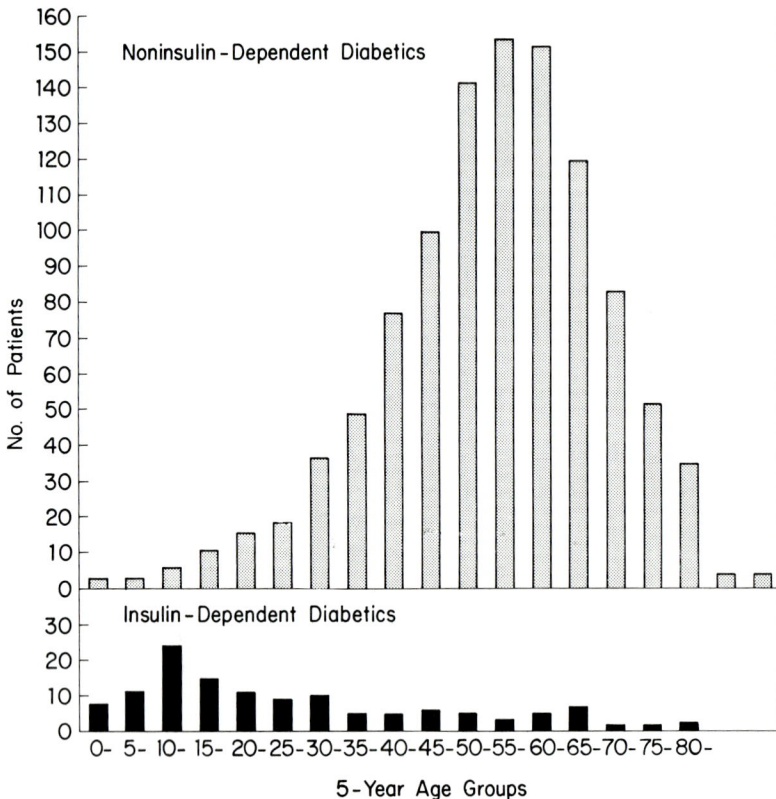

FIGURE 10.   Frequency distribution of age of diagnosis of diabetes in the diabetes clinic of King's College Hospital, London (Gamble and Taylor, 1969).

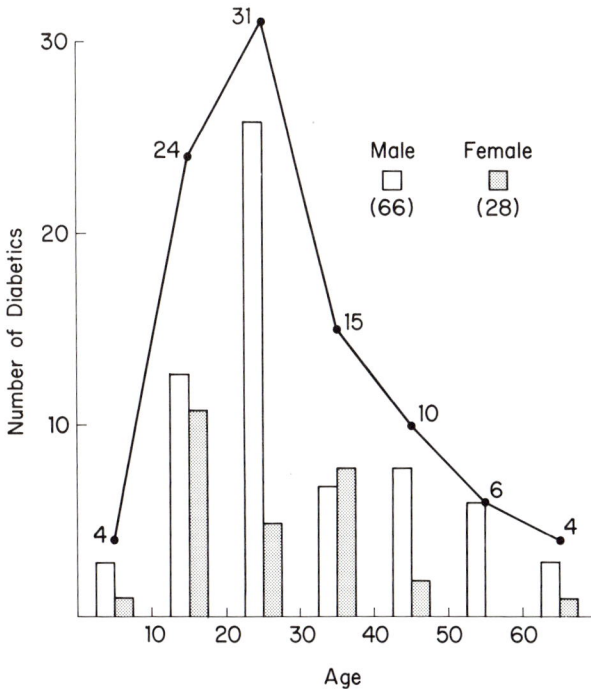

FIGURE 11. Frequency distribution of age of onset of diabetes in area of Gondar, Ethiopia (Belcher, 1973).

relation to the number at risk in that particular age group. Much of the apparent decline in old age is only the result of the smaller number at risk in old age. This is discussed more fully in the section on incidence in Chapter V, where other studies on incidence by age are reviewed, including the excellent data of Falconer, et al (1971) from Edinburgh.

In interpreting data on incidence one should also keep in mind that the duration of diabetes before discovery is often considerable and is seldom known either for individuals or populations. This interval is greatly influenced by several factors, including age, adiposity, frequency and methods of screening and detection, etc. In North America the time between onset and discovery probably averages about a decade in maturity-onset cases (Anderson, 1966), but no directly relevant data are available.

To what extent is the increasing incidence with age the effect of aging itself? It seems likely that other factors such as obesity and decreasing exercise account to some extent for the rise of incidence with age. Figure 11 shows the relationship of age to incidence in the Gondar area of Ethiopia (Belcher, 1973). It may be seen that incidence appears to *decrease* sharply with age in this very lean population. These latter data have to be interpreted with some caution because of some uncertainties and special circumstances that prevail in Ethiopia. The number of screening and diagnostic tests performed in the older segment is relatively low, and the number of middle-aged people at risk is relatively lower than in more affluent populations. Even so, the decline in incidence with age is impressive. Moreover, it was shown by Mollineaux, et al (1966) in this same Ethiopian population that the decline of incidence with aging is even greater in the poorest class. Tripathy and Kar (1966) have shown the same phenomenon in the poorest class of a community of India. Several factors could explain the disparity between Gondar and London, the main one probably being the leanness of the Ethiopians. Another related possibility is that higher levels of exercise protect the middle-aged poor in certain societies. The possibility that the association between aging and increasing incidence of diabetes may not be direct and casual deserves much more attention than it has received. The data from Ethiopia, India, and other such populations suggest the exciting possibility that age itself may have little direct influence on susceptibility to diabetes.

Apparent incidence by age is greatly affected by frequency of testing, by methods used, and especially by the diagnostic criteria employed. For these and other reasons it has been difficult to determine whether the incidence of diabetes declines, increases, or stays the same after the sixth decade. In Massachusetts it appeared that incidence declined in old age (Joslin, et al, 1936), but in Edinburgh (Falconer, et al, 1971) and in Rochester, Minnesota (Palumbo, et al, 1976), incidence did not decline in old age. In many societies old people have more tests. Also, it can be argued that a substantial portion of elderly subjects thought to have diabetes do not have true diabetes, because they do not have fasting hyperglycemia. For this reason, it would be important to know rates of fasting hyperglycemia among elderly subjects with newly discovered diabetes. Unfortunately, this rather simple counting procedure has rarely been applied. Furthermore, information is scant on risk of the specific complications of diabetes in elderly subjects with poor glucose tolerance and normal fasting blood glucose levels.

Generally, the difference between new "diabetics" and "nondiabetics" seem to narrow in old age with respect to relative risk of vascular disease and death. This is consistent with the possibility that some elderly patients labeled diabetic may not have diabetes, but there are some other possible explanations for this phenomenon. They include the much higher risk of vascular disease and death in old nondiabetics as compared to younger nondiabetics, and the relative mildness of hyperglycemia in diabetics with onset after age 60. Data of Silwer (1958) showed that the proportion of cases that were "severe" declined sharply in old age. In the sixth decade 28% of cases were severe by his criteria. In the eighth decade only 11% were severe, and in the ninth only 4%. In several populations the peak incidence of diabetes has appeared to shift with time to older age (Silwer, 1958; Hirohata, 1969). Among the possible explanations for this is the progressive increase in the frequency with which glucose tolerance tests have been performed.

The unique circumstances relating to the Pima Indian population have been exploited by Hamman and Miller (1975) who determined relationship of age to risk in a whole population. Among the special assets of their approach were unusually good baseline data and definitive testing of all subjects with glucose tolerance tests. This permitted determination of actual year of onset, which under other circumstances often precedes by a decade or more the discovery of diabetes. Their data indicated that Pimas who were 25 to 44 years of age at time of entry to the study had a higher incidence in the following eight years than those who were 45 to 74 at entry. In less obese populations onset probably occurs later than in the very fat Pimas. Middle-aged Pimas are much fatter than elderly Pimas. These and additional data on the Pimas have been summarized by Bennett, et al (1967a). Incidence of diabetes *falls* markedly with age after peaking in the fourth decade. To some degree these findings may be peculiar to this population, but they fit well the possibility that much of the relationship of age to incidence of diabetes observed in other populations may not be a direct effect of age. Much of the relationship may be the result of the association of age with other factors such as degree and duration of fatness.

Other considerations concerning the problem of defining diabetes in the elderly have been discussed in Chapter 4 in the section on diagnostic tests. Peculiar age-onset patterns attend certain special types of diabetes, including insulin-requiring diabetes not associated with ketosis, and diabetes associated with pancreatic calcification. These are discussed in Chapter 8 on special types of diabetes. Effects of age on incidence are discussed further in the section on incidence in Chapter 5.

Figure 10 also shows the distribution of age of discovery of insulin-requiring diabetes in London. Few data are available concerning the frequency of the various subelements of this or other populations of insulin-requiring diabetics (ketosis-prone cases, ketosis-resistant cases, "secondary" diabetes associated with factors such as pancreatitis, etc.). In most affluent societies a substantial portion who take insulin would not require it under optimum dietary management. In these societies most of the diabetics that really require insulin are lean patients with little or no insulin secretion and a propensity to develop ketonemia in the absence of insulin therapy. This type of diabetes often develops rapidly and, in general, the time between onset and discovery is shorter than for typical maturity-onset diabetics. Thus in the ketosis-prone cases the frequency distribution of age at discovery reflects more closely age at onset.

Full information is rarely available from whole populations, or representative samples thereof, concerning the age of onset in relation to the many important factors that deserve systematic study, such as degree of insulin dependence, adiposity, and severity of hyperglycemia with and without treatment. Much is left to be learned, but it does appear that in well-fed societies there is a fall in the incidence of insulin-dependent diabetes after it reaches a peak at about puberty. The rate probably remains above that of infancy throughout life, however. The relationship of age to risk of insulin-independent diabetes in lean persons probably varies with several factors including the definition of "lean". The very low rates of this type of diabetes in some societies suggests the possibility that risk may be lower in very lean persons than in moderately lean persons. However, rates of ketosis-resistant insulin-dependent diabetes are highest in young adults who are extremely lean. The incidence of adult-onset diabetes in lean subjects is discussed further in Chapter 8 on special types of diabetes.

Experimental data of Bjorntorp, et al (1977) are compatible with the possibility that adiposity and indolence are more responsible than aging for the deterioration of glucose tolerance in middle-age that is typical in affluent societies. Short and Johnson studied this matter and reported their results in a little-known publication of 1939. Their results in insurance policy holders suggested that most of the deterioration of glucose tolerance observed with aging was attributable to increasing adiposity and to increasing duration of this fatness. In older persons who had remained lean, tolerance was almost as good as in young lean persons. It should also be kept in mind that duration of fatness is probably an important risk factor, and this is strongly related to age. Kruse-Jarres and Werner (1973) also thought that deterioration of glucose tolerance with age was partly attributable to the incidental concomitants of aging.

In a few lean populations no deterioration of glucose tolerance with aging was observed. These included Indians studied by Tripathy, et al (1973) and Egyptians tested by Ayad (1967). On the other hand, West and Kalbfleisch (1971) observed a modest decline in tolerance with age in each of eight different lean populations. This included East Pakistan, where there was no weight gain with age. Chlouverakis, et al (1967) studied insulin secretion by age in a representative sample of a whole population (Bedford, England). In relation to their blood glucose levels the older subjects secreted more insulin. These investigators acknowledged some conflicting evidence, but concluded that diminution of glucose tolerance with age is probably mainly the result of lesser tissue response to insulin. The greater fatness of older subjects may contribute to this, but mean fatness tends to decline after the seventh decade even in affluent societies.

In affluent societies distribution of age of onset of diabetes is similar in dogs and people. In dogs, juvenile-onset diabetes (before 4 years of age) is quite uncommon; incidence then rises abruptly and persists at about the same rate in dogs from 7–12 years of age (Foster, 1975). The older dogs, are, of course, fatter. There may be some differences by breed in age of onset patterns. In Foster's study (1975), dachshunds seemed to have earlier onset than poodles.

The age-onset pattern of juvenile diabetes is discussed in Chapter 8. The effect of age on glucose tolerance is reviewed in the section on diagnostic tests (Chapter 4).

SEX

Many observations have been made on the frequency of diabetes in the two sexes in the hope of providing insights into its nature and causes. It is still widely believed that females are more susceptible to maturity-onset diabetes, and in most affluent societies there is female dominance of varying degree.

WHO, in its report of 1964, calculated an average of mortality rates for males and females in the 45 countries from which they received reports. The mean male:female ratio was 1:1.5. Before 1900, however, diabetes was observed more frequently in men in both Europe and the United States (Lepine, 1909; Joslin, 1917). Lepine (1909) cited seven different series from widely different parts of Europe in which observations were made on distribution by sex. Females constituted from 17% to 43% of cases. In England and Wales, male:female ratios were typically 2:1 before 1910 (Emerson and Larimore, 1924). But since 1930 clinicians of both America and Europe have repeatedly observed a greater frequency in females. By 1952 diabetes mortality rates were higher in females of every country from which data were available except for Japan and Italy (Hargreaves, 1958). This led many to overgeneralize and to assume a specific and special female susceptibility. This propensity has only recently been mitigated by more thorough analyses and less provincial perspectives.

Appendix 7B, at the end of this chapter, illustrates the complexity of these matters. It is clear that there are marked variations among societies in the apparent sex ratio. In Western Europe, for example, rates are substantially higher in females, while in rural South Korea males have a rate of diabetes 3.4 times higher than women (Kim, et al, 1975). Even in certain modern American communities the male:female ratio of diabetics is greater than one. Rates were somewhat higher in males of Massachusetts (O'Sullivan, et al, 1967; Garcia, et al, 1974) and in Rochester, Minnesota (Palumbo, et al, 1976). A recent study in Greece found that rates were the same in the sexes (Christocopoulos, et al, 1976).

Sex ratios have not infrequenty changed substantially over time in the same society (Harris and McArthur, 1951). In Britain and in several countries of Western Europe the apparent female preponderance has recently diminished considerably (Malins, et al, 1965; Nicholson, 1971; Nilsson, et al, 1967 in Sweden; Drury and Timoney, 1972 in Ireland). In Birmingham, England a generation ago, diabetes was decidedly more common in women; but in 1970–1972 the male:female ratio was about 1.5 for new cases from 20 to 64 years of age, and 0.75 for new cases over 64 years of age (Malins, 1974b). These changes in Britain may be the result of increasing adiposity in men and decreasing fatness in women (Malins, 1974b).

The important effect of age on these sex ratios deserves more emphasis than it has received. One of the first and best demonstrations of this was by Spiegelman and Marks in 1946. They pointed out that in both Massachusetts and the United States the rate of diabetes was only slightly greater in young women than in young men, while in the age group 40 to 69 diabetes was almost twice as prevalent in women. In still older people the female preponderance declined substantially. The same phenomenon is evident in many other societies including most European countries (WHO, 1964). In a recent study in a community in the USSR (Zybina, 1975), diabetes rates were about twice as high in women. But in the fifth decade of life rates were the same in the sexes, while in the fourth decade rates were about four times as high in women.

217

Silwer reviewed in 1958 data that had been collected up to that time on prevalence by sex in many European communities, finding that results were quite variable. Most, but not all, studies showed a female preponderance. In populations with a female preponderance in middle age, ratios regularly declined toward unity in old age. This is consistent with the possibility that female predominance is mainly the result of the greater increase in fatness in women during middle life. This trend toward increasing adiposity is usually reversed in old age in both women and men, but reversal typically begins about a decade earlier in men (West, 1973).

Vinke, et al (1958) collected data on height and weight in a large group of diabetics whom they deemed representative of the universe of diabetics in northern Holland. There was no significant difference at any age level between the sexes in the number with insulin-dependent diabetes. In the seventh decade the ratio of male to female diabetics was about 1:4, but obesity was much more common in females of this age. While not conclusive, the data suggested that the overall predominance of female diabetics of 2:1 in this population was mainly or entirely attributable to the greater fatness of the women.

In many societies the frequency of testing and clinical care varies substantially by sex. It seems very likely, for example, that the relatively low rates observed in females of certain communities in India, Iraq, Pakistan, and Ethiopia are at least in part the result of the lesser frequency of testing in women. Reed reported in 1915 that 118 of 136 Chinese diabetics in his group were men, but he concluded correctly that this phenomenon was mainly or completely the result of the lesser amount of testing that then prevailed in women. In one recent study of Hong Kong Chinese patients, known diabetes was slightly more common in females (McFadzean and Yeung, 1968). On the other hand, death certificate data of WHO for 1965 show that death from diabetes in Hong Kong was 2.65 times more common in males (Kurihara, et al, 1970). In modern mainland China rates in the sexes are similar (Chung, et al, 1962).

In several series of clinical cases from the Indian subcontinent, rates in males have been much higher in females. For example, Ibrahmin (1962) in Pakistan published data from a clinic where the ratio was about 7:1. In a series of Dutt (1927) only 4 of 300 Bengali diabetics were females, and in a group of Chakravarty (1938) only 6 of 853 were females! In several other Indian series a male:female ratio of 4:1 was typical (Shankar, 1966). When, however, comparisons are made from surveys, rates are usually similar in the two sexes. In the series of Gupta, et al (1970), for example, rates were only slightly higher in males. Subsequently, Gutpa, et al (1975) summarized sex ratios in several subpopulations of India in which results were based on surveys. The ratios of males to females varied considerably, from 1:1 to 2:1. In Bombay screenees (K.E.M. Hospital Group, 1966) rates were 3.1% in females and 2.1% in males. In a survey conducted in Hyderabad rates were 3.4% in males and 5.8% in females (Satyanarayana, et al, 1966). Campbell reported to Tulloch (1962) that 70% of his Indian diabetics in Durban, South Africa, were women.

It also seems likely that there are circumstances in which women are tested more frequently than men. Another major consideration is that differences between the sexes in adiposity vary considerably among societies. In East Pakistan, for example, little difference was observed between the sexes (West and Kalbfleisch, 1971), while in North America black females are much fatter than black males (West, 1973). In some American clinics diabetic black females have outnumbered males as much as four to one (Altschul and Nathan, 1942). In 1933, Joslin, et al reported that mortality rates from diabetes were similar for the sexes in young adult blacks insured by the Metropolitan Company, but rates were almost three times higher in middle-aged black females. Charles and Medard (1969) observed that rates of known diabetes in the poor of Haiti were much higher in women than men (4.7:1). In a small group of Yemenites of Israel (Cohen, 1961) diabetes was somewhat more common in males (14 of 325 males and 8 of 426 females). In Massachusetts Jews diabetes was twice as frequent in females as in males (Rudy and Keeler, 1939). Ajgaonkar (1970) cited higher rates in males than in females of Uganda, Ceylon, Japan, Rhodesia, and Fiji. He thought that generally in tropical countries women worked harder than men; and that this might account for their relative immunity to diabetes.

In our international studies in 11 countries (West and Kalbfleisch, 1970, 1971) we did not find any differences between the sexes in rates of diabetes that could not be explained by their differences in adiposity. In Central America diabetes was about twice as common in females, but matching for fatness corrected this difference entirely. In Malaya our rates were somewhat higher in males but the numbers of diabetics were quite small. DeZoysa reported to Tulloch (1962) that men of Ceylon were more frequently obese than women, DeZoysa (1951) had previously reported a higher rate of diabetes in men of Ceylon.

With very few exceptions, these two considerations (differences in fatness and frequency of testing) explain most or all of the deviation of the sex ratio from unity. There are some special peculiarities that deserve further study. In Japan, sex ratios have been highly variable. In some communities diabetes appears to be considerably more common in men, even when rates are determined by mass surveys (Blackard, et al, 1965; Belsky, et al, 1973). On the other hand, little difference between the sexes has been observed in other Japanese communities where rates were based on surveys (Tsuji and Wada, 1970; Sasaki, et al, 1973). Moreover, death rates from diabetes for all of Japan and for Japanese Americans seem to be very similar in the sexes (Tsuji and Wada, 1970; Entmacher and Marks, 1965). In Japan, adiposity seems to be similar in the sexes (Rudnick and Anderson, 1962).

Since data showing male predominance in South Korea (Kim, 1970, 1973, 1975) and Okinawa (Sakumoto, 1970) were based on community surveys, it is probable that the apparent male predominance in those communities is real. Among the factors associated with but not directly related to sex, that could account for some part of these variations are the differences in societies in levels of exercise in men and women. Often in surveys women receive loading doses of glucose that are the same as for men. Since the volume of distribution of the administered glucose is smaller in women, this would tend to increase

219

their blood glucose values slightly more than in men. In some circumstances this factor would be negligible, but in others it would probably be appreciable.

Another consideration is that men have a lower renal threshold for glucose than women (Gordon, 1964; Keen, 1964; Butterfield, et al, 1967; Mimura, 1970). With few exceptions surveys in Asia have used urine tests as the prime screening instrument. This would tend to increase the preponderance of males.

Evidence cited below under parity suggests that under most circumstances childbearing probably does not have much effect on risk of diabetes. In general, parity is very great in those societies (eg, Pakistan, Uganda, Iraq, India) where male:female ratios of diabetes have been low. Pyke and Please (1957) showed that higher rates in women of certain elements of the population of Britain might be due to childbearing. One reason they cited was that the higher rates of diabetes in women could not be explained entirely by their greater fatness. But subsequently, as explained above, there was a dramatic reduction in the female preponderance in Britain. In general, sex ratios of prevalence of diabetes in Britain in the 1960s were roughly proportional to the degree of fatness in the two sexes demonstrated by Pyke and Please in the 1950s. Other evidence cited by Montegriffo (1968) suggests that prior to the 1950s the considerable disparity between fatness of women and men had been narrowing in Britain.

Blackard, et al (1965) suggested the possibility that men were more susceptible to diabetes and that female:male ratios might approach or exceed unity only when women were fatter. Another complicating factor in interpreting present evidence is that women, whose weights are 100% of our standard or ideal levels for women, are substantially fatter than men whose weights are 100% of our present standard for men.

Additional details concerning mortality rates by country and sex may be found in publications of Marigo, et al (1974), Kurihara, et al (1970), Marks and Krall (1971), and the World Health Organization publications of 1964 and 1974. The 1964 publication also gives interesting details by age. It is shown, for example, that in many different Western societies female predominance is especially striking in the age group 45—64.

In the aggregate, present evidence suggests little difference between the sexes in susceptibility to typical adult-onset diabetes after corrections are made for the various factors described above, but more investigation is required with respect to some of the unexplained disparities. Sex ratios in certain special kinds of diabetes will be discussed below in Chapter 8.

Sex ratios are strongly influenced by environmental factors; and geographic variations in sex ratios are more often related to environment than to race itself. In Trinidad and in many communities of India, diabetes is more common in Indian males, but in British Guiana rates in Indian men and women were very similar, while in Durban rates were higher in Indian women (Tulloch, 1962). WHO (1964) data show little difference in diabetes mortality rates of males and females who are South African Asiatics.

It is generally accepted that in the United States diabetes is more common in women than in men. A National Health Survey confirmed this (Bauer, et al, 1967). This latter comparison was based on ascertainment by interview. In a national survey, Ranofsky (1977) found that about 60% of American patients hospitalized for diabetes were women. However, Gordon, et al (1964) found little difference in levels of glucose tolerance in men and women.

In dogs diabetes is much more common in females. Female:male ratios have ranged from 2:1 to as high as 20:1. In two of the larger and well-studied series (Krook, et al, 1960; Foster, 1975), ratios were about 2:1. In cats, diabetes is less common and epidemiologic data are few, but it appears that the disease is more common in males (Meier, 1960). Generally, female dogs are fatter than males, but data are not adequate to determine the extent to which the greater adiposity explains the higher rates in females. In a certain strain of mice, females are more resistant than males to the diabetogenic effect of a virus (Craighead, 1971). Dickie (1969) cited a few examples of the production of obesity, islet hyperplasia, and diabetes in genetically susceptible small animals by increasing or reducing sex hormones. In one strain of mice, islet-cell hypertrophy and obesity in males followed gonadectomy.

Variations and possible variations by sex in the manifestations and types of diabetes have been reviewed by Danowski, et al (1966). These will also be discussed in this volume in sections to follow (Chapters 8 and 10). Appendix 7B at the end of this chapter lists many populations in which substantial differences have been observed between the sexes in the frequency of diabetes.

PARITY

It has long been known that the first manifestations of diabetes often present themselves during pregnancy. Bose mentioned in 1895 that glycosuria occurred frequently with pregnancy, and often subsided thereafter. In 1924 Emerson and Larimore reported that in married women of New York City the rate of mortality from diabetes was about four times higher than in single women. But the difference was as great between married and single men. Mosenthal and Bolduan also noted in 1933 that married women seemed to have more diabetes than single women. The same phenomenon prevailed in Britain (Hargreaves, 1958). Joslin and his associates (1935) had also observed this, but they found that their married diabetic women weighed 20 lb more on the average than single diabetic women. No difference was found in weights of married women with and without children. They also presented data showing that in Canada mortality rates from diabetes were considerably higher in married than in age-matched single women. Munro, et al (1949) and Pyke (1956) reported from Britain results of more detailed studies on parity and susceptibility to diabetes, establishing a strong association. These and subsequent studies showed that in their populations the greater weight and age of multiparous women did not entirely account for the association between parity and risk of diabetes (Pyke and Please, 1956). This was confirmed in Britain by reports of FitzGerald, et al (1961a) and of Middleton and Caird (1968), and in Trinidad by Pyke and Wattley (1962).

Subsequent to the initial epidemiologic reports, many physiological studies

221

identified attributes of the state of pregnancy that seemed to be potentially diabetogenic. These included the identification of placental lactogen, which exerts effects similar to those of growth hormone, and the relative hyperinsulinemia required by pregnancy. Frequently fatness increases during pregnancy, placing further demands on the beta cells. The frequency with which diabetes was discovered in pregnancy also suggested that pregnancy increased susceptibility to diabetes. Response of the beta cells to tolbutamide declines substantially during the course of pregnancy (Kaplan, 1961). Tissue chromium levels were found to be lower in multiparous women (Hambidge and Rodgerson, 1969). Finally, it was noted that mild diabetes during pregnancy often disappeared after delivery.

For these reasons, it became rather generally accepted that pregnancy increased risk of diabetes and this notion is still held by most specialists in diabetes. Recently, however, a considerable body of evidence has appeared suggesting a need to reexamine this matter. Even as far back as 1947, Wilkerson and Krall had found that males in Oxford, Massachusetts had as much diabetes as females. In 1959, Vinke, et al found in Holland no relationship of parity and risk of diabetes. Steinberg (1958) had also questioned the widely held conclusion that pregnancy was diabetogenic. In 1964 Seftel concluded that in South African blacks, parity was similar in diabetics and controls. We subsequently reported results in ten populations (West and Kalbfleisch, 1970). In Central America (and in each of its six countries) there was no relationship between parity and prevalence of diabetes. Nor was there any such association in Malaya or East Pakistan. In Venezuela and Uruguay there was a relationship of parity and rate of diabetes, but there was also a relationship between parity and adiposity. In these two countries the relationship between parity and diabetes may have been partly or wholly attributable to the greater fatness of multiparous women. There was no relationship of parity and diabetes in Pima Indians (Bennett, et al, 1967). In Hong Kong, McFadzean and Yeung (1968) found parity somewhat greater in nondiabetics. In Sweden, neither Pehrson (1974) nor Lunell (1966) observed any relationship between parity and glucose tolerance. In Bedford, England, a relationship of parity and diabetes was not found (Keen, 1964). In a group of Indian women, Gupta, et al (1970) found a lower rate of diabetes in women who had not borne children, but in women who had had more than three children rates of diabetes were not higher than in women who had borne one to three children. These latter data from India were not adjusted for age or weight. Wicks and Jones found no association between parity and diabetes in Rhodesian blacks. Results of O'Sullivan, et al in Sudbury, Massachusetts (1967) were also negative in this respect as were those of Florey in Jamaica and of Dunn (1968) in the United States. On the basis of his data and wide experience in various populations of South Africa, Jackson (1961,1965) concluded that parity probably had little, if any, importance in determining risk of diabetes even though it sometimes precipitated the disease.

One of the most impressive pieces of negative evidence is the result of the US National Health Survey. In a large sample representative of the general population of the United States, there was little relationship between parity and blood glucose levels after oral glucose (O'Sullivan and Gordon, 1966). These latter data were corrected for age and skinfold thickness. Among known diabetics in the US National Survey there was a weak relationship between parity and rates of known diabetes, but these latter data were not adjusted for fatness. After analyzing their data in those with both occult and diagnosed diabetes from the national surveys, O'Sullivan and Gordon concluded that "available data seem to favor the conclusion that pregnancy plays no role in the causation or early appearance of diabetes". They did not, however, regard the present evidence as entirely decisive.

Rates of parity are very high in several populations in which the incidence of diabetes appears to be lower in women than in men (eg, India, Pakistan, Korea, Iraq, Malawi, and Nigeria).

In contrast, a few of the more recent studies tend to confirm an association of parity and risk of diabetes. Walker and Carridge in Britain (1961) found a decidedly positive association, but those data were not adjusted for age or adiposity. Harger in the United States found a strong relationship of parity and diabetes in mothers of large babies, but it was not clear whether this was attributable to a relationship of diabetes to maternal age and weight that he also demonstrated. Dreyfuss, et al (1962) found a strong association of parity and diabetes in a group of Israeli women. These data were not adjusted for age, however.

The study done by Middleton and Caird (1968) in an English community again confirmed the strong association between parity and diabetes that has usually been observed in Britain. The relationship of childbearing and fatness did not account fully for the association between parity and rate of diabetes. Frequency of family history of diabetes was not related to parity. If parity had a direct effect in producing permanent decompensation of beta-cell function, one might expect a relationship between time of pregnancy and time of onset of diabetes. This would produce earlier onset of diabetes in multiparous women. But neither Munro (1949), Pyke (1956) nor FitzGerald, et al (1961a) observed any relationship between time of pregnancy and time of onset of diabetes. In recent years the sex ratio of the incidence of diabetes in Britain has closely approached unity (Malins, 1974b). This diminishes the likelihood that parity is an important risk factor.

Both Munro (1949) and FitzGerald, et al (1961a) found the frequency of family history of diabetes declined with increasing parity, but Middleton and Caird (1968) did not. Tulloch reviewed in his book (1962) the results of several other studies on parity and diabetes. Results and conclusions were conflicting, and most of these earlier studies were difficult to interpret because of incomplete information on factors such as ages, weights, etc. A good review of Jackson (1967) on pregnancy and diabetes cites 275 references.

What is to be made of all this conflicting evidence? It may be that in very lean and in very fat populations the deleterious effects of pregnancy are relatively trivial as compared to the strongly protective effects of leanness and the profoundly disadvantageous effects of corpulence. It also seems possible that the associations between parity and risk of diabetes observed in some populations may not have a relationship of cause and effect. In some cases cited above, it is quite clear that factors such as fatness account for some or all of the relationship. In surveys in which a fixed glucose load is given, fatter women receive a slightly smaller load in relation to their extracellular space and body mass. When multiparous women are fatter, relative rates of apparent diabetes would be slightly lessened in them under these conditions. A fixed dose was used in Oxford, Sudbury, Bedford, and the US National Survey. This could also account, in part, for the disparity often observed in male:female ratios of rates of occult "diabetes" as compared to sex ratios of known diabetics. When a fixed dosage of glucose is given to all, females receive a relative larger amount in proportion to body sizes. Renal threshold for glucose is decreased in pregnancy, making likelihood of discovery greater. Also, pregnant women are especially likely to be tested for diabetes.

Another finding that fails to support the hypothesis that parity is diabetogenic is the failure in many societies to demonstrate an excess of diabetes in women. In Olmstead County, Minnesota, for example, diabetes was a bit more common in men (Palumbo, et al, 1976). This was also the case in Sudbury, Massachusetts (O'Sullivan, et al, 1967). Many other instances are given in Appendix 7B. On the other hand, it is quite possible that under certain circumstances pregnancy increased risk of diabetes. The well-demonstrated physiologic effects of pregnancy argue for this possibility. Yet it is also possible that these physiologic challenges imposed temporarily by pregnancy do not induce permanent diabetes in those not otherwise destined to do so. It might even be argued that a little exercise of this type could be good for the beta cells unless they are in some way defective.

Pregnancy and obesity have in common the imposition of additonal work for beta cells, but the nature of these challenges in pregnancy and obesity differs both quantitatively and qualitatively. Taken alone, epidemiologic evidence is not decisive in this instance. It neither establishes nor entirely exonerates pregnancy as a risk factor in diabetes. Present evidence does suggest that the effect of pregnancy is probably negligible or trivial in many societies.

EXERCISE AND NUTRITIONAL FACTORS

Exercise

Exercise is probably a potent protective factor. Indeed, it is possible that indolence is the most important of all inciting factors of adult-onset insulin-independent diabetes, particularly because of its enhancement of risk of obesity. In 1895 Bose observed: "Amongst Zemindars and Talookdars who consider it a pride and honour to lead an indolent life, diabetes is a common complaint". Sen (1893) had previously reviewed evidence in India that exercise protected against diabetes. This included observations summarized by Cheevers in 1886.

Several participants (Havelock Charles, et al) in a 1907 symposium on diabetes in the tropics cited examples suggesting that diabetes was common in indolent populations and rare in those with high levels of exercise. R. K. C. Bose (1907) reported, for example, that diabetes was rife in rich Bengali men and that they considered exercise quite undignified. It may be that the apparent increase in diabetes in recent years is due in part to indolence. In 1940 American workers of all types expended an average of 3 kcal/minute; by 1964 energy required on the job had declined to an average of 2.5 kcal/minute (Sukhatme, 1969).

Unfortunately, quantitative data on exercise are few and very difficult to gather. Also, the short- and long-term effects of exercise on carbohydrate metabolism are very incompletely understood. There are two general mechanisms by which inactivity can lead to diabetes. Inactivity favors corpulence, but there is also evidence of directly deleterious effects of indolence. It has been shown, for example, that inactivity impairs glucose tolerance (Altman, et al, 1969) and that physical conditioning improves glucose tolerance (Bjorntorp, et al, 1977). Improvement of glucose tolerance by exercise has been shown by many investigators including Cristophe and Mayer (1958). Experiments of Palmer and Tipton (1974) demonstrated that physical training in rats increased lipogenesis from glucose. Commesatti had shown in 1906 that glucose tolerance increased with exercise in rabbits. Lipman, et al (1970) found that complete bed rest for two weeks substantially reduced glucose tolerance in man. Apparently this reduction was the result of impaired sensitivity to insulin rather than reduced insulin secretion. Lipman, et al (1972) also showed that exercise at bed rest prevented deterioration of glucose tolerance, establishing that this impairment was not secondary to change in gravitational vector. There is evidence that highly-conditioned persons have excellent glucose tolerance despite low levels of insulin secretion (Irsigler, et al, 1976; Johansen and Munck, 1976).

Both juvenile and maturity-onset diabetes seems to be rare in primitive societies where high levels of energy expenditure are required to maintain life. There is a very good correlation between levels of electrical power consumption and rates of diabetes, both among countries and in specific countries over time (Joslin, et al, 1935). Interpretation of these associations is difficult mainly because of the association of industrialization and food supply. High rates of diabetes in fat Sumo wrestlers of Japan (Kuzuya, et al, 1975) suggest that physical conditioning alone provides only limited protection from diabetes in the presence of substantial obesity. However, the physical conditioning of these wrestlers is of a rather special kind and may not have the same effects of that developed by prolonged walking, herding, hunting, grinding, etc.

The development of corpulence is probably in some circumstances related more to overeating than to indolence, but in other circumstances the reverse is true (Greene, 1939; Johnson, et al, 1956; Mayer, 1965; Campbell, 1964,1970a). Exercise levels have not been measured systematically in the American Indian groups with exceedingly high rates of diabetes. Exercise levels in Oklahoma Indians appear to be about the same as in local whites, but this is difficult to assess and may be an erroneous assumption. They are certainly much less active than before their encounter with the white men. Wise, et al (1976) found no evidence in Australian aborigines that exercise levels were lower in diabetics than in nondiabetics. The diabetics were much fatter, but apparently not less active.

Insulin levels seem to be low in at least some primitive populations (Rubenstein, et al, 1969; Wapnick, et al, 1972). There are several possible reasons for this, of which one is high levels of exercise. More data are needed on insulin secretion patterns in lean indolent subjects, and in the exceptional subjects who are fat despite high levels of energy expenditure. Diabetes is fairly common in American athletes, but in many of these, special athletic prowess was developed after the discovery of diabetes. Seasonal variations in insulin secretion levels (Fahlen, et al, 1971) may have been attributable in part to seasonal variations in exercise. The impressive peculiarity of rates of diabetes in certain occupations (reviewed below) is probably to a considerable degree attributable to the exercise levels required or associated with these occupations. The same may be said of the associations of diabetes in certain circumstances with social and economic class. Dr. Joslin pointed out in 1935 the very low rates of diabaetes in agricultural workers of Britain and America. Ahrens, et al (1968) showed that even at the same weight, animals that exercised more had less body fat. This illustrates the need to use relative weight cautiously as an index of fatness. It would be of interest to examine the fatness of the various South African races after matching for relative weight. Eskimos are very lean despite moderately high relative weights (West, 1974; Schaefer, 1977).

In one of the few studies in which an attempt was made to examine the relationship of physical activity and risk of diabetes, Rao, et al (1966) found that the rate of diabetes in a group of 21,396 Indians of Hyderbad was 3.2% in the majority (18,316) who were considered "moderately" active. In 2,263 "sedentary" persons the rate was 7.9%, and 2.8% in 877 who were deemed to engage in "severe" activity. These data were not corrected for age or adiposity. In 1924 Emerson and Larimore described observations suggesting that exercise protected from diabetes. They cited, for example, low diabetes rates and high occupational exercise in certain Negro groups.

One possibility that deserves attention is that much of the strong association between adiposity and risk of diabetes is partly incidental to the relationship of corpulence and indolence. There are, however, some considerations that indicate an independent effect of obesity itself. In fat people caloric deficits alone produce profoundly normalizing effects on insulin secretion patterns; and in obese subjects with impaired glucose tolerance, tolerance is greatly improved with dieting alone. Kawate, et al (1975) found glucose tolerance much better in Japanese of Hiroshima than in those of Hawaii, even though caloric intake seemed to be higher in the leaner more active group in Hiroshima. Details will be given below concerning very sharp reductions in rates of death from diabetes in civilian populations during deprivations of war. These circumstances do not suggest that reductions in exercise occurred. Rather, the reduced levels of diabetes would appear to have been attributable to reduced food supplies. These considerations do not argue against a major role of exercise in preventing obesity, but they suggest that degree of fatness is in itself a very important determinant of risk of diabetes. Experimental work in animals confirms that exercise can mitigate adiposity even when food is not limited. Ahrens, et al (1968) showed this in rats, for example. Griffiths and Payne (1976) found exercise levels lower in children of obese than of nonobese parents.

A major problem in the epidemiologic study of indolence as a risk factor is the difficulty in measuring levels of exercise. Dawber, et al (1966) described a simple scheme for crudely measuring levels of energy expenditure by history. Recently, Montoye, et al (1977) reported on data from a whole population of adult men in whom levels of exercise as obtained by history were related to levels of adiposity, serum insulin, and glucose tolerance. No relationship was found between exercise and these variables except that glucose tolerance was somewhat better in the leanest subgroup when exercise levels were high.

Calories

Evidence linking obesity to diabetes will be discussed in detail below. In this section some observations will be cited in which food intake has been related to risk of diabetes.

Long before the days of systematic epidemiologic studies, clinicians suspected that dietary excesses enhanced risk of diabetes and that risk was minimized by dietary continence. Hindu physicians of the sixth century attributed diabetes to overindulgence in rich foods. According to Thomas Willis (1679), "the diabetes was a disease so rare among the ancients that many famous physicians made no mention of it; and Galen knew only two sick of it. But in our age, given to good fellowship and gusling down chiefly of unalloyed wine, we meet with examples and instances enough, I may say daily, of this disease". Bouchardat (1875) observed that rates of diabetes declined sharply during the seige of Paris in the Franco-Prussian War. Subsequently, similar war-related deprivations have been associated with marked declines in rates of death from diabetes. Figure 12, prepared by Joslin and presented by Himsworth (1935-1936) shows the dramatic effects of World War I in populations that were short of food, and the lack of effects in Tokyo and America where food was plentiful. In Berlin the diabetic mortality rate declined from 23.1 per 100,000 in 1914 to 10.9 in 1919! Geiger (1952) described sharp declines in rates of diabetes in Europe during the deprivations of World War I, and in Belgium and France in World War II. Gajewski (1920) reported on the decline of diabetes rates in Berlin during World War I. In World War II, similar changes were observed in Europe (Schliack, 1954) and even in the United Kingdom where the shortage was relatively mild (Himsworth, 1949a). Vartianen (1946) showed that diabetes mortality decreased in Finland during the deprivations associated with World War II. In occupied Norway diabetes mortality rates in women fell from 17.4 in 1940 to 8.9 in 1945; then they rose to 17.2 in 1949 (Akademisk Tryknings

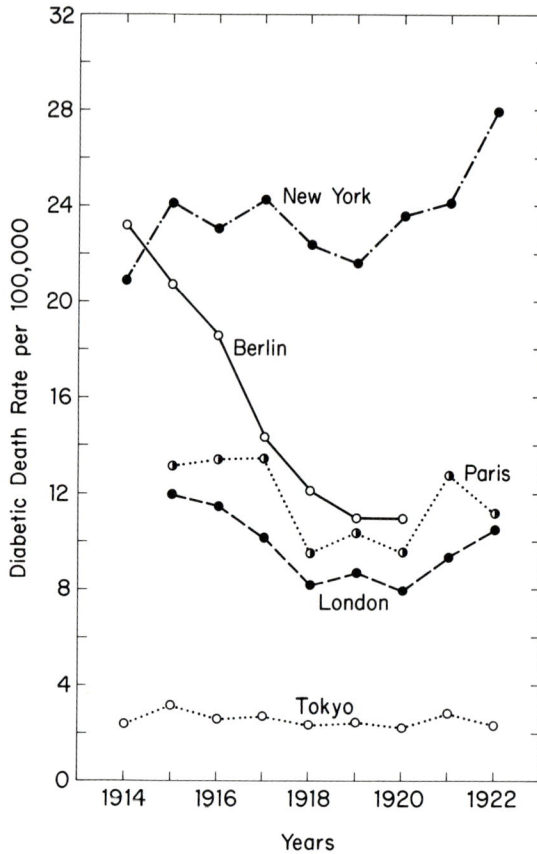

FIGURE 12. Effect of World War I on diabetes mortality rates. Data compiled by Joslin as presented by Himsworth (1935–1936).

Central of Oslo, 1954). Comparable changes occurred in men. Goto (1958) presented evidence that rates of diabetes fell sharply in Japan during World War II as a result of undernutrition. The percentages of total inpatients and outpatients who were insulin-dependent diabetics fell moderately, while the percentages of these patients who were insulin-independent diabetics declined drastically. It is probable that the favorable effects of these war-related deprivations on diabetes mortality rates are not wholly related to greater longevity of existing cases with prewar onset. Rather the data suggest a marked decline in new cases. Even so it does not seem likely that declines of this degree could be accounted for by declining incidence alone. The magnitudes of these effects suggest the exciting probability that longevity is indeed increased by dietary restriction. There are, of course, possibilities that qualitative features of diet account for part of the decline in incidence and mortality. This will be discussed below. It seems likely, however, that the major preventive factor was reduction of calories.

In 1919, Allen, Stillman, and Fitz reviewed an extensive array of evidence and concluded that gluttony was a major cause of diabetes. ". . . . A regulated mixed diet, rather than carbohydrate abstinence is recommended for prophylaxis on the same principle as for treatment". Joslin wrote a classic paper, published in 1921, incriminating obesity and dietary excess (see below). In 1924 Emerson and Larimore wrote what was probably the first paper in which the term epidemiology was applied in a study of diabetes (although Joslin had applied the word epidemic as early as 1921). Emerson and Larimore reviewed evidence linking caloric consumption to risk of diabetes. They concluded that quantitative rather than qualitative features of the diet were probably most critical. In 1935 Himsworth published a scholarly landmark paper on diet and incidence of diabetes. His main hypothesis, to be discussed later, was that a high-fat, low-carbohydrate diet was the principal culprit. On the other hand, the data that he skillfully brought together from very many sources were also consistent with an effect of total calories on risk of diabetes. He acknowledged this probability. In 1953 R. D. Lawrence concluded that diabetes was substantially more common in Sydney, Australia, than in Britain, and that the high rate in Sidney was the result of overeating.

Precise measurement of caloric consumption is very difficult both in populations and in individuals except under carefully controlled conditions. Moreover, it is seldom possible to control such conditions over long periods of time. These difficulties have limited the epidemiologic approach to the study of caloric consumption as a risk factor. There are, however, some further modern circumstances that suggest the influence of caloric consumption. Diabetes rates appeared to have increased markedly in the last generation in Japan at a time when food consumption per capita was rising sharply (Oiso, 1970). In Taiwan there has been a sharp rise in the prevalence of diabetes coinciding with an increase in daily food consumption from 1,217 kcal/person/day in 1948 to 2,509 in 1968 (Tsai, 1971). In Haiti, food consumption was found by Charles and Medard (1969) to be very low in poor people (980-1,500 kcal/person/day) and high in the affluent (more than 3,000 kcal). Diabetes rates were about 100 times as great in the rich! In Africa, and in Papua and New Guinea (Price and Tulloch, 1966) food consumption and diabetes rates have usually been quite low in rural villages. In both of these areas diabetes rates have often risen sharply in urban environments after food consumption has increased. Food consumption is still very low in many Asian countries, all of which have low rates of diabetes (Mimura, 1970). In privileged societies where diabetes is regularly common, consumption averages 3,000 kcal daily. In the developing world where diabetes is uncommon, consumption in adults averages 2,150 kcal, and in some societies it is less than 2,000 (Sukhatme, 1969).

The industrial revolution greatly enhanced rates of diabetes by increasing food supply and reducing exercise levels. To the extent that primitive populations are protected from the effects of industrialization, they are protected from

229

diabetes. The nomadic Broayas of the Sahara, for example, have excellent glucose tolerance; both obesity and diabetes are unknown. Of 161 adults tested by DeHertogh, et al (1975), none had a two-hour plasma glucose over 150 mg/100 ml, despite glucose loads that averaged about 2 gm/kg!

In some intrapopulation studies no difference has been found in caloric consumption of those with and without occult diabetes when consumption was measured by an interview technique. In a study of Baird (1972) caloric consumption was greater in diabetics than in nondiabetics, but a small group with occult diabetes ate no more than their nondiabetic relatives. In Israel men with occult diabetes and prediabetes appeared to consume a number of calories quite similar to those who did not develop diabetes during the course of a study on the incidence of diabetes by Medalie, et al (1975). In the studies of Baird and of Medalie food consumption was measured by the interview technique. This raises the possibility that fat people in some societies are less likely than lean to give a full account of their food consumption. Another possibility is that obesity under some circumstances may be more attributable to indolence than to gluttony (Campbell, 1970a). This will be discussed further below. The group of Medalie, et al (1975) did find a strong relationship in this same Israeli population between relative weight and risk of diabetes. In a small number of offspring of two diabetic parents, the group of Booyens (1970) in South Africa were unable to demonstrate any qualitative or quantitative peculiarities in food intake in either those with or those without occult diabetes. Kawate, et al (1975) found glucose tolerance better in Hiroshima Japanese than in Japanese of Hawaii, even though caloric intake seemed to be higher in Hiroshima. The people in Hiroshima were leaner and more active.

In animals susceptible to diabetes, rates have been increased and decreased in proportion to levels of food intake (Renold, et al, 1971; Wyse and Dulin, 1970). This was also demonstrated by Allen in partially depancreatized dogs (1919) and by Martinez in alloxanized rats (1946). In many of the reports of animal experiments it was difficult to determine to what degree the onset of diabetes was attributable to quantitative or qualitative dietary changes. But more recent studies, such as those of Gerritsen, et al (1974) and Grodsky, et al (1974) in hamsters, demonstrate that quantitative changes alone may greatly influence susceptibility to diabetes.

The excessive insulin secretion observed in obese human subjects is partly attributable to excessive consumption of food (Olefsky, et al, 1975). It is possible that caloric levels in infancy could affect risk of obesity or diabetes at a later time (Brook, 1972; Yudkin, 1972).

Severe diabetes is common in feed-lot sheep being fattened for market (Warren, et al, 1966). Diabetes does not develop in these animals if feeding levels are lower and fattening more gradual (Meier, 1960).

STARVATION

It was well known as early as the 19th century that starvation in lean persons could precipitate hyperglycemia when refeeding was initiated (Allen, 1913).

This was sometimes referred to as "vagabond" diabetes, and the hyperglycemia was characteristically evanescent. The possibility that severe deprivation of protein or of calories and protein may cause diabetes will be discussed in chapter 8. Most of the available evidence suggests that calorie deprivation alone, although it may produce transitory hyperglycemia during refeeding, does not cause permanent diabetes. Under at least some conditions the insensitivity of beta-cells induced by starvation can be restored by the administration of calcium (Zawalich, et al, 1977). Protein-calorie malnutrition is discussed below in the section on protein consumption.

Obesity and Leanness

It has long been known and now quite generally accepted that obesity is an important risk factor for diabetes. But even today, the very great strength of the relationship between adiposity and diabetes is not sufficiently appreciated. In the United States and in most affluent societies obesity is the main cause of diabetes. In populations where obesity is rare, diabetes is rare, despite the presence of genetic susceptibility (West and Kalbfleisch, 1970,1971). Moreover, a very substantial majority of people with gross obesity of long duration develop diabetes irrespective of race or genetic status. Evidence to this effect is cited below. In general, diabetes has been looked upon as a hereditary disorder in which obesity often plays a "precipitating" role. More recent evidence would suggest that in affluent societies obesity is more often the prime cause, with heredity frequently playing a precipitating role. In these well-fed societies a small but significant minority of adult-onset diabetics have never been fat. Even so, these "nonobese" individuals have much more fat tissue than the average of persons in the underdeveloped world where a majority of humankind reside (West, 1973). The case against fatness will, therefore, be reviewed in some detail.

Some Observations of the Past with Modern Relevance

Indian physicians observed as early as 400 BC that diabetes was a disease of the well-fed. In his essay of 1868 Brigham mentioned reports of Roberts and Prout of diabetes in very fat persons. Prout's case weighed 23 stone (322 pounds)! Bose (1895) observed in Calcutta that " . . . victims of diabetes are generally selected from the fat and robust class of men". In the landmark symposium in diabetes in the tropics published in the *British Medical Journal* (Havelock Charles, et al, 1907), there was repeated allusion to the relationship of diabetes to overeating and sloth, but not much direct emphasis on obesity. The same may be said of Allen's great book of 1913 and the vast literature it cited. One reason for the slow recognition of the importance of obesity is that, in lean societies, most diabetes is not caused by obesity. Even if risk of diabetes is increased tenfold in decidedly obese persons, the link between obesity and diabetes may not be readily apparent in communities where less than 1% are obese. In the 19th century obesity was common only in special elements of a

231

limited number of societies. Even today obesity is uncommon in many societies. The potent diabetogenic effect of obesity becomes evident when obesity becomes common.

Joslin should receive a major share of the credit for demonstrating the prime importance of obesity. In a classic but now largely forgotten paper of 1921, he assembled an overwhelming indictment against obesity. Indeed, some of this evidence was as good as or better than much of our modern epidemiologic data. He recognized the importance of separating data by age of discovery of diabetes. In contrast to most previous and subsequent studies he also took into account weight prior to the discovery of diabetes (lifetime maximum), as well as present weight. There were some imperfections in the data available to him. The numerators were his own groups of diabetic patients (not necessarily representative of the universe of diabetics in his community). His denominators were insured populations (not ideally representative of the general population). But in several respects the approaches used were commendable even by modern standards. Large numbers were used (1,000 diabetic patients and insured populations of 135,249 and 744,672). He compared the frequency distribution of weights and maximum weights of diabetics with the frequency distribution of weights of the general population (as roughly reflected by the weights of the insured population). This is one of the very few studies where degree of leanness as well as obesity was studied. He found that diabetes was considerably more common in people of average weight than in those who had always been especially thin. Although his data on the latter aspect leave much to be desired, it is difficult to find any as good in the modern era. These data do suggest strongly that the relationship between adiposity and maturity-onset diabetes is not limited to that between risk of diabetes and what we in the privileged world regard as obesity. Rather it seems likely that those of average fatness in affluent societies are more likely to become diabetic than those in the rest of the world who are of average fatness in their communities. Typcially, average weight for height in poor societies is about 80% of our standards, and in some very poor societies it is less (Whyte, 1965; West, 1973; DeHertogh, et al, 1975).

In certain respects some of our own modern data (West and Kalbfleisch, 1966,1970,1971) on leanness and risk of diabetes are not as good as the 1921 data of Joslin. In our studies in 11 countries we did not, for example, obtain information on previous or maximum weight. A significant number of our diabetics had lost substantial amounts of weight, tending to obscure to some extent the negative correlation between marked leanness and risk of diabetes. Nevertheless, some of our data did suggest that very lean people had less diabetes than those whose relative weights were normal by our Western standards (West and Kalbfleisch, 1971).

Doctor Joslin's report of 1921 showed that rates of diabetes were 6 to 12 times greater in fat people than in thin, and in certain age groups this ratio was about 40-fold! He also pointed out that the association with diabetes of several other factors was probably secondary to their association with obesity. Those mentioned included conjugal diabetes, Jewish race, affluence, middle age, mental work, and gout. Joslin was one of a very few who have appreciated that the familiality of diabetes is in part incidental to the familiality and the hereditability of obesity. It has been shown above that the association between parity and diabetes is in some societies partly or wholly incidental to the association of parity and obesity. Evidence reviewed in Chapter 9 suggests that the association between maternal prediabetes and large babies is incidental, in at least some circumstances, to the relationship of maternal adiposity and birth weight.

The earlier observations of Joslin have been largely confirmed by subsequent experiences. In 1937 the Metropolitan Life Insurance Company reported in its Statistical Bulletin on "Birth and Death". Among persons more than 24% overweight, death from diabetes was eight times that in persons of normal weight and 13 times greater than in those who were underweight!

In 1915 Kisch averred that 50% of people with "constitutional obesity" had glycosuria. Paullin and Sauls reported in 1922 the results of glucose tolerance tests in a group of 26 people not known to have diabetes who were 10% to 80% overweight. Fifteen (58%) had abnormal tolerance. In a discussion of that paper, S. R. Roberts described a man who had gangrene and diabetes at a weight of 350 lb. As a result of a diet, he lost 170 lb, later maintaining a weight between 180 and 200 lb, at which time the blood sugar had become normal.

Anders and Jameson reported observations in 1925 on 7,100 patients, of whom 1,306 were obese and 5,850 were not. Calculations from their data show that only 0.5% of their nonobese patients had diabetes while 9% of their obese patients had diabetes, a difference of 18-fold. However, these two groups were not matched for age. In 1927 Allison who served as "Physician, Ruthin Castle", reported on glucose tolerance tests in 20 people who were 40% to 130% overweight. Eight had abnormal tolerance. Allison was one of few who gathered and reported data on duration of obesity. Glucose tolerance was normal on only 1 of 11 persons who had been overweight for more than ten years! One of his cases lost 45 lb with return of glucose tolerance to normal. Henry John reported in 1929 on the results of 1,100 glucose tolerance tests on his patients at the Cleveland Clinic. He concluded that obesity was the most important determinant of risk of abnormal tolerance. By his criteria, frequency of impaired tolerance was rather common in all subgroups, but of 172 very fat people, 65.6% had impaired tolerance. In 1931 Aschner reported a study of the frequency of family history of diabetes in 500 German patients with obesity and in 500 without obesity. In obese subjects a family history of diabetes was more than four times as frequent (29.2% and 6.6%).

In an excellent but little-known publication of 1939, Short and Johnson reported on the relationships of glucose tolerance to obesity and duration of obesity in 541 insurance policyholders. Rates of abnormal tolerance were related strongly to degree and duration of obesity. Even after known diabetics were removed, 44% (20 of 45) of persons with weights exceeding 150% of ideal had impaired tolerance. In 26 persons weighing less than 95% of standard, glucose intolerance was not seen. Rates of abnormal tolerance were still higher in obesity of long duration. In those with obesity of less than five years duration tolerance was good. This phenomenon may explain why rates of diabetes are only moderately higher with obesity in some circumstances. Almost all subjects can tolerate a few years of obesity, but only a minority can withstand three decades of severe obesity without decompensation of the beta cells. More evidence to this effect is presented below.

A classic paper by L. H. Newburgh appeared in 1942 extending his report with Conn of 1939. In a series of 47 obese hyperglycemic subjects who lost substantial amounts of weight after dietary therapy, glucose tolerance returned to normal in 77%!

Rabinowitch (1949) studied a group of fat diabetics in whom 16 were able to reduce their weight with diet to less than 115% of ideal weight. Glucose became normal in half of these (8 of 16).

MODERN OBSERVATIONS

In many societies diabetes has been more common in cities than in rural areas. This is discussed later in this chapter in the section on social factors. To a considerable degree these differences may be attributable to the greater fatness of urban people. Slome (1960) showed a dramatic difference in the adiposity of rural and urban Zulus. This change coincided closely with a great increase in rates of diabetes in the recently urbanized Zulus. In a series of black diabetics in Atlanta, Bowcock (1928) reported that 92% of females were obese. Until recently, diabetes was rare in Tonga but Queen Salote (Charlotte), who assumed the throne in 1918, later developed diabetes. It was said that she weighed 270 lb. Campbell (1960) pointed out that diabetes was common in the Zulu Royal Family in whom prodigious corpulence is legendary.

Faludi, et al (1968) performed oral glucose tolerance tests on 238 obese subjects with no evident diabetes. Hyperglycemic values were found in 40.5%. In 101 others (42.5%) tests were thought to exhibit hypoglycemic values in the later stages of the procedure. These investigators thought that such responses were probably indicative of "early latent diabetes".

Recent evidence confirms that obesity *alone* can and does produce diabetes if sufficient in degree and duration. Of 106 very fat patients recently studied by Kempner, et al (1975), 63% had elevated plasma glucose levels two hours after a test meal, even though average age was only 34 years! After marked weight loss only 14% had abnormal glucose levels. Jahnke, et al (1976) studied carefully glucose tolerance in seven fat diabetics before and after marked mitigation of obesity. Beta-cell function improved dramatically in all; in three it was restored to normal. Childs (1972) also achieved spectacular success in entirely reversing abnormal tolerance in a group of fat subjects who lost weight with low-fat diets.

In fat people dramatic reversal of diabetes occurs regularly with weight loss whether the diet is low or high in carbohydrate. The recent observations of Berger, et al (1976) also suggest that beta-cell function can be restored to normal in most diabetics with substantial mitigation of obesity. These investigators found, however, that diabetes was decidedly less reversible in older persons with very severe obesity of long duration.

Apparently most adult-onset diabetes is preventable, and probably a majority is curable, provided that complete and permanent reversal of obesity is achieved.

There is much to suggest that the female preponderance in the prevalence of diabetes observed in many societies is mainly if not entirely the result of the greater fatness of women in these populations. Results of Vinke, et al (1958) in the Netherlands were typical in this respect. Rates of insulin-dependent diabetes were the same in the two sexes at all age levels. The prevalence of insulin-independent diabetes was much higher in women over 30 years of age, but these Dutch women were much fatter than Dutch men.

Hundley (1956) published a good review on obesity and diabetes. He pointed out that in Japan, people in middle age weighed no more than young adults, while older American men (increase with age of 8%) and women (increase of 15%) were much heavier than young adults. Hundley also reviewed evidence showing that in 1948 death rates from diabetes in the United States were about ten times those in Japan. Later data of Kagan, et al (1974) confirmed that glucose tolerance was better in Japanese men of Japan than in Japanese men of Hawaii and California. The Japanese-Americans were much fatter, but not as fat as white Americans. Later we showed that older adults of East Pakistan were no heavier than young adults, and that diabetes in the United States was roughly seven times more frequent than in East Pakistan (West and Kalbfleisch, 1970, 1971).

Comstock, et al (1966) studied the causes of death over a fourteen-year period in a group of 24,390 adults in Muscogee County, Georgia in whom the thickness of subcutaneous fat had been estimated by photofluorographs. The most striking association observed was that between fat thickness and diabetes. In very thin people with a trapezius fat thickness of less than 5 mm, the standardized mortality ratio for diabetes was 55 (55% of standard); in those with a thickness greater than 9 mm this ratio was 162.

Figure 13 shows in ten populations the strong correlation between rates of maturity-onset diabetes and mean percent of standard weight (West and Kalbfleisch, 1971). We also found the same strong association in intrapopulation studies (West and Kalbfleisch, 1970, 1971). For example, in Central America diabetes was three times as common in people who were slightly to moderately obese than in those with weights near standard. Many races were included in these international studies (whites, blacks, Chinese, Malays, Indians, and American Indians). After adjustments for adiposity, differences among races were very small. In no case could we identify with certainty any racial difference independent of fatness. Small differences could have been missed because of the types of data available, but the studies appeared to exclude any major racial differences in these particular populations with respect to the susceptibility to maturity-onset diabetes in subjects matched for fatness.

In various aboriginal populations of the Western Hemisphere and Oceania

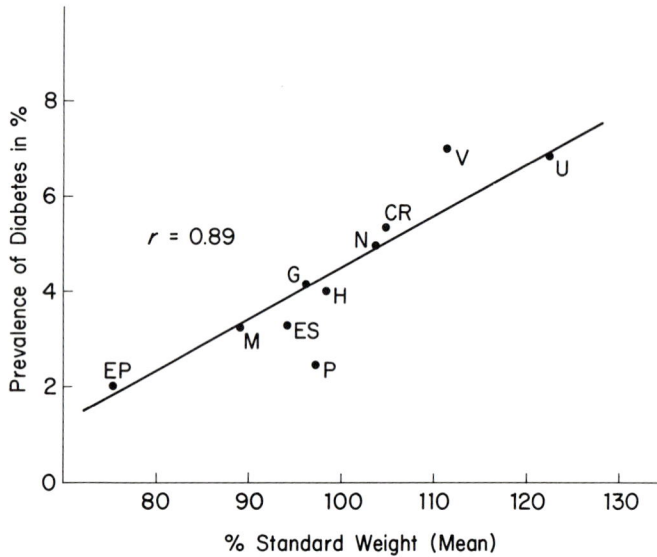

FIGURE 13. Relationship of average fatness and prevalence of diabetes among populations of ten countries (East Pakistan, Malaya, El Salvador, Guatemala, Panama, Honduras, Nicaragua, Costa Rica, Venezuela, and Uruguay, as designated by their initials; eg, East Pakistan—EP) Data apply only to persons over 29 years of age. From West and Kalbfleisch (1971).

there are very great differences by tribe and population groups in rates of maturity-onset diabetes (West, 1974). These rates of diabetes are very strongly related to the adiposity of these populations. Very fat populations of Micronesians, Polynesians, and American Indians have more than five times as much diabetes as other lean populations of these same races (West, 1974). Jackson, et al (1971) found that rates of diabetes in Natal Indians (South Africa) ranged from 1.9% in very lean subjects to 17.8% in those that were decidedly fat, a difference of ninefold. All subjects had been tested with oral glucose. Seftel (1964a) noted that about half of diabetics in India appeared to require insulin, while only about 4% of Campbell's diabetics in Natal, South Africa appeared to require insulin. This fits the possibility that the greater obesity of Indians of urban South Africa accounts for an increase of several fold in the rates of insulin-independent diabetes in those Indians whose ancestors migrated to South Africa. There are, of course, other possibilities that could account for these differences.

As shown in the section of this chapter on aging, differences in adiposity among populations probably explain why the typical sharp age-related increase of diabetes is blunted or completely absent in leaner communities such as Gondar, Ethiopia (Molineaux, et al, 1966; Belcher, 1970) and Orissa,

India (Tripathy and Kar, 1966). Even in very lean societies glucose tolerance usually deteriorates with age (West and Kalbfleisch, 1970), but this is not invariably the case (Tripathy, et al, 1973; Ayad, 1967). It is possible that a substantial portion of age-related deterioration of glucose tolerance is attributable to the increase of adiposity (degree and duration) with age. In natives of New Guinea where diabetes is quite rare, body weight in both sexes is about 25% *less* at age 60 than at age 20 (Sinnett and Buck, 1974).

In Chapter 5 on prevalence it has been shown that in the middle-aged population of the United States diabetes rates are moderate in black men and very high in black women. Figure 14 shows dramatically the reason for this. Our black men are on the whole relatively lean and our black women are quite fat. Populations in which epidemics of diabetes were associated with epidemics of obesity have included: Malta (Maempel, 1965); Mabuiag Island (Winterbotham, 1961); Hawaii (Sloan, 1963); New Zealand Maoris (Prior, 1962); many American Indian tribes (West, 1974); many groups of Jews as shown in the section on race in this chapter; Australian aborigines (Wise, et al, 1970); Sumo wrestlers of Japan (Kuzuya, 1975); and many other groups of blacks, Polynesians, Micronesians, and Melanesians (Tulloch, 1962; West, 1974).

Several recent epidemiologic studies have demonstrated the great strength of obesity as a risk factor. MacDonald and his associates (1963), in a study of 7,488 federal employees, found rates of occult diabetes were about six times higher in moderately obese subjects as compared to those of normal weight. In very fat persons (more than 149% overweight) risk was increased by a factor of about

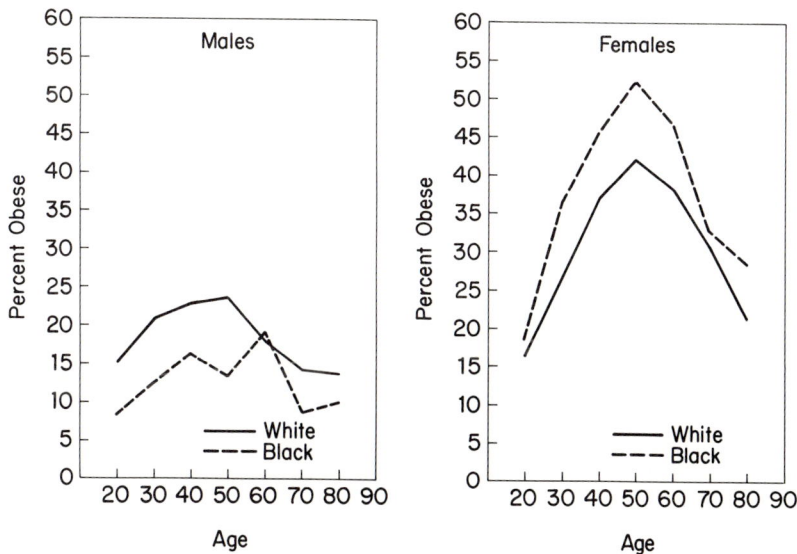

FIGURE 14. Prevalence of obesity by age, sex, and color in combined samples of populations of ten US states (US Public Health Service, 1972).

12! These latter data were not adjusted for age but in other calculations these investigators showed that at all ages of adult life, obesity profoundly influenced risk of diabetes. Rimm (1975) studied the frequency of history of diabetes in relation to degree of overweight in 73,352 members of a weight-reducing club ("TOPS"). In women 50 to 59 years of age the rate of purported diabetes rose progressively from less than 2% in the slightly obese (10% overweight) to 8% in those with marked obesity (average of 85% overweight). In 1,267 Helsinki policemen, Pyorala, et al (1974) studied the *incidence* of diabetes over a period of five years. In policemen who were 10% or more overweight the incidence of diabetes was 3.9 times higher than in those of normal weight. The prevalence of diabetes was also much greater in overweight men, by a factor of 4.3. In the Bombay area of India the K.E.M. Hospital Group (1966) did urine screening and follow-up diagnostic testing on 43,352 persons. Rates of diabetes were 2.42% in those of "average body build", 0.64 in "thin", and 7.86 in obese subjects. These data were not age-adjusted but adiposity is not so much affected by age in India as in richer countries. In Hyderabad, rates of diabetes were 1.0% in thin and 9.3% in fat persons (Rao, et al, 1966). Gupta, et al (1975) tested a group of subjects over 15 years of age in rural India. Diabetes was present in 1.3% of those with normal weight and in 20% of those who were overweight.

The study of Westlund and Nickolaysen (1972) is in some respects unique. They observed the incidence of diabetes in a representative sample of Oslo men (3,751) who were 40 to 49 years of age at the beginning of the study. Results are summarized in Figure 15. Several points deserve emphasis. Most important is the very great strength of the association of relative weight and risk of diabetes. In those who were decidedly fat the incidence was 12% in a single decade.

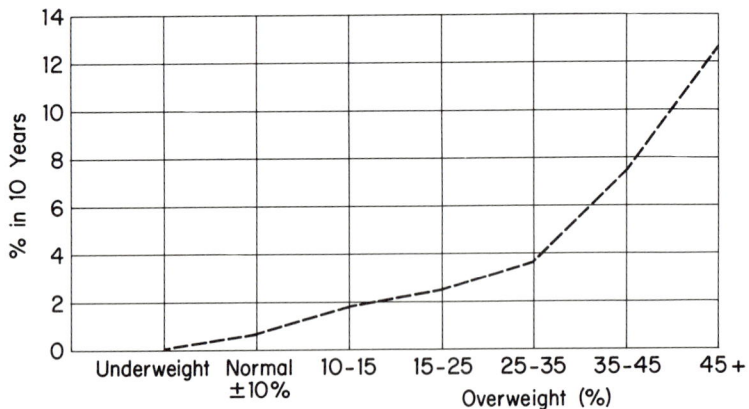

FIGURE 15. In 3,737 men of Oslo incidence of diabetes was determined prospectively for a decade. These men were 40 to 49 years of age at the start of the study. From Westlund and Nicolaysen (1972).

These data are also consistent with the possibility that a majority of very fat people will eventually develop diabetes if marked corpulence persists. In this population one cannot identify any upper termination in relationship of risk to degree of obesity. It is quite possible, even probable, that incidence would be still higher in those whose weights substantially exceeded 45% of standard (the highest figure on this chart). Also notable was the extremely low incidence of diabetes in slender men. None who was less than 90% of standard weight developed diabetes.

According to an article in *Sportsmedicine* (1974), Professor Shinkichi Ogawa of the Institute of Sport Science of the Tokyo University of Education has studied rates of diabetes in retired Sumo wrestlers. They are typically quite fat. Of 80 tested, 29 had diabetes (36%). This rate was judged to be about five times the expected rate in Japan for this age group. Only 3 of the 29 with diabetes had a family history of diabetes. Kuzuya (1975) reported similar experiences with regard to glucose tolerance in Sumo wrestlers. His data suggested that a substantial majority of these fat wrestlers will ultimately develop diabetes. This evidence is compatible with my notion that obesity is quite capable of inducing diabetes in the absence of any specific genetic trait for diabetes.

Medalie, et al (1975) studied the incidence of diabetes in a group of Israeli men. The factor most strongly associated with risk of diabetes was relative weight. In Gothenburg, Sweden fasting glucose levels and adiposity were studied in a group of 50-year-old men (Aurell, et al, 1966). Elevated glucose values were four times more common in men with trunkal skinfold thickness above the 90th percentile than in those with skinfold thickness below the tenth percentile.

In mothers of large babies Horger, et al (1975) found an exceedingly strong association of maternal weights and blood glucose levels. Rates of abnormal blood glucose at delivery were 0 for women under 150 lb (0 of 50), and 20% for those who weighed more than 199 (15 of 74). Of mothers who weighed over 249, 55% had abnormal tolerance (6 of 11).

Recently Hamman and Miller (1975) studied the incidence of diabetes in Pima Indians with corrections for initial blood glucose levels. When the baseline two-hour plasma glucose was clearly normal (less than 160 mg/100 ml), risk of diabetes was increased by a factor of 3.4 in those who had weights ranging from 125% to 150% of normal, as compared with those whose weights were less than 125% of standard. In persons whose weights were 150% or more above standard, risk of diabetes was increased by a factor of 6.4. In subjects whose baseline two-hour values were equivocal (160-199 mg/100 ml) the excessive risk relating to obesity was less. In the moderately fat persons, risk of subsequent diabetes was only 1.4 times standard, and in the severely obese it was 2.6. The Pimas are very fat: Bennett, et al (1976a) reported that in persons 35 to 44 years of age, 64% of men and 91% of women weighed more than 125% of standard.

Another way to evaluate the relationship between fatness and risk of diabetes is to examine the frequency distribution of present or previous adiposity in a population of diabetics. In most such studies in affluent societies a majority of adult-onset diabetes have been fat. Because some diabetics lose weight with treatment and some without therapy, present weight often underestimates considerably the weight at or before onset of diabetes. In Oklahoma Indians, even at discovery of diabetes, weight was often much lower than weight of a few years before discovery (at the time decompensation had probably begun). The large group of Joslin Clinic patients are not necessarily a representative sample of the general population of diabetics, but Joslin's data are in some respects best, particularly because he estimated lifetime maximum weight, a variable seldom measured by other investigators. About 80% of Joslin's 4,596 adult-onset patients were "overweight" prior to onset of diabetes (1936). Fifty percent of his diabetic men and 60% of women were at least 20% overweight. Of Joslin's Jewish women with diabetes, 94% had been overweight! It has been my experience that obese people frequently understate their lifetime maximum weight (unpublished data). The true lifetime maximum weights of Dr. Joslin's patients were probably even greater than his estimates.

The percentage of adult-onset diabetics who have been fat varies considerably, of course, by population and is low where obesity is rare in the general population. Even so, rates of diabetes are much higher in obese persons of these societies (Gupta, et al, 1975). In a recent German study (Petzholdt, et al, 1975), 85% of 1,302 diabetics were judged to be overweight.

Some negative observations and the factors to which they are attributable

The evidence cited above establishes very clearly the great strength of the association of fatness and risk of diabetes, but in a few population studies the degree of this correlation has been less impressive. Examples will be given below. There are several possibilities that may account for a masking or mitigation of this relationship. Some of these reasons have already been mentioned. First, weight loss may occur in diabetes either because of the treatment or the disease. Previous fatness is often not reflected by the present weight. This was well illustrated by observations of Tulloch (1962). Of 216 diabetic women of Jamaica who had been "overweight", only 110 were overweight at the time of their first visit for diabetes. Of 55 men who had been overweight, only 17 were overweight when they first visited for diabetes. Seftel (1964a) reported that about 70% of diabetics in a Madras clinic had been fat before onset of diabetes, but the rate of obesity was subsequently much lower among persons with established diabetes. A study of Nilsson, et al (1967) in Sweden showed that short-duration diabetics were much fatter than age-matched diabetics of long duration. Among the most informative data on this matter are some very old observations of Adams (1929). He found that 27% of his diabetics with onset between ages 41 and 60 were fat (more than 20% above ideal weight). But 74% had been fat at onset of diabetes. Seki, et al (1975) found that a substantial portion of Japanese diabetics weighed considerably less than before the onset of diabetes. In London Keen (1974a) found that, in nondiabetic persons from 40 to 70 years of age, disparity between present weight and lifetime maximum weight averaged about 10 lb. In diabetics this difference averaged about 30 lb.

Second, obesity of short duration is not so strongly related to risk of diabetes. Watson (1939), for example, found little relationship of obesity and risk of diabetes in college students. The degree of effect of duration deserves more study but it appears to be of considerable importance. A third factor that may mask the relationship of obesity and diabetes is that, compared to lean persons, overweight subjects as a group have a larger extracellular and intracellular mass (including a somewhat larger muscle mass). In screening studies in which a glucose load of fixed amount is administered to all subjects, the overweight subjects receive amounts of glucose that are smaller in relation to body size. This factor has little effect in determining relative rates of marked impairment of glucose tolerance, but it is a significant consideration when rates of mild abnormalities are compared in those whose weights are normal and excessive. A fourth factor is that the strength of association between obesity and diabetes would under some circumstances be diminished by removing from a population study those who have already developed diabetes. Obese subjects are in most circumstances more likely to be tested for diabetes. This would tend to increase rates of known diabetes among the obese, but it would tend to reduce rates of diabetes among the obese subsequently tested (eg, in screening surveys). The residual of overweight people who have escaped diabetes for decades may be a very biased sample of the universe of obese subjects.

Another consideration is that weight for height is only a crude index of fatness and may, under some conditions, be misleading (Lesser, et al, 1971; Kalkhoff and Ferrou, 1971). Bassett and Schroffner (1970) found that, in Hawaii, Chinese men were fatter than Japanese, even though weights were the same in relation to heights. Diabetics studied by Umezawa, et al (1974) were fatter than nondiabetic controls of the same weight for height.

Finally, in older age groups prevalence of the combination of obesity and diabetes is probably diminished somewhat by the excessive rates of death in obese diabetics, particularly in the very obese. This may explain why the excess of diabetes in the prospective study of Westlund and Nicolaysen (1972) was even greater than that usually shown in studies of prevalence. Incidence was increased more than tenfold in middle-aged men who were decidedly fat. Among diabetics matched for age and duration of diabetes, rates of death are probably higher in the obese than in nonobese. This would tend to diminish the apparent association of diabetes and obesity.

Taken together these considerations explain to a considerable degree the failure in some circumstances to demonstrate a strong association between fatness and risk of diabetes. On the other hand, present evidence by no means excludes the possibility that the strength of the association between obesity and diabetes may be influenced by factors that are not now appreciated or

241

understood. Among several possibilities are exercise levels, genetics, and hormonal and dietary factors. For example, some preliminary data of Booyens, et al (1970) suggest that Indians of South Africa may be unusually indolent. This might account in part for the high rates of diabetes despite weights in relation to height that are not much different than in certain white and black groups of South Africa (Jackson, 1972). It is also possible, however, that these Indians are fatter than other groups even at the same weight for height. Results of Fredman (1972) in Capetown Tamils are consistent with this possibility. The Tamils had small muscles and a high ratio of fat to muscle. A substantial majority were "endomorphic" and mesomorphism was rare. In most of our studies there was a good correlation of relative weight for height and skinfold thickness, but this relationship is not invariable (Lesser, et al, 1971). Primitive Eskimos, for example, tend to be very lean despite substantial weight for height. In some studies the relationship between obesity and diabetes has been *overestimated* because the fatter subjects were older than the lean.

In Oxford and Sudbury postprandial glucose values showed little relationship to obesity. However, diabetes rates were considerably higher in obese people when subjects in these same populations were given glucose tolerance tests (O'Sullivan, 1970). Under the conditions of his study, Medley (1965) was not able to show such effect of obesity on susceptibility to diabetes. The relationship of fatness and glucose tolerance was generally weak in the study of Nilsson (1962) in Kristianstad, Sweden. In this study, the glucose load was based on body surface area. Little relationship of diabetes and obesity was found by Grönberg, et al (1967) in Sweden. The correlation was also weak in Tecumseh, Michigan (Evans and Ostrander, 1967), where a fixed load of 100 gm was given to all subjects, and those with known diabetes were not included in this aspect of the analyses. In Bedford, Abrams, et al administered 50 gm of glucose to all subjects. Association between fatness and glucose level was weak. In women it was insignificant. Lynn, et al (1967) found that diabetes was not especially common in Italians of Roseto, Pennsylvania, despite the fact that they were rather heavy. Rosselin, et al (1971) observed higher levels of insulin in heavier men, but two-hour glucose levels were not related to an index of corpulence. Both Albrink and Meigs (1964) and Hollister, et al (1967) found a positive correlation of weight gain during adult life and blood glucose levels, but Harlan (1962) did not.

Genetic interrelationships of diabetes and obesity

In the section above on heredity, evidence is set forth that much of the family aggregation of maturity-onset diabetes is attributable to the family aggregation of obesity. The familiality of obesity has both genetic and nongenetic determinants. Observations of Joyce Baird (1973) illustrate the interrelationships of the familiality of obesity and diabetes. Rates of diabetes were determined by testing siblings of obese and nonobese diabetics. In obese siblings of nonobese diabetics rates of diabetes were highest (27.3%). In obese siblings of obese diabetics the rate of diabetes was 10.8%; in nonobese siblings of nonobese dia betics, 7.3%. Rates of diabetes were lowest (4.8%) in nonobese siblings of obese diabetics. These and the data of Köbberling (1971) are consistent with the possibility that obesity alone often produces diabetes. These data of Baird also suggest that obesity often precipitates diabetes in individuals genetically susceptible to diabetes and vice versa.

At what level of fatness does increased susceptibility to diabetes begin?

Present data are not adequate to answer this question. As indicated above, older evidence of Joslin (1921) suggested strongly that diabetes was less frequent in very lean persons than in those of typical weight.

In adults of urban India Gupta, et al (1975) found that rates of diabetes were 3.6% in those with a normal weight and only 1.5% in subjects who were underweight. The numbers for certain of the subgroups of Westlund and Nicolaysen (1972) were too small for conclusive results, but their data on incidence of diabetes also suggest that persons who are "underweight" may be even less likely to develop diabetes than persons whose weights are "normal" by traditional standards. In these middle-aged men of Oslo, none of those whose weights were under 90% of standard developed diabetes over a ten-year period. Our data were not conclusive, but they also suggested that persons of "normal" weight have a higher risk of diabetes than those who are "underweight" (West and Kalbfleisch, 1971). Comstock, et al (1966) found diabetes mortality rates only 55% of standard in those who had been very lean at the onset of a fifteen-year study. To some degree this very low susceptibility to diabetes in very lean persons may reflect superior physical conditioning as well as their leanness.

There is a wide range of adiposity among persons who are "nonobese" by standard criteria. Even in affluent societies the fat mass in this nonobese group is frequently as low as 6% of body weight and as high as 30%. Thus, differences in adiposity as great as threefold are common within this group of nonobese. In marathon runners, fat typically constitutes less than 5% of body mass (Costill, 1972), while in healthy old women whose weights are at an "ideal" level, fat may constitute more than 35% of body weight (Brozek, 1968).

DURATION OF OBESITY

A relationship of risk of diabetes and duration of obesity has been cited in some of the older studies (eg, Oglevie, 1935; Short and Johnson, 1939). Schultz (1973) reported that in children hyperinsulinism was considerably greater in obesity of long duration than in obesity of short duration. But duration of obesity in this group was also related to degree of obesity and age. In this and other studies it has been difficult to assess the independent effect of duration. In Plains Indians we were able to correct for degree of obesity, and found that diabetes was much more common in obesity of long duration (West and Mako, 1976), but these latter data were not matched for age.

In some of the populations studied by Jackson, et al (1971) in South Africa, diabetes was less strongly related to degree of obesity in the elderly than in

243

younger adults. This same phenomenon was observed by Bennett, et al (1976a) in Pimas. One possible explanation for this is that persons who are very fat tend to develop diabetes after ten to twenty years of obesity, usually between the ages of 30 and 50, while persons with mild obesity do not decompensate until they have been obese for a longer period. Elderly persons tend to weigh less than they did earlier (West, 1973). This may mask the effect of obesity on incidence of diabetes in the elderly. It can also be argued that in some circumstances many small elderly subjects thought to have diabetes do not have it. They exhibit slight hyperglycemia only because they are old, and because the glucose loads administered are very large in relation to their small extracellular volumes. Very fat people seldom survive to old age. This also tends to reduce the frequency of obesity among new diabetics who are elderly.

As pointed out above, however, there have been some populations in which glucose tolerance did not appear to decline with age (Tripathy, et al, 1973; Ayad, 1967). These have been populations in which weight did not increase with age; but in some very lean populations glucose tolerance declines with age despite lack of weight gain (West, 1970). On the other hand, old people are somewhat fatter than young adults even when matched for relative weight. It seems likely that duration of obesity is an important risk factor for diabetes, but more data are needed in determining its strength.

IS INCREASING ADIPOSITY THE CAUSE OF RISING RATES OF DIABETES?

It is rather generally believed that people of North America and Europe are fatter than heretofore, and that rates of diabetes have risen continuously in the United States since 1900. These notions may be correct but direct evidence is scant. As shown in Chapter 5 on prevalence, much of the apparent rise in frequency of diabetes is attributable to a great increase in the sensitivity and frequency of testing. Moreover, weight in relation to height has not changed much in Britain or America since the early 20th century (Montegriffo, 1968; Stoudt, et al, 1965; Metropolitan Life Insurance Company, 1970). Both men and women are substantially taller. In relation to height, men of both countries are probably a few pounds heavier, and women are about the same or a little lighter. Of course, it is possible that at the turn of the century we were more muscular and less fat even at the same weight for height. The same trend with time (men slightly heavier, women slightly lighter) has been observed recently in East Germany (Von Knorre and Bode, 1976).

ADIPOSITY, INSULINEMIA, AND FAT CELLS

There have also been some variations in results among population studies when serum insulin levels have been related to fatness. Usually, however, a positive correlation has been observed. Results of Abrams, et al (1969) in Bedford are typical in showing a rather strong association.

These results confirm those of clinical investigators, showing in obese subjects an insensitivity of muscle to insulin (Rabinowitz and Zierler, 1962; Butterfield, et al, 1965) and increased levels of circulating insulin (Karam, et al,

1963; Bagdade, et al, 1967). There is experimental evidence that insulin levels may be more influenced by fat-cell size than by cell number (Salans, et al, 1968; Sims and Horton, 1968; Bjorntorp, et al, 1971). Liver tissue also appears to be less sensitive to insulin in obesity (Felig and Wahren, 1975). Not all studies have shown a consistent relationship of degree of hyperinsulinism to degree of obesity, but these apparent discrepancies would probably be less with larger numbers and better matching for other factors such as exercise, age, and degree of hyperglycemia. The young adult obese subjects of Johansen (1973) had hyperinsulinism, but not much difference was observed in fat and lean older subjects. However, his older obese subjects were only slightly heavier than controls. These and other data do indicate that factors other than degree of obesity are of significance in determining levels of serum insulin. More data are needed to determine the influence on insulin secretion patterns of factors such as exercise, race, qualitative features of diet, and genetics.

Epidemiologic evidence is not at all conclusive concerning the relative importance of fat-cell size, and fat-cell number, and fat-mass in determining risk of diabetes. Nor is it clear whether there is a difference in risk relating to whether obesity is of late or early onset. In many populations, maturity-onset obesity has been associated with substantial increases in risk of diabetes. Risk of diabetes has not been studied much in childhood-onset obesity. It is of interest, however, that insulin levels are high in fat children, and glucose tolerance is frequently impaired (Martin and Martin, 1973; Drash, 1973a). The insulin:glucose ratios were somewhat low in the fat children of Drash who had impairment of glucose tolerance. None had developed symptomatic diabetes. In obese children studied by Brook and Lloyd (1973) there was hyperinsulinemia, and fat cells were large. Insulin levels declined sharply with weight reduction, but correlation of insulin levels with fat-cell size was weak in this study.

It is by no means certain that an increase in fat-cell number is innocuous with respect to risk of diabetes, although the relationship of risk to fat-cell size has been better demonstrated thus far. A very important issue is whether the increase in serum insulin levels is related mainly to obesity itself or to associated factors such as indolence or the increased levels of food intake. Probably all three factors (obesity, overeating, and inactivity) are significant (Grey and Kipnis, 1971; Olefsky, et al, 1975; Bjorntorp, et al, 1977).

In fat persons with borderline glucose tolerance, substantial reduction of adiposity is associated with decreased insulin secretion as well as improved glucose tolerance. These phenomena were not observed in all studies, but results have been impressively consistent in studies of the kind described below, in which reduction of adiposity was substantial and the number of experimental subjects large. The recent studies of Groothof, et al (1975) illustrate this well. After six months or more of mild but persistent caloric restriction, one of his subgroups (21 subjects) lost an average of 15.8 kg (about 35 lb). One-hour glucose levels declined from a mean of 165 to 122 mg/100 ml. Mean one-hour insulin levels declined from 370 to 181 μU/ml. This study was rather

245

unusual in several respects. Dietary carbohydrates were not sharply restricted and calories were only moderately reduced. Carbohydrate calories accounted for about 50% of energy (more than 200 gm daily) and the dietary instruction allowed a daily intake of about 1,700 kilcalories. Despite this, insulin levels declined greatly with weight reduction. It is also important that these observations after weight loss were not made during a phase of sharp weight reduction. Full details were not given but circumstances suggested that at the time of the terminal studies the weights in this latter subgroup were approximately at a plateau, and that calories were sufficient or almost sufficient to maintain weight at the new level. While not decisive, these data are compatible with the notion that obesity itself accounted for a substantial portion of the aberrations of carbohydrate metabolism.

In recent studies of Joffee, et al (1975), moderately fat African subjects had higher insulin levels than lean subjects, but a small number of very fat subjects did not. The reasons for this are not clear. The fat subjects were not drawn from the same sources as the lean. This may or may not be significant. Of several possible explanations for the relatively modest insulin levels in these very fat Africans one might consider qualitative peculiarities of diet, unusually good physical conditioning, and racial peculiarities. As pointed out by Salans, et al (1971), resistance to insulin in obesity is probably attributable to several factors, including cell size and both quantitative and qualitative features of the diet. More epidemiologic data would be useful. For example, it would be interesting to examine insulin levels in groups matched for fatness but different in exercise, sugar intake, fat intake, etc. Himsworth (1935) cited evidence that high carbohydrate regimens might increase sensitivity to insulin. Perhaps Africans who are obese are less hyperinsulinemic than fat Americans who eat more fat and less carbohydrate. Under certain short-term experimental conditions insulin levels have been higher when carbohydrates replaced other calories, even when total calories were not increased (Grey and Kipnis, 1971). But, as indicated below in the section on dietary carbohydrate, many populations on very high carbohydrate diets have relatively low levels of insulin.

In our studies in Oklahoma Indians (West and Mako, 1976) in whom obesity is rife, there was a strong relationship of adiposity and insulinemia, and we found no evidence that obesity was secondary to hyperinsulinism. Lean young adults, most of whom we expect to become fat if present trends continue, have normal insulin levels. Young and old Indians have levels of insulin secretion before and after insulin that are very similar to those of whites after appropriate matching for fatness. The deleterious effects of corpulence are dramatically evident. We recently recruited from several sites 200 subjects from the general population of Kiowas and Comanches of southwestern Oklahoma. Only those with no previous history of diabetes were tested. Age ranged from 18 to 83 years; mean age was 44. In 38 subjects who had never been fat, 37 had clearly normal glucose tolerance. One had borderline glucose tolerance (two-hour plasma glucose 155 mg/100 ml). In 104 subjects who were quite fat (weight greater than 129% of standard), 50 (48%) had abnormal tolerance. Rates of hyperglycemia were even higher in gross obesity or obesity of long duration.

246

On the other hand, Bennett, et al (1977) found that young Pima Indians had blood insulin levels higher than those of weight matched whites.

Lehtovirta's excellent review (1973) covers much of the available evidence relating to fat-cell size and number, insulin secretion patterns, blood glucose levels, and age. The role of insulin receptors has been well reviewed by Olefsky (1976).

CHILDHOOD OBESITY

Effects in adult life of childhood-onset obesity have been discussed above. In privileged societies, the adiposity of children destined to develop insulin-dependent diabetes appears to be similar to that of other children. This does not exclude the possibility that nutritional factors influence susceptibility to juvenile diabetes. Sterky (1967) found that diabetic children had more adipose tissue than nondiabetics even at the same weight for height. Nutritional factors in the etiology of juvenile diabetes will be discussed below under special types of diabetes (Chapter 8).

There also remains the possibility that fatness in adult life might be determined by fetal or infant nutrition (Brook, 1972; Yudkin, 1973; Hirsch, 1972). The main thrust of this hypothesis is that early feeding may determine the number of fat cells in adult life, and this could influence susceptibility to obesity even in adult life. But in a small series Verdy, et al (1974) found no relationship between birth weight and risk of adult obesity. It has been clearly demonstrated that fat children are likely to become fat adults, but the extent to which childhood obesity is a *direct* cause of adult obesity is not known in man.

ANIMALS

Most animal breeds that have a propensity to develop diabetes are fat (Renold, et al, 1970; Krook, et al, 1960). A significant minority are not. But even in some of those that are not grossly obese, rates of diabetes can sometimes be lowered by increasing the degree of leanness, as shown by Gerritsen, et al (1974) in hamsters. In his book of 1919, Allen described experiments in which diabetes was precipitated in animals by fattening them.

Few epidemiologic data are available in animals, but observations that have been made suggest that obesity is a major risk factor in most species. Krook, et al (1960) carried out a very interesting study in the dogs of Stockholm. Among 10,993 autopsied, 167 had diabetes. The rate of diabetes in fat dogs was about five times greater than in dogs of "normal" weight and approximately 12 times that of dogs that were especially lean! Moreover, it seems likely that diabetes had reduced adiposity in some of the dogs. Foster (1975) quotes Lavignette to the effect that most cats that develop diabetes are or have been obese. Thus both literal and figurative "fat cats" are more likely to develop diabetes. Among the fattest of domesticated animals are certain breeds of sheep fattened in feedlots. They frequently develop severe diabetes (Meier, 1960). This can be prevented by slowing the rate of feeding and fattening. Yields of insulin from pancreata of feed-lot cattle exceed those from range-fed cattle.

Anatomic Distribution of Fat

Studies of Vague (1965) had suggested that risk of diabetes might be related to the distribution of adiposity. He found that persons with a "masculine" distribution were more at risk than those with a "feminine" distribution. The masculine type had a relatively greater portion of body fat at the root of the arm, while the feminine type had relatively more at the root of the leg. Feldman, et al (1969) found that persons with a more central distribution of fat had a somewhat higher rate of diabetes than those whose fat had a more peripheral distribution. Albrink (1973) had shown previously that late-onset obesity is predominantly central. Plains Indians of Oklahoma have very high rates of obesity and diabetes. They have a distribution of fat that is markedly central (West, et al, 1974). It is not yet clear how much of this centrality is accounted for by the fact that obesity is usually of a maturity-onset type; but crude matching with whites who also have late-onset obesity suggests that the "centrality" of distribution is greater in Indians, and that the peculiar distribution is probably a racial characteristic. In general, this centrality of distribution is associated with large fat cells and lesser increases in number of fat cells or no increase.

Does Diabetes Cause Obesity?

For more than a century the possibility that diabetes might cause obesity has been occasionally considered (Brigham, 1868). Allen reviewed these arguments in some detail in his book of 1913, and concluded that evidence was quite unimpressive. Even as recently as 1949, Arthur Mirsky, a respected scholar in the field, thought it quite probable that obesity might be secondary to the diabetic diathesis. Vallance-Owen (1962) also cited this possibility. It does seem quite likely that persons with a genetic propensity for obesity are in a sense "prediabetic". Yet, taken as a whole, available evidence does not suggest any causal role for hyperglycemia in obesity. Nor is there persuasive evidence that diabetic genes cause obesity except for those genes that cause diabetes secondary to obesity. It is clear from the epidemiologic data above that populations with genetic propensities for obesity (eg, Asian Indians, American Indians, Jews) are well protected from diabetes when environmental circumstances prevent obesity.

Consumption of Carbohydrates and Sugars

History of a Controversy

The possibility that risk of diabetes is related to carbohydrate consumption has been suggested frequently. This hypothesis was based on several considerations. Although the ingestion of fat and protein also stimulates beta-cell function, the ingestion of carbohydrate presents a challenge to beta cells that is stronger, more direct, and more immediate than when protein or fat are ingested alone. Blood glucose levels are higher immediately after ingestion of carbohydrates than after other foodstuffs. Diabetes often improves after restriction of carbohydrates. In general, populations that consume more sugar have more diabetes. Diabetes rates have risen sharply in many populations at a time when sugar consumption increased substantially.

In every decade of the last 100 years there have been well-informed scholars who believed that overconsumption of sugars increased rates of diabetes, and those who believed it did not. Table 30 summarizes this history. Cheevers (1886) noted that Bengali men in whom diabetes was quite common were fond of sweets. The famous 19th century Italian physician, Cantani, believed that, because of their overly rich carbohydrate diet, Italians of Rome had higher rates of diabetes than Germans or Austrians (cited by Allen, 1913). Allen, et al (1919) mentioned that as early as 1859 Greisinger had considered consumption of sugars and starches as an inciting factor, although of secondary importance. According to Bose (1895) it was rather generally believed that diets high in sugar and starch increased susceptibility to diabetes. He expressed a contrary opinion, based on rather impressive evidence, some of which is described below. On the other hand, Mitra (1903) thought that overconsumption of "excessive sugary food" was a factor in the diabetes epidemic of Bengal. This view was shared by some of the participants in the *British Medical Journal* symposium of 1907 (Sir R. Havelock Charles, et al) and by Williamson (1918). Lepine (1909) thought that consumption of sugar was one of the causes of diabetes, while Von Noorden (cited by Allen in 1913) held the opposite view.

Both Wilcox (1908) and Morse (1913) thought sugar consumption might be a cause of juvenile diabetes. LeGoff (1911) performed a systematic survey of diabetes mortality rates and sugar consumption by locality. He concluded that the positive association observed was probably that of cause and effect. The early antisugar groups received support from an interesting source. Henry Ford (Spier, 1975) thought that granulated sugar was bad because he believed its crystals cut blood vessel walls!

On the other hand, Brigham observed in 1868 that cane cutters of the West Indies rarely had diabetes despite large amounts of dietary sugar. Sen (1893)

TABLE 30   Does Sugar Consumption Cause Diabetes? History of a Controversy

YES OR PROBABLY		NO OR PROBABLY NOT	
Greisinger (1859)	Cohen (1961)	Brigham (1868)	Mills (1930)
Cantani (late 19th century)	Campbell (1963)	Naunyn (1898)	Himsworth (1935–1936)
Mitra (1903)	Gelfand (1963)	Von Noorden (1900)	Walker (1966)
Havelock Charles, et al (1907)	Alpert (1964)	Sandwith (1907)	Tsai (1970)
Wilcox (1908)	Yudkin (1964)	Saundby (1908)	Baird (1972)
LeGoff (1911)	Ziegler (1967)	Benedict (1909)	Stare (1973)
Morse (1913)	Tsuji (1970)	Lemann (1911)	Truswell (1973)
Harris (1950)	Schaefer (1971)	Allen (1913)	Keen (1974)
Del Greco (1953)	Edginton (1972)	Joslin (1917)	Bierman (1975)
Cleave (1956)	Pfeiffer (1973)	Emerson (1924)	Medalie (1975)
	Wales (1976)	Dutt (1928)	Walker (1977)

also cited populations in which diabetes was rare despite high levels of sugar consumption. These included sugarcane-producing populations of British Guiana and Mauritius. Bose (1895) reported that in India diabetes was, in general, more common in ethnic groups on mixed diets than in those on high carbohydrate diets. In Jains consuming high-starch diets, diabetes was seen in only 2 of 5,000. In certain elements of the Calcutta population that consumed lower percentages of carbohydrate, diabetes was rife. Bose reported that Sadhus, Jogees, and Chowbays of Mattra "lived on sweets" but did not suffer from diabetes. Sandwith observed in 1907 that diabetes was uncommon in Cairo despite the popularity of dietary sugar. Benedict (1909) very much doubted that risk of diabetes was related to overconsumption of carbohydrates. Lemann (1911) shared this skepticism. He pointed to the high carbohydrate diet of American rural Negroes in whom rates of diabetes were quite low. He also mentioned that rates of diabetes were very low in blacks who worked on sugar-producing plantations and in whom sugar consumption was high. Lemann quoted Naunyn, from his book of 1898, to the effect that diabetes was not caused by excessive consumption of sweets or carbohydrates. In 1908 Saundby pointed out that some rural populations with high consumption of sugars had low rates of diabetes. Brown had mentioned in 1907 the association in China of very high levels of dietary carbohydrate and very low ratio of diabetes. Reed (1915) found diabetes to be uncommon in Chinese of lower classes despite diets very high in carbohydrate.

In his books of 1913 and 1919 Allen dealt at some length with evidence for and against the notion that eating too much sugar causes diabetes. In general he was dubious, holding the view that the particular source of excessive calories was probably relatively unimportant, even though overnutrition was very important. He left open the question of whether excessive sugar consumption might precipitate diabetes in persons predisposed to it by other factors. In 1928 Dutt challenged the notion that sugar consumption accounted for high rates of diabetes in Bengal. He cited the frequency with which he observed diabetes in patients who had "scarcely touched sugar". He also pointed out that diabetes was extremely rare in laborers of Bengal despite daily consumption of carbohydrate that often exceeded 600 gm.

Joslin (1917) and Emerson and Larimore (1924) acknowledged a general association between sugar consumption and diabetes among populations, but doubted a cause-and-effect relationship. Mills (1930a) reached similar conclusions after extensive studies. In 1935 Himsworth brought together an impressive array of evidence suggesting a negative association between total dietary carbohydrate and risk of diabetes. He and Marshall had reported (1935–1936) that before the development of diabetes, British diabetics seemed to have eaten proportionally more fat and less carbohydrate than controls. Himsworth also reviewed experimental evidence against the "sugar consumption" hypothesis. Even so, this notion continued to thrive. Seale Harris (1950) thought that overconsumption of sugar caused diabetes and said that Banting had held the same view. Several other "modern scholars who favor this hypothesis are listed in Table 30. The more recent evidence mobilized by these workers and data to the contrary will be reviewed below. But first, it is important to emphasize the need to consider separately the possible etiologic roles of sugar, of starch (high and low in fiber), of total carbohydrate calories, and of total calories.

STARCHES AND TOTAL CARBOHYDRATES

More recent epidemiologic and experimental evidence rather conclusively exonerates dietary starch as a specific risk factor for diabetes. Since early in this century total carbohydrate consumption has *declined* in the United States by about 25% (Page and Friend, 1974) at a time when diabetes rates have probably increased. Figure 16 shows in eight populations a decidedly negative relationship between rates of diabetes and percentage of calories as carbohydrate (West, 1974). A wider perspective confirms this: rates of diabetes are lowest in most of the societies where carbohydrate consumption is highest (eg, in rural Africa and Latin America, in Asia, and in other primitive areas such as New Guinea). Diabetes, for example, has been very uncommon in Korea where carbohydrates provide as much as 90% of calories (Mimura, 1970). In certain communities of Papua-New Guinea, diabetes is rare, and carbohydrates consti-

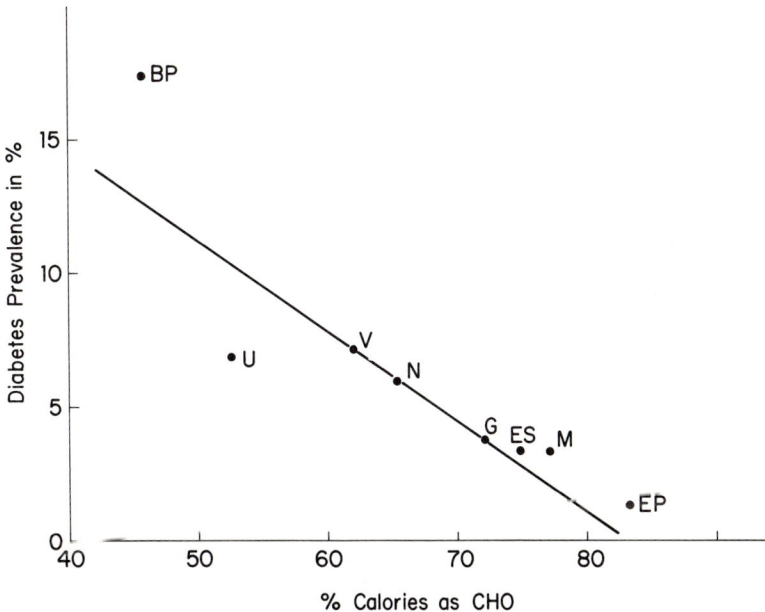

FIGURE 16. Relationship of prevalence of diabetes (two-hour blood glucose < 149 mg/100 ml) and percentage of calories as carbohydrate in eight populations. Data were limited to subjects more than 34 years of age. Populations as designated by their initials (left to right) are Bangor, Pennsylvania; Uruguay, Venezuela; Nicaragua, Guatemala, El Salvador, Malaya, and East Pakistan. From West (1974a).

tute 94.6% of calories (Sinnett and Buck, 1974). In 1955 carbohydrate consumption per person exceeded 400 gm daily in Japan (more than 70% of
calories) at a time when diabetes rates were much lower than in the United
States (Rudnick and Anderson, 1962). Chun reported in 1925 that diabetes was
rare in China (0.09% of outpatients), despite a diet in which cereals furnished
87% of calories.

Schettler (1974) reported experiences in Germany suggesting that it is
restriction of calories rather than restriction of carbohydrates that protects
against diabetes. He described experiences in two different areas immediately
following World War II before the systems for food production and distribution
had been reestablished.

> We were living in the French zone of occupation. Daily intake of calories
> was very low, about 800-1000 calories, mainly from carbohydrates. Fat
> intake was about 10 gm per day. We had no severe forms of diabetes and
> nearly no ketoacidosis. In the southern zone, the Allgau, there was a lack of
> carbohydrate. The farmers breed cattle and do not grow potatoes, corn,
> wheat, or other cereals. Total calorie intake was high, about 3000 calories
> per day. From this area very often came fat patients with severe ketoacidosis;
> diabetic complications were frequent. In my mind total calorie intake is very
> important. Under unusual conditions a diet high in calories, coming mainly
> from fat and protein, there can exist severe diabetes, although the carbohy-
> drate intake is low.

A similar experience was described by Vartiainen in Finland (1946). Carbohydrate consumption increased and diabetes rates fell during World War II.
Consumption of fat and calories had declined. Himsworth (1949a) noted a
marked fall in diabetes mortality in Britain during and immediately following
World War II. During this period caloric intake declined moderately, fat consumption declined sharply, and carbohydrate intake *increased*.

High levels of dietary starch do not, however, in themselves provide protection from diabetes. Nor do low levels of starch intake necessarily incite diabetes. Imperato studied three groups in Mali. Glucose tolerance was best in a
group in which starch intake was lowest. These Bambara farmers were slender
hard-working people whose caloric intakes were quite low. In Fiji (Hawley and
Jansen, 1971) and in Mabuig Islanders (Winterbottom, 1961) obesity occurs
commonly in certain elements of the population despite high-starch diets.
Sumo wrestlers of Japan consume high-starch diets. They are very fat and have
high rates of diabetes (Kuzuya, 1975). This and other evidence suggests that
excessive calorie consumption, irrespective of the sources of calories, may
induce obesity and increase risk of diabetes. There is no evidence, however,
that those who eat starch are particularly likely to develop obesity and diabetes
(West, 1972,1973,1974). It is even possible, as suggested by Himsworth (1935–
1936) that carbohydrate or starch have to some degree a protective effect that is
only overcome in rare situations in which total caloric consumption is high
despite high-starch diets. The fat diabetic patients of Kempner, et al (1975) and
Childs (1972) improved greatly on high-starch, low-calorie diets. In most,

diabetes disappeared. More than forty years ago Himsworth (1935–1936) presented data very similar to those in Figure 16 showing a strongly negative correlation of carbohydrate consumption and diabetes rates; but it is very hard to dispel the notion that eating too much carbohydrate causes diabetes.

SUGARS AND REFINED CARBOHYDRATES

Table 30 summarizes the conflicting citations on sugar consumption as a cause of diabetes. Opinion has been about equally divided. The issue has persisted for more than a century and the controversy thrives today. It is an issue of great practical importance. This matter was recently the subject of an excellent review by Walker (1977).

Sugars

Del Greco and Scapellato (1953) and Alpert (1955) each reported an interesting case in which diabetes developed in an adult man following massive consumption of simple carbohydrates. One, however, had pneumonia at onset of symptoms of diabetes. Both were consuming prodigious levels of calories. Diabetes disappeared in both with reduction in consumption of carbohydrates and calories. Follow-up was short, rendering it impossible to report whether these men ultimately developed sustained diabetes.

The issue of sugar consumption and risk of diabetes was revived by A. M. Cohen in 1961. He found that diabetes was common in Yemenites who had lived for long periods in Israel and very rare in new immigrants from Yemen. The most evident and dramatic difference in the contrasting circumstances of these groups was that sugar consumption was very low in Yemen and considerable in Israel (10% of calories were derived from sucrose). Cohen also produced diabetes with high-sugar diets in specially bred rats (1972). He concluded that sucrose consumption was probably of major importance in the etiology of diabetes. This opinion received support from Cleave in a series of publications beginning in 1957. Campbell (1963) observed that in African blacks a marked increase in rates of diabetes followed closely a sharp rise in sugar consumption. Gelfand and Forbes (1963) thought increasing rates of diabetes in Africans might be attributable to the rise in consumption of sugar and fat. In Australian aborigines Wise, et al (1976) found a temporal relationship of rising rates of diabetes to decreasing consumption of fiber, and increasing consumption of refined flour and sugar. Several observers noted that deprivations of war were often associated with declines in sugar consumption and lower rates of diabetes.

Yudkin (1964) examined for each of 22 countries the diabetes mortality rate for either 1955 or 1956. He then calculated the correlation of these data with levels of sugar consumption about twenty years earlier in these countries. He found a strongly positive correlation coefficient of .73. He also examined for 44 countries the interrelationship of fat consumption and sugar consumption; the correlation coefficient was 0.85. He concluded that the association of fat consumption and diabetes was incidental, while the relationship of sugar consumption and diabetes was that of cause and effect. Some problems in

253

interpreting such correlations will be discussed below. Schaefer (1971) considered the possibility that rising rates of diabetes in certain Eskimo groups might be caused by a marked increase in sugar intake. Prior found that the epidemic of diabetes in Maoris of New Zealand was temporally associated with increasing sugar consumption (1971). Zeigler (1966) concluded that rising rates of diabetes in Switzerland were caused by increases in sugar consumption. Tsuji (1970) noted the corresponding increase of diabetes and sugar consumption on the Japanese Island of Oki-Erabu. World consumption of refined sugar has increased steadily in the past several decades and is now about seven times greater than in 1900 (Aykroyd, 1974). An increase in rates of diabetes of roughly comparable degree has occurred simultaneously.

Cleave thinks that ingestion of sugars and other refined carbohydrates tends to produce diabetes. His arguments to that are well set forth in the most recent edition of his book (1974). He points out that some of the exceptions to the association of diabetes rates and levels of sugar consumption may be attributable to high levels of "refined" dietary carbohydrates other than sucrose. Cleave and others, including Campbell (1970a) think that the consumption of unnaturally concentrated carbohydrates is harmful to beta cells because it overtaxes them. Cleave and many others believe that consumption of refined carbohydrates also tends to induce obesity, thereby further increasing risk of diabetes. Similar views were expressed by Wales (1976).

It is quite conceivable that in some circumstances the apparent lack of correlation between rates of diabetes and sugar consumption might only reflect an inadequate duration of high sugar consumption. The same possibility exists with respect to obesity and diabetes. Yudkin (1967) has written an interesting historical review on changes in consumption of dietary carbohydrates.

On the basis of epidemiologic and experimental evidence to be reviewed below, several other scholars in the field have, on the other hand, concluded that sugar consumption is of little if any importance in the etiology of diabetes. The negative views of Bose, Lemann, Joslin, and of Mills and Himsworth have been mentioned above. Walker (1966), Truswell (1973), and Keen (1974) reviewed the available evidence on this issue; each concluded that the case against sugar was weak, as did an editorial in the *South African Medical Journal* (1966). Neither Stare (1973) nor Bierman and Nelson (1975) saw any reason to believe that eating sugar or other dietary carbohydrates caused diabetes. Joslin, et al (1934) examined the relationship between diabetes mortality rates and sugar consumption for 18 countries for which data were available. They also evaluated relationships over time for individual countries. They concluded that sugar consumption was "not an important factor" in the etiology of diabetes.

Keen (1974), Walker (1977) and West (1972) have pointed out the difficulties in determining whether relationships between rising sugar consumption and increasing diabetes rates are causal or coincidental. The available data on both sugar consumption and diabetes are with few exceptions imprecise. The sensitivity and reliability of data on death certificates are discussed in detail above in Chapter 6 on mortality. The sensitivity of this method varies considerably by country and in the same country over time. Among countries the correlation of both sugar and fat consumption with rate of diabetes has been fairly strong under certain circumstances, but no greater than with many other variables, such as motor vehicles per capita, number of television sets, consumption of power, and number of bath tubs. A very important consideration, often ignored, is that frequency of testing for diabetes and the sensitivity of testing methods tends to be much greater in the highly-developed countries, where sugar consumption is usually high. The degree of effect of this factor on diabetes mortality rates is not known, but it seems likely that this factor contributes significantly to the strength of the association between national diabetes mortality rates and sugar consumption. These factors probably also influence the degree of relationship between diabetes rates and other factors in intercountry comparisons (consumption of fat and fiber, obesity, economic status, etc).

Several of the scholars who have been concerned about the possible role of sugar consumption in the etiology of diabetes have cited an association between diabetes mortality rates by country and sugar consumption. Problems of interpreting such data have also been discussed above. Even with all the difficulties involved, it seemed appropriate to review more systematically and extensively the degree and consistency of the association of these two variables. Data presented by LeGoff (1911) and Yudkin (1964) showed an impressively positive correlation. Although Mills (1930a) was not impressed with the consistency of the association, his data did show a generally positive correlation between diabetes mortality rate and sugar consumption. Mills compared sugar consumption in 1927 to diabetes mortality in 1927 or to the nearest year for which data were available. Judy Stober and the author recently measured a correlation coefficient for these data of Mills (17 countries). It was rather strongly positive: r was .62. This agrees with Yudkin's findings (1964) who found a coefficient of .73 when he related prewar sugar consumption to diabetes mortality rates about twenty years later. But in general, countries with low sugar consumption have younger populations, and diabetes mortality is very strongly related to age. The correlation coefficient was, for example, quite strong (.65) between sugar consumption (1971) and life expectancy (1970) in the 46 countries for which figures were available to us. Also, when we examined the correlation of sugar consumption with diabetes mortality for specific age groups, the association was considerably weaker than for whole populations. Correlation coefficient was only .27 for sugar consumption and diabetes mortality in 50 countries when 1960 sugar consumption was compared with mortality rates of persons 45 to 64 years of age during the years 1959–1961. The morality data were from WHO (1964) and sugar consumption estimates from the *International Sugar Year Book* of 1963. Age-adjusted data for 1958–1960 were available to us on only 12 countries for which sugar consumption levels were also available (1960). Correlation coefficient for these 12 pairs was only .15 (not statistically significant).

Another problem is that sugar consumption by country is also related to wealth which, in turn, is related to other factors that might induce diabetes. We determined correlation coefficient of gross national product per capita in 1970 and sugar consumption (1971) using all countries (44) for which pairs of data were available. The correlation coefficient between affluence and sugar consumption was .56.

Another difficulty in interpreting the interesting positive correlation shown by Yudkin was that the twenty-year period between his figures for prewar sugar consumption and his diabetes mortality rates in 1957 included World War II, during which there were major changes in sugar consumption. Yudkin's strategy of examining the relationship of diabetes mortality and sugar consumption several or many years before seemed to be an appropriate approach. So the correlation coefficient was examined between sugar consumption in 1951 (*International Sugar Year Book*) and diabetes mortality in 1971 (WHO, 1974). Paired data were available for 44 countries. The correlation coefficient was quite weak (.18). These data were not age-corrected, but for reasons cited above, it seems likely that age correction would further weaken the association. The correlation between sugar consumption in 1971 and diabetes mortality in 1971 (paired data available for 39 countries) was also weak (.19). Correlation of diabetes mortality and total calories was somewhat better (.45). This latter coefficient was calculated for 18 countries where pairs of data were available. The caloric estimates were supplied by the Food and Agriculture Organization of the United Nations (FAO).

Because the very high degree of correlation found by Yudkin was unique we reexamined the original sources of data that he had used. He had related "prewar" sugar consumption in 22 populations to diabetes mortality rates about twenty years later. The mortality rates were derived from a table in Joslin's book (1959) on rates for 1956: if 1956 data were not available, the rate for 1955 was used. The prewar (World War II) data on sugar consumption were from a publication of FAO (Viton and Pignalosa, 1961). In these sources there were paired data on 37 populations, and when all available data were used the correlation coefficient was considerably less (.52) than with the 22 pairs selected by Yudkin (.73). Moreover, populations with low sugar consumption were generally younger. Thus, adjustment of mortality rates for age distribution would have further reduced the strength of this correlation. Also, the frequency of testing for diabetes was probably higher in countries with high sugar consumption; they were generally more affluent. Correction for these two factors was not possible because no quantitative data were available. But it seems likely that such adjustments would reduce the strength of the correlation between diabetes mortality and sugar consumption to insignificant or very low levels.

Although these measurements relating sugar consumption and diabetes mortality by country do not exclude the possibility of a cause-and-effect relationship under special circumstances, in the aggregate they lend little, if any, support to the hypothesis that sugar consumption causes diabetes.

The striking associations of increases in sugar consumption and diabetes over time in many societies do, however, deserve careful examination in other ways to determine the extent to which the relationship may be causal. In each of the populations in which such relationships have been perceived between diabetes rates and sugar intake (eg, Yemenites, Indians, and Zulus), other changes have also occurred. These have usually included higher caloric consumption, increased fat consumption, lower exercise levels, and increasing adiposity. For example, the "old settlers" studied by Cohen were considerably heavier than the new immigrants from Yemen, and fat consumption rose sharply in urbanized Zulus.

We studied sugar consumption and diabetes rates in 13 populations (West and Kalbfleisch, 1971; West, 1972,1974). There was generally a positive correlation. On the other hand, there were some impressive discrepancies. Sugar consumption was far higher in Costa Rica than in Malaya, but diabetes rates were about the same. Levels of sugar consumption were similar in Costa Rica and the United States, but diabetes rates were much higher in the United States. It should be pointed out, however, that an imperfect correlation between sugar consumption and diabetes rates would not exclude sugar consumption as one of several risk factors. There is, however, additional negative evidence.

In several countries rates of diabetes have not correlated well over time with levels of sugar consumption (Mills, 1930a; Keen, 1974). In certain elements of the Chinese population of Hong Kong, diabetes is common despite low levels of sugar consumption (Barnes, 1974). The considerable changes in rates of diabetes observed in Taiwan have borne little relationship to levels of sugar consumption (Tsai, 1970). Despite low levels of sugar consumption, diabetes and obesity have recently become common in women of a Fiji community (Hawley and Jansen, 1971) and in females of Tokelau (Prior, 1974). Sugar consumption is high in several countries where rates of diabetes are low. These include Nicaragua, Costa Rica, Colombia, and Mauritius (Walker, 1977).

In many American Indian tribes rising rates of sugar consumption have coincided with marked increases in rates of diabetes (West, 1974). In general, rates are low in tribes that eat little sugar and high in those that eat more. But Pimas have the highest rates of diabetes in the world despite levels of sugar consumption that are considerably less than the general population of the United States (Reid, et al, 1971). Diabetes is also rife in Kiowas and Comanches, despite levels of sugar consumption that are about the same as those in the general United States population (West, et al, 1976). In the United States (Page and Friend, 1974) and Britain (Hollingsworth, 1974) sugar consumption has changed little since 1920, but diabetes rates are probably higher now in both countries. These increased rates, however, are at least partly the result of increased frequency and sensitivity of diagnostic tests. American females are fatter than males and have more diabetes, but they eat a little less sugar than males (Page and Friend, 1974). When, however, sugar intake is expressed as percent of total calories it is very similar in US men and women. Young adults eat about twice as much sugar as middle-aged adults (Page and Friend, 1974), but have a much lower incidence of diabetes.

Campbell (1964) mentions a personal communication from Pederson indicating that "Greenlanders" had very low rates of diabetes and very high sugar consumption. It is widely believed that sugar consumption is high in Indians of South Africa in whom diabetes is rife, but data of Booyens and DeWaal (1970) and Walker (1972) suggest that their sugar intake is quite modest, much less than in Americans or South African whites, and similar to that of local urban blacks. Sugar consumption in these Indians is, however, higher than in India. Walker (1974) found little difference in sugar intake of black and white children in urban South Africa. In Lautoka, Fiji, Sorokin (1975) estimated that diabetes was about five times more common in Indians than in Fijians. Sugar consumption was the same. The Indians ate less carbohydrates, more refined cereals, less fiber, and more fat. Prior (1974) found no differences in rates of diabetes in Polynesians of Pukapuka and Europeans of Carterton, New Zealand, despite the fact that the Europeans consumed more than five times as much sugar.

Thus, there is on hand both positive and negative evidence from two kinds of epidemiologic observations. These are correlations of the two factors (sugar consumption and diabetes) among populations, and also in studies of the relationship over time in individual populations. In the aggregate, the evidence from these two approaches would appear to exclude sugar consumption as a dominant and universal etiologic factor. Evidence available from these latter two approaches neither excludes or establishes that sugar consumption may play a significant role in some circumstances. Evidence of other kinds seems to be more negative than positive.

Intrapopulation studies have been almost uniformly negative. Himsworth and Marshall (1935) found that prior to the discovery of diabetes, diabetics appeared to eat proportionately more fat and less carbohydrate than controls. Baird (1972) found in Scotland no difference in the sugar consumption of people with occult diabetes and that of controls. In England, Keen, et al (1976) studied sugar consumption and glucose tolerance in three populations with negative results. Tolerance was *better* in those who ate more sugar. Medalie, et al (1975) studied diet and the incidence of diabetes in a large group of Israeli men. Those who were later found to be diabetic had not eaten any more sugar or carbohydrate than controls. In a very small group of Indians studied by Booyens, et al (1970) in South Africa, the result was also negative. Paffenbarger and Wing (1973) interviewed 26,954 men by questionnaire concerning presence or absence of diabetes. These responses were then compared to their soft drink consumption in college as had been determined by questionnaire sixteen to fifty years earlier. No relationship was found between soft drink consumption and susceptibility to diabetes. Diabetics did drink more tea and coffee in college, and conceivably this could have led to greater sugar consumption.

We recently studied sugar consumption in 190 Plains Indians (West, et al, 1976). In 76 later found to have occult diabetes, refined sugar consumption did not differ from that of 216 found to have normal glucose tolerance. No association with sugar consumption was found with either insulin secretion or fatness. This approach would be insensitive in populations in which there was little intraindividual variation in sugar consumption. In our Indians, however, the range of variation was quite wide. Mean consumption of refined sugar (145 gm daily) was similar to the US average of 130 gm/day, but levels below 70 and above 200 were common.

There are several other difficulties in evaluating epidemiologic results in this field. Levels of sugar consumption are difficult to measure, particularly in individuals. Consumption changes over time in both individuals and societies. Differences are usually found by age and sex. In societies where sugar consumption is considerable, a substantial majority of dietary sugar is usually sucrose, but other sugars may constitute significant portions. Conceivably, there might be differences among the various sugars in propensity to enhance risk of diabetes. As has been demonstrated in animals by Cohen (1972) and others, there could be genetic differences in susceptibility to diabetogenic effects of dietary constituents.

In several parts of the world there are sugar-cane cutters who consume large amounts of sucrose (Brigham, 1968; Saundby, 1908; Lemann, 1911; Banting, 1929; Campbell, et al, 1967; Truswell, et al, 1971; Cleave, 1974). This sucrose is usually derived from two sources. They often receive allotments of refined sucrose, and they chew and ingest sugar from the cane (Truswell, et al, 1971). Quantitative data are few but it appears that rates of diabetes are quite low and sugar consumption quite high in certain groups of these cutters (Cleave, 1974). In one group studied by Truswell, et al (1971) in South Africa, sugar consumption appeared to average roughly 400 gm daily. The cutters are quite lean and exercise levels are high. Their levels of sugar tolerance are quite remarkable. Campbell, et al (1967) administered single loads as great as 450-900 gm with modest rises in blood glucose! Cleave and others have attributed the very low rates of diabetes to the slow rates at which sugar from the tough cane is mobilized and swallowed. Other possibilities are that sugar consumption is innocuous in this respect, or that it is not diabetogenic in hard-working people. Levels of serum triglycerides are low despite huge amounts of dietary sugar (Truswell, et al, 1971).

Does sugar consumption cause obesity? It is widely believed that eating sugar tends to induce obesity. Some epidemiologic experience consistent with this notion has been reviewed above. Also, the obese patients of Dunlop and Lyon (1931) were often on diets judged to be particularly high in carbohydrates. Less well known is a considerable body of negative epidemiologic evidence concerning sugar and carbohydrate consumption as etiologic agents in obesity. Some of these observations have also been cited above. This includes mention of populations in which obesity was common despite low levels of sugar consumption (eg, the women of Tokelau and certain communities of Fiji).

Walker (1969, 1974) has studied extensively the relationship of sugar consumption and fatness, and has found little evidence of a relationship of cause and effect. Both Richardson (1972) and Keen, et al (1976) found sugar consumption lower in fat people than in lean. Many fat diabetic patients maintain their weight very nicely despite low levels of sugar consumption as confirmed by their spouses. In the studies of Keen and of Richardson, sugar consumption

259

was measured by interview techniques. This raises the possibility that fat people in Britain delude the interviewers and perhaps themselves about their sugar consumption. But the same results have been found in other societies. In Israel there was no relationship between sugar consumption and relative weight (Medalie, et al, 1975). In Micronesia Hankin, et al (1970) found that weights of subpopulations were not well related to levels of sugar consumption in these various groups. In New Zealand levels of sugar consumption are very similar in whites and Polynesian Maoris, but Maoris have about three times as much diabetes (Prior, 1974). The Maoris are much fatter (Prior, 1971).

In our Plains Indians we could detect little evidence of guilt concerning obesity or sugar consumption. Most of our interviews on sugar consumption were conducted in the presence of the spouse or another member of the household who verified the validity of the responses. Even so, we could find no relationship between adiposity and sugar consumption (West, et al, 1976). Results of Ries (1973) were similarly negative in Leipzig, as were those of Nichols, et al, in Tecumseh, Michigan (1976).

All this negative evidence does not exclude the possibility that sugar consumption may under *some* circumstances increase risk of obesity. But this negative evidence does suggest a need for caution in accepting the widely prevailing notion that sugar is particularly fattening. It should be kept in mind that sugar has 4 kilcalories per gm, alcohol 7, and fat 9. I suspect that sugar consumption is poorly related to obesity in societies where there is a wide array of attractive and readily accessible dietary alternatives to sugar, particularly dietary fat. The obese patients of Childs (1972) were allowed sugar and starch freely, but lost weight very satisfactorily when fat was restricted. Hood, et al (1969) observed no effect on rate of weight loss with isocaloric reduction diets containing sucrose varying in amounts from 3% to 50% of calories. A committee of the Nutrition Council of the Netherlands concluded that eating sugar did not play a primary role in causing obesity or shortening life (Dalderup and Van Haard, 1971).

Refined carbohydrates

In 1956, Cleave put forward a concept he called the "saccharine disease". This concept has undergone some subsequent modification. Its latest description is set forth in the 1974 edition of his book. Cleave concluded that several major diseases of modern man are mainly the result of replacing more natural foods with refined carbohydrates. This book is quite interesting and full of provocative observations and useful information. Cleave has clearly recognized in this and earlier publications that a certain degree of oversimplification attends his general thesis. While having, here and elsewhere, expressed some reservations about this concept as it applies to the etiology of diabetes, it is still this writer's view that Cleave deserves considerable credit for illustrating so well the profound effects of environmental and dietary changes on disease patterns. Evidence presented on interpopulation variations in rates of colon diseases is, for example, very impressive indeed. Moreover, it is quite possible that by direct or indirect means, refinement of carbohydrates may *under certain conditions* enhance susceptibility to diabetes. As shown by Cleave and others, dramatic increases in rates of diabetes have often followed increases in the consumption of refined carbohydrates. This requires an evaluation of the possibility that this association reflects cause and effect. The need for systematic investigation is also suggested by the vast numbers of people to whom this question applies.

One of several problems has been that the marked changes in rates of diabetes have also been preceded by other changes that might account for them. Among the changes that often attend the rising rates of consumption of refined carbohydrates are decreasing exercise, increasing consumption of dietary fat, increasing availability of other nutrients, rising affluence, and greater adiposity.

Cleave (1974) concluded that the imperfect correlations between diabetes rates and the consumption of sucrose might be explained by a deleterious effect of other "refined carbohydrates". No precise definition, however, has been offered for *refined*. Cleave did make clear that he was mainly referring to refined sugars and to processed flour from which fiber has been removed, but in one communication (1974a) he included rice. It does not seem likely that the gut or the beta cells recognize the previous state of the nutrients offered. Rather, the potentially significant considerations would appear to include factors such as caloric density and chemical and physical composition at the time of consumption. It is quite true that, in general, carbohydrates are less readily absorbed in their natural state. On the other hand, certain natural and unrefined carbohydrates such as orange juice and honey would be expected to produce sharper rises in blood glucose than bread from refined flour. Also, many types of cooked starches are very rapidly absorbed even though they have not been "refined". Cleave and Campbell (1969) believe that the rates at which the carbohydrate calories are consumed may be important. They point out that the need to chew natural foods may be protective because rates at which the nutrients are presented to the stomach is slowed.

This is only one of several interrelated factors that might contribute to an enhanced risk of diabetes with consumption of refined carbohydrates. Ingestion of refined carbohydrates might produce diabetes because of deleterious effects of dietary sucrose or other sugars; or because of increases in carbohydrate calories, total calories, or caloric density; or because of a paucity of dietary fiber. Conceivably, risk of diabetes might be affected by the rate at which certain nutrients were absorbed from the gut. While it is possible to examine each of these several possibilities, it is very difficult to evaluate together the effect of a heterogeneous group of factors called "refined carbohydrates", even if a more specific definition can be developed for "refined". It is not possible to measure quantitatively in any satisfactory way the total consumption of "refined carbohydrates". What unit of measurement could be used? One can only determine this element by element (eg, how much sucrose, how much fiber, or how much low-fiber flour). One could express each element (sucrose, maltose, flour, etc) in calories or percent of calories, but the diabetogenic effect per calorie might be different with the various types of refined carbohydrates. For this reason the evidence on effects of dietary sugar and dietary fiber are reviewed here in separate sections.

Evidence cited above strongly suggests that diets made up mainly of rice have no particular propensity to induce diabetes. But Cleave and others have raised some important issues that require further evaluation. (1) Does rapid absorption of carbohydrates tend to induce diabetes? On a theoretical basis one could argue that this exercise of the beta cells was either exhausting or conditioning. (2) To what extent does the availability of concentrated readily absorbable carbohydrate enhance risk of obesity? Epidemiologic evidence concerning these two questions is not at all conclusive, as pointed out in the section above on sugars, and in that below on fiber.

Frequently the experimenter may find in epidemiologic data valuable clues to guide the course of his laboratory investigations. Similarly, the epidemiologist often benefits by determining the degree to which epidemiologic observations correspond with experience in the laboratory. The question whether eating sugar enhances risk of diabetes is so important that a review of experimental evidence is in order. The discussion of experimental data will follow the review of epidemiologic evidence in this section on nutritional factors.

Dietary Fiber

Maimonides in his 12th-century work on general health measures, advised: "bread should be made of coarse flour; that is to say, the husk should not be removed and the bran should not be refined by sifting". Publications of Cleave have been cited above, suggesting the possible deleterious effects of substituting concentrated carbohydrate for high-fiber foods. Less well known are earlier exhortations of Dr. John Kellogg, who invented some of our most popular breakfast cereals. In 1918 Kellogg warned of the dangers of "concentrated" foods and advocated diets containing generous amounts of fruits, cereals, and bran (Bale, 1976).

Trowell (1973,1975) has recently published good reviews showing some strongly negative relationships between dietary fiber and rates of diabetes. In Australian aborigines, Wise, et al (1970) found that rising rates of diabetes coincided with decreases in consumption of high-fiber cereals. Sorokin (1975) found in Lautoka, Fiji, that the natives had much less diabetes than the local Indians. The Indians ate much less fiber, but they also ate more fat, less carbohydrate, more refined flour, and the same amount of sugar as the natives. We did not measure dietary fiber systematically in any of our worldwide studies, but crude estimates suggest to me a general correlation (negative) between dietary fiber and diabetes rates among the populations we studied (West and Kalbfleisch, 1971). Central Americans, for example, consume more fiber than North Americans and have lower rates of diabetes. Conceivably, a protective effect might be direct, resulting from a lower rate of absorption of dietary carbohydrate (Westhuizen, et al, 1972), or incidental to a lesser susceptibility to obesity when calories are less concentrated (Heaton, 1973; Trowell, 1974). Cleave (1974) also cited evidence of this negative association between diabetes and dietary fiber.

Malins (1974), however, wasn't impressed by the consistency of the relationship between diabetes rates and fiber consumption over time in Britain. Eastwood, et al (1974) have challenged the assumption that dietary fiber has declined substantially in Britain. We have not measured fiber consumption systematically in Oklahoma Indians in whom diabetes rates are exceedingly high (West, 1974), but it appears that levels of dietary fiber are about the same as in local whites. James (1974) has suggested that deleterious effects of removal of fiber might be related to the incidental removal of zinc, leading to zinc deprivation. There are some other apparent exceptions to the generally negative relationships between dietary fiber and rates of diabetes. It seems likely that levels of dietary fiber are substantial in the Mabuiag Islanders, who have high rates of diabetes (Winterbotham, 1961). Few data have been published on levels of fiber consumption in lean rice-consuming Asian populations in whom rates of diabetes are low. Fiber consumption may be relatively low in some of these groups. Some primitive and lean Eskimo groups with low rates of diabetes consume very little complex carbohydrate (West, 1974). These exceptions do not exclude the possibility that high-fiber diets might have a protective effect under some circumstances. One problem in evaluating dietary fiber as a protective factor is that among populations it also has direct and coincidental associations (both positive and negative) with other factors that may protect against or cause diabetes. These include exercise levels (generally positive), total dietary carbohydrate and dietary starch (generally positive), fat consumption (usually negative), sugar consumption (generally negative), calorie consumption (usually negative), adiposity (generally negative).

Burkitt, Walker, and Painter (1975) recently reviewed evidence implicating fiber removal in the etiology of nine common diseases. Diabetes was not included.

The case for fiber removal as a possible risk factor in obesity has been well set forth by Heaton (1973). James and Cummings (1974) point out, however, that evidence is quite incomplete with respect to the establishment of fiber removal as an etiologic agent in obesity. It was found by Jeffrys (1974) that the presence of fiber either facilitated or inhibited glucose absorption, depending on the type. Reilly and Kirsner (1975) pointed out how little is known about dietary fiber and its effects. One of the many problems is that of classification and definition of the many fibers (Trowell, 1976). Van Soest and McQueen (1973) have written on the chemistry and estimation of fiber. Trowell, et al (1974) and Cleave (1974) have compiled a limited amount of information about dietary fiber consumption in various populations and in certain populations over time. Connell (1976) and Bing (1976) have reviewed some of the recent work on dietary fiber. Few data are available *within* populations on consumption of dietary fiber and risks of obesity and diabetes. Westhuizen, et al (1972) point out that factors other than fiber content also determine rate and completeness of digestion of unrefined carbohydrates. Southgate, et al (1976) showed that adding substantial amounts of fiber to the diet increased loss of calories in stools by only trivial amounts.

Dietary Fat

Himsworth (1935-1936) brought together an impressive array of evidence suggesting the possibility that risk of diabetes was positively related to fat consumption and negatively related to carbohydrate consumption. These data included both laboratory and epidemiologic observations. This hypothesis has received some support from modern experimental data to be discussed below. However, by 1949 Himsworth was considering the possibility that the relationship of diabetes to fat consumption might be mainly incidental to other factors such as its general association with greater caloric intake. In Asian countries and rural populations of Africa and Latin America, fat consumption and diabetes rates are low. Hargreaves (1958) cited evidence that had led him to suspect that risk of diabetes was increased by consumption of animal fat.

In our epidemiologic observations we have also found a generally positive association of fat consumption and diabetes rates. But in contrast to the association of diabetes and adiposity that persists in both inter- and intrapopulation analysis, the relationship between fat consumption and diabetes rates was quite variable in our intrapopulation observations. In Montevideo, rates of diabetes were much higher than in rural Uruguay, but levels of fat consumption were about the same. Fat consumption is, by international standards, high in most primitive Eskimo groups, averaging about one third of calories, but diabetes rates are very low (West, 1974). Prior to 1940 diabetes was rare in Iceland (Albertsson, 1952), despite high levels of dietary fat. Diabetes rates were apparently low in the Masai of East Africa (Orr and Gilkes, 1931), despite high levels of fat consumption. In Israeli men levels of fat consumption were not significantly elevated in those later found to have diabetes (Kahn, et al, 1971; Medalie, et al, 1975). Diabetes rates rose sharply in Japan after World War II during a period when fat consumption increased by a factor of 2.4 (Oiso, 1970).

It seems likely that fat consumption favors the development of obesity under certain conditions (Childs, 1972), but a specific and direct effect on increasing risk of diabetes remains to be demonstrated in humans. Some animal data relating to this issue will be reviewed below. As in the case of the other dietary factors, interpretation is complicated by the association of fat consumption of populations with other variables that may induce or protect against diabetes. With a few exceptions, levels of caloric intake are high, for example, and exercise levels low in populations that consume high amounts of fat. Yudkin (1964) showed the close association between fat consumption and sugar consumption among 22 selected populations.

In carp, diabetes has been produced by feeding certain oxidized oils. This can be prevented by feeding alpha-tocopherol. These studies from Japan have been summarized by Wolf (1976).

Dietary Protein

Protein consumption by country relates to diabetes rates about as well as any of the other nutrients mentioned previously. Yet the notion that protein consumption causes diabetes has not been popular, probably because it has been difficult to explain a basis of the diabetogenic effect of protein. Also there is epidemiologic evidence that is inconsistent with this possibility. Levels of protein intake were about the same in rural and urban Uruguay, but diabetes rates were much higher in the urban population. Primitive Eskimos consume very great amounts of protein and have low rates of diabetes. Yet some animal studies, to be described below in the section on experimental studies, are consistent with the possibility that high-protein diets might in some circumstances be more diabetogenic than alternative regimens.

Protein deficiency is probably not a major cause of diabetes except in special circumstances (eg, in diabetes secondary to pancreatic fibrosis and calcification). This is discussed in detail in the section of Chapter 8 on that subject. However, in both children and adults, protein-calorie malnutrition impairs glucose tolerance (Pimstone, et al, 1972; Pitchumoni, 1974; Smith, et al, 1975). Nevertheless, rates of both childhood- and adult-onset diabetes tend to be low in communities where protein consumption is low. Data of Pimstone, et al (1972) showed that in children impairment of glucose tolerance secondary to protein-calorie malnutrition was usually corrected promptly with improved nutrition.

Other Nutrients

In 1959 it was demonstrated by Schwarz and Mertz that a deficiency of a chromium-containing factor could impair glucose tolerance in rats. Subsequently their group and many others have explored further the possible role of chromium deficiency in human diabetes. Much of this work was well summarized by Hambidge (1973). Tissue chromium levels are lower in older people, multiparous women, and, generally, in societies that consume more processed food. Under some conditions impaired tolerance of malnourished infants is restored by feeding chromium. In older subjects with clinical diabetes or impaired tolerance, results have been variable with chromium supplements. Data in animals and men are suggestive enough to require intensive follow-up of these findings. There are, however, some negative findings that also deserve attention. According to Hambidge (1973), tissue levels of chromium are very low in Nigeria (where diabetes rates are also quite low).

Data on chromium levels in foods have been published by Toepfer, et al (1973). Beef has considerable chromium, but diabetes is very common in beef-eating populations. Beer is also high in chromium. In both beer and beef, the chromium is in a biologically effective form. Ordinary American white bread also contains considerable levels of biologically active chromium. Diabetes is rife in Oklahoma Indians who drink beer and also in those who do not. In some foods high in chromium the element is not in a form that is biologically effective. It has been shown by Toepfer, et al (1973) that after alcohol extraction there is a good correlation between chromium concentration and biologic activity. The activity appears to be effected by facilitating the action of insulin at the cell membrane.

In the study of Sherman, et al (1968) there was no effect of chromium feeding in adult diabetics. This study was more carefully controlled than others reporting positive results. Nevertheless, the possibility cannot now be excluded that long-term deficiency of a chromium-related factor might increase susceptibility to diabetes under certain circumstances. It is clear that modern processing of cereal foods substantially reduces available chromium. Conceivably, the association of sugar intake and diabetes could be attributable to the lower levels of tissue chromium in those who substitute refined flour and sugar for "natural" cereals. Most of the evidence cited above against the "dietary sugar hypothesis" could also be used against the chromium-deficiency hypothesis. It would be of interest to know the levels of tissue chromium in some of the special populations that have very high or low rates of diabetes. Glucose ingestion usually lowers serum chromium levels, but no data were available to me on the acute effects of oral ingestion of starch or other nutrients that also stimulate beta cells.

Under some conditions deficiencies of other metals, including iron and zinc, have produced aberrations of carbohydrate metabolism in animals. There is as yet no evidence that these deficiencies have significance in human diabetes. On the other hand excesses of iron are of significance, and will be discussed in Chapter 8 on special types of diabetes. These include hemochromatosis and thalassemia (Lassman, et al, 1974). Coelingh-Bennick and Schreurs (1975) and Spellacy, et al (1977) have reported greatly improved glucose tolerance after large doses of pyridoxine in gestational diabetics, but Perkins (1977) observed no beneficial effect. Podolsky (1971) reviewed the relationships of diabetes to trace metals.

Protein-calorie malnutrition may impair glucose tolerance both in infants (Hambidge, 1973) and in adults (Smith, et al, 1975). It is not yet clear whether this produces changes leading to clinical diabetes. The possible connection between malnutrition and diabetes secondary to pancreatic fibrosis is discussed in Chapter 8 on special types of diabetes. This latter discussion also includes the possible role of cassava consumption in the etiology of pancreatic disease.

In hyperaldosteronism and with administration of certain diuretics, impairment of glucose tolerance may result from low levels of serum potassium. Deficiencies of dietary potassium may increase susceptibility to diabetes under certain conditions, but there is little evidence to suggest this as an etiologic factor of primary significance.

The effects of alcohol on carbohydrate metabolism are highly variable depending on circumstances. Alcohol can indirectly increase risk of diabetes in two ways. Pancreatitis is much more common in heavy drinkers. Alcohol consumption may also enhance risk of obesity, although this is not well established. In the United States and other affluent societies, there is very little epidemiologic data on the relationship of diabetes rates to mild, moderate, or heavy drinking. Klatsky, et al (1977) found a variable relationship of alcohol intake and adiposity depending on sex and race. This association was not impressively positive. Gerard, et al (1977) found a negative association between glucose tolerance and level of alcohol consumption as ascertained by dietary history. Katsumata and Yamada (1964) increased rates of diabetes in albino rats by feeding diets high in alcohol. In certain African communities some alcoholic drinks are very high in iron. This may lead to hemochromatosis as discussed below.

Meal Frequency

Under certain experimental conditions (Cohn, et al, 1965), animals may gain more weight on "gorging" regimens than when consuming the same number of calories in more frequent meals ("nibbling"). On the other hand, in mice studied by Petersson and Hellman (1962) obesity and diabetes were prevented by a regimen that limited consumption to one meal daily with no limitation of the size of the single meal, and no qualitative difference in diets of "nibbling" mice with unlimited access and the mice that were required to "gorge" on a single meal. Woods, et al (1976) provided unlimited food to rats during a single two-hour meal. These rats subsequently weighed less than rats that had had continuous access to the same nutrients.

Fabry, et al (1964) studied meal frequency by history in residents of Prague. He found a negative relationship between meal frequency and frequency of both obesity and abnormal glucose tolerance. It may also be noted, however, that a regimen of one or two meals daily is common in certain populations of Africa and Asia in which both diabetes and obesity have been rare (Osuntokun, et al, 1971; Chun, 1925).

Experimental Evidence

Diabetes has been produced in goldfish by feeding 100% of calories as glucose (Sterne, et al, 1968). In several special animal breeds that are especially susceptible, rates of obesity and diabetes have been higher with diets containing concentrated simple carbohydrates than with vegetable or grain rations or other regimens. In most of these circumstances production of diabetes has required production of obesity (Renold, et al, 1971). Cohen, et al (1966,1967), however, produced diabetes with very high sucrose diets in genetically-selected rats without increasing body weights. Subsequently, diabetes was also produced with sucrose feeding in genetically-selected rats by Vrana, et al (1973) and by Laube, et al (1976). Laube, et al (1976) found that, although weight was not greater in sucrose-fed rats, their adiposity was greater.

Typically, the high-sugar regimens that have produced diabetes in animals have contained a substantial majority of calories as sugar. These are levels far higher than are consumed by any human population. Sucrose constituted only about 10% of calories, for example, in the Yemenites who were long-term residents of Israel. It is, of course, conceivable that the levels observed where sugar is popular and widely available (eg, 10% to 30% of calories), if sustained for twenty to fifty years, could be diabetogenic. A few individuals in affluent societies do consume very large amounts of sugar, some as much as one third of total calories. Risk of diabetes in this small minority is not known precisely, but such data as are available give little evidence of increased susceptibility (see above).

Occasionally diabetes has been observed in persons who have been drinking large amounts of sugar-containing soft drinks (Del Greco, 1953), but it is usually difficult to exclude the possibility that this consumption was the result of polydipsia rather than the cause of diabetes. Bisht, et al (1971) found no difference between diabetics and nondiabetics in taste threshold for sucrose.

Taken as a whole, work in animals demonstrates better a resistance, rather than a susceptibility, to diabetes in animals fed large amounts of sugar. Allen in his books of 1913 and 1919 summarized the experience of many workers who had failed to induce diabetes by feeding or injecting sugars. Interest was revived subsequently by the report of Dohan and Lukens (1948), who induced "diabetes" and hyperglycemia in cats by injecting large amounts of glucose intraperitoneally. These results were widely misinterpreted and overinterpreted by those who did not read details that were carefully and fully recorded by the authors. These results could be used better to argue the resistance rather than the susceptibility to massive glucose infusions. Twenty-seven cats received the injections, but only one had hyperglycemia that persisted after the infusions. This animal had a blood sugar of 58 mg/100 ml after thirty-two days of massive glucose infusions! The infusions were resumed on the 33rd day and continued through the 39th day, then stopped. Mild fasting hyperglycemia continued at a level of about 200 mg/100 ml for twenty-two days, at which point the animal was sacrificed. The cats were very sick from these infusions, with anorexia, weakness, ataxia, and weight loss not attributable to the mild hyperglycemia. Several died from the toxicity of this regimen. The one cat that had persistent hyperglycemia after termination of injections was quite ill, exhibiting weakness, depression, and a blood urea nitrogen of 105 mg/100 ml. It and a few of the other cats exhibited some hydropic degeneration of beta cells. Eight additional cats were similarly treated after half of the pancreas had been surgically removed. In only two did hyperglycemia continue after injections were stopped; and in one of these, blood glucose values returned to normal in fifty days. The second animal died after eight days of persistent hyperglycemia. The recovery of the aforementioned cat after fifty days suggests the possibility that the other two cats (one partially pancreatectomized and one intact), in whom hyperglycemia persisted eight and twenty-two days before death, might have recovered if they had survived the very toxic regimen to which they were subjected. Dohan and Lukens also reviewed the work of several other scientists who had tried unsuccessfully to produce diabetes by feeding or injecting large amounts of sugars.

Astwood, et al (1941) gave huge amounts of intravenous glucose to dogs (12 gm/sq m/hr) with no untoward effects, even over long periods of continuous infusion. Yoshikawa (1954) studied the effect of intraperitoneal glucose injections in cats and rabbits. One of five cats became hyperglycemic after a course of glucose injections in large amounts, and another cat with partial pancreatectomy developed diabetes after such injections. In 9 of 30 rabbits diabetes developed after such injections, but all had been pretreated with alloxan. It was not possible to determine from these data the extent to which glucose injections alone contributed to the development of diabetes, although it does appear that they enhanced susceptibility in these circumstances.

Under certain conditions female Holtzman albino rats exhibit a stronger preference for sugar and sweetness than males (Valenstein, et al, 1967). This deserves further study in other animals and humans, but American males eat more sugar than females (Page and Friend, 1974). When expressed as percent of total calories, sugar consumption is very similar in US males and females. Obese humans do not exhibit the marked temporary decline in preference for sweetness that develops in lean subjects immediately after consuming a large amount of sugar (Cabanac and Duclaux, 1970). It is not yet clear whether this peculiarity is a cause or an effect of obesity. Vartiainen (1967) studied craving for sugar in rats and found evidence of a genetic factor. Nordsiek (1972) has written a good summary on consumption of sugar and sweets and the factors that affect them. A detailed discussion on sugar consumption and its effects may be found in the book edited by Sipple and McNutt (1974).

Diabetes has been produced much more frequently in animals by feeding fats (Katsumata, 1970,1970a; Kaku, 1971; Zaragoza, et al, 1969), than by feeding carbohydrate or sugars. Usually these high-fat diets involve a lowering (either absolute or relative) of dietary carbohydrate (Katsumata, 1970, 1970a; Zaragoza, et al, 1969; Young, 1950). Haist, et al (1940) found that feeding fat exclusively to dogs seemed to have a protective effect on beta-cell function. These dogs had borderline pancreatic compensation, artificially induced by pancreatectomy of pituitary extracts. But this diet tended to produce anorexia. The ameliorative effects may have been attributable to reduced caloric intake. Diabetes has also been produced occasionally by increasing dietary protein (Petersen, et al, 1974; Young, 1950; Levine, 1974). Yakote, et al (1970) produced diabetes in carp on a high-protein regimen, but they thought the diabetes was probably attributable to an oxidized oil that was also in the diet. There were no sugars in this regimen; less than 20% of calories were carbohydrate, and protein supplied about 60% of calories (Yakote, 1973). In the rats of

269

Martinez (1966), in which 95% of the pancreas had been removed, rates of diabetes were enhanced by overfeeding with any of the major nutrients, but diabetes was induced most expeditiously with high-fat diets (Martinez, 1946; Houssay and Martinez, 1947). Florence and Quarterman (1972) studied in rats the effect of substituting sugar for starch. At first when rats were young, glucose tolerance was better during sucrose feeding, but later as rats aged there was no difference with the two regimens. Coltart and Crossley (1970) fed very high-sucrose diets (75% of calories in a fat-free regimen) to baboons for thirteen weeks. Fructose tolerance declined but glucose tolerance improved. Bennett and Coon (1966) fed to dogs diets containing 54% sucrose for nine to eleven days. Tolerance to glucose remained unimpaired.

Cohen (1977) has recently reported that, in genetically susceptible rats, diabetes is produced by high-fructose diets as well as by diets high in sucrose. Since beta cells are not stimulated by fructose, this finding lends no support to the notion that diabetes is produced in these animals by postprandial surges of the blood sugar that overtax the beta cells. Most animal species in which diabetes is common are quite fat (Herberg and Coleman, 1977). Cameron, et al (1976) produced obesity and diabetes in KK mice by feeding monosodium glutamate. Uram, et al (1958) found under certain conditions that rats had better glucose tolerance on high-starch regimens than on high-sucrose diets, but effects varied greatly depending on factors such as other dietary character- istics and duration of experiments. Diabetes was not produced by any of the regimens. Matsuo, et al (1970) studied the effects of synthetic diets in KK mice and CRK mice. Increases in adiposity were observed with diets high in sucrose, but also with diets high in either fat or starch. High-fat diets produced greatest adiposity. In KK rats diabetes was produced with all three of the synthetic diets. Hyperglycemia was more prompt and greater with a high-starch regimen than with an otherwise equivalent diet high in sucrose. None of the diets produced diabetes in the CRK mice.

Sand rats eat a vegetable diet in their native habitat. When caged and fed Purina Laboratory Chow containing high amounts of simple carbohydrate, they become fat and often develop diabetes. Most of this increased susceptibility to diabetes is attributable to the dietary change, but caging itself is partly respon- sible. Even those captive animals fed vegetables not uncommonly develop diabetes (Hackel, et al, 1965). It has now been shown repeatedly that under- feeding with no qualitative changes in diet can protect susceptible animals from diabetes (Wyse and Dulin, 1970; Gerritsen, et al, 1974; Grodsky, et al, 1974). Petersson and Hellman (1962) prevented the development of diabetes in obese hyperglycemic mice by limiting feeding to one meal period daily. There was no qualitative change in these diets, nor were calories limited in the one meal.

Under some conditions serum insulin levels are raised by feeding of sugars in animals and man, but effects on serum insulin and glucose tolerance are highly variable depending on the duration of experiments and the experimental conditions.* Under isocaloric conditions and when sugar is substituted for starch in amounts ordinarily consumed in affluent Western societies (140 gm daily), there is probably little, if any, effect on insulin secretion (Mann and Truswell, 1971). Anderson, et al (1973) fed very high-sucrose diets to human volunteers for periods up to ten weeks. Glucose tolerance improved. Restriction of carbohydrate regularly improves glucose tolerance in fat subjects, but in most circumstances this improvement has been the result of concomitant reduction in calories.

Eaton and Kipnis (1969) found that under certain conditions glucose feeding lowered serum insulin levels of rats. In the human subjects of Swan, et al (1966) there was little difference in acute insulinemic effects of sucrose and starch. Forster, et al (1970) compared the effects of starch syrup and glucose on insulin secretion and blood glucose levels using doses of 50, 100, and 300 gm. At each dosage results were "largely independent" of the type of carbohydrate.

The effects of qualitative changes in diet on adiposity has also been highly variable depending on many factors. But dietary fat has more frequently produced obesity than the other major dietary constituents (Schemmel, et al, 1969; Renold, et al, 1971). Kramer, et al (1969) have cited evidence consistent with the possibility that dietary fat may have a diabetogenic effect independent of its effect on increasing adiposity. Some of the results of Himsworth (1935), of Zaragoza (1970), and of Brunzell (1971) are consistent with this possibility, although it is difficult at times to determine whether potentially deleterious effects of dietary manipulation are the results of too much fat or too little carbohydrate. One of the greatest problems in interpreting results of dietary experiments relating to major sources of calories is that in changing a particular constituent, a second confounding variable must be created. One must change caloric intake or make reciprocal alterations in the consumption of one or more of the other constituents.

Fidler, et al (1973) gave huge amounts of intravenous glucose (856-1150 gm/day) to human subjects for periods up to seven weeks without untoward effects. R. A. Jackson, et al (1972) studied peripheral utilization of glucose in human subjects. It was impaired in both liver and muscle after a phase of carbohydrate restriction. The effects of dietary sucrose have been recently reviewed by Bender and Damji (1972). Rupe and Mayer (1967) described evidence that ingestion of sucrose may induce endogenous release of glucose into the blood.

In some circumstances caloric density of the available food may be a significant factor in determining risk of obesity, but in general, animals and man appear to adjust rather well to alterations of caloric denisty, being much more sensitive to caloric value than to density unless caloric density is very low

---

*References: Yudkin, 1972; Szanto and Yudkin, 1969; Gray and Kipnis, 1971; Fry, 1972; Pfeiffer, 1973; Anderson, et al, 1973; Dunnigan, et al, 1970; Mann and Truswell, 1971; Brunzell, et al, 1971; Himsworth, 1935; Kelsay, et al, 1974; Farquhar, et al, 1967; Swan, et al, 1966; Genuth, 1976; Boozer and Mayer, 1976.

(Petersson and Baumgardt, 1971). Richter, et al (1945) reported some interesting results in rats. On unlimited self-selection diets, rats did not develop diabetes, but diabetes was produced on certain fixed combinations of the same nutrients.

Cleave (1974) believes that high levels of sugar consumption do not induce diabetes if rates of absorption are relatively slow, as in sugarcane-chewing cane cutters. He and others have thought that the repeated abrupt absorption of simple sugars might eventually exhaust overworked beta cells. The attraction of this hypothesis has been somewhat diminished by demonstrations that mixed meals, containing carbohydrate with protein or fat or both, produce greater surges of insulin secretion than carbohydrate alone (Rabinowitz, et al, 1966; Dobbs, et al, 1975). For example, Dobbs, et al (1975) found that ingestion of fat with glucose markedly increased beta-cell response to glucose. Also, obesity appears to produce a much greater challenge to beta cells than high-carbohydrate diet. Several populations consuming high-carbohydrate diets have been found to have low serum insulin levels (Rubenstein, et al, 1969; Wicks and Jones, 1973). Pima Indian women eat less sugar than US whites (Reid, et al, 1971), but have high insulin levels (Bennett, et al, 1976a). Our fat Kiowas and Comanches consume amounts of sugar that are quite similar to those consumed by US whites, but serum insulin levels in these Indians are very high (West, et al, 1977). Bjorntorp, et al (1971) found levels of insulin secretion better related to fat-cell size than to fat-cell mass or age. Ditschuneit (1970) and Salans, et al (1970) have reviewed evidence bearing on the interrelationships among diabetes, hyperinsulinism, and obesity. Most evidence suggests that hyperinsulinism is secondary to overeating and obesity, but there is some evidence that hyperinsulinism may in some circumstances be primary (Joffee, et al, 1975; Mahler, 1971,1974; Olefsky, et al, 1974). Recent work of Genuth, et al (1976) and of Boozer and Mayer (1976) suggest that obesity in OB/OB mice is not primarily attributable to the hyperinsulinism present in these animals.

It is clear that under certain short-term conditions, high-sucrose diets can increase serum insulin levels in man even when calories are not increased (Labbe, et al, 1976). It is not clear under what circumstances and to what extent this is disadvantageous, and what happens over long periods (years) of high-sucrose diet when feedings are isocaloric. In Oklahoma Indians plasma insulin was unrelated to level of sugar consumption (West and Mako, 1976). Another uncertainty is the extent to which high-sucrose diets (unlimited in calories) increase risk of obesity in man. In some circumstances sucrose appears to be more fattening in animals than starch (Allen, et al, 1966), while in other circumstances starch is more fattening than sugar (Ahrens, et al, 1968).

In general, experimental data do not give much support to the notion that consumption of sucrose or other sugars is an important risk factor in human diabetes.

Several recent clinical studies show that diabetes in obese persons can often be completely reversed with mitigation of obesity. These include observations of Davidson (1977), of Savage, et al (1977), of Groothof, et al (1975) and of Kempner, et al (1975).

Summary and Conclusions on Nutritional Factors

Obesity is the most important nutritional factor in the etiology of diabetes. In societies where obesity is rare, other factors account for most cases of diabetes. But in most of the affluent world, including Europe and North America, obesity is the most important environmental risk factor for diabetes. Indeed, there is some evidence that its importance equals or exceeds the strong influence of diabetes-related genetic factors. More data are needed, but it appears that a majority of grossly obese persons develop diabetes if obesity persists for more than thirty years. It is quite possible that much of the famililiy of diabetes is the result of familiality of obesity. This familial aggregation of obesity has both environmental and genetic determinants. There is a strong association of degree of adiposity and risk of diabetes. Very lean persons seem to have a lower risk of adult-onset diabetes than persons of standard weight for height. In comparison to persons of standard weight, moderately obese subjects have diabetes about four times more frequently, while risk is increased about tenfold in grossly obese persons. Epidemiologic evidence to this effect receives strong support from laboratory investigations in animals and man. Most of the marked differences in rates of adult-onset diabetes observed among populations and intrapopulation subgroups have been attributable to differences in adiposity, including differences among races and between sexes. It is not yet clear to what extent obesity is the result of indolence or of excessive consumption of calories. Both factors appear to be important.

Qualitative dietary factors conceivably may induce diabetes either directly or by enhancing susceptibility to obesity. But for the most part, epidemiologic data are inconslusive with respect to specific dietary elements as causal agents in diabetes. The factor most widely suspected is sucrose. Both positive and negative epidemiologic evidence has been reported. Many diabetologists believe that overconsumption of sucrose may be a significant factor in the susceptibility to diabetes, and many have a contrary view. On the whole, the negative evidence is more impressive in this respect than the positive, but more evidence is needed. The question should remain open for the present. Several intrapopulation studies have failed to show a relationship between sugar consumption and fatness. It has also been suggested that other concentrated, quickly absorbed, "refined" carbohydrates might increase risk of diabetes. Present evidence is inconclusive. Another possibility is that removal of dietary fiber enhances risk of diabetes and obesity, but no decisive epidemiologic evidence is available in support of that hypothesis.

There are few modern adherents to the notion that dietary fat is diabetogenic, but it is conceivable that risk of obesity is increased when attractive sources of dietary fat are widely available. In animals, diabetes has been produced by diets high in fat, by high-sugar diets, and by diets high in protein or starch. But in animals high-fat diets have been more frequently effective in inducing diabetes than those high in the other major nutrients. Epidemiologic evidence in support of fat or protein as directly diabetogenic agents is unimpressive. It is possible that concentration of calories in foods consumed is of some importance but there is evidence against, as well as for, this possibility. High rates of diabetes have been observed in populations on high-sugar, high-protein, high-fat, and high-starch diets. High rates of diabetes have not been observed in any lean population. These considerations suggest that qualitative features of diet are not critical, while caloric intake in relation to energy expenditure is very important.

Excessive consumption of iron sometimes causes diabetes by inducing hemosiderosis or hemochromatosis. Consumption of alcohol sometimes causes diabetes indirectly by inducing pancreatitis. Youth-onset diabetes associated with fibrosis and calcification of the pancreas (Chapter 8) is closely associated with consumption of cassava. This dietary factor may induce diabetes either by pancreatic toxicity or by protein deprivation, or both. In animals, severe deficiency of chromium may impair glucose tolerance. Evidence from clinical and epidemiologic studies in man does not yet answer the question of whether chromium deficiency is a significant cause of diabetes in man.

The possible roles of nutritional factors in typical juvenile-type diabetes are discussed in Chapter 8. Below is a list of nutritional factors that have been considered to have possible etiologic significance in diabetes.

1. *Generally acknowledged:* excessive calories (obesity); excessive alcohol consumption (pancreatitis); excessive iron consumption (hemo-chromatosis);

2. *Widely suspected as etiologic or contributing factors:* deficiency of potassium (as during diuretic therapy); protein deficiency (eg, deficiency of sulfur-containing amino acids as a cause of fibrosis of pancreas);

3. *Other possibilities being considered:* sugar consumption; fat consumption; low carbohydrate consumption; low levels of dietary fiber; deficiencies of chromium, zinc, iron, and pyridoxine; infrequent feeding ("gorging" rather than nibbling); cassava consumption; low dietary fiber.

SOCIAL AND ECONOMIC STATUS

There is a considerable amount of information on this subject in the 11th edition of Joslin's book (1971), particularly in chapters of Marks and Krall (1971) and of Entmacher and Marks (1971).

Ancient Hindu physicians described diabetes as a disease of the rich (Christie, 1811). Nineteenth-century physicians of Europe also recognized the association between affluence and diabetes that prevailed at that time. Von Noorden was quoted later by Lemann (1921) to the effect that " . . . wealth and culture increase liability tenfold". It has been widely told that Disraeli considered the appearance of diabetes in the early history of the Jews as a mark of their precocious cultural attainment. In 1893 Sen reported that death rates from diabetes in Calcutta were about 20 times higher in Hindus than in Moslems!

The many editions of Joslin's book beginning in 1916 are rich in information concerning socioeconomic status and diabetes. Joslin's interpretation of these associations was that they were mainly incidental to the relationship between socioeconomic status and fatness, a view that receives considerable support from modern evidence. Lambert reported in 1908 that diabetes was not rare in affluent Chinese even though it was exceedingly rare in poor classes. In one such group of Nanking, only one of 24,000 patients had known diabetes! In 1914, the special correspondent from India reported to the *British Medical Journal* that diabetes was rife in the educated class of Madras.

In 1919 Delangen observed that in Batavia, Java diabetes was a disease of the idle rich. Emerson and Larimore published a good review in 1924 of relationships that had been observed between social status and risk of diabetes. Among American enlisted men in World War I, rates of diabetes, expressed as number per thousand per annum, were 0.16 for whites, 0.13 for blacks, 0.18 for Hawaiians, 0.05 for Filipinos, and 0.08 for Puerto Ricans. The rate was considerably higher in officers, but they were older.

The British have collected over the years some interesting data on these social variables. Collins (1927) summarized some age-adjusted data from England and Wales for 1910–1912. Diabetes mortality rates in unskilled workers were only 44% as great as in professional and salaried workers. A table summarizing data for 1930–1932 from England and Wales was presented in a more recent publication of Harris and McArthur (1951). In men, rates of diabetes mortality were about 2.5 times higher in the "upper classes" than in the "lower classes". In females there was little relationship between social class and diabetes mortality rates. Data collected subsequently (to be described below) suggest that to some extent these differences were attributable to differences between the sexes in the relationships of social class to fatness. In general, poor Englishmen are very lean, while poor English women are fatter than poor men. Himsworth (1935-1936) cited diabetes mortality data by class for England and Wales. There was little difference by class for adults less than 55 years of age, but in persons 55 to 64 from the highest of five classes, diabetes was three times more common than in the lowest of five classes (data for 1921-1923).

Emerson and Larimore (1924) showed that in the United States diabetes mortality rates for 1919 were higher in high-income states and lower in low-income states.

Even in the modern world, rich people living in poor countries usually have much more diabetes than the poor of those countries. In Haiti, for example, the well-off have more than ten times as much diabetes as the poor (Charles and Medard, 1969). One problem in interpreting data on diabetes rates in rich and poor is that occult diabetes in most circumstances is more likely to be discovered in the rich because they are tested more frequently. Under some conditions, however, it has been possible to compare rates while controlling this variable. We determined rates by class in Central America under conditions where all subjects had tests of glucose tolerance (West and Kalbfleisch, 1970). In those with moderate income and relatively privileged social status, diabetes was about four times more common than in the poor. This may have been attributable entirely to the leanness of the poor. In a Bombay survey (K. E. M. Hospital Group, 1966), diabetes was four to six times as common in the upper-income group as in the poor. On the other hand, extreme poverty may in some circumstances increase risk of diabetes secondary to fibrosis and calcification of the pancreas, as indicated in Chapter 8.

Among ten countries, we found a close relationship of prosperity and diabetes, up to annual income levels of about $800 per person (West and Kalbfleisch, 1970). In more affluent societies the relationship of risk of diabetes and economic status becomes inconsistent. Diabetes mortality rates are, for example, about five times higher in Belgium than in Norway despite roughly comparable levels of socioeconomic status (WHO, 1974). Indeed, in many circumstances, poorer people have higher rates of diabetes. In Africa, rich generally have more diabetes than poor; in Capetown, however, the situation is reversed in some areas. In certain groups of Indians, for example, Jackson (1972) found the poor had more diabetes than the more affluent. In Capetown whites rates of diabetes were similar in the different classes. In Capetown Indians rates were similar in poor and upper-class Indians. In contrast, diabetes was about 20 times more common in the rich Tamils of Pondicherry, India, than in the poor of that community (Datta, 1966). In a Hyderabad survey of Rao, et al (1966), rates of diabetes were 2.4% in poor and 7.2% in rich. Pell and D'Alonzo (1968) found little relationship between income level and rates of diabetes in American employees of the Dupont Company. The rate of diabetes was, however, somewhat lower at the very highest salary level.

Data of the Metropolitan Insurance Company on diabetes-related mortality show that rates are somewhat higher in men of lower income than in those of greater income. In women, these differences are great; those with lower income have very high rates of diabetes. In females from 55 to 64 years of age mortality rates were 13.8 for a group from the middle and upper levels of income and 33.3 in women with lesser incomes. There is now a considerable amount of evidence that these findings reflect the corpulence of poor women now prevailing in many segments of US society (West, 1973).

Kitagawa and Hauser (1968) studied the relationship in the United States population between educational attainment and death rates from diabetes. In men there was little relationship between these two variables, but in women rates of diabetes were 3.5 times higher in the least educated as compared to the most educated. In 1973 an interview survey was conducted on a representative sample of the United States population by the National Center for Health Statistics. Among persons with a family income exceeding $10,000 per year, the rate of known diabetes was 1.37%; in persons with family income of less than $5,000 it was three times as high (4.02)! This is probably because poor

American women are now considerably fatter than women who are not poor. In persons 45 to 64, rates of diabetes were also related inversely to level of education of the head of the household. When this education was less than nine years, 7.7% had diabetes, while only 3.1% had diabetes when education of the head of household had exceeded twelve years.

In a survey of 1971-1972, the National Center for Health Statistics found that in persons 20 to 44 years of age, the rate of obesity in those above the poverty level was 17.0% for white men and 18.6% for white women; 11.3% for black men and 25.0% for black women. For those below the poverty level the rate of obesity in this age group was 9.3% for white men, 25.1% for white women; 10.9% for black men and 35.0% for black women. These results are consistent with the possibility that the US poor now have more diabetes because poor women have become very fat.

Urban-Rural Status

Emerson and Larimore (1924) indicated that in Prussia diabetes was apparently about three times as high in the urban population as in the rural. It is possible that some of this difference was the result of more frequent testing in the cities. In American draftees of World War I there was little difference in rates of diabetes in those from rural and urban areas, but rates were twice as high in draftees from New York City as in those from elsewhere. (Emerson and Larimore, 1924). Silwer (1958) reviewed observations in Europe on urban-rural status and prevalence of diabetes. In his study in Kristianstad, Sweden, little difference was observed with respect to this variable. He cited several other studies showing higher prevalence in urban areas, but pointed to the difficulties in determining whether these differences were real or only apparent. Horstman (1950) thought that the rural paucity was real in Denmark. Interestingly, he found that on the Island of Fyen diabetes was apparently more common in smaller towns than in the largest city (Odense).

Occupation

Bouchardat (1875) concluded that at least 1 in 20 of distinguished Frenchmen was glycosuric in the fifth and sixth decade of life. He mentioned particularly members of learned societies, legislators, successful businessmen, and high-ranking army officers.

The participants in the 1907 Symposium on Diabetes in the Tropics (Havelock Charles, et al) mentioned repeatedly the association of diabetes with social, economic, occupational, and educational status. Diabetes was thought to be rare in Nepal, although common in high officials. In Bengal difference by caste and religion were cited. Chunder Bose observed that: "What gout is to the nobility of England, diabetes is to the aristocracy of India". Some of the symposium participants thought that diabetes might be precipitated by mental work. Mitra had considered this possibility in 1903. Even in those days, however, some observers including Joslin thought that the association of

277

mental work and diabetes was not that of cause and effect. Joslin, et al (1935) cited evidence that diabetes was uncommon in farm laborers and miners. They also found a general association by regions of the United States between income and diabetes rates.

A report of Bertillon from France in 1912 includes the following passages:

> Diabetes is very common among the following occupational groups:
>
> 1. In the learned professions, especially among lawyers and doctors. Pharmacists and clergymen have lower, though high rates. Lastly, teachers, architects and musicians have average rates.
> 2. Occupations exposed to alcoholism: Innkeepers, brewers, and maltsters.
> 3. Butchers.
> 4. Certain other professions (dyers, commercial travelers, commercial clerks, railway clerks).
>
> "On the other hand, diabetes is very uncommon in the following occupational groups:
>
> 1. Coachmen and drivers, nonwithstanding they are proverbial drunkards.
> 2. Hand laborers of all kinds, such as dock laborers, porters, general laborers, although drunkenness is very common among them.
> 3. Railway workmen (workers on the road bed, guards, porters), but railway clerks and also engineers and firemen rise to or above the average.
> 4. Persons engaged in agriculture (except farm tenants, who are less favored than domestic servants on the farm), gardeners and farm laborers.
> 5. Several other manual occupations carried on in the open air (masons, shipbuilders).
> 6. Miners and quarrymen (except lead miners).
>
> We find only average or insignificant figures in the metal working and textile industries, sedentary occupations and those pursued on the water".

In 1912 Hoogslag, a Dutchman, observed that:

> Captains of passenger steamers are peculiarly predisposed, as they have to preside at meals and get little exercise. Lipogenous diabetes is found in the rich and poor alike, in children and especially in brain workers and in those with much responsibility.

At a Boston station, Blotner and Hyde (1943) studied rates of diabetes in World War II inductees. There was little difference between those who did heavy and light work. It should be kept in mind that these conscripts were young.

Emerson and Larimore (1924) also did an interesting analysis of diabetes mortality rate by occupation in New York City. In interpreting the latter data two points are to be kept in mind: the number of persons at risk was estimated only crudely, and results of this kind are profoundly affected by age distribution. In 1920, for example, diabetes death rates in New York City were 5.8 per 100,000 population for persons 20 to 44 years of age, and 81.7 in those over 44.

Even so, some of the occupation-related data are impressive. Rates were very low in chauffeurs (10 per 100,000) and tremendously high (180) in bartenders. I am sorry to report that the quite extraordinary rate in bartenders was almost matched by the rate in clergymen (120)!

In 1930 the US Bureau of Labor issued a report on causes of mortality and occupational status based on experience of the Metropolitan Insurance Company. Numbers were rather small for some of the occupations but the results were interesting, particularly because they were well documented with respect to age distribution. In general, those in sedentary occupations, such as merchants and storekeepers, had rates well above the standard, while those in occupations requiring hard labor had rates well below the standard. Iron foundry workers had a rate only 27% of standard, while merchants and storekeepers had a rate that was 203% of standard. It seems probable, however, that testing for diabetes was more common in the more affluent element who generally pursued occupations that were physically less demanding.

Dutt (1927) commented on the extreme rarity of diabetes in manual laborers of Bengal. He estimated that he saw about 10,000 diabetics per year. He could recall seeing only one diabetic laborer during a five-year period.

Marks and Krall (1971) have reviewed some of the modern data on the relationship of diabetes mortality rates to occupational status. Among their resources were results from the US National Center on Health Statistics. The differences among occupations were modest for the most part. Lowest rates were in carpenters (61% of standard) and highest in cooks (225% of standard). They also summarized data by class and occupation from Britain for a more recent period (1949-1953). These differences by class have become much smaller than heretofore. Interestingly, mineworkers had the lowest rate (67% of standard) and their wives had the highest (205% of standard). In general, rates were higher in men of higher class; the reverse was true in women. These and all the other data above on rates of diabetes by occupational status should be interpreted in the light of the fact that diabetes rates are affected profoundly by age and that few of the presently available data have been corrected completely for age. Tsuji, et al (1966), for example, found that occult diabetes was about half as common in farmers as in a group of business employees, teachers, and public officials; and that diabetes in the latter group was about 14 times as frequent as in fabric workers. These data are interesting but difficult to evaluate without information on other characteristics, especially age.

Wadsworth and Jarrett (1974) found youth-onset diabetes somewhat less common in offspring of manual workers, but they pointed out that rates of ascertainment might have been lower in these families of relatively low income. Johnson, et al (1956) measured exercise levels, relative weight, and caloric intake for each of several occupations. It seems quite likely that differences in exercise explain at least some of the differences in rates of diabetes in occupational groups. Christau, et al (1977) observed that childhood-onset diabetes, was less common in affluent sections of Copenhagen than in the less privileged areas.

279

Marital Status

Marks and Krall (1971) presented age-adjusted data of the National Center for Health Statistics on marital status and diabetes mortality in whites. In men age 15 and over, rates were 20.0 in single men, 13.5 in married men, 21.9 in widowed, and 26.6 in divorced men. In women, rates were 12.9 for the single, 17.7 for the married, 22.2 for the widowed, and 15.8 for the divorced. Some other data on diabetes and marital status have been cited above in the section on parity as a risk factor.

MENTAL STRESS AND NERVOUS SYSTEM DYSFUNCTION

No generally recognized definition exists for the term *stress*. This makes even more difficult evaluations of the possible significance of psychologic or mental stress as an etiologic factor in diabetes.

Allen, et al (1919) cite a report by Trincavella (1476-1568), a Venetian, of a case of diabetes attributed to persecution and grief. Thomas Willis observed in the 17th century that prolonged sorrow could cause diabetes. In his review of 1868, Brigham mentioned reports of Rayer of onset of diabetes after a fit of anger, and of Landowzy concerning diabetes following violent grief. Brigham also mentioned reports of onset of diabetes after hemiplegia, apoplexy, and epileptic convulsions. Claude Bernard had demonstrated in 1859 that lesions in certain parts of the brain produced hyperglycemia. In 1911 Cannon described "emotional glycosuria", attributing it to the increased release of epinephrine. In 1952 Hinkle and Wolf demonstrated some impressive physiologic and biochemical effects of life stress in diabetic patients (eg, ketonemia). Since central nervous system signals play a role in the control of insulin secretion, it is conceivable that subtle aberrations of brain or autonomic function might cause diabetes. Another possibility considered is that long-standing occult elevations of catecholamine secretion might induce diabetes by mechanisms similar to those that prevail when pheochromocytomas induce diabetes.

It does not seem likely, however, that central nervous system lesions are of substantial importance in producing permanent diabetes. Joslin reported in 1921 that during World War I, despite stress of maximum degree, glycosuria was observed in only 2 of 40,000 American soldiers in a hospital center in France. The profound anxieties of civilian populations in Nazi-occupied territories during World War II were attended by substantial *declines* in the incidence of diabetes. Hyperglycemia following subarachnoid hemorrhage is quite common but seldom persistent (Hallpike, et al, 1971).

In a detailed review Treuting (1962) cited many reports linking onset of diabetes to emotional trauma, but pointed out the difficulties in interpreting these temporal associations. He concluded that the available evidence was not decisive with respect to the etiologic importance of emotional factors. This issue has also been reviewed by Marks, et al (1971) and Kravitz, et al (1971), whose conclusions were similar to those of Treuting. Several studies have shown that under certain conditions stress may lower the blood glucose.

Simonds (1977) found little difference between diabetic and nondiabetic children with respect to their psychiatric status. Although the personality traits and psychologic status of selected groups of diabetics have been studied, no data are available in representative samples of diabetics and nondiabetics from a population. Stein and Charles (1971) studied the family background of groups of adolescent diabetics and another group of adolescents. There was a significantly higher incidence of loss and family disturbance in the families of the diabetic children. It is not known whether the findings in these families were representative of those in the entire universe of families of adolescent diabetics in this population, nor whether the results in the control group were representative. As indicated in the review of Treuting (1962), evidence is quite conflicting concerning the psychologic status of juvenile diabetes. The same conflict has persisted in more recent studies (Kravitz, et al, 1971).

Hoffer and Osmond (1960) have cited evidence that rates of diabetes are unusually low in schizophrenia. This may be attributable, at least in part, to weight loss that commonly occurs late in the course of schizophrenia.

OTHER FACTORS ASSOCIATED WITH EXCESSIVE RATES OF DIABETES

Some have thought that the incidence of diabetes was increased after trauma. This subject has been reviewed by Marks, et al (1971) with generally negative conclusions.

Reports on the relationship of diabetes and gout have been quite conflicting. Some, but not all, investigators have found high rates of gout in diabetics, or higher rates of diabetes in those with gout. To some extent this relationship can be explained by the increased rates of both gout and diabetes when obesity is present. In Israel Herman, et al (1976) found serum uric acid levels slightly lower in diabetics than controls, but uric acid values were slightly higher in "prediabetics" than controls. These "prediabetics" had had normal screening tests for diabetes, but were later found to be diabetic in the course of longitudinal studies. The greater fatness of these subjects did not entirely explain their higher uric acid levels. A good detailed review on gout, hyperuricemia, and diabetes has been published by Podolsky (1971). These relationships deserve further investigation, but present evidence does not suggest that diabetes is caused by hyperuricemia or gout.

It has long been known that Dupuytren's contracture is common in diabetics (Podolsky, 1971). The significance of this association is unknown. Past studies have not been well designed to elucidate the strength or significance of this relationship.

There have been reports of excessive rates of diabetes in patients with cancer of the uterus. But in the study of Kessler (1970), where numbers and controls were in general more satisfactory, there was no increase in risk of death from uterine cancer in diabetics. For obvious reasons, diabetes is especially common in patients with cancer of the pancreas. Binazzi, et al (1975) demonstrated a high frequency of abnormal glucose tolerance in patients with psoriasis, but an excess of clinical diabetes was not shown in this study.

Taste blindness has been quite common in certain groups of diabetics (Terry, 1950). Terry found, for example, that taste blindness was present in 22 of 99 diabetics (19%) and in 49 of 632 (8%) of those with no apparent diabetes. The significance of this association is unknown. It may be the result of diabetic neuropathy.

Walsh, et al (1975) reported on eight patients (all females) with diabetes and hyperparathyroidism. They pointed out that diabetes had not seemed to be unusually common in other groups of patients with hyperparathyroidism, and suggested a need for further investigations of the strength and significance of this association. In the section on juvenile diabetes in Chapter 8, associations are described between diabetes and certain conditions linked with autoimmunity. These include pernicious anemia, adrenal and parathyroid atrophy, and Hashimoto's disease of the thyroid gland. In all of these conditions rates of diabetes appear to be excessive, probably because the autoimmunity is frequently multiglandular, and sometimes includes the beta cells.

Many studies have reported a strong association between cholelithiasis and diabetes. For example, cholelithiasis has usually been found more commonly at autopsy in diabetics than in nondiabetics. This literature has been reviewed by Jenson (1971) and by Goldstein and Schein (1963). Cholelithiasis and diabetes are both common in pancreatitis. Epidemiologic data on the association of diabetes and gallbladder disease are few. Although it is possible that gallbladder disease causes diabetes or the reverse, it seems more likely that the association is mainly the result of factors such as obesity that increase risk of both these disorders. Epidemiologic data could elucidate the strength and character of this relationship.

The association between diabetes and tuberculosis is very strong. In some societies tuberculosis is still a leading cause of death in diabetics. Among the few epidemiologic studies of this association was that of Oscarsson and Silwer (1958) in Kristianstad, Sweden. They also included in their publication an excellent review of the literature, beginning with observations of Avicenna (980-1027). In the 19th century tuberculosis was typically found to be present in about one quarter of known diabetics, and in some European series as many as one-third had tuberculosis. In more recent times rates of tuberculosis have typically been about two to three times higher in diabetics than in the general population. The study of Oscarsson and Silwer was of particular interest because of the rarity of data on diabetes and tuberculosis in a general population. They found tuberculosis rates to be about two to five times higher in diabetics than in general population, the degree of excess varying by age group. In general, excesses were greater in younger age groups. Risk of tuberculosis was higher in patients with severe diabetes and with diabetes of long duration.

Not surprisingly, rates of diabetes have usually been found to be excessive in groups of patients with tuberculosis. Even though rates of tuberculosis are still excessive in diabetes, tuberculosis is no longer a major cause of morbidity and mortality in diabetics of the advanced countries. In their excellent review on tuberculosis and diabetes, Younger and Hadley (1971) pointed out that in recent years the prevalence of tuberculosis in Joslin Clinic patients was only 0.1%, and death from tuberculosis had become rare. However, tuberculosis when present still tends to be more advanced in diabetics. The mechanisms for the increased susceptibility of diabetics to tuberculosis are not known. One suggestion has been that tissue glycerol levels are higher in diabetics. It does appear that the association between diabetes and tuberculosis is mainly the result of the increased susceptibility of diabetics to tuberculosis rather than the reverse.

Bisalbuminemia appears to be less rare in diabetics than in nondiabetics (Vladutiu, 1976).

FACTORS ASSOCIATED NEGATIVELY WITH DIABETES

Some important protective factors have been discussed above (eg, leanness and physical activity).

Some have thought that cancer was less common in diabetics than the general population (Rostlapil, 1974). But previous comparisons are difficult to evaluate because of problems in appropriately matching data from diabetic and nondiabetic groups. Among the more satisfactory data were those of Kessler (1970) in the Joslin Clinic patients. From mortality data there was no evidence of a generally protective influence of diabetes against cancer nor of the reverse relationship. On the other hand, death rates from cancer of the lung were impressively low in diabetics. This deserves further study. Among the possible explanations suggested by Kessler was that the percentage of Jews (in whom lung cancer is uncommon) was much higher in this group of diabetics than in the control group. He also pointed out that the diabetics might have smoked less. In British diabetics, there was a paucity of lung cancer and emphysema (Armstrong, et al, 1976).

Peptic ulcer appears to be uncommon in diabetics. In the study of Pell and D'Alonzo (1968) nondiabetics had duodenal ulcer twice as frequently as a well-matched group of diabetics. No significant paucity of gastric ulcer disease was found in the diabetics. Jenson (1971) has reviewed additional evidence indicating a protective effect from peptic ulcer of diabetes. In general, gastric acid secretion is less in diabetics, a factor that may account for the lower risk of peptic ulcer. Peptic ulcer is particularly uncommon in American Indians of Arizona in whom diabetes is rife (Sievers, 1973), but this relative immunity to ulcer disease was probably present before the recent epidemic of diabetes, and may not be secondary to the diabetes. On the other hand, Buckley (1967) has cited evidence suggesting that hyperglycemia itself may have a protective effect against peptic ulcer. Westlund (1969) examined the association of peptic ulcer and diabetes in his study in Norway of death certificates. No significant relationship was evident.

Hoffer and Osmond (1960) reviewed some reports suggesting low rates of diabetes in schizophrenics. They noted that in schizophrenics of New York mental hospitals the death rate from diabetes between 1930 and 1939 was only 11.9 per 100,000, while it was 89.8 in general hospitals. Data of this kind are difficult to interpret, but several other observers have commented on the apparent paucity of diabetic schizophrenics. This deserves further study. Late in the course of schizophrenia weight loss is common, which would tend to prevent diabetes. It is also conceivable that the same metabolic aberration that leads to schizophrenia could protect against diabetes.

7A
APPENDIX

SUMMARY OF REPORTS OF HIGH
AND LOW RATES OF DIABETES

Low Rates

19th-century sugarcane cutters of West Indies (Brigham, 1868)

Poor of London and Berlin before 1900 (Lemman, 1911)

Eskimo (Heinbecker, 1928; Scott and Griffith, 1957; Schaefer, 1968; Mouratoff, et al, 1967)

North American Indians before 1940 and in some present tribes (West, 1974)

Many other populations prior to 1920 (see text)

Jewish Yemenites and Kurds (Cohen, 1961)

Primitive Micronesians, Melanesians and Polynesians (Tulloch, 1962; West, 1974)

Algeria (Lebon, et al, 1953)

Morocco (Bacque, 1964)

Rural blacks of South, East, West, and Central Africa (Tulloch, 1962,1964); (text cites many specific populations)

High Rates

Many tribes of American Indians (West, 1974; Cohen, 1954)

Rich Indian men of Bengal (Cheevers, 1886)

Many populations of immigrants from India (Cosnett, 1957, and many others); see text on Indians of South Africa, East Africa, Figi, Saigon, Singapore, etc

Malta (Saundby, 1909; Lepine, 1909; WHO, 1964; Maempel, 1965)

Uruguayans of Montevideo (West and Kalbfleisch, 1970)

Many groups of Polynesians and Micronesians (Sloan, 1964; Prior, 1962; West, 1974; Zimmet, et al, 1976)

US black women (see text)

Malays of Capetown (Marine, et al, 1969)

Many groups of Jews (Joslin, 1923, including Sephardic Jews of Rhodesia (Krikler, 1969)

Low Rates (Continued)

Poor whites, blacks, and Indians of Central America (West and Kalbfleisch, 1970)

Blacks of rural US prior to 1924 (Williamson, 1909; Emerson and Larimore, 1924)

British Honduras (Williamson, 1909)

Bahamas (Tulloch, 1962; Hoffman, 1922)

Grenada (Hoffman, 1922; Tulloch, 1962)

Haiti, Jamaica, British Guiana, and Cuba before 1922 (Hoffman, 1922)

Rural and poor of India (Sen, 1893; Patel and Talwalker, 1966)

Broayas of the Sahara (DeHertogh, et al, 1975)

Chinese and Malays of Singapore (Cheah, 1975)

Philippines (Concepcion, 1922; Entmacher and Marks, 1965)

Thailand (WHO, 1956,1974)

Burma (Entmacher and Marks, 1965)

Papua and New Guinea (Tulloch, 1962; C. H. Campbell, 1963)

Natives of rural Fiji (Williamson, 1909; Cassidy, 1967)

South Korea (Entmacher and Marks, 1965; Kim, 1970)

Viet Nam (Montel, 1924; Hai, et al, 1965)

East Pakistan (Bangladesh) (West and Kalbfleisch, 1966)

Japanese of hilly districts of Kii peninsula (Miyamura, et al, 1975)

Yemen (Cohen, 1961; Tulloch, 1962)

Jordan (WHO, 1962)

Affluent societies during war-related famines (Joslin, 1923; Goto, 1958; and others)

Tulloch (1962) also received reports that diabetes was uncommon in Surinam, Seychelles, St. Helena, Muscat, and Dominican Republic

High Rates (Continued)

Welsh (Ashley, 1967)

Luxenbourg, Belgium, and Holland (WHO, 1964)

Urbanized Australian Aborigines (Wise, 1970)

Mabuiag Islanders of Torres Straits (Collins, 1968)

Chinese-American men (Entmacher and Marks, 1965)

Japanese of town in Kii peninsula (Miyamura, et al, 1975)

High frequency "legendary" in certain special groups, including Sumo-wrestlers of Japan (Kuzuya, et al, 1975) and Royal families of Polynesia and Melanesia

7B

MALE-TO-FEMALE SEX RATIOS IN ADULT-ONSET DIABETES

SOME POPULATIONS WITH HIGH MALE:FEMALE RATIOS

Most populations in the 19th century (Joslin, 1923; see also text)

Most rural African black communities; ratios of 2:1 have been typical (Tulloch, 1962,1966) but ratios are now reversed in some modern urbanized groups

Africans of Malawi, 4:1 (Goodall and Pilbeam, 1964)

Ethiopians, 2:1 (Belcher, 1970)

Kenya, 2:1 (Steel, 1974)

Nigeria, variable ratios; as high as 2:1 in some groups (Osuntokun, 1971)

Uganda, variable ratios; Otim (1975) reported 1.5:1 in a group of clinic patients

Ceylon, 2:1 prior to 1951 (DeZoysa) but this ratio has recently declined to unity (Weerasinghe, 1967)

Trinidad, 3.8:1 in young adult blacks (Poon-King, et al, 1968)

SOME POPULATIONS WITH LOW MALE:FEMALE RATIOS

US blacks, see text; ratios of 1:3 are typical

Haitian poor (blacks), 1:4.7 (Charles and Medard, 1969)

Barbados (blacks), about 1:2 (WHO, 1964)

Ghana (blacks), variable ratios; in one group of older diabetics Dodu (1959) found ratio of 1:2

Trinidad (blacks), 1:2 (Poon-King, et al, 1968)

Libyans, about 1:4 (Mekkawi, 1972)

Sweden, variable ratios; Larsson (1967) found 1:2

Malta, about 1:2 (WHO, 1964)

Belgium, Holland, Luxembourg, about 1:1.8 (WHO, 1964)

UK, variable (see text); WHO (1964) data on mortality for 1959-1961 showed ratio of about 1:2 for Scotland and for England-Wales

SOME POPULATIONS WITH HIGH MALE:FEMALE RATIOS (Continued)

Hong Kong, variable ratios (see text); death certificate data suggested strong male dominance (2.65:1)

Iraq, 2:1 (WHO, 1964)

Yemen, 3:1 (Tulloch, 1961)

Jordan, 2:1 (WHO, 1964)

Japan, variable ratios (see text); some studies report male preponderance as great as 2:1

Okinawa, about 4:1 (Sakumoto, et al, 1970)

Korea, variable ratios (see text); some studies (Kim, 1970, 1973) show rates as high as 3:1

Indians and Pakistanis, highly variable by circumstance (see text); in some clinic populations of Indian subcontinent ratios exceeding 4:1 have been observed. Most screening surveys reveal little difference between sexes. In immigrant Indians of South Africa, Trinidad, Fiji, East Africa, ratios are highly variable but male predominance has been observed in some circumstances. In Malawi it was 2:1 in clinical cases of Goodall (1964)

SOME POPULATIONS WITH LOW MALE: FEMALE RATIOS (Continued)

Europe; WHO report of 1964 by country on death certificates for 1959-1961 showed consistent trend of female predominance; ratios averaged about 1:1.6

USSR, about 1:2 in Ulan-Ude (Zybina, 1975) Central America, about 1:2 (West, 1970; WHO, 1964)

Capetown Indians, variable, but Jackson, et al (1970) reported a ratio of 1:1.8 in one group

Cuba, about 1:1.5 (Mateo de Acosta, et al, 1973)

US Indians, ratios of 1:1.5 are typical (West, 1974)

US Whites, variable ratios; in Massachusetts one study showed 1:2 (Joslin, 1933). In national survey of 1964-1965 it was 1:1.3 (MacDonald, 1967). In some communities there has been slight predominance of males. In Massachusetts Jews there was female predominance of 2:1 (Rudy and Keeler, 1939)

Hanuaba, New Guinea, 1:3 (Price & Tulloch, 1966)

Thailand, about 1:2.5 (Vannasaeng, et al, 1976)

Urbanized aborigines of Australia, 1:2 (Wise, et al, 1970)

Polynesians, variable ratios; a decided female predominance in some groups (Prior, 1971)

Micronesians, variable ratios; striking female predominance in some groups (Reed, et al, 1973)

A slight female predominance prevailed in whites of New Zealand, Australia, and South Africa

8
CHAPTER

Special Types of Diabetes

TYPICAL JUVENILE-ONSET DIABETES

Childhood-onset diabetes received attention in several previous chapters, and its morbid effects on the vascular and nervous systems are discussed in Chapter 10. This section will review the etiology, prevalence, and incidence of this most typical type of youth-onset diabetes.

Most cases of juvenile-onset diabetes are severe. In the earliest stages these children often have some endogenous insulin that mitigates the typical clinical expressions of severity, but after the disease is established, beta-cell decompensation is usually complete or virtually complete (White, 1965). The complete absence of endogenous insulin leads to ketonemia and severe hyperglycemia. Insulin therapy is then required to prevent severe symptoms and profound biochemical aberrations. Because typical juvenile-onset diabetes is relatively uncommon in all societies, epidemiologic data have been few and difficult to gather. Of historical interest are the pioneer papers of Wilcox (1908) and Morse (1913), who reviewed evidence available up to that time on juvenile diabetes. They pointed to the very considerable contributions in the latter part of the 19th century by Kulz in Germany. Among the best general sources of information on juvenile diabetes are the Joslin text (Marble, et al, 1971), the book of Sussman (1971), and the volume edited by Laron and Karp (1972).

This type of diabetes has a strong genetic background. Data in identical twins suggest that in Western societies about half of unaffected identical twins eventually develop insulin-dependent diabetes if their twin has typical juvenile diabetes (Tattersall and Pyke, 1972). It is often mistakenly assumed that this conclusive evidence of an underlying genetic basis precludes an environmental influence in cases in whom the genetic diathesis exists, but this is not necessarily the case. Consider, for example, the very specific genetic defect that induces hemolysis secondary to a deficiency of glucose-6-phosphate dehydrogenase. If an identical twin exhibits hemolysis of this kind, his identical twin would invariably exhibit hemolysis provided that environmental factors were also identical. But removing fava beans from the diet (or discontinuing an offending medication) would prevent completely the clinical manifestations or completely reverse them. Because of these considerations one could easily make the mistake of assuming that this hemolytic disorder was either "100% genetic" in etiology or that it was "100% environmental," depending upon one's frame of reference.

In juvenile diabetes it will be appropriate to look for environmental factors that may alone or together produce diabetes in individuals with no genetic defects relating specifically to diabetes. On the other hand, it is possible, even likely, that youth-onset diabetes secondary to specific genetic defects is also susceptible to environmental influences. In hamsters with a genetic diathesis for diabetes, diet modification has, for example, delayed onset and prevented ketosis-prone diabetes (Gerritsen, et al, 1974). In Israel (Cohen, 1970) juvenile diabetes has apparently increased considerably during a period when marked changes were occurring in diet and other environmental circumstances. It will therefore be appropriate to study systematically the effect of environmental factors.

Most children with typical youth-onset diabetes have demonstrable islet-cell antibodies at the time of diagnosis (Irvine, 1977). Such antibodies are much less frequently demonstrable at the time of diagnosis in adult-onset insulin-dependent diabetes.

Diagnostic methods and criteria in children have been discussed in Chapter 5 on diagnostic methods.

Prevalence and Interpopulation Comparisons

Rates of prevalence for juvenile-onset diabetes are difficult to determine. Because the disorder is infrequent, large population samples are required, and it is difficult to obtain a representative sample when numbers so large are needed. Table 31 summarizes information on approximate rates of prevalence in most of the populations where estimates have been made. Methods of ascertainment are not precisely comparable in these populations. For this reason differences of moderate degree are not necessarily significant. Rates of juvenile diabetes are not so much affected as maturity-onset rates by interpopulation differences in frequency and types of testing. But occult juvenile diabetes is not so rare as was once supposed. In Dayton, Ohio, Sharkey, et al (1950) performed urine tests after a carbohydrate-rich meal in 38,528 schoolchildren.

He found 18 new cases of diabetes (0.5 per 1,000). This figure is roughly one third of the rate of known diabetes for American schoolchildren, and it exceeds the rate of known cases in some populations.

In a 1973 questionnaire survey by household, of a representative sample of the US population, it was found that the rate of known diabetes in children less than 17 years of age was 1.3 per 1,000 (data of the National Center for Health Statistics cited by Bennett, et al, 1976). In children 6 to 16 years of age it was 1.7 per 1,000. These are probably the best data available on national prevalence, but circumstances of these estimates do not preclude a modest degree of error. In a similar sample of 1964-1965 the rate was 1.3 per 1,000 for persons under 25 years of age. This suggests the possibility that juvenile diabetes is becoming more common. But probably the increase was apparent only. The method of questioning for presence of diabetes was more detailed in 1973.

It would appear that juvenile diabetes is about equally common in the United States and Sweden (Silwer, 1958; Sterky, 1963). Rates were found to be somewhat lower in Britain, as shown in Table 31. But differences are modest and could be partly or even wholly attributable to differences in method of ascertainment or other factors such as frequency of testing.

Some of the best data on prevalance and incidence of diabetes, including juvenile diabetes, are those of Silwer, et al (1958) in Kristianstad, Sweden, and of Falconer, et al (1971) in Edinburgh. Both of these publications report comprehensive community surveys. Details are given below under incidence of juvenile diabetes. Prevalence of juvenile diabetes can be compared in three populations in which methods seemed to be comparable. In Berne, Switzerland, Teuscher, et al (1976) found the rate of diabetes to be 0.06% (184 in 310,000) in those under 20 years of age. In Edinburgh the rate for this age group was 0.15% (221 in 145,000). In Kristianstad the rate was 0.21% (181 in 88,000). Teuscher, et al (1976) found rates were five times higher in a mountainous district than in Berne. But these high rates were only slightly above those found in Kristianstad, Sweden by Silwer (1958) and by Gorwtiz, et al (1976) in Michigan.

It is possible that juvenile diabetes is now more common in Europe than prior to 1920 but evidence is inconclusive. Joslin noted in 1921 that in six series reported by European authorities the relative frequency of onset in the first decade of life averaged only 0.7% of all cases of diabetes. It is not clear, however, how much this rate was affected by local propensities in the referral of children with diabetes either to pediatricians or to internist diabetologists. None of the authorities cited by Joslin was a pediatrician. Another factor strongly affecting prevalence prior to the discovery of insulin was the very short life of most juvenile-onset cases. Available data do not permit a precise determination of prevalence trends over time in the United States. In New York City diabetes mortality rates in children rose only slightly between 1866 and 1920, during a time when diabetes mortality rates increased 16-fold for persons over 44 years of age (Emerson and Larimore, 1924). But mortality rates constitute a very imprecise measurement of the prevalence of juvenile diabetes for

291

TABLE 31　Prevalence of Youth-Onset Diabetes

Investigators and Year of Report	Population	Ages	Rate per 1,000	Method of Ascertainment
Nat'l Health Survey of 1935–1936 (Spiegelman and Marks, 1946)	US (representative sample)	0–15	0.38	Household interviews
Nat'l Center for Health Statistics (Bauer, et al, 1967)	US (representative sample)	0–24	1.3	Household interviews, 1964–1965
Nat'l Center for Health Statistics (1973)	US (representative sample)	0–16	1.3	Household interview method, 1973
Sultz, et al, (1968)	Erie County, NY	0–16	0.6	Count of known cases including records
Gorwitz, et al (1976)	Michigan schoolchildren	5–18	1.6	Questionnaire survey of school personnel
Kyllo (1978)	Minnesota	6–18	1.89	Known cases
Palumbo, et al (1976)	Rochester, Minn schoolchildren	5–18	1.0	Survey of clinical records
Guell R (1974)	Cuba	0–14	0.13	Registry
Falconer, et al (1971)	Edinburgh	0–9	0.13	Comprehensive survey for known cases
		10–19	0.93	Diagnosed cases
Beardmore and Reid (1966)	North Hamptonshire, England	5–16	0.8	Diagnosed cases
Wadsworth and Jarrett (1974)	Britain	11	0.1	Diagnosed cases in a cohort
		17	0.5	
		25	3.4	
National Child Development Study cited by Wadsworth (1974)	Britain	7	0.2	Questionnaire
		11	0.5	
Teuscher (1975)	Canton of Berne, Switzerland	0–19	0.59	Known cases plus urine screening
Schliack (1973), cited by Wadsworth (1974)	East Germany	0–9	0.2	Diagnosed cases
		10–19	0.8	
		20–29	1.6	
Lestradet	France	0–19	0.3	Registry (insulin-treated only)
Fromantin, et al (1971)	Vincennes, France	19–20 (men only)	1.2	History and urine screening in 98,770
Rostlapil, et al (1976)	Czechoslovakia	0–15	0.39	Registry

Investigators and Year of Report	Population	Ages	Rate per 1,000	Method of Ascertainment
Kruger (1965)	Schwerin, E. Germany	1–9	0.16	Urine screening in 102,219
Pinelli (1976)	Venice, Italy	0–13	0.26	
Silwer (1958)	Kristianstad, Sweden	0–4	0.1	Comprehensive survey for known cases
		5–9	1.3	
		10–19	1.7	
Holmgren, et al (1974)	Vasterbotten County, Sweden	0–15	2.2	Known cases
Sterky (1963)	Stockholm	7–14	1.44	Diagnosed cases
Christau, et al (1976)	Denmark	0–29	0.7	Registry
Koivisto, et al (1976)	Finland	0–19	0.22	
T. Cohen (1970)	Israel	2–16	0.16	Diagnosed cases
	Father born in Asia or Africa	2–16	0.09	
	Father born in Europe, "America", or Israel	2–16	0.24	
Hososake and Matsuyama (1966)	Kitayushu City, Japan	1–15	0.1	Urine screening of 44,144
Miki and Maruyama (1970)	Japan	0–15	0.025	Survey estimate of diagnosed cases
Mimura, et al (1975)	Kumamoto, Japan	6–15	0.115	Urine tests on 250,000
Proust and Smithurst (1968)	Australia	20 yr old males	3.7	Interview and screening registration for national service
	Canberra and Toowoomba	0–19	1.0	Screening survey
Sathe (1973)	India		Rare	
West (1974)	American Indians and Eskimos		Uncommon	
Tulloch (1962); Seftel (1964)	Primitive blacks of several areas and in Chinese Indians and Malays of Singapore		Rare	
Tsai (1971)	Taiwan		Rare	
Hai et al (1965)	Viet Nam		Rare	
Mekkawi and Aswad (1972)	Libya		Rare	
Wang (1937)	Chinese		Rare	
McFadzean and Young (1968)	Hong Kong Chinese		Rare	
Cassidy (1967)	Indians and Melanesians of Fiji		Uncommon	
Belcher (1970)	Ethiopia		Uncommon	
Jarrett and Keen (1975)	Malta, Ceylon, Cook Island Maoris, and Trinidad blacks		Uncommon	

several reasons, as indicated in Chapter 6 on mortality. It is possible that a moderate increase has occurred in the United States in the past 50 years but this is by no means certain. Data on prevalence of youth-onset diabetes were quite limited in all countries prior to very recent years. In England and Wales the annual number of deaths of diabetic children did not vary significantly between 1948 and 1972 (Smith and Hudson, 1976). Data from Michigan and Erie, Pennsylvania suggest a modest increase in recent decades in the incidence of juvenile diabetes (North, et al, 1977). Data from Minnesota do not (Polumbo, et al, 1976).

There are some real differences among populations in rates of youth-onset diabetes. Rates in the United States appear to be roughly seven times higher than rates in Israel and as much as 14 times greater than rates in Japan (Table 31). Mortality data for Japan suggest a smaller disparity of roughly five to one. Data of the British Registry (Bloom, et al, 1975) suggest that there may be valid differences of modest degree by region in Britain, and that rates in Britain may be slightly higher than those in Ireland.

Rates of childhood-onset diabetes in certain populations are probably even lower than in Japan, although part of the apparent paucity could be the result of insensitive systems of ascertainment in these poorer societies. Rates of diabetes are not well established for young children in the various parts of India but onset before age 16 has been found to be rare in varying degrees in several communities (Sathe, 1973). In a town in the north of India, Berry, et al (1966) did not find a single case of glycosuria among 1,984 subjects 10 to 19 years of age. In several Indian series of diabetics less than 1% have had onset before age 16 (Viswanathan, et al, 1966; Patel, et al, 1966). Although adult-onset diabetes is not common in Bombay by Western standards, these cases constituted 99.7% of all cases seen in a clinic series (Patel, et al, 1966b). Only 18 (0.3%) of 5,481 had had onset of diabetes before age 16. Only 2 of these 18 had a family history of diabetes. Cassidy (1967) reported a series of 340 Indian diabetics in a community of Fiji. Only one had onset in the first decade. Jackson, et al (1971) commented on the rarity of insulin-dependent diabetes in adolescent Indians of South Africa.

In primitive African populations, juvenile diabetes is rare (Dodu, 1958; Tulloch, 1962). In a hospital serving a population of about 800,000 black South Africans, Seftel (1964) reported that no cases had been observed with onset prior to age 14! Clinicians who work at this Baragwanath Hospital are quite well informed about diabetes and would not be likely to overlook cases. In a large population of Haiphong, Viet Nam only two cases were observed in five years (Hai, et al, 1965). Striker was told in 1945 by two prominent Guatamalan pediatricians that juvenile diabetes was "extremely rare" in that country. In 1960 C. E. Field reported to Tulloch (1962) that juvenile diabetes was rare in Asians of Singapore (Chinese, Malays, and Indians). In Israel, Cohen (1970) found that the rate of diabetes was much lower in children whose parents were born in Asia and Africa (0.09 per 1,000) than in those whose parents were born in Europe or North America (0.24). Juvenile diabetes has been rare in many other populations, including several tribes of American Indians (West, 1974),

Taiwan (Tsai, 1971), China (Wang, 1937), Ethiopia (Belcher, 1970), and Libya (Mekkawi and Aswad, 1972). Among 1,085 cases of diabetes in Chinese in Hong Kong only two began in the first decade of life (McFadzean and Yeung, 1968). In a diabetic clinic of Indonesia with 2,401 patients, only 0.2% had had onset in the first two decades of life (Tjokroprawiro, 1976). Childhood diabetes has also been reported to be especially uncommon in Malta and Ceylon, in Trinidad blacks, and in Cook Island Maoris (Jarrett and Keen, 1975a), but detailed data are not available.

Childhood diabetes seems to have been extremely rare in Japan prior to the most recent generation. In the 1923 edition of his book, Joslin cites a personal communication from Muryama and Yamaguchi, indicating that only 1.1% of their cases had had onset prior to age 20, and only 0.2% in the first decade of life. In considering this it should be kept in mind that adult-onset diabetes was then quite uncommon in Japan. In 1920 the diabetes mortality rate was 23.0 per 100,000 in New York City and 2.0 in Tokyo. Iwai reported in 1916 a series of 608 Japanese diabetics. None had had onset in the first decade of life. These considerations and other evidence suggest that the incidence of juvenile diabetes in the early 20th century was at least ten times greater in the US than in Japan, and possibly as much as 100 times higher. Differences in frequency of screening and diagnostic testing may have accounted for some of the apparent differences, but in general, medical practice in Japan was at a fairly sophisticated level by standards of that period. Evidence on the previous rarity of juvenile diabetes in Japan was also cited by Isoda (1947) and Blackard, et al (1965).

Tsuji, et al (1966) found occult diabetes in 1.6% of a group of 8,047 rural Japanese, but none of 1,069 high school students had glycosuria. Only two of 1,671 subjects 10 to 19 years of age had glycosuria, and neither had occult diabetes when follow-up testing was performed. One indirect index of the prevalence of juvenile diabetes is the diabetes mortality rate in the fourth decade, at which time death from recent-onset diabetes is rare and death from childhood-onset diabetes is very common. Data reviewed by Kurihara, et al (1970) and by Kuzuya and Kosaka (1970) suggest that death rates from diabetes are at this period of life about three or four times as prevalent in the United States as in modern Japan. Moreover, as indicated in Chapter 6 on mortality, deaths of diabetics in Japan are more likely to be ascribed to diabetes than are deaths of U.S. diabetics. In an apparently representative group of Japanese diabetics studied by Mimura (1970) only 2 of 556 were children. Five older diabetics had had onset in childhood. Only 1.3% of all diabetics had onset prior to age 15.

The prevalence figures given above include not only typical cases of juvenile diabetes, but also those with mild hyperglycemia. Even in Europe and North America a significant percentage are atypical cases of the type to be discussed below. In the National Survey of 1964-1965, published by the National Center for Health Statistics (Bauer, 1967), 68.5% of diabetics under 25 years of age were known to be taking "insulin only" (no other antidiabetic medication). Even in typical juvenile diabetes, remission for months or a few years is

295

common in the early stages. It may be assumed, therefore, that many of those not taking insulin will later develop manifestations of more typical character and degree. In the Michigan questionnaire survey of Gorwitz, et al (1976), 69.3% of diabetic schoolchildren were known to be taking insulin. Status was not known for all of the remainder, so the actual percentage taking insulin was somewhat greater. In Stockholm schoolchildren all of 147 cases were receiving insulin, but 19 were receiving less than 20 units (Sterky, 1963). It is not clear whether this paucity of cases treated without insulin indicates a significant peculiarity of disease pattern or only a difference in therapeutic approach. One case was receiving only 4 units.

One of the few studies in which age of onset was recorded in a whole population was that of Falconer, et al (1971) in Edinburgh. Of 2,932 diabetics 27 were less than 10 years of age, but 62 had had onset in the first decade (2.1% of all diabetics). Of all living diabetics, 7.2% had had onset in the first two decades. Only 76 were under 20 years of age, but 211 had developed diabetes prior to age 20. Thus the number of juvenile-onset diabetics was almost three times as great as the number of juveniles with diabetes. In Kristianstad (Silwer, 1958) about 14% of all living diabetics had developed their diabetes in the first two decades. Prevalance of diabetes was about 2% at age 70 and 0.2% at age 20.

The portion of juvenile-onset cases is quite small when expressed as a percentage of all those who will *eventually* develop diabetes. In most affluent populations this ratio is probably about 1 in 30. Grönberg estimated lifetime risk of clinically detected diabetes in Sweden as about 8% (4.8% in males and 10.3% in females). This risk was roughly 40 times as great as the risk of developing diabetes in the first two decades.

Incidence

Data on incidence are rather limited. Although ascertainment in the British Registry system of Bloom, et al (1975) is not yet ideal, the data for its first two years provide a rough index of incidence for children under 16 in Britain and Ireland. The rate for the two-year period was 7.67 per 100,000 at risk (0.08 per 1,000); circumstances suggest that the actual rate is somewhat higher. Data gathered by Falconer, et al (1971) in Edinburgh permitted crude estimates on age-specific incidence in childhood. During the first five years of life, incidence was roughly 0.03 per 1,000 annually. In the age group 5 to 9 it was about 0.07; and from 10 to 14, roughly 0.12 per 1,000. These rates for Edinburgh were similar to those obtained by the British Registry cited above. Silwer (1958) did not compute incidence from his excellent data in Kristianstad. But prevalence seemed to be somewhat greater than in Edinburgh, suggesting that incidence was probably greater also. In Edinburgh prevalence was 0.13 per 1,000 in the first decade, in Kristianstad about 0.6. In the second decade prevalance was 0.9 per 1,000 in Edinburgh and 1.7 in Kristianstad. In Edinburgh there were 221 diabetics in whom onset had occurred in the first two decades of life; in Kristianstad, 181. But the population at risk was considerably greater in Edinburgh. In that city there were roughly 145,000 persons under age 20, while in

Kristianstad there were only about 88,000 in this age group. The total populations were estimated to be 468,000 in Edinburgh and 260,000 in Kristianstad. The data suggest that the incidence of childhood diabetes over a period of three decades was about one third greater in Kristianstad, and considerably greater in more recent years. The data also suggest that the incidence for the second decade was formerly greater in Edinburgh than in Kristianstad. In Kristianstad there were only 44 persons over 19 years of age who had had onset in their second decade. In Edinburgh there were 112. Among the interesting possibilities is that considerable fluctuations in incidence may have occurred over time in one or both of these populations.

Recently a registry system has been established in Denmark, apparently with excellent success. In a sample (one third) of all Danes under 30 years of age, ascertainment was said to be "complete" (Christau, et al, 1976). Annual incidence in this age group was 13.2 per 100,000 or 0.13 per 1,000 (474 cases in a five-year period in a population at risk of 716,245). There was a striking peak at ages 12-14 (Christau, 1977). These data could not be compared directly to those from Edinburgh or Michigan, but it appears that rates in Denmark may be a little less than in Michigan (Gorwitz, et al, 1976) and somewhat greater than in Edinburgh. Probably completeness of ascertainment is now best in Denmark.

Seasonal variations of incidence will be discussed below under infection.

Gorwitz, et al (1976) found 277 new cases in a one-year period (1972) in a survey of 1,710,212 Michigan schoolchildren (0.16 per 1,000). This survey was intensive but not complete. Note that rates in schoolchildren would be expected to be considerably higher than in all children, because of the very low rates in preschool ages. In a study in Canberra, Australia (Proust and Smithurst, 1968) the annual incidence of diabetes in schoolchildren during a four-year period was only 0.03 per 1,000. In the report of the National Diabetes Commission, Bennett, et al (1976) estimated that the annual incidence of diabetes in the segment of the US population under 17 years of age was very roughly 20,000 new cases per year or about 0.3 per 1,000. It would appear that juvenile diabetes is more common in the United States than Australia, but it is quite possible that the apparent differences are partly attributable to differences in methods and criteria of ascertainment.

Age of Onset

Figures on age of onset from the Joslin Clinic are of interest because the series is so large and well-studied, but it should be kept in mind that this is a selected sample. Incidence by age in the group of juvenile-onset cases who came to this renowned clinic may or may not differ appreciably from that in the general population of New England or the United States. Incidence in the yough-onset Joslin patients rises with age, reaching a peak at age 11 (White and Graham, 1971). Peak frequency of onset for girls is highest at age 10, and for boys at 13. There is a definite decline during the years 15-19. It is important to consider here that the Joslin Clinic is not just a pediatric unit. Thus, a decline in incidence after age 14 is more likely to reflect a real reduction than one found on a pediatric service. The peak rate of onset early in the second decade is in the Joslin series as high as the incidence in the fourth decade (White and Graham, 1971). Diabetes may be found in earliest infancy but all series have shown a much lower rate in the first five years than in the second.

Figure 17 summarizes results of Bloom, et al (1975), who are conducting a study of juvenile diabetes in Britain and Ireland using a registry system. As in Denmark (Christau, 1977) these British data suggest a plateau in incidence between the fourth and eighth years before a sharp rise with a peak during ages 10-13. As in the Joslin series a sharp decline occurs in the rates at 14 and 15. Gorwitz, et al (1976) found a very similar distribution of age of onset in Michigan schoolchildren. In the large series of Danowski (1957) there was also a decline in incidence at ages 14 through 16. Peak frequency occurred in ages 9 through 13 but there was also a peak only slightly lower at ages 5 and 6. The fall in incidence after age 14 observed by several groups is probably a real decline. But more data are needed to confirm this phenomenon and measure its degree. Children in the "teen-age" groups with new diabetes may be identified less frequently by counts in systems that practice either mainly adult medicine or exclusively pediatrics.

Data of Silwer (1958) from Kristianstad, Sweden showed that incidence was about six times more frequent in the second five years than the first five years of life.

Mimura (1970) collected 202 cases from the Japanese literature and from his own experience in whom information on age of onset was available. Incidence

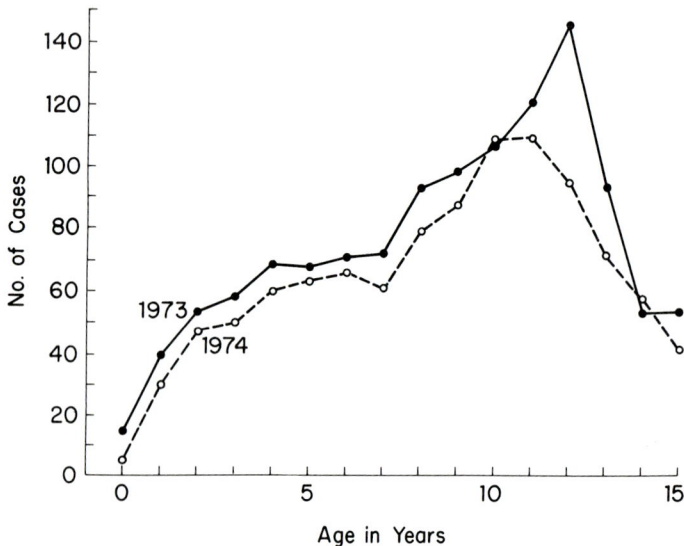

FIGURE 17.   Age of onset of diabetes in children of Britain and Ireland as ascertained by a Registry system (Bloom, et al, 1975).

was greatest at age 10 (24 cases) and at age 13 (32 cases). At age 14 there was a sharp fall (16 cases). At age five there were only ten cases.

Francois, et al (1972) reported a series of 552 cases with onset of diabetes before age 15, of whom 14 (2.5%) had onset in the first year of life. In the Joslin Clinic patient onset occurred in the first year of life in 0.5% of juvenile-onset cases, and 0.05% of all cases (White and Graham, 1971). Onset in the first six months of life is very rare (Cornblath and Schwartz, 1976). Guest (1947) found a case in an infant nine days old. Most cases with hyperglycemia in very early infancy have only transient diabetes (Cornblath and Schwartz, 1976), usually lasting only a few days or weeks. Five such patients have been followed for periods of three to twenty-five years with no evidence of subsequent diabetes. Gilly, et al (1972) summarized reports on 32 such cases. Birth weight has often been low in babies with transitory diabetes and hyperglycemia is often severe. The causes of this syndrome are poorly understood.

Sex, Height, Weight, and Growth

In most series the number of boys and girls has been very nearly equal. In the United States national sample of 1964-1965, there was no significant difference in rates for boys and girls. Rates for the sexes are also very similar in Denmark (Christau et al, 1977). In the British Registry study (Bloom, et al, 1975) rates were very similar in boys and girls. In children under 5, incidence was very slightly higher in boys; the reverse was true in children 5 to 10. Differences (male predominance) will be described below in certain special circumstances (eg, in societies where substantial portions of cases are attributable to pancreatic fibrosis and calcification). In the patients of Doctor Priscilla White, peak onset was at age 10 for girls and at age 13 for boys (White and Graham, 1971). This corresponds fairly well with the beginning of puberty and growth spurt for the two sexes, but in Britain (Bloom, et al, 1975a) this difference between boys and girls was not observed, and in general, patterns of onset in Britain do not suggest a relationship of risk of diabetes with either puberty or growth spurts.

In the Stockholm series of Sterky (1963), diabetic boys were slightly shorter than controls but diabetic girls were not. The Swedish diabetic girls were a bit heavier than controls. In the follow-up study (Sterky, 1967), the diabetic boys grew at a faster rate in the late phase of growth, so their final height was only 3 cm. less than controls. Moreover, there were only 21 in the control group. This difference, therefore, may or may not be significant. In both boys and girls skinfold thickness was greater in diabetics, even when weight for height was matched. Final development of bones in Weil's diabetic children (1967) was not different from that in nondiabetic siblings, but rates of development in both groups was somewhat slower than in a control group. In Canada, Birkbeck (1972) found growth and skeletal maturity normal in a group of juvenile diabetics. He concluded that growth was impaired only when control was decidedly poor. In a group of Japanese juvenile diabetics studied by Izumi, et al

299

(1976) growth was retarded in the subgroup who had had diabetes more than four years.

The best controls available are identical twins. In those of Tattersall and Pyke (1973), final height was 2.25 inches greater in the 12 nondiabetic twins of juvenile diabetics. No effect of prediabetes was seen on height in these studies. Birth weights were the same in twins discordant for diabetes (Pyke and Tattersall, 1976). Danowski's diabetic boys and girls weighed slightly less than control groups (1957). The heights and weights of the Joslin Clinic diabetic children were close to the norms for children of comparable age, but prediabetic children seemed to have been a bit tall for their age (White and Graham, 1971). Birth weights of juvenile diabetics were similar to those of nondiabetics, as were those of the series of Danowski (1957). Apparently, interference with growth of substantial degree is only observed with decidedly suboptimal treatment. Jivani and Rayner (1973) found that heights of diabetic children in Birmingham, England, were normal at onset of diabetes, but growth was subnormal in the ensuing three years. No relationship was observed between rates of growth and degree of "control." It is well known, however, that prior to the availability of long-acting insulin, marked retardation of growth sometimes occurred with prolonged gross hyperglycemia. This condition was known as diabetic dwarfism. In 1927 Morrison and Bogan reported that bone age was somewhat advanced at onset of childhood diabetes. With childhood diabetes of long standing, bone age was retarded.

Brown and Thompson (1940) measured growth and intelligence in a group of juvenile diabetics in Minnesota. They found no differences in these respects between diabetics and nondiabetics. No distinctive traits of personality were found in these juvenile diabetics.

In girls treated by White (1972), menarche occured earlier in those with diabetes of short duration than in those with onset of diabetes in early childhood. Tattersall and Pyke (1973) observed age of menarche in two pairs of identical twins. Menarche was, in each instance, considerably later in the diabetic than in the nondiabetic twin.

Although grossly obese children often have abnormal glucose tolerance and hyperinsulinemia (Paulsen, et al, 1968), only a very small portion of children with clinical diabetes are fat. This is consistent with the notion that more than a few years of obesity are required to produce gross decompensation if beta cells are unaffected by other factors. Few data are available on long-term risk of diabetes in fat children. Mouriquand (1920) stated that half of cases of lifelong "inherited" obesity become diabetic before age 40, but details were not given concerning the basis for this conclusion.

Etiologic Factors

GENETICS

The role of genetics has been discussed above in the section on heredity in Chapter 7. Rates of diabetes in identical twins of diabetics have been studied by many observers. Rimoin and Schimke (1971) and Frias and Rosenbloom (1973) have reviewed these reports. But data are rather few on twins of juvenile-onset cases. Observations of Tattersall and Pyke (1972) suggest that long-term concordance may be as low as 50%. Moreover, T. Cohen (1970) reported no instances of diabetes among 201 siblings of Israeli children with diabetes! Only 11% of the British Registry cases (Bloom et al, 1975) had first-degree relatives with known diabetes. In diabetic Michigan schoolchildren 9.6% gave a history of diabetes in parents or siblings or both. In Joslin Clinic patients 9% of offspring had juvenile diabetes when one parent had juvenile diabetes, but this high rate was probably attributable in part to the methods of ascertainment (White, 1974). Concordance has not been studied in any substantial series of twins of juvenile diabetics of less privileged societies. It is quite possible that environmental factors raise or lower rates of concordance in identical twins of juvenile diabetics. Farquhar (1969) studied the offspring of 329 diabetic mothers of whom 293 (89%) were taking insulin at the time of delivery of the offspring. Follow-up examinations were conducted in 260 surviving offspring for periods of one to nineteen years. Only 2 of 260 had developed diabetes (0.77%). Even so, this rate was judged to be about 22 times as great as the rate of juvenile diabetes in the general population of children of comparable age. Results were similar in a study of Yssing (1975) in Copenhagen. After fifteen to twenty-six years, 1% of children of such diabetic mothers had developed diabetes. This rate was deemed to be about 30 times greater than that expected in a group with this age distribution. Hansen and Degnbol computed the risk of developing insulin-dependent diabetes prior to age 30 when the propositus was an insulin-dependent diabetic with onset before age 20. Risk was 5.4% in offspring, 5.9% in sibs, and 1.5% in nephews.

Most of the recent evidence cited in the previous section on genetics suggests that the genetic mechanisms for juvenile- and maturity-onset diabetes are separate. It is apparent that both environmental and genetic factors are important in growth-onset diabetes (Frias and Rosenbloom, 1973; Pyke, 1977; Barosa, et al, 1977). The special genetic features of atypical mild childhood diabetes will be discussed below. Neel (1977) has published a good succint review on the genetics of juvenile diabetes.

Many reports have been made concerning possible prediabetic stigmata before the onset of childhood diabetes. This subject is discussed in Chapter 9 on prediabetes. The histocompatibility antigens are discussed in this chapter in the section below on infection and immunity.

RACE AND NUTRITION

Geographic differences in the prevalence of growth-onset diabetes have been reviewed above. The degree and basis of these differences are not clear. Low rates of typical juvenile diabetes are probably real in Eskimos (West, 1974) in at least some American Indian populations (West, 1974), and certainly in Japanese (Blackard, et al, 1965). It is rare in some populations of Indians (Sathe, 1973), Ethiopians (Belcher, 1970), Fijians (Cassiday, 1967), Chinese of Taiwan (Mimura, 1970), and other populations (Tulloch, 1962). Neither racial nor environmental factors can be excluded as explanations of the low rates.

Among several series from different parts of India there has been considerable difference in the percentage of cases with onset under 16 years of age. In a large series of Patel, et al, from Bombay (1966b), only 0.3% were juvenile-onset cases, while 2.3% of a large series of Vaishnava, et al (1974) from New Delhi had onset in childhood. Any combination of several factors would account for these differences, including nutritional factors. All the reports from India suggest a rate of childhood-onset diabetes considerably lower than in the United States or Europe. This could be attributable to racial or environmental factors. Also rates of ascertainment are probably lower in India. Even so, it does not seem likely that this explains the paucity of juvenile-onset cases.

In Japan rates of juvenile diabetes have probably increased in the last generation at a time when diet was changing substantially (Tsuji and Wada, 1970). Little is known about rates of childhood onset of diabetes in Indians, Chinese, and Japanese who live in Western societies. This information would be of considerable interest. Mortality from diabetes in the age group 15-44 is about the same in Indians and whites of South Africa (WHO, 1964). Evidence cited below indicates clearly that Africans lose immunity to juvenile diabetes when they live in affluent Western societies. This could be related to nutritional factors but could also be related to immunologic factors such as differences in degree and timing of exposure to certain viruses.

As explained above, rates of juvenile diabetes are probably increasing in Israel (T. Cohen, 1970), and they may be higher in Europe than they were prior to 1920. Conceivably, underfeeding in fetal life, infancy, or childhood could under certain circumstances be protective (Brook, 1972; Yudkin, 1973). But Laron and Kauli (1972) found skinfold thickness the same in diabetic and nondiabetic children of Israel. Rates and severity of insulin-dependent diabetes have been modified by dietary manipulation in hamsters, in which diabetes is not associated with obesity (Gerritsen, et al, 1974; Grodsky, et al, 1974). These effects appeared to be the result of quantitative rather than qualitative dietary changes. It should be kept in mind that the range of adiposity of "nonobese" children and adults is very great. We found that the average thickness of fatfolds in children of East Pakistan was only about one third as great as those of typical "nonobese" American children.

The apparent rarity of diabetes in primitive black populations has been cited above. Although available evidence is not conclusive, black American children probably had in the past less diabetes than whites. Bowcock reported on blacks of Atlanta in 1928. He had seen one female with onset of diabetes in the first decade of life, but no males with onset in the first two decades. Altschul and Nathan reported in 1942 on a series of 622 black diabetics seen in Harlem Hospital in New York City. Not a single one of 126 males had had onset in the first decade of life, and only two males had developed diabetes prior to age 20. One of the 496 females had onset in the first decade, and 6 of 496 in the second. Prior to 1942 rates of ascertainment in US black diabetic children were probably lower than in whites, but these observations do suggest that juvenile diabetes was probably less common in blacks than in whites. The young black soldiers of World War I probably had less diabetes than white soldiers (Emerson and Larimore, 1924). Diabetes in young men of this age is usually insulin dependent.

In the study of Gorwitz, et al (1976) in Michigan schoolchildren, diabetes was only half as prevalent in black children as in whites. They considered the possibility that schools with more blacks did not report as thoroughly as other schools. MacDonald (1975) found that in black children diabetes was less frequently a cause for admission to a St. Louis hospital than in white children (10.7 per 1,000 in whites and 3.8 in blacks). Rosenbaum (1967) reported that only half of juvenile diabetics seen in Charity Hospital, New Orleans, were black, even though 80% to 85% of all children attended were black. In the National Survey of 1964-1965 the prevalence of diabetes for those less than 25 years of age was 8.3 in whites and 3.4 in nonwhites. More than 90% of "nonwhites" were blacks. Because the number of nonwhite children in the sample was small (and because of other factors), it is not entirely certain that this apparent difference between whites and nonwhites was real. In the 1973 National Survey the sample size for nonwhite children was again considered too small for precise measurement of prevalence, but in this survey the prevalence in those under 17 years of age was 1.4 per 1,000 for whites and 1.3 for nonwhites.

It seems probable that environmental differences between the races are diminishing in the United States. Studies in recent years have shown little difference in the adiposity of American white and black children (US Dept. of Health, Education, and Welfare, 1972; Johnston, et al, 1974; Hamill, 1972). Neither is there much difference between fatness of poor black children and black children who are not poor. American black children are now much heavier than children of Egypt and very much heavier than children of India (Hamill, 1972). It is conceivable that the apparent rise in juvenile diabetes in US blacks to some extent relates to an increase in adiposity. MacDonald (1975) found obesity more common in black diabetic children (38%) than in white (6%). He also found mild diabetes more commonly in the black juvenile diabetics.

Epidemiologic data on feeding in infancy and risk of later juvenile- and adult-onset diabetes are quite incomplete, but juvenile- and maturity-onset diabetes of the typical types are usually not common in populations where infants have received a low caloric ration. Rates of juvenile- and adult-onset diabetes also correspond fairly well with height, in interpopulation comparisons. This could reflect the association between final height and feeding in infancy and childhood. Evaluation of these possibilities by epidemiologic approaches is quite limited by difficulties in ascertaining true rates of juvenile diabetes. Wilcox (1908) cited experiences that led him to believe that juvenile diabetes may sometimes be caused or precipitated by overconsumption of sugar. Morse (1913) also thought that increased consumption of sugar might be a significant etiologic factor. Wales (1976) cited indirect evidence suggesting the possibility that sucrose feeding might increase risk of juvenile diabetes, particularly when combined with generous amounts of dietary fat (eg, in sweetened milk). Karam, et al (1976) thought that risk of childhood-onset diabetes might be increased by overfeeding. Direct epidemiologic evidence is quite sparse and inconclusive on sugar consumption as an etiologic factor in juvenile diabetes. These issues are reviewed in detail in the section on nutritional factors in Chapter 7.

DesChamps, et al (1977) found that glucose tolerance was almost as good in obese children as in lean children. But insulinemia was considerably greater in the fat children. Others have found impairment of glucose tolerance more commonly in obese than in lean children (Rosenbloom, et al, 1973).

Possible nutritional aspects of youth-onset diabetes in patients with pancreatic fibrosis and calcification will be discussed below, in this chapter.

Infection and Immunity

Infection

It is clear from experimental and clinical evidence that some viruses can produce diabetes. This subject was well summarized by Gamble and Taylor (1976), Maugh (1975, 1975a), Maclaren (1977), and in an editorial (*The Lancet,* 1976). Present epidemiologic data are, however, not adequate to determine whether infection is a common or rare cause of juvenile diabetes. The agents that are capable of producing diabetes in animals or man include the viruses of mumps, rubella, Coxsackie B4, foot-and-mouth disease, Venezuelan encephalitis, and encephalomyocarditis. Some of this experimental work suggests the possibility that clinical expression might follow by months or years the initial contact between virus and the affected tissues.

At least occasionally, mumps causes diabetes by producing pancreatitis. A case was reported by Harris in 1899 and five cases were reported by Patrick in 1924. In 1922 Farnham was able to cite from the literature 119 cases of mumps pancreatitis. It is also clear that mumps pancreatitis may occur without evident parotitis (Rennie, 1935). Gunderson observed in 1927 that mortality rates from diabetes in children seemed to be greater two to four years after epidemics of mumps. Melin and Ursing (1958) reported on an epidemic of mumps in which 4 of 40 cases developed diabetes. More recently, Sultz and co-workers (1975) observed that the incidence of diabetes in the Buffalo, New York area seemed to rise about four years after national epidemics of mumps. Block, et al (1973) reported a case of severe diabetes secondary to mumps with complete recovery.

Gamble, et al (1973), however, observed no increase in the immunologic manifestations of mumps in children with recent onset of diabetes. He found evidence of Coxsackie B4 antibodies more frequently in children over 10 years of age with recent onset of diabetes. Controls under 10 had B4 antibodies as frequently as diabetics of comparable age. Moreover, Dippe and associates (1974) found no evidence of increased rates of diabetes in a population that suffered a widespread epidemic of B4 Coxsackie virus. Hadden, et al (1973a) found no increase in the immunologic manifestations of Coxsackie infections in 60 new diabetics. Nelson, et al (1975) were not able to implicate viral infections as a cause of diabetes in their studies of 30 identical twins with juvenile diabetes. These subjects were studied for immunologic responses to mumps, cytomegalovirus, rubella, Coxsackie types B1 through 5, and mycoplasma. Huff and associates (1974) performed extensive virologic studies in nine new cases of juvenile diabetics that had been part of an unusual geographic cluster. Results were equivocal and did not clearly implicate any specific virus.

In 44 individuals between 20 and 30 years of age with the congenital rubella syndrome, Forrest and her associates (1971) found four had abnormal glucose tolerance and one diabetes. Peculiarities of insulin secretion were observed in others. Although not entirely conclusive, these results are consistent with the possibility that congenital rubella infection may cause aberrations of beta-cell function long after initial contact with the virus. Monif (1973) has recovered rubella virus from the pancreas as long as three years after birth. In a subsequent follow-up of the series reported in 1971 by Forrest, et al, Menser and co-workers (1974) reported that 5 of 50 cases of congenital rubella had developed diabetes from fifteen to twenty-nine years after birth. On glucose tolerance testing with insulin measurements in additional 13 of 45 tested were thought to have "features of latent diabetes." It is also possible that this high rate of peculiarities in beta-cell function could be at least in part attributable to factors other than infection of beta cells. Other possibilities include an indirect or direct effect of fetal maternal rubella on the development of cells and enzymes at other sites.

Interesting differences by season have been observed in the onset of juvenile diabetes. Gamble and Taylor (1969) found that in London youth-onset diabetes was discovered much less commonly in April through June. It was especially common in July, in October, and in winter. They estimated that, on the average, onset of symptoms occurred about one month prior to these times of discovery. These authors reported that a similar pattern had been observed in Birmingham, England. In cases with discovery prior to age 30, 35 were found in winter, 20 in spring, 21 in summer, and 44 in autumn (data for 1960–1966 compiled by FitzGerald and Malins). Bloom and associates (1975) found no significant seasonal variation in onset of symptoms of cases with onset before age 5 compiled by the British Registry. In children who became diabetic between the ages of 5 and 16 the rate of onset of symptoms in winter was more than twice as common as in summer. The incidence pattern by season for children for all ages was very similar in 1973 and 1974, as shown in Figure 18. There was no difference in prevalance of family history of diabetes in those with summer and winter onset. Because of the large numbers and the method of collection, these data from the British Registry are among the best available in several respects, including the matter of seasonal variation. Preliminary data from this Registry project were also summarized by Gamble (1974). Gamble pointed out that, prior to the availability of vaccine, poliomyelitis rates were low in some of the same countries that had low rates of diabetes. This was compatible with the possibility that early exposure to certain viruses might engender an immunity not

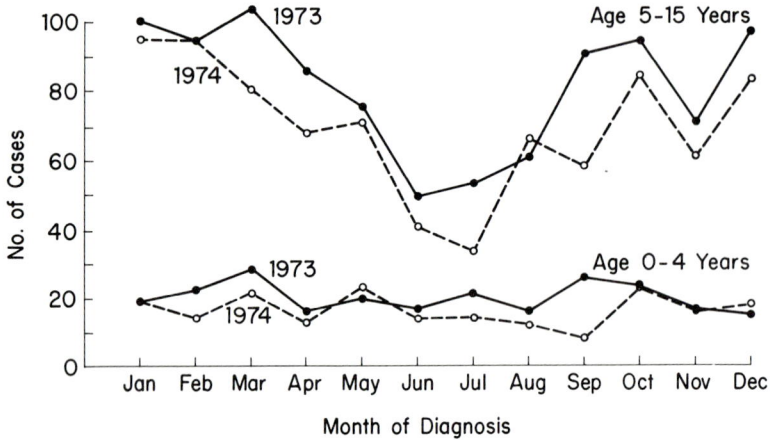

FIGURE 18.   Month of diagnosis of diabetes in British and Irish children as ascertained by the Registry system. On the average, symptoms had begun a month earlier (from Bloom, et al, 1975).

enjoyed by children who were protected from early exposure. Further, Gamble showed that British children who started school at less than 5 years of age seemed to have a different age-incidence pattern than children who started school later. The children who began school early had onset of diabetes less frequently between ages 9 and 14. Gamble pointed out, however, that the two groups of children also differed in respects other than age of starting school.

Danowski's cases (1957) exhibited little variation by season in onset of symptoms except that rates were high in January and low in May. In the youth-onset cases of the Joslin Clinic, onset was also common in January (White and Graham, 1971), but onset in July was also especially common. In a small series, Spencer (1928) had also observed a greater number in summer than in winter. Adams had analyzed patterns of onset by month in 1926. In these Minnesota cases incidence was greatest in September and lowest in May and June. It will be interesting to see how seasonal patterns of incidence differ by geography, climate, race, and in the same locality over time. Some of the seasonal variations in these different series is probably attributable to precipitation of diabetes by infection not involving the pancreas in patients already destined to become diabetic. Very frequently there is a history of infection, particularly upper respiratory infection, at or just prior to onset of diabetic symptoms (John, 1934). Such infections were noted near onset of diabetes in 42% of Danowski's cases (1957). Since infections tend to intensify the diabetic state, their presence at onset may reflect only an unmasking of the diabetic state, rather than a specific etiologic role of infection. It is a little difficult to compare some of the series because some authors recorded month of diagnosis and others recorded month of onset of symptoms. Danowski (1957) recorded both. Duration of symptoms had been less than one month in most cases but some had had symptoms many weeks or months. This raised the average to eighty-two days. More than 90% were symptomatic; 93 of 513 had acidosis at discovery.

In a small series in Kentucky, McMillan et al found differences in seasonal patterns with age of onset. In children with onset after age five, there was a paucity of new cases in summer, but in children who were older at onset, discovery was frequent in July. The new Danish registry found frequency lowest in May through July (Christau, et al, 1977).

In a small series of 30 identical twins with juvenile diabetes, Nelson, et al (1975a) found that twins concordant for diabetes had onset more frequently in January through March than did the diabetics whose twins were not diabetic. Gleason et al (1977) studied month of onset in 1178 youth-onset cases in Massachusetts. No significant seasonal variations were demonstrable.

In an epidemiologic study in dogs, Foster (1975) found that onset of symptoms was most common in winter and spring, but in entire bitches, symptoms began somewhat more frequently in summer and autumn.

In England, Coxsackie B4 infections occur most commonly in autumn (Gamble et al, 1973) at a time when onset of childhood diabetes is not especially common (Bloom, et al, 1975). Rates were, however, high in October in the London cases studied by Gamble and Taylor (1969). In the diabetics with Coxsackie antibodies the seasonal pattern for onset of diabetes was similar to that of all patients (high rates in winter and low in spring), but onset of diabetes was less common in the autumn in those with Coxsackie antibodies. The effects of this or other viruses might, of course, be a delayed one. In mice hyperglycemia began about twelve days after inoculation (Taylor, 1974). A delay might occur if a virus-mediated hypersensitivity were the etiologic mechanism. In the patients of King's College Hospital, London, there was a rather good correlation between the incidence of Coxsackie B4 infections and insulin-dependent diabetes when the data were expressed as new cases per year (Gamble and Taylor, 1969). But these authors called attention to problems in interpreting the significance of this association, including the small number of diabetes cases. Fahlen, et al (1971) found insulin secretion in normal Swedes was somewhat greater in winter than in summer.

The significance of the occasional association of onset of diabetes with infectious hepatitis has been discussed above under liver disease. Webb, et al (1976) and Yoon and Notkins (1976) demonstrated that genetic factors in mice determined the capacity of the beta cell to support growth of a virus.

The case for viral etiology in human diabetes is diminished by failure to culture any virus from the pancreas in any diabetics. MacLean and Sullivan (1929) studied glucose tolerance in 17 children with acute infection. Despite these infections, glucose tolerance was good, suggesting that most children have a considerable reserve of beta-cell function.

Immunologic factors

There is a considerable amount of evidence suggesting that immunologic factors may be of importance in the etiology of juvenile diabetes. Excellent reviews of this subject have recently appeared (Bastenie and Gepts, 1974; *The Lancet*, 1974; Christy, et al, 1977). Reviews on histocompatibility antigens are cited below.

Warren (1927) and LeCompte (1958) observed lymphocytic infiltrations of the pancreatic islets frequently in children who died soon after the onset of diabetes. This had also been observed before the discovery of insulin (LeCompte, et al, 1966). Lymphocytic infiltration has been reported in only two adults with insulin-dependent diabetes (LeCompte and Legg, 1972), but is not uncommon in children who die in the first year of the disease (Gepts, 1965). Renold and associates (1964) observed lymphocytic infiltrations after sensitizing heifers to beef insulin. Such infiltrations were later produced in other animals by the injection of insulin from both homologous and heterologous sources, usually without producing diabetes. But diabetes was produced in a few rabbits by this means (Karam, et al, 1969). LeCompte, et al (1966) noted the similarity of lesions induced by these methods and the pancreatic lesions sometimes observed in early juvenile diabetes. Excessive rates of diabetes have been reported in several diseases in which autoimmunity appears to play a role, including pernicious anemia, idiopathic hypoadrenocorticism, Hashimoto's thyroiditis, and hypothyroidism (Bastenie and Gepts, 1974; *The Lancet*, 1974). Drash (1971) found that 15% of his cases of juvenile diabetes had antibodies to either thyroid, gastric, or adrenal tissue as compared to less than 1% in controls. Maturity-onset diabetics had no increase in the frequency of these antibodies (Goldstein, et al, 1970). Other workers have also found these antibodies with especially high frequency in insulin-dependent diabetics (Bastenie and Gepts, 1974). Gastric parietal-cell antibodies have also been found more often in typical adult-onset diabetes than in controls (Bastenie and Gepts, 1974).

Persons with certain inherited histocompatibility antigens appear to be more susceptible to some of the autoimmune disorders and viral infections. These include antigens HLA-B8 and HLA-BW15, the genetic potential for which is located on the sixth pair of chromosomes. Finkelstein and co-workers (1972) found no increase in the frequency of the presence of these two antigens in juvenile diabetics, but several others have found that insulin-dependent diabetics have these antigens more frequently than controls (Singal and Blajchman, 1973; Nerup, et al, 1974; Cudworth and Woodrow, 1975). Nerup, et al (1974) concluded that those with HLA-B8 had a risk of insulin-dependent diabetes about twice that of controls. Risk was judged to be elevated by a factor of 2.8 in those with W15. Cudworth and Woodrow (1975) lumped data from three centers. They saw no evidence of heterogeneity. In the combined data increased relative risk for those with HLA-B8 was 2.12 and 2.60 for W15. No link was found between these antigens and maturity-onset diabetes. In the subjects of Cudworth and Woodrow HLA-B8 was present in 31.8% of controls and 54% of juvenile diabetics. In controls 12% had W15, while 18% of juvenile diabetics had W15. The modest degree of these differences indicates a need for larger numbers of controls and diabetics, but the associations are impressive.

In 18 patients with congenital rubella and manifestations of diabetes or "latent diabetes" Menser, et al (1974) found no increase in the frequency of W15, but 50% (9 of 18) had B8 as compared to 24% of controls. Rolles, et al (1975) found in Birmingham, England that 26 (46%) of a group of 56 diabetic children had the B8 antigen. In these children onset of diabetes was more frequent in October through February. This followed about two to three months behind the peak onset period for Coxsackie B4 infections. Seasonal patterns of onset of diabetes seemed to be different for the children without HLA-B8. There were no cases in January and rates were highest in spring and in February. Numbers in both these groups were small, however (26 with B8 and 30 without). In a series of Barbosa, et al (1977) there was no significant difference in season of onset in children with and without this antigen.

Nerup, et al (1975) found that antigens LD-8a and W15a were more strongly associated with juvenile diabetes than was BW15. As compared to controls, relative risk of juvenile diabetes for those with W15a was 4.5, for LD-8a it was 3.7. Sixty-six percent of their juvenile diabetics had either islet-cell antibody or antipancreatic cell-mediated immunity. Islet-cell antibody was found in 36% of those without LD-8a and in 75% of those with that antigen. Antibodies to Coxsackie B4 were more frequent in those with LD-8a. Apparently risk of juvenile diabetes is even greater in those with both BW15 and B8 than in those who have only one of these antigens (Nerup, et al, 1976).

Menser and associates (1975) have noted that the frequency of both HLA-B8 and juvenile diabetes is very low in Eskimos. They considered the possibility that paucity of the B8 antigen in Eskimos explained the absence of diabetes in Eskimos who had antibodies to Coxsackie B4. The frequency of various histo-compatibility antigens have been measured in more than 50 populations in widely separated parts of the world (Bodmer and Bodmer, 1973). Some of the sample sizes are very small but it is clear that there are substantial interpopulation differences. In many groups HLA-B8 was not observed, while rates as high as 16% were seen in Oxford and the Hebrides. Generally, rates were higher in white Caucasians of Europe, low in Mongols, and intermediate in the Middle East. On the Indian subcontinent rates were highly variable by subgroups. Rates around the world for BW15 ranged from zero to 44% with no consistent pattern by race in the groups tested. Rates were, however, relatively low in the black and Arab groups tested. In Japan B8 is rare, but BW15 is common. In a small group of Japanese juvenile diabetics the frequency of BW15 was not excessive, but the frequency of BW22j was decidedly excessive (Wakisaka, et al, 1976).

Nelson, et al (1975) studied rates of the presence of histocompatibility antigens in identical twins in whom diabetes had been found in one or both before the age of 45. In diabetic twins with later onset, no peculiarities were found in the frequency of these antigens. In 38 twin pairs with early onset who were concordant for diabetes, rates of B8 and BW15 were elevated in a degree roughly comparable to that observed in juvenile diabetics of the combined series of Cudworth and Woodrow (1975) described above. The results in 31 youth-onset discordant pairs were different. They had no greater incidence of the B8 antigen than controls, but the frequency of BW15 was higher than in controls. In a small series, Barta and Simon (1977) found among juvenile diabetics no increase in the frequency of BW15, a mild excess of those with B8, and a very great excess of those with both B8 and BW15 antigens. In a small series Barbosa (1977) observed no relationship between the frequency of the presence of the B8 antigen and the season of onset of insulin-dependent diabetes. Cudworth et al (1977) found an excess of those with BW15 among those with onset in winter but not in autumn. The September 1976 issue of *Diabete et Metabolisme* has several other reports on the histocompatibility antigens in juvenile diabetes.

Schernthaner, et al (1976) found in a small series that HLA-B7 was *less* common in juvenile diabetics than in controls, as did Van dePutte, et al (1976) and Cudworth and Woodrow (1976). Ludwig, et al (1975) measured the frequency of histocompatibility antigen T3 in siblings and other relatives of juvenile diabetics. They found a significant increase in the frequency of T3 in these family members as compared to controls. In siblings of juvenile diabetics, intolerance to intravenous glucose was especially frequent in those with T3. They pointed out the need for more data because of the modest numbers in their preliminary studies. Cattaneo, et al (1976) found that the number of "T" lymphocytes was reduced in juvenile diabetics but not in maturity-onset diabetics.

Nerup, et al (1976,1977) found that the frequency of Dw3 and Dw4 antigens were much more frequent than in controls (Dw3 was 6.4 times as frequent and Dw4 was 3.7 times as frequent). Ludwig et al (1977) observed an excessive frequency of the Cw3 antigen in insulin-dependent cases.

The possibility has been suggested that genetic recombinations in the HLA region might be especially common in insulin-dependent diabetics but recent observations of Barbosa (1977), of Nerup et al (1977) and of Hsu et al (1977) were negative in this respect.

In small series of Patel et al (1977) the prevalence of the HLA-B8 and BW15 antigens appeared to be somewhat excessive in both blacks and Mexican-Americans with insulin-dependent diabetes. In Japan, Nakao (1977) found an association of insulin-dependent diabetes with HLA-B12 but not with B8 or BW15. In the general population of Japan, where juvenile-onset diabetes is rather uncommon, the frequency of HLA-B8 is also very low (Kawa et al, 1977). In Japanese insulin-dependent diabetics the frequency of HLA-B22 was excessive (Kawa et al, 1977).

According to J. A. W. Smith (1975), approximately 80% of children with celiac disease have B8 antigen, and diabetes is especially frequent in celiac disease.

Lendrum, et al (1976) measured islet-cell antibodies in youth-onset diabetics. When diabetes was of recent onset, 59% had these antibodies. Rates were much lower in youth-onset cases of longer duration. Only 1 of 51 maturity-onset cases with insulin-independent diabetes had these antibodies. Christy, et al (1976) reported similar results. The frequency of islet-cell antibodies seemed to be especially frequent in subjects with the HLA-B8 antigen, but numbers of cases were small.

Irvine, et al (1977) studied immunologic factors in 972 diabetics. Islet-cell antibodies (ICA) were observed in 60% of insulin-dependent diabetics tested during the first year of known diabetes. When insulin-dependent diabetes had been present ten to twenty years, only 5% had these antibodies. In 157 first-degree relatives of those with ICA, only three (2%) had such antibodies. Of the diabetics who did not require antidiabetic medication, none had ICA. But Del Prete et al found ICA rather commonly in insulin-independent diabetes. Irvine et al (1971) showed that ICA were especially likely to persist in patients with HLA-B8 and A1 antigens. Cudworth et al (1977) were unable to demonstrate a relationship of the presence of islet-cell antibodies with either HLA phenotype or viral antibodies. From their data, Buschard et al (1977) concluded that islet-cell antibodies were probably not a causal agent in diabetes.

Woodrow (1975), Cathelineau (1976), Nerup (1976, 1976a), and Christy, et al (1977) have recently reviewed the interrelationships of genetic and immuno-logic phenomena in the etiology of juvenile diabetes.

The meaning of all these interesting observations on the histocompatibility antigens is not at all clear. In certain instances these antigens may affect responses to viruses. On the other hand, the association with juvenile diabetes might be indirect. The relationship might be the result of geographic proximity in the chromosome of separate genetic materials controlling histocompatibility and risk of diabetes. These relationships between immunologic characteristics and insulin-dependent diabetes are impressive, but considerably more data are needed to ascertain their etiologic significance.

Associations of diabetes with blood groups have been discussed in Chapter 7 under race. No consistent pattern has been observed.

Congenital aplasia of the pancreas

This is a very rare cause of diabetes (Kriss, 1927). Warren, et al (1966) pointed out that some of the cases with very small amounts of pancreatic tissue may have represented atrophy rather than aplasia.

Hormonal factors

The possibility that endocrine factors other than insulin may be of some etiologic importance has been extensively investigated. These matters receive well-deserved attention in the standard texts and reviews on diabetes. The possibilities considered have included aberrations of the secretion of growth hormone and glucagon (Johansen, et al, 1974) and of epinephrine, cortisol, and sex hormones. Suffice it to say that epidemiologic data are few in support of any of these possibilities. Height, growth, and sexual development of juvenile diabetics have been discussed above. Campbell (1963) has described certain stigmata in young adult Indian diabetics, fitting the notion that hypersecretion of adrenal steroids might be involved. These include centrally distributed adiposity and hirsutism; but elevated levels of such hormones have not been demonstrated. Hormonal factors are discussed further in Chapter 9 on prediabetes.

ADULT-ONSET DIABETES IN THE LEAN

Rather little systematic study has been devoted to the epidemiology of either insulin-dependent or insulin-independent diabetes of maturity onset in lean persons. One reason for this is that the universe of such patients is not neatly separated from other types of diabetes. No generally accepted definitions exist for either *lean, adult, diabetes,* or *insulin-dependent.* These problems of definition and standardization are discussed in some detail in the section on classification (Chapter 3). The development of the capacity to measure secretion of insulin, even in patients who take insulin (Rubenstein, et al, 1975), will be helpful in some aspects of the classification problem. When used in this discussion without definition, "insulin-dependent" means that insulin is required to relieve symptoms of hyperglycemia even with optimum diet therapy. Some suggestions concerning more specific definition are set forth below. Chapter 3 provided a simplified clinical classification showing the general relationships of insulin-dependence to clinically detectable factors, such as degree of glycosuria, fatness, response to diet, and presence or absence of ketonuria. The following presents a classification of adult-onset diabetes by clinical type:

1. *Typical obese diabetics:*
   usually asymptomatic with appropriate diet therapy
   in most western societies this group constitutes about 60–90% of all
   adult-onset cases

2. *Obese insulin-dependent diabetics:*
   very uncommon in all societies

3. *Lean insulin-dependent diabetics:*
   hyperglycemia severe or considerable even with optimal diet
   common among diabetics with onset in third and fourth decades
   less common but not rare in those with onset in later life
   a. ketosis-prone
   b. not ketosis-prone

4. *Lean insulin-independent diabetics*
   hyperglycemia mild
   asymptomatic even when insulin not given
   frequency not precisely established
   prevalence rates affected greatly by definition of "diabetes", "lean",
   and "insulin-dependent"

Study of the insulin-dependent adult-onset group is important for several reasons. It will elucidate further the effects of heredity and adiposity in the etiology of diabetes. It is not clear to what degree the genetic mechanisms for insulin-dependent adult-onset diabetes correspond to those for either (a) typical childhood-onset diabetes, (b) typical maturity-onset diabetes of the obese, or (c) maturity-onset insulin-independent diabetes in lean adults.

In only a few genetic or epidemiologic studies have observations taken into account the need to distinguish the different types of maturity-onset diabetes. Among the few informative data are those of Gamble and Taylor (1969), who separated their cases systematically into those considered to be insulin dependent and insulin independent (Figure 10). The criteria for this separation were not given, nor was it clear what portion of each subgroup was or had been obese. However, data of these kinds suggest that in Western societies the incidence of insulin-dependent diabetes may not change greatly by decade during adult life. This incidence rate is probably somewhat lower than in school-age children. Vinke, et al (1958) classified their cases (2,112) into two classes, *diabete gras* and *diabete maigre*. Criteria of classification were incompletely defined, but in general those with *diabete gras* were fat and insulin independent, and those with *diabete maigre* were lean and insulin dependent. All cases were at least 13 years of age. The prevalence of *diabete maigre* varied little with age, although it was somewhat more common in the seventh decade. About half of the males and one fifth of the females were deemed to have *diabete maigre*. All cases below 30 years of age had *diabete miagre*. In the middle aged and elderly of affluent societies the incidence of insulin-independent diabetes is several times greater than that of insulin-dependent diabetes. It is quite evident, however, that this ratio is greatly influenced by environmental factors. In societies where obesity is rare, a much greater portion of adult-onset cases are insulin dependent even though their number is probably smaller. In most circumstances the number who take insulin is much greater than the number who would *need* insulin with optimal long-term diet therapy.

Interpopulation comparisons are made very difficult because the portion who take insulin is such a poor index of the number who are truly insulin-dependent in the sense that the term is usually applied. Moreover, the level of this disparity is highly variable. In some circumstances many patients with generous levels of endogenous insulin are also given insulin therapy because of hyperglycemia attributable to excessive caloric intake. In other circumstances such patients are given oral antidiabetic agents. Lean persons with mild hyperglycemia are sometimes given insulin, sometimes oral agents, and sometimes neither. Counts have been made in many groups of diabetics concerning the number who take insulin. But these reports seldom include enough supporting data to permit estimates of how many of those taking insulin are truly insulin dependent. Also, there are often appreciable numbers of insulin-dependent patients among those not taking insulin. In the survey of the US National Center for Health Statistics it was found that 28% of all diabetics took insulin (Bauer, 1967). Rough extrapolations from those data suggest that about

313

24% of adult-onset cases were taking insulin. The portion taking insulin was considerably greater prior to introduction of oral agents. One of the few studies of a representative group of diabetics was that of Silwer (1958) in Kristianstad, Sweden. These data were gathered before the introduction of oral agents. About two thirds of adult-onset cases were then taking insulin. In the relative corpulent Western societies there is a sharp decline in the fifth decade in the percentage of all diabetics who require insulin. After that time there appears to be a further but more gradual decline in the percentage taking insulin (Silwer, 1958). It is not yet clear whether this represents a decline in the incidence of insulin-dependent diabetes or only a rise in the prevalence of insulin-independent diabetics. Among other factors that affect this ratio of insulin takers to all diabetics are the number in whom diabetes grows worse, and the disinclination of physicians to give insulin in older subjects. Nilsson, et al (1967) showed that the portion requiring insulin increased with duration of diabetes.

Levels of endogenous serum insulin have not been reported in a representative group of diabetics taking insulin, nor in a representative group not taking insulin. In the absence of these or other data it is not possible to estimate with precision what percentage of diabetics taking insulin are truly insulin-dependent. The problem of defining insulin-dependence is discussed further in Chapter 1.

Another difficulty of classification is that persons who were fat before the discovery of diabetes may lose sufficient weight to change their classification from "obese" to "nonobese." One method of taking this into account is to measure and analyze using both current weight and lifetime maximum weight. The latter can be estimated with a moderate degree of accuracy in some populations, but with only mediocre precision in others.

Even with all these problems of obtaining optimum data, it would be highly desirable to have more systematic observations on the characteristics of the universe of adult-onset diabetics. Key data include age of onset or of diagnosis; present and previous fatness; level of glycemia with and without therapy; type of therapy including dosage of insulin, family history of diabetes, and type of diabetes; and fatness of family members with diabetes. More observations are needed of the kind made by Köbberling (1971). He measured fatness systematically in a large group of diabetics. He found a strongly inverse relationship between fatness of the diabetic probands and risk of diabetes in their siblings. More data are also needed in which rates of various complications are compared for the different types of diabetics, with appropriate control of variables such as age, duration of diabetes, age of onset of diabetes, fatness, levels of blood glucose and lipids, among others. Most evidence suggests that increased risk of death is not as great in insulin-independent diabetes as in insulin-dependent diabetes. This is probably attributable to the lower degree of hyperglycemia, but evidence is quite incomplete in this respect. It has been argued, for example, that atherosclerosis may be enhanced by elevated levels of insulin (Mahler, 1973; Stout, 1973,1975). These matters are discussed in detail in Chapter 6 on mortality and in the section on vascular disease in Chapter 10.

Preliminary results in a small number of cases suggest that the frequency of certain histocompatibility antigens may be excessive in groups with adult-onset insulin-dependent diabetes, as it is in typical insulin-dependent diabetes with onset in childhood. The frequency of these antigens is not excessive in typical maturity-onset insulin-independent diabetes of the obese. More data are needed to confirm and extend these preliminary observations in insulin-dependent adult-onset diabetes (Cudworth and Woodrow, 1976). Irvine (1977) and others have shown that islet-cell antibodies are present much more frequently in insulin-dependent than in insulin-independent diabetes.

MILD DIABETES WITH ONSET IN YOUTH

There are several distinct types of mild diabetes with onset in youth. Some of these persons are fat, some have specific genetic syndromes (Rimoin and Schimke, 1971), some are lean with no family history of diabetes, some have hyperinsulinism (Drash, 1973), some have hypoinsulinism (Fajans, et al, 1976), and some have a family history of mild youth-onset diabetes (Tattersall, 1974). This heterogeneity of pathogenesis and expression has seldom been sufficiently appreciated. Attempts to simplify have led to use of the term *maturity-onset diabetes of youth* (MODY). The discussion below will stress the disadvantages of attempting to lump this group of disorders into one group under a single designation.

In 1928, Cammidge described cases of mild hyperglycemia with a familial background. He thought that the inheritance was of dominant type. These observations and conclusions received little attention in the subsequent thirty years. In 1960 Fajans and Conn presented evidence showing that abnormal glucose tolerance and mild fasting hyperglycemia were not as rare in the young as was generally believed. Fajans and his associates (1976) have subsequently studied 78 patients with onset of mild diabetes between the ages of 9 and 35. Twenty-nine of these have exhibited fasting blood glucose levels over 120 mg/100 ml, while the remainder have had "abnormal" glucose tolerance tests. Only 18 of 78 were obese. In general, the nonobese had low serum insulin levels. Follow-up studies have been performed for at least several years in most, in one case for twenty-two years. Only a few subjects have exhibited decompensation to ketosis-prone diabetes; none of this latter subgroup had elevated serum insulin levels at the time of first testing. Johansen (1973a) also found that young latent diabetics who later developed dependence on insulin had initially exhibited low or delayed secretion of endogenous insulin when challenged with glucose.

Mild Youth-Onset Diabetes with Dominant Heredity

Tattersall (1974) presented strong evidence that his cases of youth-onset mild diabetes were primarily the result of a dominant genetic trait. He described detailed data on the families. Of 69 offspring each of whom had a mildly diabetic parent, 33 were diabetic and 36 were nondiabetic. In these families, diabetes was almost always mild, and onset usually occurred in the second or third decade of life. Twenty-three of the cases with onset under 30 years of age were studied in some detail. Despite onset in youth, severe ketosis was never observed. Insulin secretion was measured in four cases, in each of whom secretion was subnormal but present. Many of these cases were followed for years or decades with no evidence of further decompensation of beta-cell function.

Johansen and Gregersen (1977) described a family in which mild diabetes appeared to be inherited by a dominant mechanism.

In both the cases of Tattersall (1974) and of Fajans, et al (1976), vascular complications were infrequent, even with diabetes of long duration. Retinopathy was present in only 5 of 12 long-duration cases of Tattersall (all ages), despite an average duration of known diabetes averaging thirty-seven years. Fourteen of the cases with onset before 30 years of age had retinal examinations. Average duration of diabetes was twenty-four years. Only two had retinopathy. None of Tattersall's cases had proteinuria.

In 77 of the patients of Fajans, et al (1976), muscle biopsies were performed to determine status of the capillary basement membranes. Approximately 25% had membranes that were considered abnormally thick. Large-vessel disease had also been uncommon in patients with this disorder. None of the patients of Tattersall had died of vascular disease.

The reasons for this immunity to the vascular lesions of diabetes are not known. One possibility is the mildness of the hyperglycemia. Some of the patients of Tattersall also had renal glycosuria, a trait that would also tend to lower blood glucose levels.

Character, Prevalence, and Heterogeneity of Mild Youth-Onset Diabetes

The frequency of mild hyperglycemia with onset in youth is not well established in any population. The rate would be very greatly affected by criteria of definition. If only cases with fasting hyperglycemia were included, rates for this condition would probably be less than 1 per 1,000 in the second decade. If, on the other hand, the criterion is the result of glucose tolerance above the two standard-deviation range, the rate would be about 22 per 1,000. The very great disparity between the numbers of children and young adults with "abnormal" tolerance and the number of young adults with fasting hyperglycemia suggests that only a small minority of the subjects with "abnormal" glucose tolerance and normal fasting glucose levels will develop fasting hyperglycemia and the syndrome described by Tattersall (1974). It is not yet known what portion of those who later develop this syndrome of Tattersall (1974) are drawn from those who have normal glucose tolerance in most or all of childhood, and what percentage are drawn from the group of children described by Fajans and Conn (1960), who have "abnormal" tolerance but normal fasting hyperglycemia.

316

Priscilla White (1974) had also found "abnormal" glucose tolerance to be very common in children of diabetic parents. This rate (23% of children of diabetic mothers) is probably about ten times greater than the number who will develop typical juvenile diabetes, and probably more than 100 times as great as the number who may be expected to develop the specific syndrome of Tattersall. Although siblings and offspring of youth-onset diabetes develop juvenile diabetes much more frequently than controls, in most studies rates have been less than 5%. For example, Farquhar (1969) found only two cases of diabetes in 260 children of mothers who had diabetes at delivery, despite follow-up periods as long as seventeen years. A substantial majority of these mothers had insulin-dependent diabetes. Drash (1971) indicated that several investigators had determined rates of chemical diabetes in siblings of juvenile diabetics. Rates of "chemical diabetes" ranged from 15% to 35%. It is of importance that the parents of Tattersall's cases also had the very special type of diabetes described above. Thus, children and young adults with abnormal tolerance or mild fasting hyperglycemia are not likely to have this syndrome of Tattersall if their parent or parents have either of the more common types of diabetes. Nor is this syndrome likely in such children with no family history of diabetes. It is evident that there are multiple causes of the youth-onset mild fasting hyperglycemia that does not progress. It also seems very clear that there are multiple causes for mild abnormalities of glucose tolerance in childhood and youth (Fajans, et al, 1976). On the other hand, the cases of Tattersall (1974) with fasting hyperglycemia regularly had a family history of this type of diabetes. The frequency of this latter disorder would be increased by more widespread testing of blood glucose levels in children and young adults, but in older adults who are more frequently tested the syndrome is also rather uncommon.

It is not clear yet whether rates of this special type of familial mild diabetes are similar in various populations. It is uncommon but not rare in England, the United States and Denmark (Johansen, 1973a). Mild diabetes has also been observed in the second and third decades of life in other societies, including Japan and India, but it is not known whether these cases are of the same etiologic type as those observed in the West. Data on family history are sparse except for the white groups that have been studied (Tattersall and Fajans, 1975). Data are often available on rates of family history of diabetes, but only rarely on the particular type of diabetes in the family member.

One very crude way to estimate the rate of mild diabetes with onset in youth is to determine among young diabetics the portion of cases who do not take insulin. Such figures must be interpreted with caution. Many of such cases are typical juvenile diabetics in the early stages. Also, as pointed out by Tattersall, insulin is not infrequently given to cases with mild hyperglycemia. The portion of youthful diabetics on insulin varies widely. Of the 147 juvenile diabetics studied in Stockholm by Sterky (1963), all were taking insulin. Of 39 school-age diabetics in North Hamptonshire, England, all 39 were taking insulin (Beardmore and Reid, 1966). In the National Health Survey of 1964–1965 (Bauer, 1967), only 73.2% of the diabetics under 25 years of age were

317

reported to be taking insulin. This ascertainment was by questionnaire method with interview of the diabetic or members of his household. It is quite possible that the actual rate of insulin administration is somewhat higher. In a survey of 2,816 Michigan schoolchildren with diabetes by questionnaire method answered by school personnel, 15.5% were reported not to be taking insulin (Gorwitz, et al, 1976). In 6.3% no information was provided on insulin therapy, and in 8.9% the respondent said he was unable to ascertain this information. In 69.3% the child was reported to be taking insulin. Wadsworth and Jarrett (1974) did a follow-up study to age 26 in a cohort of 5,362 British children. Only one was found to have diabetes while still in school but by age 26, 15 more were found to have diabetes. Of these 15, 14 were found to be diabetic in some kind of screening program. Eight of the 16 were taking insulin at age 26.

The subject of "chemical diabetes" in childhood was reviewed in detail at a 1971 conference. The results presented were summarized by Rosenbloom, et al (1973). As explained above the group of children with "chemical diabetes" are a very heterogeneous group with respect to adiposity, serum insulin and glucose levels, genetic make-up, etc. Rosenbloom summarized results of follow-up of varying duration (one to seventeen years) by nine different investigators in children with "chemical diabetes". Twenty-one of 198 had later developed "overt diabetes mellitus". Among the different investigators, the rate of progression from "chemical diabetes" to "overt diabetes" ranged from zero to 100%.

Drash (1973) studied asymptomatic children with abnormal glucose tolerance. He found that their blood insulin levels were as high as or higher than controls despite the absence of obesity. But in proportion to the levels of glycemia, the insulin levels appeared to be similar to those of controls. Results of Rosenbloom (1973) were similar to those of Drash in asymptomatic children with abnormal glucose tolerance. On the other hand, most of the cases of Fajans, et al (1976) had insulin levels that were low in relation to plasma glucose levels, although some were normal or high.

It is not clear whether oral medications or *qualitative* dietary changes prevent progression of mild hyperglycemia in lean youthful patients (Rosenbloom, 1973). In general, results are unimpressive with these two approaches. Insulin therapy frequently produces remissions in patients with typical juvenile diabetes, but few data are available concerning its effect on mild hyperglycemia with onset in youth. Not much is known of the natural history of mild hyperglycemia in obese children. It does appear that children with normal fasting glucose levels and abnormal glucose tolerance tests seldom develop severe diabetes rapidly (Fajans, et al, 1976).

The problem of standardization of methods and criteria for testing and evaluating glucose tolerance is discussed in Chapter 5 on diagnostic methods. Many of the children thought to have mild abnormalities of glucose tolerance are probably normal. This is because some criteria have classified tests outside the range of two standard deviations as abnormal. This latter method of assigning normal range rests on the dubious assumption that about 2% of children have occult diabetes. Another problem is that the reproducibility of results with such tests is not very good. In children with "abnormal" glucose tolerance and normal fasting blood glucose values the risk of developing clinically significant diabetes is not known.

Need for Standardization of Definitions and Nomenclature

Tattersall in his report of 1974 called his syndrome "mild familial diabetes with dominant inheritance". The term most commonly used for mild hyperglycemia with onset in youth is one that has been applied by Fajans and his associates, who included Tattersall (Fajans, et al, 1976). It is maturity-onset diabetes of youth (MODY). Various objections could be raised to this or to alternative suggestions. The designation "maturity-onset" tends to suggest that such patients are characteristically fat and hyperinsulinemic, but they are usually not obese and most are not hyperinsulinemic (Fajans, et al, 1976; Johansen, 1973a). Another problem is that cases in the MODY group are of mixed etiology and character. Arguments could be made for using the term "youth-onset mild hyperglycemia" to designate the entire group of types that in the beginning exhibit mild hyperglycemia.

Those patients that also have specific features described by Tattersall (1974) deserve a separate designation. These special manifestations include evidence of this same type of diabetes in family members, nonprogression of the degree of hyperglycemia, as well as absence of a susceptibility to ketosis. The original title presented by Tattersall in 1974 does not include allusion to the propensity for onset in youth, although he made this clear in his description. One reason for this was that occasionally this type of diabetes was not discovered until the fourth or fifth decade of life. Another problem of nomenclature is that there may be other types of diabetes with dominant inheritance. The several possibilities of designation do not appear to include any brief title that is adequately descriptive. Among the more cumbersome designations that would include the basic elements of the disorder described by Tattersall would be "mild nonprogressive youth-onset diabetes with dominant inheritance". These difficulties suggest alternatives such as Tattersall syndrome, Cammidge-Tattersall syndrome, Tattersall-Fajans syndrome, etc. Pyke (1977) has used the designation "Mason diabetes", because the first family studied by Tattersall have this name.

Of crucial importance is the mitigation of confusion that has risen and is likely to arise when the following designations are used without definition or standardization of definition: *chemical diabetes, youth, mild, hyperglycemia, maturity-onset, obese, abnormal glucose tolerance, family history, clinical diabetes, ketosis, latent diabetes.* Even if international agreements cannot be reached on such definitions, the interpretation and value of reports will be greatly enhanced if each author describes specifically what he means by each of the above terms. The recent report of Fajans, et al (1976) is a good model in several of these respects. It was made clear how many cases had fasting hyperglycemia and how many had abnormal tolerance, and to what degree; the ages of discovery were indicated and obesity defined; specific supplemental information was given on factors such as serum insulin, subsequent ketosis, duration of follow-up, type of treatment. Of particular importance in such reports is the separation of those with and without fasting hyperglycemia. A definition of fasting hyperglycemia is also desirable. Unfortunately, few data are available on the frequency distribution of the fasting blood glucose in *general* populations either in children or adults. As pointed out previously, information has rarely been given on type of diabetes in family members. This is quite important.

Fajans, et al (1976) have proposed a working classification of youth-onset diabetes into Types I, II, and III, and have set forth criteria for attempting these delineations. They admit several problems in identifying and classifying certain of these patients, particularly at the time of onset. Essentially, Type I includes persons who are typical juvenile diabetics. Those designated Type II have the special features described by Tattersall (1974), and those with Type III require insulin but are not ketosis-prone and do not have relatives with youth-onset mild hyperglycemia. It may be kept in mind that there are still other types of youth-onset diabetes, including the J-type of ketosis-resistant patients with both moderate and with severe hyperglycemia, cases with calcification of the pancreas, obese children with mild hyperglycemia, those with other genetic syndromes, cystic fibrosis of the pancreas, etc. Some lean children with mild diabetes have low serum insulin and in some insulin levels are normal or high, even though clinical manifestations are similar. It is probably a mistake to try to combine etiologic, biochemical, and clinical parameters in a general classification scheme, even though there is some degree of correspondence in these. For example, those patients with the syndrome of Tattersall do indeed regularly have mild diabetes, low insulin levels, and relatives with a similar condition. But there are several other causes of low insulin levels, and several other causes of mild diabetes. Moreover, these various factors used in definition often change with stages of the disease (eg, serum insulin levels, requirement for insulin, severity of hyperglycemia). Classification is also made more difficult by our incomplete knowledge of the strength and character of the relationships between these various factors.

Below is a classification of youth-onset diabetes. Acquisition of additional knowledge will doubtless alter this scheme considerably, making it in some respects simpler and in other respects more complex.

1. *Typical juvenile diabetes:* severe glycemia, ketosis-prone, insulin-dependent, usually lean; manifestations may be milder in the early stages of this disease

2. *Syndrome of Tattersall:* familial (dominant) nonprogressive mild hyperglycemia

3. *Other mild hyperglycemias*

   a. Obese or lean

   b. Hyperinsulinemic, hypoinsulinemic, or normoinsulinemic

   c. With or without fasting hyperglycemia

   d. With or without other hereditary stigmata (eg, cystic fibrosis)

   e. With or without a family history of typical juvenile or typical maturity-onset diabetes

4. *Malnutrition diabetes:* extremely lean, typically from very poor families

   a. Pancreatic fibrosis-calcification syndrome, usually resistant to insulin and to ketosis but not always. Onset of diabetes usually in second or third decade; usually extremely lean

   b. Without evident pancreatic fibrosis or calcification
     J-type diabetes (resistant to insulin and to ketosis)
     Other types (ketosis-prone, insulin-independent, insulin-dependent but not insulin-resistant)

5. *Transient neonatal hyperglycemia*

6. *Congenital absence of the pancreas* (very rare)

J-TYPE DIABETES AND OTHER KETOSIS-RESISTANT, INSULIN-DEPENDENT TYPES

In 1955 Hugh-Jones reported from Jamaica that, of a consecutive series of 215 diabetics, 13 had a peculiar type of diabetes. They required high dosages of insulin but were resistant to ketosis. With few exceptions these cases were quite lean, and onset of diabetes had occurred between the ages of 10 and 40. Hugh-Jones selected the designation "J-type" for such cases (for Jamaica). This nomenclature has since gained rather general acceptance, despite the unfortunate and confusing correspondence of the letter J in both Jamaica and juvenile. Far better designations would have included "H" for Hugh-Jones, "T" for tropical, or "M" for malnutrition (see below).

In an addendum to his report, Hugh-Jones mentioned personal communications to him of descriptions of such cases from Malaya and Nigeria. Subsequently, there have been many additional reports of this syndrome from widely scattered parts of the tropics (Tulloch and McIntosh, 1961), including Indonesia, Ghana, South Africa, Fiji, Congo, Brunei, New Guinea, Kenya, Tanganyika, and Nyasaland. More recently such cases have been described in Pakistan (Ibrahim, 1962), and extensive experiences with this condition have been recorded in India (Ahuja, et al, 1965; Patel and Talwalker, 1966; Kar and Tripathy, 1967).

A standard definition has not been developed for the syndrome. This has produced some difficulties. Tulloch and McIntosh (1961) found in Jamaica that many of the "insulin-resistant cases" described by Hugh-Jones were not really a peculiar type of diabetes. Rather, they were very poorly treated cases of an ordinary type. This led Tulloch and McIntosh to question the existence of a truly peculiar type of diabetes. Also, Campbell (1960) reported from South Africa that most of the cases thought originally to be of the J-type were responsive to oral agents and not really insulin-dependent. In Uganda, Shaper (1958) noted that some of the insulin-dependent cases resistant to ketosis did not require large dosages of insulin. In at least some of the groups of diabetics in the tropics, a portion of the patients resistant to insulin or to ketosis, or both, were not exceptionally lean. It also became apparent that in some groups, a portion of J-type patients had calcification or fibrosis of the pancreas (Zuidema, 1959; Geevarghese, 1968). Finally, in tropical societies and elsewhere, both lean and well-fed diabetics were found who exhibited no ketosis despite severe hyperglycemia (hyperosmolar nonketotic coma). And this latter condition has been observed in both youth-onset and maturity-onset diabetes.

It is therefore apparent that considerable heterogeneity exists with respect to the background of all of the features described by Hugh-Jones (ketone resistance, insulin resistance, age of onset, and degree of leanness). On the other hand, experience subsequent to 1955 does suggest grounds for designation of at least one special type of diabetes. These cases have four striking features that occur together with sufficient frequency to warrant designation as a specific type: resistance to ketosis, resistance to insulin, extreme leanness (probably with marked underfeeding in infancy and childhood, and onset of diabetes in youth (usually between the ages of 15 and 40). There are two possibilities concerning future nomenclature. Using the term J-type diabetes would have advantages but also two disadvantages. One, cited above, is the potential for confusion because J suggests both Jamaica and juvenile. Another problem is that the syndrome described immediately above is defined somewhat differently than the original description of Hugh-Jones. An alternate designation might be "ketosis-resistant diabetes associated with childhood malnutrition," or KR-M, or simply M (for malnutrition).

Ketosis-prone diabetes does occur in societies where infant malnutrition is rife. Moreover, well-fed persons may have resistance to both insulin and ketosis. But the association is very striking between severe childhood malnutrition and the portion of youth-onset diabetics who are insensitive to insulin and resistant to ketosis. Ahuja, et al (1965) found that many young Indians with insulin-dependent diabetes remained free of ketosis even after withdrawal of insulin for one to four weeks. These investigators also demonstrated resistance to insulin in a large subgroup of such patients. Tripathy, et al (1976) studied in Cuttack, India, the frequency of resistance to ketosis in two groups with youth-onset diabetes. In one group, all subjects were extremely lean (weight less than 76% of standard). Resistance to ketosis was common (35%) in this group. In those with higher relative body weight, resistance to ketosis was rare (0.7%). Most of the later group were also lean, but none was extremely lean. In the study of Vaishnava, et al (1974) in northern India, almost half of insulin-dependent diabetics with onset prior to age 40 were resistant to ketosis. Of these 903 ketosis-resistant patients, 91.4% were asthenic (underweight) and 95% were poor. In the same series only 36% of the ketosis-prone patients were poor by these standards, and only 32% of the insulin-independent diabetics were poor. Studies in a group of ten ketosis-resistant cases showed a striking depression of the usual rise in free fatty acids when epinephrine was administered. This defect was also reported by Malik, et al (1974) and by Hagroo, et al (1974).

A family history of diabetes was observed in only 3.3% of the ketosis-resistant cases of Vaishnava, et al (1974). Both Hugh-Jones and Campbell (1960) had reported a high rate of positive family history in "J-type" diabetics. But Campbell's group of cases were quite different in some respects from the syndrome described above. For example, most of his cases were not insulin-dependent. As mentioned earlier, the group of Hugh-Jones now appears to have been heterogeneous. Kar and Tripathy (1967) found a positive family history of diabetes in only 1 of 31 malnourished diabetics with onset in youth who were resistant to ketosis and insulin. Moses and Ghandi (1973) reported that only 15% of their Indian diabetics with onset under 30 years of age were ketosis-prone!

As pointed out by Kar and Tripathy (1967), several groups of such patients have contained an excess of males. But in most urban centers in the tropics the number of young women available for examination is often relatively small. It is, therefore, difficult to determine the extent to which the excess of male diabetics is real. It might be significant that females tend to have a somewhat greater amount of body fat.

In the group of Kar and Tripathy, 39.7% of young insulin-dependent diabetics were ketosis resistant. Average insulin requirement was 97.5 units daily despite the very small body mass in these ketosis-resistant diabetics. In this study, diabetes resistant to insulin and ketosis was most common when discovery of diabetes occurred between ages 15 and 25. In an earlier report on diabetes in the very poor, Tripathy and Kar (1966) showed a very impressive peak in the incidence of diabetes in early adult life, with substantially lower rates after age 25 and very low rates prior to age 15. Almost all those with onset during this peak (ages 15–25) had diabetes resistant to insulin and to ketosis. Only one of these cases had pancreatic calcification; and calcification was also uncommon in the group of Vaishnava et al, (1974). On the other hand, resistance to insulin and to ketosis is common in youth-onset diabetes with calcification (Geevarghese, 1968). In regions where calcification is common it is possible that some of those without demonstrable calcification do have extensive pancreatic fibrosis. It does not seem likely, however, that pancreatic fibrosis is fundamental in the etiology of the resistance to ketosis and insulin.

It appears likely that undernourishment in youth or early childhood (or both) leads to physiologic changes that account for the time of onset and three cardinal features: diabetes, insensitivity to insulin, and resistance to ketosis. The studies of Vaishnava, et al (1974,1976) have provided useful insights concerning one aspect of this peculiar syndrome. The fat cells are unresponsive to a stimulus that usually incites release of the free fatty acids, the building blocks for ketones. Other studies of this kind are needed. Qualitative features of diet may be of some significance. Tulloch and McIntosh (1961) produced ketosis by feeding fat in three J-type diabetics. Snapper (1941) reviewed evidence indicating that vegetable fat was less ketogenic than animal fat. In the environments in which this syndrome is common, diets are usually low in calories and fats, and a majority of fat is usually of vegetable origin. Ketosis has also been rare in Eskimos whose dietary fats are highly unsaturated. Do long-term differences in amounts or character of dietary fat affect the capacity of fat cells to respond to ketogenic stimuli? Present data do not exclude this possibility, but it is also possible that the aberrations are due to other dietary factors such as calorie or protein deprivation, either at the time fat cells are developing or later. In diabetic hamsters propensity to ketosis is greatly inhibited by isocaloric low-fat diets (Gerritsen, 1976).

It would also be of interest to know whether these cases have as much glucagonemia as typical cases of juvenile diabetes. Low levels of glucagon would probably tend to protect from ketosis (Schade and Eaton, 1975). However, Barnes, et al (1975) found no correlation between glucagon levels and ketone levels in a group of British insulin-dependent cases.

Conceivably alpha-cell function might be impaired by malnutrition or by previous malnutrition. Malnutrition could also produce peculiarities of liver function. The liver is a major site of action of insulin. It would be interesting to know more about the sensitivity of liver, muscle, and fat to the various functions of insulin in the ketosis-resistant cases. Hugh-Jones found liver tissue normal on biopsy of three of his J-type cases, and Tulloch and McIntosh (1961) reported eight negative biopsies. The latter authors also reported normal glycemic response to glucagon injections in J diabetics. They also thought insulin binding and insulin-disappearance time were, in these cases, similar to those in other types of insulin-dependent diabetes. Alford, et al (1970) found growth-hormone levels normal in six J-type diabetics. Data on levels of serum insulin in this syndrome are contradictory (Krishna Ram, 1976). The mechanisms for resistance to insulin and to ketosis remain to be established. Krishna Ram (1976) has reviewed the present status of knowledge on this subject.

It should also be kept in mind that the relative frequency of a certain type of diabetes within a group of diabetics does not necessarily reflect well its prevalence in the total population. Suppose, for example, that the rate of insulin-dependent ketosis-resistant diabetes was the same in two communities. Suppose further that typical ketosis-prone diabetes was ten times more prevalent in one of these populations. In these circumstances the ratio of ketosis-prone cases to ketosis-resistant cases might be 10:1 in one population and 1:1 in the other despite an identical prevalence of ketosis-resistant cases in the two general populations. Typical ketosis-prone juvenile diabetes appears to be uncommon in most, if not all, of the underfed societies in which ketosis-resistant cases constitute a substantial portion of insulin-dependent cases.

DISEASES OF THE EXOCRINE PANCREAS

Pancreatic Calcification and Fibrosis

In most societies pancreatic calcification is uncommon, even in diabetics. Calcification of the pancreas is usually largely confined to the small portion of diabetics in whom diabetes is secondary to severe chronic relapsing pancreatitis. These are often alcoholic men of middle age. But in a few poor societies, calcification of the pancreas is common in adolescents and young adults. Indeed, in some geographic areas a substantial portion of all diabetics have demonstrable pancreatic calcification.

Cases of pancreatic calcification had been reported from India as early as 1937 (Kini). In 1954 Elizabeth and Stephen reported from Vellore on nine cases observed at autopsy. Five of these had died before age 30 and one had had known diabetes. The first clear description of the syndrome of calcification and diabetes was published by Zuidema in 1955. This classic paper described seven young Indonesian patients with pancreatic calcification. Six were discovered in a single year, and of the seven, six had diabetes. The first of these seven cases had been discovered in 1939 by a Professor Bonne at autopsy in a 19-year-old girl with severe diabetes of brief duration. The sudden increase in the number of such cases in this Bethesda Hospital of Jakarta appeared to coincide with the employment of roentgenography of the pancreas as a common procedure in young diabetics. Zuidema also noted that adolescents and young adults constituted an unusually large segment of the population of diabetics in Java. The age at discovery of calcification ranged from 15 to 28. None consumed alcohol; all had diffuse calcification; three were females and four were males. Symptoms, signs, and laboratory evidence of insufficiency of pancreatic exocrine function were minimal, and biliary disease was not observed. Only one complained of abdominal pain. Insulin requirements were high, and in the absence of therapy blood glucose levels were very high. There was, however, little tendency to ketosis. Emaciation was severe. Weights were recorded in five patients, and ranged from 57 to 74 lb! In some cases a hard pancreatic mass was palpated. All were poor and gave histories of diets deficient in protein.

Zuidema also studied six other young diabetic patients with features very similar to those with pancreatic calcification. Although these patients did not have pancreatic calcification, all had some evidence of insufficiency of pancreatic exocrine function and low levels of duodenal lipase. Zuidema concluded that most cases of diabetes in young poor Javanese were probably the result of pancreatic disease of which calcification was the end stage.

Three of the six diabetics with calcification had enlargement of the parotid glands, a finding that has been observed in many areas of the world where nutrition is very poor (Pitchumoni, 1973). A subsequent report by Zuidema (1959) included 45 patients from 12 to 45 years of age with evidence of pancreatic disease of whom 18 had calcification, 43 diabetes, and 16 parotid enlargement. This group included six of the seven cases with calcifications that had been reported previously plus other cases encountered from 1953 to 1957. Changes in scalp hair were noted in 15. These hair abnormalities were similar to those in patients who have or have had protein deficiencies. There were 32 males and 13 females. Other features of these 45 cases and the 18 with calcification were much the same as in the smaller initial group. Bilateral cataracts were observed in 15 of these 43 young diabetics.

Since the first report of Zuidema in 1955, very similar cases have been observed commonly in several other widely separated societies. These have included Uganda (Shaper, 1960), the Congo (Bourgoignie, 1962), southern India (Geevarghese, et al, 1962), Nigeria (Kinnear, 1963; Olurin and Olurin, 1969), Madagascar (Merlihot, 1963), and Ceylon (Rajasuriya, et al, 1970). Pancreatic calcification has also been observed with significant frequency in diabetics of Malawi (Goodall and Pilbeam, 1964) and in Singapore (Fung, et al, 1970). Kinnear (1963) found pancreatic calcification in 75% of Nigerian juvenile-onset cases. It is now evident, however, that these high rates of pancreatic calcification in young diabetic adults are not typical even in very poor societies. In an extensive experience with South African black diabetics, Seftel (1964a) had not observed any such cases. Tulloch (1962) observed pancreatic lithiasis only occasionally in Jamaica. Wicks and Jones (1974) found that pancreatic disease was not uncommon in Rhodesian black diabetics, but pancreatic calcification was rare. In Rhodesia only 1% of African diabetics had pancreatic calcification (Gelfand and Forbes, 1963). Calcification was also rare in Senegal (Sankale, et al, 1970). Only 1 of 37 black diabetics in Tanzania had roentgenographic evidence of calcification (Haddock, 1964). In young Indian diabetics calcification of the pancreas is common in Cuttack, Madras, and Hyderabad (Sathe, 1973), and extremely common in the state of Kerala (Geevarghese, 1968), but much less common in other parts of India (Geevarghese, 1968). In New Delhi, Vaishnava, et al (1974) found evidence of pancreatic calcification in only 2 of 84 young diabetics. Campbell and McNeil (1958) reported only one case of pancreatic lithiasis among 405 Indian and black diabetics seen in Durban, South Africa.

Knowledge of this condition has been extended by the reports of Geevarghese, described below, including his book of 1968, in which he describes 400 such cases in Kerala state of India. In a recent abstract (1976), he alludes to 1,080 cases!

Although epidemiologic data are quite incomplete, it appears that degree of undernutrition is not the sole determinant of risk of pancreatic fibrosis and calcification. Geevarghese, et al (1969) believe that nutritional deprivations, including protein deficiency, have been at least as great in certain parts of India, where calcification is less common, as in Kerala where it is rife. Association between consumption of cassava (manioc, manihot, or tapioca) and rates of pancreatic calcification is very impressive. Cassava is consumed in generous amounts by all populations in which high rates of calcification have been reported. McGlashan (1967) studied this association in Central Africa where cassava consumption is highly variable. Among populations served by hospitals in which diabetes was rare only 2 of 32 groups were cassava eaters. But half (12 of 24) of the populations served by hospitals in which diabetes was common were cassava eaters.

Cassava is very poor in protein, lacks essential sulfur-containing amino acids, and may contain pancreatic toxins (Banwell, et al, 1967; Geevarghese, 1968; Terra, 1964; Pitchumoni, 1973). Hydrocyanic acid is concentrated in the outer skin of the cassava tuber. Methods of preparation and cooking affect the chemical composition, as do other factors such as part of the plant consumed, its age, type of cassava, soil, and climate (Terra, 1964). Typically, tapioca consumed has only about 0.4% protein, of relatively poor quality. Susceptibility to pancreatic toxins is in some circumstances influenced by nutritional status. Hydrocyanic acid is detoxified by the enzyme rhodenase in the presence of sulfur-containing amino acids. Quite possibly, low levels of these amino acids could increase susceptibility to a toxin in cassava. Pitchumoni (1973) has published an excellent review of nutritional factors in pancreatic disease. Other toxic effects of cassava have been demonstrated in animals and man (Montgomery, 1965; Osuntokun, 1970). These include neuropathy in man. Chandraprasert, et al (1976) recently described six typical cases of this syndrome in Thailand, but no information was given concerning cassava consumption. Cassava is produced in Thailand, but little is eaten by some elements of the population.

Secretion of insulin is impaired in both children and adults by protein-calorie malnutrition (Smith, et al, 1975; Pitchumoni, 1973), but, as pointed out above, it seems likely that additional factors such as toxicity are required to produce pancreatic calcification. Because of the very close association between cassava consumption and protein malnutrition, it has been difficult to determine whether in man cassava consumption can produce pancreatic disease in the absence of protein deficits. Also, it is difficult to find populations where protein makes up so small a percentage of the diet, as in societies that consume high levels of cassava. Even in populations that consume very low levels of protein, the quality of protein is likely to be better than that of cassava. Further study is needed. Circumstances in India and Uganda are well suited to such investigations.

Zuidema (1959) presented evidence that in Indonesia fibrosis is associated with calcification and precedes it. This has been confirmed elsewhere in areas where calcification is common. In Kampala, Uganda, Parson, et al (1968) found extensive pancreatic fibrosis in 17 of 56 consecutive autopsies of diabetics. Calcifications were often present when fibrosis was advanced. Pancreatic fibrosis was noted in 8.2% of all autopsies (78 of 955), but only 7 of these 78 had massive fibrosis with calculi, Pancreatic fibrosis is also common in cases of starvation, kwashiorkor, and cirrhosis. In the same institution, Banwell, et al (1963) studied a typical group of 30 African diabetics from 15 to 60 years of age. Twelve had calcification of the pancreas and eight more had impressive evidence of impairment of exocrine function. In comparison with diabetics without disease of the exocrine pancreas, the diabetics with pancreatic disease had more frequently: abdominal pain, parotid enlargement, skin changes, hair changes, bulky stools, stool fat of more than 8 gm daily, abnormalities of duodenal mucosa on biopsy, impairment of D-xylose excretion, abnormal secretin-pancreozymin tests, and emaciation. Sonnet, et al (1966) studied 20 Congolese diabetics who had pancreatic calcification, with similar results. They had found calcification in the roentgenograms of ten of a consecutive series of 75 African diabetics (15%). Control observations suggested that only 0.3% to 0.4% of the general population had such calcifications. They had one case in which small calcifications were found at autopsy despite a previously normal roentgenogram. From this and other evidence it is clear that a small degree of calcification is frequently not apparent with x-ray examination. Studies of the liver in this and other series showed varying degrees of biochemical and morphologic dysfunction. It does not appear, however, that liver dysfunction plays a major etiologic role in the pathogenesis of this disorder. A substantial percentage have liver function that is normal or near normal. In some of these societies (eg, Uganda) alcohol consumption may contribute significantly to the development of this syndrome, but in none of these areas does alcohol consumption appear to play a major etiologic role.

Sonnet, et al (1966) pointed out that this kind of pancreatic dysfunction may increase iron absorption, and thereby further enhance pancreatic fibrosis. A majority of their African diabetics without calcification (10 of 16) also had evidence of dysfunction of the exocrine pancreas, while a control group from this population did not. These authors concluded that a majority of their Congolese cases of diabetes were probably secondary to pancreatic disease. Only one with pancreatic disease had marked steatorrhea, but 13 of 20 with pancreatic calcification had excessive stool fat detectable with microscopic techniques. In these populations with high rates of pancreatic disease dietary fat is typically quite low. In most, calorie consumption is also low. These factors may account, at least to some degree, for the mildness of the clinical manifestations of pancreatic exocrine dysfunction. George, et al (1971) studied exocrine function in 15 young Indian patients with pancreatic calcification. Protease and lipase secretion seemed to be more diminished than amylase secretion. Volume of pancreatic juice was markedly reduced but bicarbonate concentration was well preserved. George was impressed that this pattern of disturbed function was different from that usually seen with other types of pancreatic disease, such as the type of pancreatitis commonly seen in the West.

Sonnet, et al (1966) reported that acute hemorrhagic pancreatitis and typical chronic relapsing pancreatitis had not been observed in their Congolese. In the Congolese cases with pancreatic calcification, there was no evidence of familial aggregation. In the series of Geevarghese (400) there were seven families with two or more cases. In addition there were 14 other families in which a relative had evidence of either growth-onset diabetes or pancreatic calculi. Geevarghese was not certain whether this moderate degree of family aggregation was the result of genetic or environmental factors.

Typically about one third to one half of the diabetics with pancreatic calcification have painless parotid enlargement. The cause is unknown. Parotid enlargement has also been seen frequently in malnourished people without diabetes or evident pancreatic disease, as well as in cirrhosis. In some of the pancreatic diabetics of Geevarghese (1968) the enlargement subsided. In some of these, enlargement later returned. It was not clear whether improvement was related to therapy. Parotid biopsy in 12 cases showed increase in connective tissue in one, round-cell infiltration in three, and normal gland in the others. In eight patients with parotid enlargement, sialograms showed no enlargement of the ducts. Conceivably, it may be significant that both pancreatic and parotid cells secrete bicarbonate while the sublingual gland does not. The sublingual gland is apparently unaffected in this syndrome. Alappatt and Anathachari (1967) studied parotid enlargement in some detail in 23 Indian diabetics with pancreatic calcification. Studies of secretory activity and sialography were performed in all, and 14 parotids were biopsied. No qualitative peculiarities of secretion or morphology were observed. Findings were consistent only with functional and structural hypertrophy. Fain had noted an association of parotid enlargement and cassava consumption in 1947. Parotid enlargement has been observed occasionally in diabetics of populations in which pancreatic calcification does not appear to be endemic (eg, in Hong Kong; McFadzean and Yeung, 1968).

Levine, et al (1970) found parotid enlargement common in Pima Indians in whom diabetes and obesity were rife and pancreatic calcification rare. Lawrence, et al (1976) have reported that in rats and some other species the salivary glands contain measurable amounts of insulin and glucagon.

History of abdominal pain was not common in Indonesian diabetics with pancreatic calcification described by Zuidema (1959). In other populations abdominal pain has been common in such cases. This is especially so in the huge series of 400 cases reported by Geevarghese (1968) from the Kerala area in India. In his series 95% gave a history of abdominal pain. In addition to the 400 cases with calcification, Geevarghese has observed 115 other diabetics under the age of 30 with evidence of disease of the exocrine pancreas. Many of these complained of abdominal pain. In patients with calcification, onset of abdominal pain often antedated the discovery of diabetes or its symptoms by many years. Onset of pain in early childhood was common. Onset of pain was also frequent in each of the first four decades of life and rare thereafter. Occasionally pain began after the discovery of diabetes.

Zuidema (1955) was impressed with the resistance of these patients to insulin. All but 1 of 37 cases observed by Olirun and Olirun (1969) in Nigeria required insulin and "most of them needed high doses". On the other hand, it is now apparent that insulin requirements are frequently moderate in such patients. In the series of Geevarghese only 28% required more than 80 units. He did note a requirement of greater than 200 units in 7 of his 400 cases. He and others found that diabetes was often "brittle" and hypoglycemia common. Considering, however, that these are thin young diabetics, often treated in primitive conditions, it is not surprising that hypoglycemia is rather common. It is conceivable that destruction of glucagon-producing alpha cells could enhance susceptibility to hypoglycemia.

The reasons for the resistance to ketosis are not entirely clear. Among the possible contributing factors are the extremely small amounts of adipose tissue, the high-carbohydrate low-fat diets, and small residuals of endogenous insulin. Although reports subsequent to those of Zuidema have confirmed that most diabetics with this syndrome are not prone to ketosis, it is now clear that ketosis is not uncommon. It was very common in Uganda (Parson, et al, 1968). In India 18% of the cases of Geevarghese (1968) had ketosis. More data are needed, but in at least some of these geographic areas there does not seem to be much difference in propensity to ketosis between the group with this syndrome and age-matched diabetics without evident disease of the exocrine pancreas. In the series of Vaishnava (1974) from New Delhi, among all insulin-requiring diabetics with onset between ages 16 and 19, there were 150 ketone-resistant cases and 160 ketosis-prone patients. Calcification of the pancreas was rare in this population of diabetics.

This syndrome has been seen more commonly in males but sex ratios in the different series have varied substantially. Moreover, in at least some of these populations there is a considerable male dominance among all patients (diabetic and nondiabetic), particularly among young adults, In the Congo the ratio of males to females with this syndrome was 5:1 (Sonnet, et al, 1966). In Ceylon there were eight males and ten females among the group who were not alcoholic (Rajasriya, et al, 1970). The ratio observed by Geevarghese (1968) is typical (252 males and 148 females). It is interesting that the type of pancreatitis more commonly observed in the West is also more frequent in males. The basis of the relatively higher rates in males is not understood for either of these pancreatic diseases. Higher rates of alcoholism in males do not explain entirely their increased susceptibility to pancreatitis. Fibrosis-calcification syndrome occurs in a much younger age group than does pancreatitis. In the series of Geevarghese there was little difference in the numbers of males and females in cases with onset of diabetes in the first two decades. Among cases with later onset there were about twice as many males. To some degree, the latter difference may be due to the lesser propensity of adult Indian females to seek medical attention. It is also possible that young adult African female cases come to attention less frequently than males.

A peculiar cyanotic hue of the lips and face has been observed in cases of chronic pancreatitis. A similar discoloration was observed by Geevarghese (1968) in 22% of his Indian diabetics with pancreatic calcification. This was especially common in dehydrated patients.

Two of the cases of Parson, et al (1968) had microscopic evidence of glomerulosclerosis, and 7% of the cases of Geevarghese had proteinuria. "Retinal aneurysm" was observed in four of the cases of Geevarghese. It is not clear how many of his 400 cases had examinations of the retinae and how many had examinations for urine protein. Because of the relatively short duration of diabetes in all of the reported series, it is not possible to determine whether microvascular manifestations are as common as in diabetics without disease of the exocrine pancreas. It is clear, however, that microvascular lesions occur in such patients. Another problem is that cataract often precludes evaluation of the retinae in the small percentage of cases with duration of diabetes as long as ten years. In a series of autopsy cases from Uganda reported by Parson, et al (1968), none of 17 cases had had known diabetes as long as nine yars and only two had had known diabetes longer than three years. Causes of death were not significantly different in those with (17) and without (37) pancreatic fibrosis and calcification. Glomerulosclerosis was not more common in diabetics without pancreatic fibrosis and calcification (4 of 37) than in those with gross pancreatic lesions (2 of 17).

Both Geevarghese (1968) and Parson, et al (1968) were impressed with the rarity of atherosclerotic disease in patients with this syndrome. But coronary arteries were also unaffected in Parson's Ugandan diabetic cases without pancreatic fibrosis or calcification. None of the patients of Geevarghese had evidence of peripheral vascular disease. Among the factors that may account for the paucity of atherosclerotic disease are low-fat diet, impairment of fat absorption, youth, and short duration of diabetes.

Table 32 summarizes the characteristics of this syndrome, including some of its clinical, pathologic, biochemical, and epidemiologic features. No general agreement has been reached concerning definition and nomenclature. Among the possibilities are that a designation could be derived from its etiology, its pathology, its clinical expressions, or the name of the person or persons who have described it. Oridinarily etiologic or pathologic terms are preferable but there are problems here. Associations with protein malnutrition and cassava consumption are strong, but the roles of these and other etiologic factors are not yet clear. Although these cases regularly have pancreatic fibrosis followed by

TABLE 32   Syndrome of Zuidema (Pancreatic Fibrosis-Calcification and Youth-Onset Diabetes)—"Type Z" Diabetes

Characteristic	Frequency or Description
Pancreatic fibrosis	Probably in all cases
Pancreatic calcification	In advanced cases (probably 35% to 50% of those with overt diabetes)
Onset of pancreatic disease	Probably in childhood in most cases
Onset of symptoms of diabetes	10 to 50 years of age; peak onset 15–35
Abdominal pain	Frequently present
Other clinical manifestations of pancreatic exocrine dysfunction	Usually mild except for emaciation
Laboratory evidence of disturbed exocrine function	Present but often mild
Emaciation	Usually
Insulin required	Usually; often more than 60 units daily
Hyperglycemia	Moderate to severe
Resistance to ketosis	Most cases resistant but ketosis not rare
Susceptibility to hypoglycemia with insulin therapy	Common
Parotid enlargement	Common
Male:female ratio	Variable but averages about 1.5:1
History of protein deprivation in childhood	Common
Clinical signs of previous or present severe protein malnutrition	Common
History of cassava consumption	Very common
Alcholism	Not especially common
Biliary disease	Rare
Atherosclerosis	Rare
Neuropathies	Very common
Microvascular disease	Occasionally

calcification, similar pathologic changes are also seen in unrelated conditions leading to diabetes, such as chronic relapsing pancreatitis. Nor is any one of the clinical features of this syndrome sufficiently specific to stand alone as a short designation. One possible compromise is the term "Z-type diabetes" (after Zuidema). This would be consistent with a developing convention for using letters in describing other types of diabetes such as J-type of Hugh-Jones, ID for insulin-dependent, K-P for ketosis-prone. The shortest descriptive designation might be "diabetes with youth-onset pancreatic fibrosis or calcification". The disadvantages of that designation are acknowledged. All things considered, the designation "Z-type" appears preferable, at least until the pathophysiology is better understood.

In Durban, South Africa, Dayal, et al (1976) performed tests of endocrine and exocrine function in a series of 42 cases in whom pancreatic calcification had been found. The distribution of causes of calcification in this group probably differ from those in Kerala, India, and other places where the calcification syndrome accounts for a substantial portion of all diabetes. In Durban it was found that 28 of these 42 cases had diabetes, and there was a close correspondence between the degree of endocrine and exocrine insufficiency. In general, onset of diabetes occurs at a later age in cases of this type as compared to those described by Zuidema and Geevarghese.

Cancer of the Pancreas

Marble and Ramos (1971) have published a good summary of the interrelationship of diabetes and cancer of the pancreas. Cancer of the pancreas is not an important cause of diabetes in any society for three reasons: it is only moderately common, most of its victims do not become diabetic, and average life expectancy is short. The neoplastic lesion usually begins in and involves the head or body of the pancreas. The tail of the gland is rich in islets, so the unaffected portions of the gland are usually able to produce an adequate insulin supply. Nevertheless, data reviewed by Marble and Ramos (1971) suggest that cancer of the pancreas is roughly three times as common in diabetics as in nondiabetics. It does not seem likely that diabetes causes cancer of the pancreas. Rather, it would appear that cancer of the pancreas increases risk of diabetes, even though most persons with cancer of the pancreas do not become diabetic.

Pancreatitis and Other Disorders of the Exocrine Pancreas

A discussion of the etiology and manifestations of these disorders is beyond the scope of this book. Many other sources of detailed information are available. As pointed out by Verdonk, et al (1975) rates of diabetes in series of cases of pancreatitis have varied widely depending on many factors. Rates of diabetes have ranged from 2% to 18% in acute pancreatitis and from 25% to 48% in chronic pancreatitis. Rates of pancreatitis in groups of diabetics are even more variable. In most of the large series reported from the United States, those with clinically apparent pancreatitis account for less than 2% of all cases of diabetes.

Of the diabetic inpatients seen by the Joslin Clinic, only 0.18% had evident pancreatitis. In contrast, laboratory evidence of minor deficiencies of exocrine function have been found in a majority of some groups of diabetics (Chey, et al, 1963; Vacca, et al, 1964). Bock, et al (1967) studied a group of South African diabetics, none of whom were alcoholic. Abnormal exocrine function was found in 10 of 46 (22%). This group of 46 included 7 whites, 7 Bantus, and 32 "coloured" patients. Harano, et al (1976) have recently presented evidence that to some extent these aberrations of exocrine pancreatic function may be secondary to poor metabolic control of diabetes.

Blumentahl, et al (1963) in St. Louis examined the pancreas at autopsy in 281 diabetics, and found histologic evidence of pancreatitis in 11.2%. In controls the rate was 5.3%. It is not possible from the above and other data to determine with precision the frequency with which pancreatitis plays a role in the etiology of diabetes in the United States or other affluent societies. It seems likely, however, that pancreatitis plays an important part in substantially less than 10% of American cases of diabetes. In communities with high rates of alcoholism pancreatitis probably accounts for a higher percentage of cases. In Rhodesian blacks with diabetes, calcification of the pancreas is rare but pancreatic disease is very common. Of 107 diabetics studied by Wicks and Jones (1974) diabetes was clearly secondary to pancreatic or liver disease in 34, and circumstances suggested that some of the remaining patients also had pancreatic disease. The causes of this pancreatic disease are not yet clear.

Donowitz, et al (1975) have reported high serum glucagon levels in acute pancreatitis, and suggested that this might help to precipitate diabetes in some cases of acute pancreatitis. Diabetes is not uncommonly the result of a combination of factors (eg, pancreatitis and genetic diathesis for diabetes). Some cases of minimal pancreatitis have diabetes and some with very severe pancreatitis do not. In general, however, there appears to be an association of extent of pancreatic damage and risk of diabetes. Few data are available on insulin and glucagon secretion in patients with varying types and degrees of disease of the exocrine pancreas. In a study of Keller, et al (1965) patients with pancreatic diabetes had as much or more serum insulin as normals. But they probably did not have as much insulin as controls would have had at comparable levels of serum glucose.

Pancreatitis is a common cause of diabetes in dogs (Anderson and Streafuss, 1971; Cotton, et al, 1971a), and frequently the pancreatitis is not recognized until autopsy.

The manifestations of diabetes in those with gross pancreatic disease are of great interest because of controversies and uncertainties as to whether vascular lesions or neuropathy are the direct result of either hyperglycemia or insulin insufficiency (relative or absolute). These matters will receive detailed discussion in Chapter 10 under sections relating to the specific lesions in question (eg, atherosclerosis, glomerulosclerosis). Available evidence is still quite incomplete, but, on the whole, existing data suggest that microvascular disease is common in such cases when duration of diabetes exceeds ten years (Verdonk, et al, 1975). Neuropathy has not been well studied in diabetes with pancreatitis, but it is exceedingly common in diabetics with pancreatic calcification (Geevarghese, 1968).

The role of viral pancreatitis in the etiology of juvenile diabetes has been discussed earlier in this chapter. Many different types of pancreatic lesions have produced diabetes by destroying beta cells. In privileged societies the most common cause of this type is pancreatitis. Diabetes may also be produced by neoplasm of the pancreas, or by surgical removal of the pancreas or a large part thereof. Geevarghese (1968) has reviewed in detail diabetes secondary to pancreatic diseases including cancer, worm infestations, hemochromatosis, cystic fibrosis, and various types of pancreatitis. Many different drugs are toxic to the pancreas, and such toxicity is occasionally a cause or precipitating cause of diabetes. Some of these are listed in Table 5 on the etiologies of diabetes. The book of Dreiling, et al (1964) contains an excellent review and discussion of the many factors that may cause pancreatitis or pancreatic toxicity.

Amyloidosis of the pancreas has been observed frequently in diabetic animals, including dogs, cats, and cattle (Meier, 1960; Warren, et al, 1966a). Fibrosis of the pancreas has many causes. Fibrosis has been described in a patient with alpha-l-antitrypsin deficiency in whom there was impairment of glucose tolerance (Freeman, et al, 1976). Fibrosis of the pancreas is very common in patients with fatty or cirrhotic livers (Woldman and Segal, 1959). The sequence and nature of this relationship is incompletely understood. It is probable that the pancreatic fibrosis may account to some degree for the frequency of diabetes in patients with fatty or cirrhotic livers, even in the absence of hemochromatosis.

HEMOCHROMATOSIS AND HEMOSIDEROSIS

The mechanisms by which hemochromatosis causes diabetes are not entirely clear. In hemochromatosis there is excessive iron in the blood, liver, skin, pancreas, and other tissues. At least some of these patients have a genetic defect leading to excessive absorption of iron. Excessive consumption of iron or repeated blood transfusions may also lead to excesses of iron in many tissues (hemosiderosis) including liver and pancreas. Thus hemosiderosis and hemochromatosis are closely related conditions having certain characteristics in common. This has lead to disagreements about definition and classification. Both hemosiderosis and hemochromatosis are associated with excessive tissue iron and excessive rates of diabetes. But in most societies less than 1% of all diabetics have excesses of tissue iron. The subject of hemochromatosis and diabetes has been well reviewed by Jenson (1971). According to Allen (1913), "bronzed diabetes" was first described by Trousseau in 1869.

The percentage of hemochromatosis cases with diabetes varies greatly by circumstances, criteria, etc, but roughly half are diabetic and a substantial majority will eventually become diabetic. In the series of Stocks and Powell (1973) 63% had abnormal glucose tolerance; and 81% had impaired tolerance in the large series (130) of Simon, et al (1973). In 115 patients studied by Dymcock, et al (1972), 63% had "clinical diabetes" and one third of the remainder had abnormal glucose tolerance.

Pancreatic fibrosis of varying degree is present in hemochromatosis. It was commonly believed that diabetes was primarily the result of this fibrosis, but more recent evidence leaves this in some doubt. Iron overload has often failed to produce pancreatic fibrosis in animals. Under some conditions pancreatic disease including fibrosis may increase iron absorption (Davis and Badenoch, 1962), but there is also evidence that pancreatic disease does not regularly increase iron absorption (Murray and Stein 1966; Balcerzak, et al, 1967). It is not clear, therefore, whether, in hemochromatosis, pancreatic fibrosis is primary, secondary, or both. Another possibility is that excessive iron is toxic to beta cells. Therapeutic depletion of body iron has not improved glucose tolerance with regularity (Balcerzak, et al, 1968), but the toxic effects appear to be reversible in some circumstances. In a large series Dymcock, et al (1972) found that glucose tolerance improved in 40% after removal of iron by repeated venesection. Their observations suggest that propensity to diabetes may be influenced by both the liver disease and the pancreatic fibrosis. Also, they found that family history of diabetes was less common in those that had no diabetes despite hemochromatosis. Occasionally, manifestations of hemochromatosis appear only after the discovery of diabetes, but more commonly diabetes seems to develop after the establishment of hemochromatosis.

Patients with thalessemia have iron overload because of destruction of red cells and the blood transfusions made necessary by this destruction. Rates of diabetes are high in these patients (Lassman, et al, 1974). This suggests that excessive iron intake itself is capable of causing diabetes. On the other hand, in studying relatives of patients with hemochromatosis, Balcerzak, et al (1968) found abnormal glucose tolerance as commonly in those with normal iron stores as in those with excessive iron. Results of Saddi and Feingold (1974) were similar in this respect. Prevalence of diabetes in the parents of patients with hemochromatosis and diabetes was high even though serum iron levels were normal in these parents. Rates of diabetes were significantly lower in parents of hemochromatosis patients without diabetes. No difference was found in iron levels of hemochromatosis patients with and without diabetes. Data of present and previous fatness were not given for the hemochromatotics or their parents. This would be of interest, since it is possible that the familiality of fatness and the effect of fatness on susceptibility to diabetes might explain these interesting findings to some extent.

Bierens de Haan, et al (1973) found that apparently healthy relatives of hemochromatotics often had impaired glucose tolerance, but this seemed unrelated to levels of serum iron. There was no evidence of resistance to insulin, but with glucose challenge there was a delay in rise of serum insulin. Stocks and Powell (1973) observed one patient whose glucose tolerance and sensitivity to insulin improved after therapeutic diminution of iron stores, but they found no significant difference between groups of treated (iron depletion)

335

and untreated patients with respect to glucose tolerance and insulin sensitivity. It was their impression that diabetes was probably caused by the toxic effects of excessive iron rather than by a direct effect of a genetic aberration.

The situation is further complicated because patients with both hemosiderosis and hemochromatosis often have liver cirrhosis, a condition frequently associated with diabetes in patients without excessive tissue iron. Thus liver dysfunction could also play a role in the etiology of diabetes in those with hemochromatosis or hemosiderosis. Finally, certain nutritional deficiencies may increase iron absorption.

Seftel reported in 1960 results of studies in 20 consecutive autopsies of Bantu diabetics. Four had heavy deposits of iron, and pathologic changes indistinguishable from those seen in hemochromatosis. Bothwell (1969) has reviewed the subject of hemosiderosis and hemochromatosis in Bantu. In many Bantu communities iron consumption is high. Local beer is often very high in iron, having been prepared or stored in receptacles containing iron. In some Bantu communities as many as 20% of diabetics have excessive levels of iron in their tissues or blood, and the frequency of elevated serum iron is considerably higher in diabetics than in these general populations. Data are rather incomplete but it appears that in some communities "iron toxicity" may account for 10% to 20% of all cases of diabetes. Hemochromatosis is also a fairly common cause of diabetes in Ghana (Dodu, 1958).

Iron-related diabetes seems to be more frequent in Bantu men than in Bantu women. Data are quite incomplete but, in general, Bantu men consume more beer and more iron than women. Also, women are protected to some extent by menstruation. To some degree, higher rates of hemochromatosis in men may have contributed to the high ratios of male to female diabetics that have been observed in some societies. In privileged societies, hemochromatosis is far more common in men than in women, but the condition is so rare that sex ratios in groups of diabetics are little affected. Only 0.16% of the Joslin Clinic diabetics had known hemochromatosis (Jenson, 1971). Of 48 cases with both these diseases, 45 were males and 3 were females.

More information is needed on the histologic status of the pancreas in Bantu diabetics with and without hemosiderosis. In communities where iron consumption is high more data are also needed on serum and tissue iron levels in Bantu diabetics as compared to nondiabetics from these communities.

The frequency of vascular lesions and other manifestations of diabetes in patients with hemochromatosis will be discussed in Chapter 10.

LIVER DISEASE

It has long been known that rates of diabetes were disproportionately high with certain diseases of the liver. This association has sometimes been referred to as "hepatogenous diabetes". Naunyn used this expression as early as 1906.

In Allen's book of 1913 there was considerable discussion of these links between diabetes and liver disease. Even now, however, the nature and strength of these associations between diabetes and liver diseases have not been well defined. Since the liver is a site of major importance for both the intake and output of glucose, it is not surprising that aberrations of liver function affect susceptibility to diabetes.

In hemochromatosis the accompanying cirrhosis may play a role in the susceptibility to diabetes in these patients. Persons with cirrhosis have both impaired glucose tolerance and clinical diabetes more frequently than the general population, but interpretation of these associations is difficult. Patients with cirrhosis are often poorly fed, often have associated pancreatic disease and other complicating disorders such as potassium depletion, usually have low levels of exercise, and sometimes have elevated growth hormone levels. Control data are few on rates of impairment of glucose tolerance in groups with characteristics matching those of the cirrhosis patients. Cirrhosis patients are more often tested for diabetes than the general population.

Megyesi, et al (1967) performed glucose tolerance tests on 28 unselected patients with chronic liver diseases. Thirty-two percent had diabetes and 25% more had impaired glucose tolerance. Only 43% had normal tolerance. The researchers thought that the high frequency of diabetes was probably due to an insensitivity to insulin in cirrhosis. Some evidence compatible with that concept was presented. They pointed out that the insensitivity to insulin was not confined to liver tissue. These authors also reviewed previous observations of others concerning liver disease and diabetes. Stocks and Powell (1973) demonstrated abnormal intravenous glucose tolerance in 12 of 21 (57%) of a group of cirrhotic patients. These cirrhotics also exhibited insensitivity to insulin. Some authors think that diabetes is now more common in patients with liver disease than it was formerly, but the increased frequency and sensitivity of diabetes testing in patients with liver disease may account for all or part of the apparent increases.

Harold Conn and his associates (1969) studied 240 cirrhotic patients and an age-matched series of 411 inpatients. Diabetes was found in 16.7% of cirrhotics and 7.1% of controls. They attributed the higher diabetes rates to a combination of several factors. They and others found diabetes more common in patients who had undergone operations to produce portal-caval shunts. Family history of diabetes was also less frequent in the diabetics with shunts than in cirrhotic diabetics without shunts. In a control group of diabetics without liver disease, a positive family history of diabetes was more frequent than in the diabetics with cirrhosis. Otherwise, the characteristics of diabetes were similar in the two groups. Usually diabetes had been discovered prior to cirrhosis. This has been the case in most such series, but not invariably so. In the study of Conn, et al, there was little difference in the clinical features of cirrhosis in those with and without diabetes, except that shunt procedures had been performed more commonly in the diabetics. This publication of Conn contains a good review of the associations between liver disease and diabetes including a bibliography of 79 publications on liver disease and diabetes.

Lickley, et al (1975) demonstrated that oral glucose tolerance was impaired in otherwise normal dogs after surgically-induced portal-caval shunts. Intravenous tolerance was not impaired.

Rates of liver disease have seldom if ever been measured in a representative sample of all diabetics. It seems likely that liver disease accounts for only a very small proportion of diabetes. In a series of 18,439 diabetics of the Joslin Clinic, only 0.78% were known to have cirrhosis (Jenson, 1971). With very poor control of severe diabetes, liver enlargement is common, but liver disease is rarely seen as a direct complication of diabetes. The cause of hepatomegaly in prolonged severe uncontrolled diabetes is incompletely understood. Fatty infiltration and increased glycogen have been observed.

Muting and Kaufmann (1975) performed glucose tolerance tests in 2,600 patients with histologically confirmed liver disease. Tolerance was frequently impaired with acute liver disease but usually returned to normal. Manifest diabetes was present in 7.2% with chronic persistent hepatitis, and in 16.3% with chronic progressive hepatitis. In both these latter conditions 30% had "latent" diabetes. Highest rates of hyperglycemia were observed with high degrees of fatty liver and those with active cirrhosis accompanied by portal hypertension. More than half of the latter patients had latent or manifest diabetes.

Westlund (1969) found in diabetics of Oslo, Norway that cirrhosis was cited on the death certificates of diabetics with a frequency 3.4 times greater than on certificates of age-matched members of the general population. Sasaki, et al (1975) found cirrhosis to be excessive in decedent diabetics by a factor of 2:1. The results of Kessler (1971) were different in follow-up studies of Joslin Clinic patients. In this group cirrhosis was not cited on death certificates with greater frequency than in a control population. Nor was liver disease especially common in the diabetic decedents of Pennsylvania (Tokuhata, et al, 1976).

Burch and Rowell (1967) thought that the propensity to both diabetes and cirrhosis might be the result of a common genetic defect and presented some indirect evidence consistent with this possibility. There is little direct evidence to support this hypothesis.

Woldman and Segal (1959) in an autopsy study in Cleveland, Ohio demonstrated a very strong relationship of liver disease and fibrosis of the pancreas.

Diabetes is common during and shortly after hepatitis. In Nigeria nine such cases were seen in a single epidemic of hepatitis (Adi, 1974). But all of these latter episodes of hyperglycemia were temporary. Permanent diabetes does sometimes follow hepatitis, possibly with a frequency greater than with other infections, but present data are not sufficient to establish this with certainty. Only 0.17 of the diabetics of the Joslin Clinic had hepatitis at the time they were being seen for diabetes (Jenson, 1971). This author observed two cases of hepatitis in diabetic spouses who had been sharing the same insulin syringe and needles!

338

9

PURPORTED MARKERS
OR STIGMATA OF PREDIABETES

It is now generally accepted that the term prediabetes designates a stage prior to any evidence of hyperglycemia. Many of the groups whose characteristics have been studied at a time prior to the discovery of diabetes contain two subgroups, one with prediabetes and one with early diabetes. Circumstances of such studies are often such that the ratio of these subgroups in the total study group is not known. Much recent evidence, some of which will be reviewed below, suggests that most stigmata thought to be associated with prediabetes are actually associated only with early diabetes. Among the factors purported to be associated with prediabetes are propensity to have large babies, increased risk of morbidity and mortality of the fetuses and infants of prediabetic mothers, hypoglycemia, qualitative and quantitative aberrations of insulin secretion, and abnormalities of the vascular and neurologic systems. Very commonly, apparent differences between prediabetic groups and control groups have not been confirmed with more extensive experience. A common cause of such premature conclusions has been inadequacy of control data (quantitative or qualitative).

The "markers" under discussion here do not include factors known to cause diabetes, such as obesity. Also, this discussion will concern mainly those factors that may be detected or measured by ordinary clinical procedures. The study of the more occult immunologic and biochemical stigmata that might be related to prediabetes are no less important. But a thorough review of these is beyond the scope of a presentation on epidemiology. The section on juvenile diabetes in Chapter 8 does review some of the available evidence concerning the histocompatibility antigens. Since genetic factors are important in diabetes it seems very likely that potentially detectable aberrations would be present before hyperglycemia. Discovery of such peculiarities would be useful in several ways. Knowledge of this kind would probably provide important clues concerning the mechanisms by which genetic or other factors lead to hyperglycemia. These potentialities have led to extensive searches for markers of prediabetes. To date no marker has been found that is sensitive and specific. It is now clear, moreover, that diabetes has many causes and that many different genetic mechanisms may produce diabetes. Thus, a "universal" marker will not be found. Nevertheless it might be possible to find one or more prediabetic distinctions for some of the most common causes of diabetes. But progress will not be served by uncritical acceptance of purported markers without appropriate proofs. The evidence related below is largely negative with respect to these purported markers, but the search should go on.

In the sections on vascular diseases in Chapter 10, certain negative evidence is reviewed concerning the possibility of an association of prediabetes with either microvascular or macrovascular disease. Soeldner, et al (1976) found "no clear-cut differences" between prediabetics and a control group when they were tested with a number of procedures. Elevated lipid levels were somewhat more common in the prediabetics but this may not have been the result of their prediabetic status. Although matched for age and weight, they were not drawn from the same universe as the controls. No conclusive evidence has been presented that the prediabetic state is an independent risk factor for either microvascular or macrovascular disease. Nilsson et al (1967), in a well-controlled study, found no differences in responses to neurologic tests between those with and without a family history of diabetes.

LARGE BABIES

It was suggested by Skipper in 1933 that the propensity to have babies with high birth weights might be present even before the discovery of diabetes. In 1945 Herbert Miller reported that, many years before the discovery of diabetes, a group of diabetic women had babies whose weights at birth were greater than those of nondiabetic women. He also presented evidence that this difference was not entirely explained by the greater fatness of the diabetic mothers. Data presented by Nathanson (1950) indicated that birth weights of more than 4.5 kg 10 lb were uncommon (1.8% in an American community). Frequency of babies of this weight has been much greater in mothers later found to be diabetic. In the study of Malins and FitzGerald (1965), for example, it was 12%. These observations on high birth weights prior to the discovery of maternal diabetes have been confirmed by many other investigators. It is, therefore, still generally believed that prediabetes is associated with a propensity to have large babies.

But more recent evidence and review of older data suggest that the excessive weight is probably attributable to factors other than prediabetes, mainly occult hyperglycemia and obesity. This conclusion is also supported by demonstrations of the strong associations of maternal adiposity and birth weight (Horger, et al, 1975) and evidence that hyperglycemia itself increases birth weight. For example, Mintz, et al (1971) showed that fetal weight was increased in monkeys whose mothers were made diabetic by streptozotocin. On the basis of his studies, Hagbard (1958) concluded that fetal abnormalities observed prior to the discovery of diabetes were probably not related to the prediabetic state, but rather to factors such as maternal occult hyperglycemia. Data of Nilsson (1962) also suggested that the propensity to have heavy babies was not due to prediabetes itself, but rather was coincidental to other factors such as maternal adiposity. Pirart (1955) studied babies of mothers who later developed diabetes. He found no difference between weights of babies of mothers who had a family history of diabetes and mothers who did not. He thought that maternal adiposity explained much of the apparently excessive weights of babies of mothers who later developed diabetes.

Lubetzke, et al (1973) found no difference in the birth weights of babies of diabetic women, obese women without diabetes, and obese women with diabetes. O'Sullivan, et al (1966) showed that insulin therapy reduced birth weights of children of mothers with gestational diabetes. They found that relationship of maternal glycemia and birth weight was limited to the highest 5% of glucose values. In the studies of O'Sullivan, et al (1966), birth weights of infants of mothers with mild abnormalities of glucose tolerance were compared with those of a control group. In a subgroup of these potential diabetics who received antidiabetic therapy (diet and insulin) during the last part of pregnancy, the number of large babies was not significantly different than in the control group. Hadden and Harley (1967) found no relationship of birth weight and glucose tolerance in 625 patients with no previous diagnosis of diabetes.

In Israel, Weitz and Laron (1976) studied height and weight in children of various ages. A small series of children of diabetic mothers were somewhat taller than those of mothers with no apparent diabetes. This was particularly notable in children with mothers of European and American origin and in those whose mothers had youth-onset diabetes. No peculiarities were observed in fatness of the children of diabetic mothers. In contrast, Hagbard, et al (1959) and Farquhar (1969) found children of diabetic mothers to be shorter and heavier than controls.

The studies of Pehrson (1974) are of particular interest because of their design, the large number of subjects tested, and the scope of the variables measured. He performed intravenous glucose tolerance tests on an unselected group of 1,002 pregnant Swedish women. It was therefore possible to examine more satisfactorily the relationships among factors such as maternal weight and age, birth weight, parity, and family history of diabetes. There was an inverse correlation between glucose tolerance and both birth weight and birth weights of previous babies. But this was rendered insignificant after corrections ahd been made for maternal age and weight. Pehrson's publication (1974) also contains an excellent review of maternal prediabetes and the fetus.

Birth weight increases with maternal age up to about age 40 (Horger, 1975). I have not been able to find any report linking high birth weight and early diabetes in which it was possible to exclude the possibility that the association was attributable to maternal age, maternal adiposity, maternal hyperglycemia, or a combination thereof. It does not seem likely that increased birth weight is a manifestation of prediabetes.

Results of studies of Malins and Fitzgerald (1965) are typical of most others in showing that babies of diabetic fathers have birth weights that approximate those of babies of nondiabetic fathers. In a few series, babies of diabetic fathers were heavier than controls (Jackson, 1954; Pirart, 1955; Kellack, 1961) but it was not possible to exclude the possibility that these associations were the result of other associated factors such as excessive adiposity in mothers of the children of diabetic fathers.

EXCESSIVE FETAL AND NEONATAL MORBIDITY AND MORTALITY

It has also been demonstrated in many circumstances that, prior to the discovery of maternal diabetes, fetal and neonatal morbidity may be excessive (Miller, et al, 1945; Gilbert and Dunlop, 1949; Moss and Mulholland, 1951). It is widely believed that this is a manifestation of prediabetes, but there is little evidence to support this view. Rather, it appears that these associations, observed prior to the discovery of diabetes, are the result of maternal hyperglycemia (early diabetes) and other factors such as the higher rates of obesity in mothers with early diabetes and prediabetes.

In 1939 Allen reported higher rates of fetal loss in women in whom diabetes was not discovered until later. This was confirmed by others in some other circumstances (eg, Gilbert and Dunlop, 1949; O'Sullivan, et al, 1966). Under other conditions fetal loss was not excessive in studies of babies born more than five years prior to the discovery of diabetes (Herzstein and Dolger, 1946; Pirart, 1955; Hagbard, 1958; Malins and FitzGerald, 1965). Sotto, et al (1958) found no relationship between maternal glucose tolerance and fetal wastage in women without clinical diabetes. Herzstein and Dolger (1946) observed no difference in fetal mortality between offspring of mothers who later required insulin therapy and offspring of mothers whose later diabetes did not require insulin. Dahlberg (1947) found no evidence of increased rates of stillbirth before the discovery of diabetes. On the other hand, well-designed studies of O'Sullivan and associates showed that gestational diabetics had higher rates of fetal loss than a control group. These investigators (Dandrow and O'Sullivan, 1966) reported that perinatal mortality was much higher in diabetics than in those with gestational diabetes. They pointed out that it was not clear to what extent the increased risk of perinatal mortality in gestational diabetes was due to disturbed glucose tolerance itself or to other factors such as the greater age and adiposity of the patients with abnormal tolerance. Their later, more detailed analysis (O'Sullivan, et al, 1973) showed that obesity accounted for a small fraction of this risk of perinatal mortality, while maternal age had a more substantial effect. In women less than 25 years of age, slightly abnormal tolerance was not associated with increased perinatal mortality.

Hadden and Harley (1967) studied glucose tolerance during pregnancy in 625 women judged to have a high risk of diabetes on the basis of several criteria. Fetal loss was only slightly higher (10.8%) in those with abnormal glucose tolerance than in those with normal tolerance (6.2%). The difference was not statistically significant. In patients of Karlsson and Kjellmer (1972) with known diabetes perinatal mortality ranged from 3.8% in those with very slight maternal hyperglycemia to 23.6% in those with substantial hyperglycemia. These and other studies suggest that risk of fetal and infant mortality is very low in early diabetes when fasting blood glucose levels are normal or very near normal. O'Sullivan, et al (1971) observed a statistically significant decline in perinatal mortality when mothers with gestational diabetes were treated during pregnancy with insulin and diet. Others have observed favorable results on fetal outcome after treating pregnant patients who have mild aberrations of carbohydrate metabolism (Hoet, 1954; van der Linden and Mastboom 1971; Botella-Lluisa and Perreion, 1969; Serr, et al, 1972; Khojandi, et al, 1974).

On the basis of his studies, Hagbard concluded that fetal complications observed prior to the discovery of diabetes were probably the result of early diabetes and its concomitants rather than prediabetes. From their data on mothers with mild glucose intolerance, Haworth and Dilling (1975) concluded that in patients without clinical diabetes documentation of degree of intolerance was of little value in predicting fetal outcome.

Goldman (1974) agreed with others that congenital malformations were more common in children of diabetic mothers, but his studies gave no support of a relationship of prediabetes and congential malformations. Oakley, et al (1972) have reviewed evidence from their studies and other sources showing that fetal hyperinsulinism and fetal hypoglycemia are the result of maternal hyperglycemia.

Beta-cell hyperplasia has been described in dead newborn of mothers later found to be diabetic, but present data are not adequate to establish whether this develops while maternal glucose tolerance is still normal.

Gabbe et al (1977) found no evidence of increased mortality in a group of 261 infants of mothers with mild intensively treated diabetes.

In the aggregate the evidence above gives very little support to the notion that the prediabetic state produces untoward effects on the fetus or infant. Rather, it seems likely that the morbidity sometimes seen prior to discovery of diabetes in the mother is the result of early diabetes or of incidental concomitants of early diabetes or prediabetes.

343

HYPOGLYCEMIA

It is widely believed that hypoglycemia is a manifestation of the prediabetic state. Evidence to be reviewed below does not, however, appear to be conclusive. The condition may not exist. Two points should be made at the outset. First, Seltzer, et al (1956), whose observations drew attention to the association of hypoglycemia and early diabetes, did *not* suggest that hypoglycemia was a manifestation of prediabetes. Their patients who developed low blood glucose levels after oral glucose already had hyperglycemia during the two-hour period immediately following glucose ingestion. Second, it is appropriate to examine separately the question whether hypoglycemia attends prediabetes for each of the two different types of diabetes (juvenile-onset and maturity-onset) since their pathogenesis is probably different in at least some respects. In both types, it has been suggested that hypoglycemia may be a manifestation of prediabetes or early diabetes.

In 1924 Seale Harris first described what is now called reactive or functional hypoglycemia. His patients had low blood glucose values a few hours after eating, and characteristic symptoms. One of these patients also had hyperglycemia immediately after oral glucose. Harris suggested that this might be an early stage of diabetes. In a 1945 paper Mirsky mentioned, as though it were common knowledge, that certain obese patients tended to develop hypoglycemia in the course of a six-hour period after ingestion of carbohydrate. No evidence was cited in support of this concept, but more recently data have been reported purporting to show that fat people frequently have reactive hypoglycemia (Faludi, et al, 1968). In 1953 Skillern and Rynearson presented two cases with hyperglycemia in the initial phases of glucose tolerance tests and low blood glucose levels in the later stages. In 1953 O. P. Allen reported that symptoms suggestive of hypoglycemia were very common in his diabetic patients in the early stage of diabetes. He described four typical cases in whom diabetes had been preceded by weight gain and symptoms he thought to be characteristic of hypoglycemia. He also reviewed retrospectively 1,207 cases of diabetes. He thought that 54.8% had exhibited these features prior to the discovery of hyperglycemia. It should be mentioned, however, that hypoglycemia was not documented in a single one of the 1,207 cases, nor in any of the four cases described in detail.

Seltzer, et al (1956) described 110 cases (70 males and 40 females) with mild "hyperglycemia" who also had low blood glucose values in the later stages of their glucose tolerance tests. Criteria were well defined. One-hour venous whole blood glucose levels of 160 mg/100 ml or greater and two-hour values 120 mg/100 ml or greater were considered "abnormal". Values of 50 or below were considered low. Eight subjects had fasting values from 100 to 120, but the remainder had fasting levels below 100. Forty-four percent had a family history of diabetes, 69% were thought to have symptoms characteristic of hypoglycemia, and 34% were obese. Symptoms usually improved after restriction of carbohydrate to 150 gm daily. This rather impressive evidence gave strong support to the concept that hypoglycemia was a not infrequent manifestation of early diabetes. Other subsequent observations were compatible with this possibility. It was found that blood insulin levels were frequently high two to three hours after oral glucose in early diabetes. On the basis of his experience Kryston (1975) concluded that reactive hypoglycemia was also a sign of prediabetes (as well as early diabetes). Faludi, et al (1968) concluded that reactive hypoglycemia was especially common in obesity.

But in recent years several considerations have suggested a need to reexamine this matter. In a very extensive experience in performing glucose tolerance tests in offspring of two diabetic parents (West, 1960), I did not recognize any cases of symptomatic hypoglycemia. Although the question is still in some dispute, most evidence now suggests that insulin levels are usually normal or low in early diabetes after appropriate corrections are made for both fatness and blood glucose level. The possibility remains, however, that a certain subgroup of prediabetics and early diabetics have elevated values. Yet in the twenty-year period following the report of Seltzer, it has not been demonstrated by any controlled study that hypoglycemia is more common in early diabetes or prediabetes than in subjects matched for characteristics other than glucose tolerance. Although decisive evidence is not at hand, there is a considerable amount of negative evidence. There is a remarkable paucity of data on blood glucose levels two to five hours after carbohydrates in *representative* samples of general populations or in representative samples of prediabetics and early diabetics. It is clear, however, that two-hour blood glucose levels above 120 mg/ 100 ml (West, 1966) and one-hour blood glucose levels above 160 are quite common in the general population of America (West, 1966) and Britain (Jarrett and Keen, 1975a), and that levels below 50 during the third and fourth hour are exceedingly common (Burns, et al, 1965; Hofeldt, et al, 1975; Cahill and Soeldner, 1974; Jung, et al, 1971).

With few exceptions "low" glucose levels in the range of 40–50 mg/100 ml after oral glucose do not produce symptoms. Fabrykant had shown in 1955 that symptoms after oral glucose were frequent in the absence of hypoglycemia, and that persons with low values after glucose were frequently asymptomatic. It is also evident that a large fraction of those Americans who complain of symptoms suggesting hypoglycemia do not have hypoglycemia as a basis for these symptoms (Editorial, *JAMA,* 1973). In the study of Jung, et al (1971) there were 285 adult females, of whom 18% had blood glucose values below 60 mg/100 ml in the course of a five-hour glucose tolerance test. In women less than 46 years of age, postglucose levels less than 60 were seen in 31% of those weighing more than 145 pounds. These investigators were not able to ascertain from their data whether low values in the later stages of the test were more common in subjects with mild hyperglycemia at one and two hours. Farris (1974) tested a group of 451 young men (US Army inductees) who had exhibited glycosuria when given 100 gm of oral glucose. On the follow-up test 8.4% of these men had two-hour *plasma* glucose values less than 50 mg/100 ml.

Hofeldt, et al (1974) studied insulin levels in 16 subjects of the type described by Seltzer (1956) who had mild hyperglycemia and reactive hypo-glycemia. Insulin levels were not different than those of weight-matched controls. Luyckx and Lefebvre (1971) had studied insulin levels in ten such patients of whom nine were obese and one lean. Insulin levels in the course of glucose tolerance testing were not different from those of control subjects.

Jackson, et al (1974) performed prolonged glucose tolerance tests in a population of Tamils in which rates of diabetes, and presumably prediabetes, were exceedingly high. Eleven subjects with normal glucose tolerance tests subsequently became diabetic. None had had reactive hypoglycemia during the course of the studies. Low blood glucose values were no more common in subjects with two diabetic parents than in controls. Park et al. (1972) performed 5-hour glucose tolerance tests in 84 "genetic prediabetics" and 123 controls. No difference was found in the frequency of hypoglycemia in these two groups. Studies of Köbberling and Creutzfeldt (1970) were not designed with this issue in mind, but they are impressively negative in this regard. They published results of glucose tolerance tests in 276 close relatives of diabetics in each of whom glucose tolerance was abnormal by any one or more of the commonly employed standards. Only 1 of 276 had a three-hour whole blood value less than 50 mg/100 ml. In collaboration with Arthur Rubenstein (West and Mako, 1976), we measured insulin and glucose levels at one and two hours after 75 gm of oral glucose in 76 adult offspring of two diabetic parents. After correction for adiposity there was no evidence of hypersecretion of insulin, and no symptoms or complaints suggestive of hypoglycemia observed between the second and fourth hour.

Sisk, et al (1970) performed duplicate oral glucose (100 gm) tolerance tests in 96 prisoners. In 19 of the subjects, three-hour whole blood glucose levels were less than 50 mg/100 ml in the course of one test, but not in the other. One subject had a low three hour value with both tests. In six tests three-hour values were less than 40 mg/100 ml. None of these subjects had high values at one or two hours and the mean values at one and two hours were *less* in "hypogly-cemic" subjects than in the others. No mention was made by these authors of any complaints suggestive of hypoglycemia. These results suggest that a very large percentage of normal subjects would have "low" values either with repeated testing or continuous blood glucose analysis.

In discussion of Seltzer's original paper (1956) Leon Smelo mentioned that he and Seale Harris had observed frequently patients with mild hyperglycemia immediately after oral glucose together with reactive hypoglycemia. It was, however, then his impression that in subsequent years the rate of development of clinical diabetes was not more frequent than in the general population. I have observed two cases with pancreatic disease and no family history of diabetes that exhibited mildly elevated two-hour values and subsequent plasma glucose values less than 50 mg/100 ml (without symptoms).

The data of Seltzer, et al (1956) established that blood glucose levels below 50 mg/100 ml were common in persons with slight elevations of one- and two-hour values. This has been confirmed subsequently by others including Sussman, et al (1966). Although suggestive, these data did not, however, establish that low values or symptoms were more common in early diabetes than in normal subjects matched for other characteristics. Seltzer and his associates did not purport to show that reactive hypoglycemia attended prediabetes. Present evidence can neither confirm or entirely refute that adult prediabetics have reactive hypoglycemia with unusual frequency. Negative evidence is at present more impressive than the positive. Considerations outlined above suggest strongly the need for well-controlled studies.

Hypoglycemia also has been described as an early manifestation of juvenile diabetes, but present evidence is inadequate to evaluate the strength and significance of this relationship. In a 1964 paper Lloyd mentioned a few previous reports of hypoglycemia prior to juvenile diabetes. He also described a child who had seizures from fasting hypoglycemia, and who later developed hyperglycemia. Insulin therapy was not required. The child had synalbumin insulin antagonism. Yalow and Berson studied insulin levels in nine children with idopathic hypoglycemia and found them normal. Sperling and Drash (1971) had two patients with idiopathic hypoglycemia of infancy who developed diabetes in childhood. One had severe and one mild diabetes. Rosenbloom and Sherman (1973) studied the families of ten children with idiopathic hypoglycemia. They thought that the frequency of diabetes and impaired glucose tolerance was probably higher than usual in these relatives. They also found abnormal glucose tolerance was frequent in the hypoglycemic children (8 of 20) during periods when intermittent hypoglycemia was occurring and after remission. Burkeholder, et al (1967) studied 138 siblings of juvenile diabetics. Twenty-five (19%) had abnormal glucose tolerance, of whom one later developed clinical diabetes. One of the children with abnormal tolerance had a three-hour value in the hypoglycemic range, but these authors were not certain whether low values at three hours were any more frequent in these siblings than in the general population of children. The child with the low three-hour value was the identical twin of a juvenile diabetic. Chutorian, et al (1973) reported four cases in children of mild abnormality of glucose tolerance associated with "reactive hypoglycemia". After oral glucose, symptoms suggestive of hypoglycemia occurred at the time of lowest plasma glucose values, but the "low" plasma glucose levels were not demonstrated to be outside the normal range, and serum insulin levels were not abnormal. All children improved after restriction of dietary carbohydrate.

Drash (1973) studied children with diabetic relatives and asymptomatic mild hyperglycemia. They all had levels of serum insulin higher than normal (although perhaps not higher than in nondiabetics with comparable blood glucose levels). But studies of insulin levels in identical twins of juvenile-onset diabetics do not show a consistent pattern of disturbed insulin secretion (Johansen, et al, 1974). A majority of studies suggest that these "prediabetics" have normal insulin secretion patterns.

Although the observations above suggest the possibility that hypoglycemia in childhood may sometimes be a manifestation of prediabetes, present evidence is indirect and incomplete. The link between hypoglycemia and propensity to slight impairment of glucose tolerance is rather impressive, but the association between hypoglycemia and subsequent typical clinical juvenile diabetes is not yet well documented.

SECRETION OF INSULIN AND OTHER HORMONES

A treatise on epidemiology cannot do full justice to the subject of secretion of insulin and other hormones; nevertheless an attempt to summarize is in order. It has been suggested that prediabetes and early diabetes are characterized by levels of insulin secretion that are, in relation to serum glucose levels, low, high, and normal! The conflicting evidence relating to this subject has been reviewed by Johansen, et al (1974). The conflict of evidence and opinion has prevailed for the early stages of both juvenile-onset and maturity-onset diabetes. Workers finding low values in prediabetes include Cerasi, et al (1973), Colwell and Lein (1967), and Tan, et al (1977). Those finding elevated levels include Lowrie, et al (1970). A majority of investigators, including Pyke, et al (1970), found insulin levels normal in prediabetes. Prediabetics and "controls" have seldom been derived from the same element of the population.

In collaboration with Arthur Rubenstein and Mary Mako, we recently measured insulin secretion after oral glucose in 73 offspring, whose parents were both diabetic, in a population of Kiowa and Comanche Indians. Insulin levels before and after glucose were the same as in an equally fat group of controls. Savage, et al (1975) studied insulin levels in Pima Indians who were confirmed prediabetics. They had normal glucose tolerance but later developed diabetes. Insulin secretion was the same in these prediabetics as in matched Indians who did not develop diabetes.

The heterogeneity of diabetes may explain some of the conflicting evidence, but methodologic disparities are probably also contributing factors. When evaluated in the aggregate, evidence currently available does not clearly establish that aberrations of insulin secretion are common in prediabetes.

Vallance-Owen (1962) has described an insulin antagonist associated with plasma albumin that he finds more commonly in nondiabetic close relatives of diabetics than in controls. This work has been confirmed in some respects, but most scientists in the field are still skeptical of the sensitivity and specificity of this factor as a marker of prediabetes. Wahren, et al (1973) have presented evidence that nondiabetic identical twins of insulin-dependent diabetics may have abnormally low hepatic glucose output under certain conditions. Among several other possibilities is that there might be genetically determined qualitative peculiarities of insulin production or secretion in the prediabetic state. But, thus far, claims concerning such peculiarities have not been generally accepted. Pozefsky, et al (1973) found sensitivity to insulin normal in muscle tissue of prediabetics.

Aberrations of glucagon (Day and Tattersall, 1975; Kirk, et al, 1975) and growth-hormone secretion (Johansen, et al, 1974) have been reported in close relatives of diabetics, but results with respect to secretion of those hormones in the prediabetic state are inconclusive (Johansen, et al, 1974; Unger, 1976; Sherwin, et al, 1976). In Pima Indians Aronoff, et al (1976) found glucagon levels normal in adult offspring of two diabetic parents. White and Graham (1971) thought that prediabetic children might be a bit taller than usual, but prediabetic identical twins of Pyke (1973) were not unusually tall.

OTHER FACTORS

Schnider, et al (1977) using sensitive methods found no evidence of proteinuria in prediabetics (nondiabetics whose parents were both diabetic). Some have suggested that prediabetics were more sensitive to the acute hyperglycemic effects of glucocorticoids. This is discussed, mostly in a negative vein, under tests for diabetes (Chapter 4). Herman, et al (1976) found in Israel that the incidence of diabetes was excessive in men with high uric acid levels. This was only partly explained by the greater fatness of these men. They had been screened for diabetes initially with negative results, but glucose tolerance tests were not performed at the time of the negative screening results. The men with unequivocal hyperglycemia had *lower* uric acid levels than those who did not have or develop diabetes. The meaning of these interesting findings is unclear. Loffer found an excessive frequency of abnormal glucose tolerance in a group of pregnant women who had had early menarche. There were no evident associated factors that explained this relationship.

SUMMARY

Many claims have been made for genetic markers or clinical stigmata of prediabetes. Some are still rather widely accepted, but evidence with respect to the sensitivity and specificity of these stigmata leaves much to be desired. Indeed, in many instances it is now clear that the purported marker is only a stigma of early diabetes, not prediabetes. In view of the mounting evidence of the marked etiologic heterogeneity of diabetes, including the multiple genetic mechanisms, it is hardly surprising that a specific genetic marker has not been found.

Specific Morbid Effects (Complications)

INTRODUCTION AND METHODS

Traditionally, the pathologic manifestations of diabetes have been referred to as "complications". With increasing frequency the appropriateness of this term is being challenged, mainly because the most important of these morbid changes seem to be inherent parts of the hyperglycemic state. Particularly, there is now much evidence to suggest that the microvascular and neurologic lesions ought to be considered manifestations of diabetes rather than "complications". Tuberculosis is a complication of diabetes, but glomerulosclerosis is, for example, a manifestation.

At first, epidemiologic studies were concerned mainly with the occurrence of diabetes and the factors associated with its presence or absence. Increasingly, the individual manifestations are becoming objects of epidemiologic study. It is now clear that outcome with respect to each of the major manifestations is highly variable. In one diabetic, retinae are severely diseased at the time of discovery of mild diabetes, while another diabetic has no evidence of retinopathy after forty years of severe diabetes. One diabetic has severe lipemia, another does not. Basic and clinical studies have contributed much to the understanding of the various manifestations. Despite decades of study, however, certain questions of critical importance have remained unanswered. The extent to which hyperglycemia itself causes microvascular and macrovascular lesions is still not clear. Some think duration of diabetes unimportant in determining risk

351

and degree of atherosclerosis, but others disagree. Some believe that certain of the neuropathic lesions are a direct result of a genetic aberration and not the result of hyperglycemia, while others have reached opposite conclusions. Arguments about whether hyperglycemia is a direct cause of the vascular lesions received detailed attention in the 1913 book of Allen. More than half a century later this controversy continues, leaving the clinician uncertain about the value and priority of attempts to control the blood glucose.

These issues that seemed at first so simple were unyielding. It became evident that clinical studies in groups of patients would continue to supply inconclusive and conflicting results unless they incorporated some of the approaches that had traditionally been employed in epidemiology. Groups of patients studied were usually unrepresentative of the universe of diabetics and nondiabetics from which they were derived. Characteristics of the controls seldom matched satisfactorily those of the diabetics with which they were compared. Definition of terms such as *diabetes, control of diabetes, duration of diabetes, hypertension,* and *hypertriglyceridemia* were often vague or unstandardized. Standardization of method was rare; description was often incomplete. Rates of retinopathy in one study would be based on chart review, in others by clinical examinations of varying degrees of sensitivity and specificity. Some of these problems have been well summarized by Danowski, et al (1966) and by Kaplan and Feinstein (1973, 1974).

Another factor that suggested the potentialities of epidemiologic approaches was recognition that rates and degrees of some of the major manifestations differed not only among individual diabetics, but among groups of diabetics. This had been known for a long time, but little appreciated until recently. It is now evident, for example, that the major problem of diabetics in affluent societies (ischemic heart disease) is in many populations of diabetics a problem of modest or little importance. At first, it was widely believed that this happy immunity was conferred by race. But recent evidence indicates that these differences in manifestations are mainly determined by environmental factors, suggesting great potential for their prevention or mitigation.

Many types of epidemiologic study have application and potential in the investigation of these diabetes-related lesions. These approaches include both intra- and interpopulation studies, case-control designs, prospective and retrospective studies, and studies concerning the sensitivity and specificity of various indexes of these lesions. Another important role of epidemiology will be to promote and assist the development of definitions, conventions, and standardized methods. With increasing frequency, more sophisticated analytic techniques, such as multivariate procedures, are being employed to determine, for example, the extent to which observed associations are independent, or to help in establishing whether these associations are coincidental or possibly causal. Some of the questions to be addressed have been suggested above. Many more will be cited below.

The experience gained by the University Group Diabetes Program in developing standardized methods will be useful in the future. These methods have been well described (University Group, 1970a). Among other standards and procedures that will be helpful are those described in the WHO manual on cardiovascular survey methods prepared under the guidance of Rose and Blackburn (1968).

ATHEROSCLEROSIS AND RELATED DISORDERS

Introduction

Discussion in this section will include all diabetes-related disease of the heart and arteries. Discussion of disease of capillaries and kidney arterioles will be reviewed in the section on microvascular disease. The main macrovascular problem is atherosclerosis, but some additional factors contribute or may contribute to the cardiovascular toll in diabetics: fibrosis and calcification of arterial walls; myocardial fibrosis; aberrations of fibrinolysis, platelet function, and blood viscosity; and hypertension and enzymatic, metabolic, or neurologic abnormalities that affect cardiovascular function.

Although the degree to which the presence of diabetes accelerates atherosclerosis is still in some dispute, it is now generally accepted that in man rates at which atherosclerosis develops are increased in diabetes. This has been established by several lines of evidence in animals and in man. Excellent reviews on the relationship of diabetes and atherosclerosis have been published by Bradley (1971), Tzagournis (1975), Jarrett and Keen (1975), Stamler (1975), Stout, et al (1975), Ostrander and Epstein (1976), and by Alberti and Hockaday (1975). Epstein (1973) has written a very good succinct review of some relevant epidemiologic evidence. Scott (1975) and Jarrett (1977) have published good summaries on coronary disease and diabetes. Accounts of the degree and character of the intensification of atherosclerosis in diabetes will be provided below. Epidemiologic studies have shown that both the incidence and prevalence of large-vessel disease is increased substantially in diabetes (Keen and Jarrett, 1973). It has also been shown in many studies that hyperglycemia is more frequent in subjects with manifestations of atherosclerosis than in those without such stigmata. In a majority of these reports controls are decidedly suboptimal, but some of these results are quite persuasive (Wahlberg, 1966; Keen and Jarrett, 1973). Stamler (1975) has pointed out that evidence of a causal association between very mild hyperglycemia and large-vessel disease is less conclusive than for unequivocal diabetes and macrovascular disease.

Anatomic studies by pathologists have yielded somewhat variable results with respect to the degree of intensification of atherosclerosis in diabetes. Atherosclerosis is very greatly intensified in the lower legs of diabetics; elsewhere the disparity between diabetics and nondiabetics tends to be less. In the coronary arteries, atherosclerosis has usually been found to be about twice as great as in nondiabetics (Bradley, 1971). Several observers, including Knowles (1975), have commented on the regularity with which severe atherosclerosis is

353

observed at autopsy in young adults with diabetes of long duration. Because of the differences by anatomic region, separate sections will review the problems of heart disease, cerebrovascular disease, and peripheral vascular disease. Clinical studies in most populations also show that morbidity from atherosclerosis is substantially increased in diabetics (Bradley, 1971). Data on mortality have shown the same phenomenon, as indicated above in Chapter 6.

Here are listed some known and possible etiologic factors in diabetic macrovascular disease.

1. Hyperglycemia (direct or indirect effects, osmotic, enzymatic, etc.)
2. Hyperlipidemia (elevations of cholesterol or triglyceride and associated lipoproteins)
    a. Deficiency of alpha-lipoprotein cholesterol
3. Therapeutic diets high in saturated fat
4. Hypertension
5. Obesity
6. Physical indolence (poor physical condition)
7. Hyperinsulinemia?
8. Hypercoagulability (eg, aberrations in amounts or functions of fibrinogen or platelets)
9. Microvascular disease (interfering with nutrition of walls of large vessels)?
10. Genetic defects (may underlie directly both enhanced rate of atherosclerosis and hyperglycemia)
11. Elevations or aberrations of glycoproteins?
12. Therapy with sulfonylureas and biguanides?
13. Neuropathy (affecting nutrition or metabolism of vessel walls)
14. Other metabolic effects of relative or absolute insulin deficiency
15. Increased blood viscosity?
16. Other factors not peculiar to diabetes (eg, smoking)

History

Prior to the discovery of insulin, only a few had recognized the link between arteriosclerosis and diabetes, for several reasons. Survival of diabetics was shorter before insulin and antibiotics. In most general populations arteriosclerosis and atherosclerosis were less common than they are today. Clinical methods for recognition of both arteriosclerosis and diabetes were much less sensitive. Yet the special propensity of diabetics for large-vessel disease had been noted by a few, well before it became generally recognized. In his review of 1868, Brigham mentioned cases of diabetes with occluded cerebral arteries, and others with unexplained sudden death. But he also quoted Bence-Jones to the effect that cataract seemed to be the only long-term untoward manifestation of diabetes! Bose observed in 1895 that angina was especially common in diabetics. Johann Baptista Helmont (1578-1644) recorded a case of lipemia in diabetes. By the time the link between lipemia and atherosclerosis had been established it was well known that lipemia was common in diabetes (Allen, 1913). In 1922 Allen published a review of diabetic lipemia with 377 references! Allen (1913) also mentioned observations of Kleen in 1900, and of Falta a few years later, that suggested the particular susceptibility of diabetics to atherosclerosis. Kleen was far ahead of his time in recognizing the relationship of atherosclerosis and gangrene. Janeway had recognized the association of diabetes and heart disease in 1916, and Levine in 1922.

The course of enlightenment concerning the association of diabetes and arteriosclerosis is well documented in the successive editions of Joslin's book (1916-1971). As recently as 1923 the usually perceptive Joslin had not appreciated that arteriosclerosis was enhanced by diabetes. He had seen 84 cases of gangrene, but had not yet realized its relationship to arteriosclerosis. Nevertheless, in 1923 he placed in special italics what he considered to be a very important observation: that Muryama and Yamaguchi had not observed gangrene in a series of 49 fatal cases of diabetes in Japan. Although he was a quarter century behind Kleen in recognizing the importance of arteriosclerosis, he was a quarter century ahead of Western diabetology in recognizing the great significance of the paucity of arteriosclerosis in some populations of diabetics. By 1925 he had recognized the strong association between diabetes and arteriosclerosis and quickly became a leader in demonstrating the strength and significance of the link.

Although the importance of arteriosclerosis (particularly atherosclerosis) in diabetes was not generally appreciated until the late 1930s, much impressive evidence was presented in the 1920s. An especially notable year in this process of recognition was 1924, when Fitz and Murphy showed the association in an autopsy study, and Allen observed that atherosclerosis was almost invariably excessive after ten years of diabetes. In the same year Woodyatt described the frequent association of arteriosclerosis with diabetes. The excessive prevalence of calcification of vessels in diabetics was also described in 1924 by Labbe and Lenfantan; and Gray reported that lipemia declined with insulin therapy.

A leading pioneer in the field was Rabinowitch of Montreal (1927, 1931, 1934, 1944). In 1934, Rabinowitch, et al demonstrated a high rate of cardiovascular disease in a very large series of 1,500 diabetics, and they identified an effect of duration of diabetes on the frequency of such lesions. Rabinowitch also called attention to the early age of onset of atherosclerosis in diabetics and to the capabilities for identifying manifestations of atherosclerosis in life. By 1927 he had recognized the important relationship between the elevated blood lipid levels of diabetics and their susceptibility to atherosclerosis. He recommended in 1931 a high-starch low-fat diet, controlled in calories, and provided considerable documentation in support of this recommendation. Although still not accepted unanimously, this type of regimen was endorsed by the American Diabetes Association (Bierman, et al, 1971) on the 40th anniversary of its promulgation by Rabinowitch! Others had previously suggested similar regimens, but the observations and explanations of Rabinowitch in this regard were probably the most lucid and perceptive of those offered in the western world during or before that period. Even though he believed in the utility of controlling hyperglycemia, he suggested that control of blood lipids might be even more important in preventing macrovascular lesions of diabetes. Very recent observations tend to support this notion. As shown below, in many populations a majority of diabetics die from atherosclerosis even though hyperglycemia is moderate, while in other groups atherosclerosis is rare despite severe hyperglycemia. In 1927 Joslin reported a personal cmmunication from Rabinowitch concerning a diabetic with profound hyperlipidemia. The concentration of fat in the blood was 18% (18,000 mg/100 ml)! With insulin therapy, about 1 lb of this fat disappeared from the blood overnight (about 500,000 mg). The remaining pound of excess fat also disappeared promptly with continued therapy. Posttreatment levels were normal. Allen, et al (1919) mentioned that rice diet had been advocated for diabetes by von During of Amsterdam in 1868!

In 1933, Lehnherr reported that aortas of diabetics had more lipid and more calcium than those of nondiabetics. Both Rabinowitch (1944) and Albrink, et al (1963) cited some evidence suggesting that atherosclerosis had become more common in diabetes during the course of the 20th century. More recent landmark observations included a series of reports of E. T. Bell and his associates Nathan and Clawson between 1932 and 1952 on atherosclerosis observed at autopsy in diabetics; and the worldwide pathology studies of Robertson and Strong (1968) showing the regularity with which excessive atherosclerosis occurred in diabetics of several races under a variety of geographic and environmental circumstances.

Population studies of the association of diabetes and atherosclerosis, a very recent development, will be reviewed below.

Toll and Cost

Diabetes-related macrovascular disease has become one of the major human problems. It is an important problem in most populations, significant even in those that are relatively poor (eg, India). In the more affluent half of humankind diabetic macrovascular disease is among the top four causes of death. The recent (1976) Report of the US National Commission on Diabetes shows that conventional methods of gathering and reporting mortality statistics greatly understate the importance of diabetic large-vessel disease in the United States. When more appropriate methods of analysis are employed, the toll probably exceeds 60,000 per year. About half of diabetics in the western world have clinically detectable and clinically significant large-vessel disease (details below). Roughly three quarters of American diabetics die from large-vessel disease, and the toll is similar in many other Western countries.

In the United States alone the costs of this morbidity and mortality total several billion dollars yearly (US National Commission on Diabetes, 1976). Details will be given below for each of the three major types of macrovascular disease (heart, brain, and legs). One of the several challenges for epidemiology in this field will be the more precise measurement of the direct and indirect costs of these lesions. In general about half the cost of large-vessel disease in diabetics is secondary to diabetes; the balance is attributable to the background of large-vessel disease in the general population. Some of the major problems in estimating this cost are discussed below. Other aspects of the economic costs of diabetes have been reviewed in Chapter 2.

Epidemiologic Studies

Pioneering observations were published in 1953 by Aarseth (Oslo) and by Lundbaeck (Aarhus, Denmark). But the association between atherosclerosis and diabetes did not receive much attention in epidemiologic studies prior to 1960. From the other lines of evidence it had been clear for decades that atherosclerosis was especially common in diabetics. It had become apparent by the early 1960s, however, that laboratory and clinical investigations had left many important questions unanswered. Studies of groups of diabetics from clinics and nondiabetic "controls" were usually difficult to evaluate because of incomplete matching for characteristics that also influenced the degree of atherosclerosis and other types of arteriosclerosis. Results of the earlier studies differed greatly concerning the strength of the association between atherosclerosis and diabetes. It was not clear to what extent this relationship was affected by other factors such as age, sex, degree of glycemia, fatness, lipidemia, type of treatment, type of diet, blood pressure. It became evident that only the types of controls and strategies used in epidemiologic investigations would suffice to elucidate these matters. In the last several years a considerable amount of systematically collected data has been accumulated that has yielded some answers and a better delineation of the relevant questions.

In the sections that follow, details will be provided on each of the different arteriosclerotic lesions. That discussion will also review interrelationships among diabetes, the other risk factors for arteriosclerosis and the different manifestations of arteriosclerosis. In this section a general account will be given of epidemiologic studies that have examined the association of diabetes and arteriosclerosis (mainly atherosclerosis). Two common approaches have been to examine and compare the occurrence of the manifestations of arteriosclerosis in diabetics and nondiabetics, and to study the occurrence of diabetes in groups with manifestations of arteriosclerosis. In certain population studies it has been possible to do both.

Among the first studies of diabetes and vascular disease in a general population was that of Lundbaeck in Aarhus, Denmark. This study confirmed the very strong relationship of diabetes and arteriosclerosis. Details of these results are cited below in the sections on heart disease, leg-vessel disease, and microangioathy. Aarseth (1953) performed detailed studies in 312 diabetics of Oslo. He found a marked excess of myocardial infarction and other heart disease, particularly in the diabetic women. Rates of leg-vessel disease were also quite excessive. More than half the diabetics had electrocardiographic abnormalities and about two thirds had roentgenographic evidence of arterial calcification. Another early community-wide study was that of Sievers, et al (1961) in Lund, Sweden. They examined rates of diabetes in a large and representative group of patients with myocardial infarction. Age-specific levels of diabetes were not known precisely in this population; but fairly satisfactory approximations were available, suggesting that rates of diabetes were excessive in those with myocardial infarction by a factor of about 5. Excesses in rates of infarction were greater in diabetic women than in diabetic men. Nilsson, et al (1967) conducted an excellent study of rates of vascular disease in a large and representative group of 598 diabetics in Kristianstad, Sweden. Calcifications of leg vessels were twice as common in diabetics of short duration than in nondiabetic controls, and four times as common in diabetics of long duration. The same relationship was found between diabetes and arcus senilis, and in the same degree.

Studies of Keen, et al (1965) in Bedford, England and of Epstein, et al in Tecumseh, Michigan (1965) showed that this association between macrovascular disease and diabetes prevailed in whole populations. In both of these studies, the original demonstrations linking hyperglycemia and large-vessel disease through cross-sectional studies of prevalence were later supported by prospective data on incidence of manifestations of atherosclerosis (Jarrett and Keen, 1975; Epstein, 1973). Results of O'Sullivan, et al (1970) were similar in Sudbury, Massachusetts, with respect to incidence and prevalence of vascular lesions in hyperglycemic subjects. Other population-based studies showing associations between diabetes and macrovascular disease have included those of Medalie and his associates (1973, 1976, 1977) in Israel; Westlund (1969) in Norway; Wahlberg (1966) in Stockholm; Romo (1972) and Pyorala (1975) in Finland; Welborn, et al in Australia (1968); Pulumbo (1976) in Rochester, Minnesota; Bengston (1973) and Elmfeldt, et al (1976) in Göteborg, Sweden; Harrower and Clarke (1976) in Edinburgh; Jackson in South Africa (1972); Krolewski et al (1977) in Poland and West and Kalbfleisch in Central America (1970). It appears also that rates of large-vessel disease are higher in Japanese diabetics than in nondiabetics of that country (Kato, et al, 1974; Hashimoto, et al, 1974), but data from some population studies in Japan were not entirely conclusive in that respect (Freedman, et al, 1965). Details concerning many of the studies cited in this paragraph will be provided below.

The extensive studies of Dawber and Kannel and their associates in Framingham, Massachusetts did not at first give primary attention to hypergly-cemia as a risk factor in vascular disease. But more recently they have gathered some very useful data of this type (Garcia, et al, 1974). They measured only the random blood glucose, and the total number with occult and known diabetes was modest; but in many respects the design and circumstances were propi-tious for examining questions concerning the effects of hyperglycemia. They have found in studies of both prevalence and incidence a strong association between hyperglycemia and risk of vascular disease of the heart, brain, and legs. Details will be discussed below, including evidence that the effect of diabetes was to a considerable degree independent of other risk factors.

Two studies in populations of employees have been particularly informative. In well-matched groups of diabetics and nondiabetics who were employees of the Dupont Company, Pell and D'Alonzo (1963, 1968) found that manifesta-tions of macrovascular disease were much higher in diabetics. Studies of Stamler (1975) in gas company employees of Chicago have addressed the question of what level of glycemia is required to increase risk of large-vessel disease. The results are in some respects still inconclusive, but they indicate that risk is not substantially increased in those who have slight or equivocal hyperglycemia. Results in Bedford (Jarrett and Keen, 1975) also show a much higher risk in those with unequivocal diabetes than in those with borderline glucose values. Hyperglycemia itself as a cause of increased atherosclerosis in diabetes will be discussed below, as well as the relationship of degree of glycemia to risk of macrovascular disease.

Some of the basic and clinical studies relating to these issues have been cited above in the section on history. Others are described in the excellent reviews of Bradley (1971), Stout, et al (1975), and Hockaday and Alberti (1975). The very important evidence from mortality studies is described in Chapter 6.

Considered in the aggregate, the epidemiologic evidence appears to warrant several generalizations. Rates of atherosclerosis are increased in diabetes. In most circumstances, this association is partially the result of the greater preva-lence in diabetics of other risk factors such as hypercholesterolemia and hypertension. Probably hyperglycemia is itself an independent risk factor. The increased hyperlipidemia in diabetes is to a considerable extent due to the diabetic state itself, although in many circumstances underlying factors com-mon to both also contribute, such as obesity and hyperinsulinemia. In diabetes generally, rates of coronary disease are considerably increased, cerebrovascular disease is usually moderately increased, and peripheral vascular disease is greatly increased. But many factors may influence the degree to which each of these lesions is increased in diabetes. These include age, sex, duration of diabetes, and many other factors known and unknown. In general, the enhancement of atherosclerosis by diabetes has been small in the elderly. Among possible reasons for this are the mildness of hyperglycemia and the high rates of atherosclerosis in nondiabetics of this age group.

One problem in determining the effect of diabetes on rates of vascular disease

359

is that data on smoking have seldom been gathered. In Massachusetts and Oxford, England diabetics smoke less than nondiabetics (Armstrong and Doll, 1975). This is also true in Poland (Czyzyk and Krolewski, 1976).

Causes of Excessive Atherosclerosis in Diabetes

Much remains to be learned and epidemiologic approaches have considerable potential. It is, however, clear that several different factors contribute (see list on page 354).

In many of the studies, even those in large populations, inadequate numbers have been a problem. In the excellent studies in Tecumseh, Framingham, and Bedford, there have been only a few hundred subjects with unequivocal diabetes. Unless numbers are large, formidable problems arise when one needs to examine for the independent effect of each of several factors, such as sex, age, age of onset of diabetes, level of glycemia, blood pressure. For some purposes populations of diabetics in the thousands will be needed to discern the nature of the interrelationships of these factors.

One possibility that deserves further exploration is that of synergism of risk factors, a phenomenon that has been well documented in the general population (Stamler, 1975). In diabetes it is conceivable, for instance, that hyperinsulinemia is in itself relatively innocuous, but is deleterious when accompanied by hyperglycemia or certain types of hyperlipidemia. Epidemiologic studies to test hypotheses of this kind generally require larger numbers of diabetics than have been tested in previous projects. More evidence is also needed regarding the levels at which increased risk of vascular disease begins. In diabetics, for example, not much is known concerning the levels of blood pressure or cholesterolemia at which increased risk of vascular disease begins. Critical levels of blood glucose have been discussed above. Evidence cited below on geographic differences suggests that hyperglycemia itself is only mildly atherogenic in subjects with very low levels of serum cholesterol. In general, it appears that risk factors for atherosclerosis are similar in diabetics and nondiabetics, but more confirmation is needed. Already there is evidence of some divergence in this respect. In some circumstances, for example, the protective effects of female sex are completely absent in diabetes (Bradley, 1971).

The relative importance of the various risk factors is not the same in the lesions of the brain, heart, and leg. For example, hypertension is especially important in cerebrovascular pathology. This deserves further study in diabetes. Jackson, et al (1970) found, for example, that Indian diabetics in South Africa had high rates of coronary disease but relatively modest rates of peripheral vascular disease. These differences in the three major lesions will be discussed further below in the sections on morbidity of the heart, brain, and feet.

Hyperlipidemia

I believe the chief cause of premature development of arteriosclerosis in diabetes, save for advancing age, is an excess of fat, an excess of fat in the

body, obesity, an excess of fat in the diet, and an excess of fat in the blood.
With an excess of fat diabetes begins and from an excess of fat diabetics die,
formerly of coma, recently of arteriosclerosis.

E. P. Joslin (1927)

Joslin's prescient views on the significance of blood lipids were not widely
accepted for many years. Although it is now known and generally accepted
that excessive serum lipids are a factor of major importance in the enhancement of atherosclerosis, there is still considerable uncertainty concerning the
extent to which differences in rates of atherosclerosis in diabetics and nondiabetics are attributable to this factor.

The degrees of these aberrations of lipid metabolism are strongly influenced
by the levels of insulin insufficiency and glycemia, and are therefore often
greatly mitigated by effective therapy of hyperglycemia. In some studies
"treated" patients have had levels of blood lipids that were not much different
than before treatment, but it is likely that this was because blood glucose levels
were not substantially reduced. In some animal experiments hyperglycemia
has not produced or aggravated hyperlipidemia, but in other studies, particularly in those more closely related to man (eg, monkeys), hyperglycemia
usually intensifies lipemia and atherosclerosis (Howard, 1974). Martin and
Hartroft (1965) studied atherosclerosis in diabetic and nondiabetic rats fed
high-lipid diets. Atherosclerosis was greater in the diabetics. At least part of
this excessive atherosclerosis was secondary to the higher serum lipid levels in
the diabetics, but it was not possible to determine whether hyperglycemia also
contributed directly to this enhancement. Bennion and Grundy (1977) demonstrated clearly the very substantial effects of mitigation of hyperglycemia in
normalizing cholesterol metabolism.

Diabetes is associated with increases in the frequency with which several of
the blood lipid components are elevated. Abnormal lipoprotein patterns produced by diabetes may be of Types I, II, III, IV or V (Frederickson, 1971).
Elevations of both low- density and of very-low-density lipoproteins are common. With insulin deficiency chylomicrons are usually increased. Shafrir
(1975) and Hayes (1977) have reviewed on hyperlipidemia in diabetes. Lopes-
Virella, et al (1977) found in diabetics that less cholesterol was bound to high
density lipoprotein, although HDL levels were normal. The degree of this
abnormality is related to degree of hyperglycemia.

In Framingham (Garcia, et al, 1974), however, cholesterol and triglyceride
were not much different in treated diabetics and nondiabetics, and these
modest differences did not appear to explain the greatly increased risk of
vascular disease in the diabetics. In diabetic women, serum triglyceride was
not a significant risk factor after taking into account levels of cholesterol in
high density lipoproteins (Gordon, et al, 1977). Diabetic women had low levels
of cholesterol in their high density lipoproteins. Lundbaeck and Peterson
(1953) found no significant difference in blood cholesterol levels of old nondiabetics and those of age-matched treated diabetics. In the study of Kenien, et al
(1977) serum lipids of diabetic children were very similar to those of their

361

nondiabetic sibs. In 654 British diabetics Lewis and Symonds (1958) found high rates of vascular disease, but no relationship between vascular disease and level of serum cholesterol. Results of Aarseth (1953) in Oslo were also negative in this respect. In Central America we found cholesterol levels somewhat higher in diabetics than in nondiabetics, but it was not clear whether this difference was attributable to diabetes (West and Kalbfleisch, 1970). In Tecumseh (Ostrander, et al, 1973), higher levels of serum lipids did not appear to account entirely for the much greater rates of large-vessel disease in persons with hyperglycemia. In Oslo serum cholesterol values were not higher in treated diabetics than in nondiabetics (Westlund and Nicolaysen, 1972). In Bussleton (Bowyer, et al, 1974) cholesterol levels in diabetics were not significantly different from those of nondiabetics. There is, however, a large body of evidence from other sources in animals and in man suggesting that levels of serum cholesterol are generally somewhat higher in diabetics and that levels of triglyceride are usually considerably higher (Wilson, et al, 1970). The degree of these differences is related to effectiveness of treatment of diabetes. In well-treated groups of diabetics, serum lipid levels are not much higher than in the general population. Chase and Glasgow (1976) found levels of serum cholesterol and triglyceride excessive in juvenile diabetics.

Pyke, et al (1977) studied serum cholesterol levels in 19 pairs of identical twins discordant for diabetes. During the first 10 years of diabetes, cholesterol levels were slightly greater than in nondiabetic twins, but values were a bit lower than controls in long-duration diabetes.

Freedman, et al (1965) found that Japanese women with diabetes had serum cholesterol values considerably higher than nondiabetic controls. In Australian aborigines serum cholesterol levels were significantly higher in diabetics than nondiabetics, but the difference was of mild degree. Triglyceride levels were considerably higher in the diabetics. In Stockholm juvenile diabetics (Sterky, et al, 1963) cholesterol values were somewhat higher than in controls, but triglycerides were not significantly elevated in these treated diabetics. In 300 diabetic Plains Indians of Oklahoma we found serum triglyceride levels elevated considerably, but triglyceride values were not elevated above those of nondiabetic controls in diabetics with fasting blood glucose levels below 150 mg/100 ml. Nilsson, et al (1967) observed in Kristianstadt, Sweden, that arcus senilis was four times more frequent in diabetics than in an age-matched element of the general population. This was a large representative sample (598) of diabetics. Mean serum cholesterol was 184 mg/100 ml in controls, 194 in short-duration diabetics, and 202 in long-duration diabetics. In diabetics of populations consuming low-fat diets, atherosclerosis is minimal but somewhat greater than in nondiabetics of these populations (Robertson and Strong, 1968). Details on the profound geographic differences in the degree of atherosclerosis in diabetics will be provided below in the section on that subject.

A very substantial majority of diabetics under treatment have "normal" serum lipid levels by conventional standards. But these criteria are inappropriate, in that they were based on the faulty reasoning that values typical in

Western societies are normal. It is now quite clear that persons with typical cholesterol values of 225 mg/100 ml are much more likely to have or develop atherosclerosis than persons with cholesterol levels of 175. Thus the appropriate question is not what portion of diabetics have, by these faulty standards, "abnormal" serum lipid levels. The main issues are the extent to which diabetics have higher levels than nondiabetics, the degree to which those levels are lowered by treatment of diabetes, and the effect of lowering these lipid levels. A better basis for defining normality would be the range of lipid values in societies where morbidity from atherosclerosis is quite rare.

Triglyceride levels tend to be considerably elevated in untreated diabetes. However, the extent to which serum triglyceride is an independent risk factor is unsettled (Brunzell, et al, 1975; Levy, 1973; Nestel, et al, 1974; Kannel, 1978). Carlson and Bottiger (1972) and Albrink (1973) believe that it is; and Stamler (1973) thinks it probably isn't. The major difficulty here is that serum triglyceride levels so often correspond with cholesterol levels. Blackburn (1974) also found present evidence inconclusive with respect to serum triglyceride as an independent risk factor. Nikkila (1973) has reviewed the subject of triglyceride metabolism and diabetes.

There is some evidence suggesting that neither triglyceridemia nor hyperglycemia alone is in itself profoundly atherogenic. Bantu diabetics have considerable glycemia and triglyceridemia but very little atherosclerosis (Shapiro, et al, 1973). Serum cholesterol levels are low. In their study in Hawaii of Japanese and Hawaiian males, Chung, et al (1969) were unable to detect any association between coronary disease and levels of serum triglyceride independent of diabetes. In contrast, Santen, et al (1972) and Reinheimer, et al (1967) found in diabetics a strong association between the presence of hypertriglyceridemia and manifestations of atherosclerosis. Fraser, et al (1973) did not find a positive relationship between the two variables in a small group of diabetics. Among many possibilities is that the apparent effect of triglyceridemia is dependent on, or synergistic with, other factors to which it is sometimes linked, such as hyperinsulinemia, obesity, physical indolence, decreased fibrinolysis. The peculiarly severe intensification in diabetes of the occlusive vascular disease below the knees deserves special attention (Barner, 1976). These differences by anatomic region in the effects of diabetes on atherogenesis suggest that there may be variations in the relative importance of inciting factors in different parts of the arterial tree. It is possible, for example, that triglyceridemia may be more important as a risk factor for gangrene than for coronary disease.

Epidemiologic approaches have special potential in elucidating these interrelationships because of the need to control for several variables simultaneously. This is harder to do when groups of diabetics to be studied are drawn from groups of clinic patients and the controls from other elements of the population. Some of the apparent conflict in previous results has been the result of failure to measure, control for, or take into account factors such as age, glycemia, duration of diabetes, adiposity, exercise, and serum insulin levels.

It is possible that study of epidemiologic moieties other than cholesterol and triglycerides will be productive. This includes the various lipoproteins. Levels of serum triglyceride in diabetics have corresponded well with the levels of very-low-density lipoproteins. And, in general, the concentrations of triglyceride and cholesterol seem to reflect about as well the status of lipid metabolism as do elements that require more complex procedures; at least in so far as epidemiologic studies are concerned. Several investigators have, however, shown a strongly inverse association between risk of coronary disease and levels of cholesterol in serum lipoprotein of high density (Kannel, 1978). Lopes-Virella and Colwell (1976) found that these lipoproteins were particularly low in diabetes, and degree of deficiency was apparently well related to degree of metabolic decompensation. There was no evidence of a qualitative peculiarity of the carrier apoprotein (alpha-lipoprotein).

Vuayagopal, et al (1973) thought dietary fiber might lower serum lipids but this requires further study. Other investigations have been negative in this respect.

Qualitative dietary factors have a particularly important influence on postprandial triglyceride levels, while fasting levels are more related to total calories consumed. Fasting levels are, however, affected to some extent by qualitative features of diet such as alcohol consumption. Also, the concentration of triglycerides is quite variable in the various types of lipoprotein complexes. For these reasons the significance of postprandial and fasting triglyceridemia is in some respects different. It is also quite possible that the atherogenic effects of postprandial and fasting triglyceridemia are not the same. It is therefore important to recognize these considerations in designing and interpreting epidemiologic studies in which levels of serum triglyceride are measured.

Therapeutic diets high in fat

As indicated above, it seems probable that the low-carbohydrate, high-fat diets prescribed traditionally in the West for diabetes have increased rates of atherosclerosis. Little direct evidence is available in this regard, however. Another factor of importance is that diets high in saturated fats are traditional in most of the affluent populations of the West. In the Occident most diabetics have been on high-fat diets for many years before they develop diabetes. Very commonly dietary fat has been further increased after diabetes has been discovered. It was widely believed previously that high-carbohydrate diets would produce hypertriglyceridemia, but it now appears that triglyceride levels are lower on high-starch diets, provided that calories are controlled (Kiehm, et al, 1976; Schellenberg and Schlierf, 1976).

Adiposity, Insulinemia, and Exercise

Several investigators have considered the possibility that the increased propensity of diabetics to atherosclerosis might be secondary to the hyperinsulinemia that often attends diabetes or its therapy. The case for this possibility has been well set forth by Stout, et al (1975) and by Mahler (1973). Stout and others have shown that under some conditions insulin has a direct local effect in enhancing atherogenesis. Although severely diabetic patients have little or no endogenous insulin, they usually receive therapeutically amounts even larger than normal persons produce. Almer (1975) and others have reported that in obesity there is impairment of certain functions that inhibit clot formation, including fibrinolysis. Most fat diabetics have generous amounts of insulin in their blood, often more than lean normals. In certain animals (eg, rabbits) insulinopenia decreases atherogenesis and insulin administration enhances atherosclerosis. Under some conditions mitigation of hyperglycemia fails to mitigate atherosclerosis in diabetic animals. In man there is in many circumstances a strong association between serum insulin and serum triglycerides. In certain types of patients Eaton and Nye (1973) reduced serum triglyceride levels by suppressing insulin secretion with diazoxide. This group included fat and lean subjects and some with and without glucose intolerance. But Wales (1976) found that triglyceride levels in untreated diabetics were not related to levels of serum insulin.

Reinheimer, et al (1967) observed a relationship of weight gain to frequency of large-vessel disease in diabetics. In several epidemiologic studies manifestations of large-vessel disease have been more common in fat than in lean persons (Dyer, et al, 1975; Kannel, et al, 1967), but it is not yet clear to what extent, if any, these excesses are the result of intensification of atherosclerosis in obesity.

Despite the evidence cited above several considerations militate against hyperinsulinemia and obesity as major causes of the association between diabetes and atherosclerosis. Results in Bedford, England were consistent with the possiblity that the greater frequencies of manifestations such as angina in the obese are mostly or entirely secondary to deleterious effects of obesity other than increased atherosclerosis (Keen, et al, 1972). For example, in hyperglycemic people electrocardiographic abnormalities characteristic of ischemic heart disease were not more frequent in fat than in lean subjects. Results in Framingham were similar (Kannel, et al, 1967). Fat people had more angina but not more myocardial infarction.

In Bantu diabetics both serum insulin levels and rates of macrovascular disease are low (Wicks and Jones, 1973). But in American Indian diabetics rates of large-vessel disease are low despite high levels of serum insulin and adiposity (West, 1974). Rates of morbidity from atherosclerosis are not much enhanced by obesity alone in the absence of diabetes, hypertension, or hypercholesterolemia (Keen, et al, 1974; Chapman, et al, 1971). Obese nondiabetics have very high levels of insulin.

Bjurulf (1959) found atherosclerosis somewhat greater at autopsy in fat people, but this may have been caused by associated factors such as lipemia. In the international cooperative project no relationship was found between obesity and pathologic evidence of atherosclerosis (Montenegro and Solberg, 1968). In Oslo diabetics, Aarseth observed no relationship between adiposity and calcification of vessels. Christensen, et al (1968) found insulin reduced in a group of patients with ischemic heart disease and abnormal glucose tolerance. In the Oslo study of Westlund and Nicolaysen (1972) overweight had no independent effect on mortality or mycardial infarction until weight reached 145% of standard. Blackburn (1974) has reviewed other evidence suggesting that the independent effect of obesity on the enhancement of atherosclerosis is weak or negligible.

Gross hyperlipemia is common in lean diabetics with low insulin levels (before any treatment is given). In some animal studies hyperlipemia has been reduced by giving insulin. In monkeys, Howard (1974) found a strongly inverse association between triglyceride levels and serum insulin levels. Kalant, et al, (1964) found that insulin deficiency increased atherosclerosis in rats on a high-fat diet. In monkeys and other animals atherosclerosis has been reversed or prevented by administration of insulin (Armstrong, 1976). In persons with type IV hyperlipoproteinema Gleuk, et al (1969) found that normal, low, and high levels of serum insulin were about equally common. Persons with beta-cell tumors and very high levels of serum insulin tend to have low serum triglyceride levels. Elkeles, et al (1971) found more vascular complications in diabetics with low insulin levels than in those with high levels. Nikkila, et al (1965) observed no relationship between serum insulin and serum lipids in coronary disease. In women of Göteborg, Sweden who had had myocardial infarction, "very low" early response of insulin secretion to intravenous glucose was more common than in controls (Bengston, 1973). Hyperinsulinemia was not more common in infarct patients.

Possibly some of the association between adiposity and triglyceridemia may be due to lower levels of exercise in fat people. Truswell and Mann (1971) found an inverse relationship between exercise levels and triglyceridemia. Hoffman, et al (1967) demonstrated that certain lipoproteins were lower in well-conditioned men. In the study of a representative sample of the population of Bedford, England, Abrams, et al (1969) observed that triglyceride levels were strongly related to blood glucose and less strongly related to blood insulin. Epstein (1973) has considered the possibility that both low and high blood insulin levels may enhance atherogenesis. Blackburn (1974) reviewed positive and negative evidence linking physical indolence to coronary disease. He found present data inconclusive concerning the importance of exercise as a protective factor.

Goodkin, et al (1975) examined the relationship of insulin dosage to mortality in juvenile-onset diabetics. No significant difference was found between those taking large dosages (75–100 units daily) and those who took small dosages (25–50 units).

These conflicting considerations do suggest the need for more epidemiologic studies, particularly in groups that have not been treated with insulin, with appropriate control for age and duration of diabetes.

In considering the effect of obesity on atherosclerosis it is important to keep in mind that obesity may, in an indirect manner, increase the toll from diseases relating to atherosclerosis. There is considerable evidence to suggest that even when levels of atherosclerosis are the same in fat and lean, the fat element of the population has more angina, more congestive heart failure, and more hypertension. Studies in diabetics of the effect of overweight on mortality have usually been difficult to interpret because of inadequate matching for factors such as age, age of onset of diabetes, type of therapy, and degree of hyperglycemia.

In Rochester, Minnesota, survival of fat diabetics was better than that of lean diabetics (Palumbo, 1975). Insurance company data also show this, but it should be kept in mind that glucose levels are higher in lean diabetics, and that groups of fat and lean diabetics also differ in other respects. Interpretation of any differences in outcome require taking into account these differences in other characteristics.

Levels of exercise have seldom been compared in diabetics and nondiabetics. It seems likely, however, that obese diabetics are relatively indolent. It also seems probable that this indolence would usually tend to promote higher serum insulin levels. (Bjorntorp, et al, 1972). Cooper, et al (1976) demonstrated a strongly negative relationship between physical fitness and several risk factors for vascular disease, including fatness, blood pressure, and serum levels of cholesterol, triglyceride, and glucose. But others have found little relationship between physical fitness and manifestations of atherosclerosis. Positive and negative evidence on physical conditioning as a negative risk factor for macrovascular disease has been reviewed by Blackburn (1974).

DIRECT EFFECT OF A GENETIC TRAIT

It has been frequently suggested that the increased risk of both large- and small-vessel disease might not be secondary to hyperglycemia but, rather, the result of an underlying genetic defect causing both vascular disease and hyperglycemia. This hypothesis is still under consideration and investigation (Vracko and Benditt, 1974; Medalie, et al, 1975; Rosenbloom, 1977). Much recent evidence is negative. As indicated above there are many different genetic mechanisms that cause diabetes. The two main types of diabetes appear to have different genetic mechanisms, but both are attended by high rates of atherosclerosis. In many different circumstances artificially-induced beta-cell destruction has been attended by acceleration of atherosclerosis. This has not been seen in all animals, but is quite striking in monkeys (Howard, 1974). Large-vessel disease is frequent in certain kinds of "secondary" diabetes such as hemochromatosis (Dymcock, et al, 1972). Two of the most severe cases of atherosclerosis I have seen were in patients with no family history of diabetes who had diabetes secondary to Cushing's syndrome.

It has sometimes been found that nondiabetic relatives of diabetics have excessive rates of atherosclerosis (Reaven, et al, 1963; Ueda, et al, 1975; Krolewski, et al, 1977). I am not aware of any such results in a study with adequate controls for age and other characteristics (eg, serum lipids, adiposity, fat intake) that might influence rates of morbidity from atherosclerosis. Several

367

negative studies have been reported. Harvald and Hauge (1963) found no evidence of increased vascular disease in nondiabetic relatives of diabetics. Sterky (1962) did not find vascular disease unusually common in relatives of juvenile-onset diabetics. The studies of Ricketts, et al (1966) were negative in prediabetics. On the basis of his studies, Ferrier (1964) concluded that arterial disease of the leg was not a feature of prediabetes. Katterman and Köbberling (1970) found lipids normal in a large series of nondiabetic relatives of diabetics. Brunzell, et al (1975) showed that the genetic mechanisms of diabetes and hypertriglyceridemia were probably separate. Patel and Talwalker (1966) found serum lipids normal in "prediabetics".

In 76 adult offspring of two diabetic parents we found no evidence of aberrations of insulin secretion, and triglyceride levels were not different from controls (West and Mako, 1976). Nor was there any other evidence of increased large-vessel disease in this group, all of whom had chest roentgenograms and electrocardiograms. In a cooperative Japanese study (Ueda, et al, 1975) risk of myocardial infarction was even more strongly related to family history of diabetes than to diabetes. But it was not clear to what degree, if any, this relationship was independent of other factors such as adiposity, hypercholesterolemia, hyperglycemia, hypertension, and cigarette smoking.

Excessive consumption of saturated fat and calories sometimes leads to adiposity, hyperlipidemia, vascular disease, and diabetes. In that sense there is a link between prediabetes and vascular disease. But it does not seem likely that a specific genetic trait directly causes both large-vessel disease and diabetes.

Microvascular Disease and Neuropathy as Causes of Atherosclerosis

It has been suggested that disease of the small vessels might enhance atherosclerosis by interfering with the blood supply to the walls of large vessels. Although this is conceivable, there is little direct evidence to this effect. In Japan microvascular disease is rife in diabetics, but manifestations of atherosclerosis are relatively uncommon. Microvascular disease as a possible contributing factor in directly impairing coronary flow will be discussed below in the section on heart disease. Neuropathy has seldom been considered as an etiologic agent for atherosclerosis, but this, too, is a possibility. Conceivably nutrition and metabolism of the vessel walls could be dependent to some extent on the integrity of afferent or efferent neurologic communication. Epidemiologic study of links between neuropathy, and its possible effects and causes, has been greatly handicapped by the paucity of field methods for reliably measuring its presence and degree. This is discussed below in the section on neuropathy. In a section below on heart disease other mechanisms are discussed by which neuropathy may impair cardiac function.

Hypertension

Jarrett and Keen (1975) have recently reviewed the role of hypertension in diabetic vascular disease. Other good reviews on this subject include papers of Christlieb (1973) and Vaishnava and Bhasim (1968). Most studies have found an increased frequency of hypertension in diabetes. A substantial majority of this excess is probably attributable to an increased frequency in diabetics of traits known to cause hypertension. These include a few uncommon disorders such as pheochromocytoma, hyperaldosteronism, and hypersecretion of the adrenal cortex. The most important causes of the excessive rates of hypertension in diabetics are probably obesity and kidney disease, the latter factor confined mainly to diabetes of substantial duration. In childhood-onset diabetics hypertension is rare at onset, with frequency starting to rise abruptly after ten years of diabetes; after thirty years of diabetes about half have hypertension (Christlieb, 1973).

Aarseth (1953) found that the excessive rate of heart disease in diabetes was strongly related to hypertension. Vaishnava and Bhasim (1968) cite 17 different reports on the frequency of hypertension in groups of diabetics. Prevalence of hypertension ranged from 10.5% to 68%. None of these groups could be considered a representative sample of all the diabetics in the general population from which they were derived. Many different variables could account for these interpopulation differences, including salt intake (Meneely and Dahl, 1961; Freis, 1976), duration of diabetes, frequency of renal disease and of obesity, and differences in methods for ascertaining and defining hypertension.

The large group of diabetics (662) studied by Pell and D'Alonzo (1967) were particularly well matched (for age, sex, and occupational functions) with their nondiabetic fellow employees of the Dupont Company. Rates of hypertension were 54% higher in the diabetics. This excess was partly but not wholly explained by the greater adiposity of the diabetic. Rates of atherosclerotic disease were greater in diabetics even after correction for blood pressure level. It did appear that the excessive rates of heart disease in diabetics were in part the result of their greater blood pressure. Even prior to the diagnosis of diabetes the diabetics had higher blood pressure levels than nondiabetics. The deleterious effects of hypertension were of approximately equal degree in diabetics and nondiabetics. Garcia, et al (1974) found in Framingham that blood pressures were somewhat greater in diabetics than in the general population, but this did not account for much of the excessive rate of large-vessel disease. The disparity in blood pressure level between diabetics and nondiabetics was greater in women (Garcia, et al, 1973).

In Tecumseh (Epstein, et al, 1965), persons with newly discovered diabetes had blood pressure levels somewhat higher than age-matched nondiabetics. But the number of new diabetics was small and the association between levels of glycemia and blood pressure was statistically significant only in women. Nilsson, et al (1967) found in their well-controlled study in Sweden that mean systolic blood pressure was 146 mm Hg in controls, 157 in diabetics of short duration, and 159 in diabetics of long duration. In Bedford (Jarrett and Keen, 1975), persons with occult hyperglycemia in certain age groups had higher blood pressure than nondiabetics. The degree of difference was somewhat greater in men. The greater fatness of those with borderline or abnormal glucose tolerance contributed to the differences but did not account for them entirely. Similar results were found in a study of London civil servants by

Jarrett and Keen (1975), but in persons with previously diagnosed diabetes, blood pressures were not excessive in this population. Stamler and his associates (1975) found in gas company employees that the greater fatness of those with glucose intolerance did not account entirely for their higher blood pressures.

The cooperative study in Japan (Ueda, et al, 1975) found that hypertension was a risk factor for myocardial infarction, but not as strong as diabetes, hypercholesterolemia, or smoking. Kato (1976) found that diabetes was a strong risk factor for myocardial infarction in Japanese, but not so strong as hypertension or hypercholesterolemia. In the Japanese diabetics studied by Baba (1976), mortality was excessive only in those with hypertension. However, Baba also cited evidence of Kagan indicating that high stroke rates in Japanese might not be entirely attributable to hypertension. Blood pressures in Japanese of California were higher than those in Hiroshima, but stroke was more common in Hiroshima. In Busselton, Australia (Welborn, et al, 1968) there was no relationship between blood glucose and blood pressure, but both factors were associated with increased risk of coronary disease. Westlund and Nicolaysen (1972) found in Oslo that blood pressure was only weakly related to glycemia. In the geographic pathology studies of Robertson and Strong (1968) a pronounced effect of diabetes on atherosclerosis was observed in persons who were not hypertensive.

In 19 diabetics studied by Pyke, et al (1977) blood pressure levels were not significantly different than those of their nondiabetic identical twins.

Under the circumstances of their study Jarrett and Keen (1976) observed no effect on blood pressure with phenformin therapy. A larger and different dosage regimen appeared to raise blood pressure significantly (UGDP, 1975).

Blood pressure was notably low in diabetics who had survived forty years or more, as reported by Oakley, et al (1974). In a group of Japanese diabetics and controls studied by Wada and Shigeta (1966), ischemic heart disease was quite excessive in diabetics, but most of this seemed to be due to the greater frequency of hypertension in these diabetics.

Severe vasculitis of the type seen in malignant hypertension is less common in diabetics than in nondiabetics. Malignant hypertension is particularly rare in diabetics (Christlieb, 1973; Osuntokun, 1972). Indeed, it seems likely that diabetes protects against some of the deleterious effects of hypertension by mechanisms not yet fully explained (Christlieb, 1973).

Risk of cerebrovascular disease is strongly related to blood pressure in diabetics as well as nondiabetics (Vernet, et al, 1975). Vernet also found that rates of coronary disease were higher in diabetics when hypertension was present.

More evidence is needed concerning the interrelationships of hypertension, diabetes, and atherosclerosis. The following tentative conclusions are offered. A substantial majority of the excess of hypertension is accounted for by the association of diabetes with factors known to cause hypertension (eg, glomerulosclerosis and obesity). In most populations blood pressures are to some degree excessive in diabetics and probably contribute significantly to the excess of large-vessel disease in diabetics. Hypertension is probably not the major cause of the excessive large-vessel disease in diabetics.

HYPERGLYCEMIA

It seems possible that hyperglycemia itself enhances atherogenesis, but the mechanism and degree of this effect are uncertain. Some scholars are even skeptical that hyperglycemia has any directly deleterious effect in this regard. This skepticism is based on several considerations. Under some experimental conditions in certain animals, hyperglycemia has little if any effect on atherogenesis. In some circumstances it has seemed that the frequency and severity of associated factors, such as hypertension and hyperlipidemia, are adequate to account for the higher rates of atherosclerosis in diabetes. In several studies (eg, Weaver, et al, 1970; Pirart, 1977), rates of atherosclerosis seemed about the same in maturity-onset diabetes of short and long duration. Many studies have shown that rates of atherosclerosis are at least as high in maturity-onset diabetes as in childhood-onset cases, despite the greater glycemia in the latter. These comparisons have not usually been corrected to take into account the profound effect of age itself on atherosclerosis. In the University Group Diabetes Study (1971) no beneficial effect on incidence of vascular disease was observed in patients treated with insulin, even though blood glucose levels were lower than those in control groups. In the study of Hadden, et al (1973) degree of hyperglycemia was a much weaker risk factor for vascular disease than other recognized risk factors. A bibliography of 130 citations covering the literature on this controversial subject has been published by the National Library of Medicine (1971) covering the years 1968 through 1971.

Despite the rather considerable amount of negative evidence, a causal role of glycemia cannot be excluded. Although mainly indirect, there is also a large amount of evidence suggesting that hyperglycemia enhances atherosclerosis. This review will ignore much important evidence from basic and clinical studies (Cahill, et al, 1976), concentrating primarily on epidemiologic data.

Data of insurance companies are impressive in this regard. They correct nicely for age in a way seldom possible in other circumstances. They show that while death rates are higher in older than in younger diabetics, the mortality-risk ratios (based on experience in age-matched diabetics and nondiabetics) are much higher in younger diabetics who typically have greater glycemia (Goodkin, et al, 1975). Details covering these data of insurance companies are reviewed in Chapter 6 on mortality. These data also show an effect on mortality of duration of diabetes that is independent of age. They demonstrate that risks of death and vascular death are greater in patients who require insulin than in those who do not. In general, patients requiring insulin have lesser levels of endogenous insulin and higher levels of blood glucose. Patients judged at outset (prospectively) to have "good" control of hyperglycemia had much lower death rates than those judged initially to have had "poor" control, even after matching for other characteristics (Goodkin, et al, 1975). Since about 75%

of American diabetics die of large-vessel disease, the excessive rates of mortality of diabetics reflect rather well their excessive rates of severe large-vessel disease.

When appropriate corrections are made for other factors, rates and amounts of vascular disease appear to be influenced by duration of hyperglycemia, although this relationship is difficult to verify in some circumstances because of many confounding variables. In the section below on leg-vessel disease, data are reviewed showing positive relationships between arterial disease and duration of diabetes. In one subgroup of 96 long-duration diabetics studied by Bradley (1971), coronary disease was responsible for death in 100% of those who died (45 deaths)! Many, including Bradley (1971) and Knowles (1971), have commented on the very extensive degree of atherosclerosis seen at autopsy in young diabetics of long duration. In most of these persons serum lipid levels are within "normal" limits. Such cases are commonly observed with no evident risk factors other than hyperglycemia. (Engle, et al, 1974). Data of Goto, et al (1975) and of Hayashi, et al (1975) in Japan also suggested an effect of duration of diabetes on risk of ischemic heart disease. On the other hand, hyperglycemia does not appear to be severely deleterious when serum cholesterol levels are very low (as in rural Africans). Atherosclerosis in young diabetics is also intensified frequently by hypertension, but the degree of atherosclerosis seems to exceed that seen with hypertension in young nondiabetics. Under geographic factors (below) much additional evidence is cited suggesting that hyperglycemia itself may contribute to the enhanced rate of atherosclerosis in diabetes.

In old diabetic woman, Vernet, et al (1974) found greater rates of vascular disease in insulin-dependent than in insulin-independent diabetes. In Framingham (Garcia, et al, 1974) and in Poland (Krolewski et al, 1977), the same phenomenon was observed. After matching for other characteristics, increased risk of vascular disease was considerably greater in patients taking insulin. Haywood and Lucena (1965) also observed this in Birmingham, England. In the studies of Grönberg, et al (1967) in Sweden, mortality ratios were only slightly excessive in elderly diabetics, but very excessive in young diabetics in whom the degree of hyperglycemia was greater. Similar results were obtained in Warsaw by Krolewski et al (1977).

In Busselton, Australia (Welborn, et al, 1969), hyperglycemia increased risk of vascular disease substantially, and this increase was independent of other major risk factors. In Framingham (Garcia, et al, 1974; Kannel, et al, 1976), the effect of hyperglycemia was not entirely independent, but was substantially so. This was also true in Tecumseh (Epstein, 1973) and in London civil servants studied by Fuller, et al (1975). In Israel it appeared that the effect of hyperglycemia on incidence of angina was to a considerable degree independent of other known risk factors (Medalie, et al, 1973). In the studies of Pell and D'Alonzo (1970), some of the excessive risk of vascular disease in diabetics was explained by the frequency of known risk factors such as hypertension, but some of the excess was unexplained by factors other than hyperglycemia. In a cooperative study of coronary disease in Japan (Ueda, et al, 1975), the strength of diabetes as a risk factor slightly exceeded that of hypercholesterolemia. Racic, et al (1976) found in Yugoslavian males a positive association between hyperglycemia and coronary heart disease. The strength of the association increased with degree of hyperglycemia. The extent to which this association was independent of other known risk factors was not indicated. The Coronary Drug Project Research Group (Klimt, et al, 1977) found a significant association between mortality and blood glucose level. Part, but not all, of this relationship was explained by an excess of other coronary risk factors in those with elevated glucose levels.

Consistent with the hypothesis that degree of glycemia is of importance is the typical finding that degree of excess of vascular disease is small in very early diabetes (a circumstance in which glycemia is usually slight). Insurance company data show this, for example (Goodkin, et al, 1975). In the studies of Pyorala, et al (1975), no excess of risk was observed in diabetics over 69 years of age. These elderly diabetics typically have mild hyperglycemia. In the section below on peripheral vascular disease several examples are cited showing a relationship of duration of hyperglycemia to leg-vessel disease.

Recent data of the WHO cooperative autopsy study also suggest the possibility that hyperglycemia is an independent risk factor for atherosclerosis (Kagan, et al, 1976). In diabetics the degree of excessive coronary atherosclerosis was equivalent to that seen with hypertension (Zdanov and Vihert, 1976). Excess of coronary disease was somewhat greater in the diabetics who had had diabetes more than ten years and in those who took insulin injections.

There are many possibilities to explain the apparently independent effect of hyperglycemia in enhancing macrovascular disease. They include a direct effect of hyperglycemia on rate of atherogenesis; a deleterious effect on coagulation, vessel-wall metabolism, or nutrition; or osmotic effects. Clements, et al (1969) have demonstrated effects of hyperglycemia on the "polyol pathway" in walls of large vessels. The demonstration that the relationship of hyperglycemia and large-vessel disease is independent of the other major known risk factors does not establish a direct causal effect of hyperglycemia itself. It may be, for example, that relative insulin insufficiency leads by separate mechanisms to both hyperglycemia and macrovascular disease. But a direct effect of hyperglycemia seems quite possible.

It is possible that some of the differences among populations observed in rates of certain complications of diabetes are attributable to differences in blood glucose levels. Unfortunately, hardly any information is available on the frequency distribution of blood glucose values of groups of diabetics. A few data are available on clinic populations (eg, Horiuchi, et al, 1970; John, 1950), but it is not certain to what extent these are representative. In the Pimas, data are available on the distribution of two-hour values (Table 20; Figure 6), but few data are available for comparison.

At what level of glycemia does increased risk begin?

This has been studied extensively with inconclusive results. This subject has been reviewed by Stamler (1975). Many studies have shown high rates of macrovascular disease in subjects with mildly abnormal glucose tolerance. Controls are decidedly suboptimal in most of these. This subject was also reviewed by Wahlberg and Thomasson (1968). Among the better studies of this kind were those of Wahlberg (1966). Rates of impaired glucose tolerance were much higher in patients of Wahlberg with coronary and peripheral vascular disease than in "control" patients matched for age. But these differences could have been attributable to other confounding variables. Relationships of impaired tolerance to vascular disease have also been shown in population studies (Epstein, 1973; Jarrett and Keen, 1975). Yet it has been difficult to determine whether the association of slightly impaired tolerance and atherosclerosis is one of cause and effect. This is mainly because of the higher rates of other risk factors in persons with poor tolerance (eg, physical indolence, obesity, hyperlipidemia, high blood pressure). In both Bedford (Jarrett and Keen, 1975) and Tecumseh (Ostrander, et al, 1973) rates of macrovascular disease were excessive in persons with borderline glucose tolerance. But in Israel Schor, et al (1975) found no excess of myocardial infarction until random blood glucose levels reached 140 mg/100 ml. It is not yet clear whether "abnormal" glucose tolerance is an independent risk factor *in persons with normal fasting blood glucose levels.*

Other Risk Factors

Many other factors known or unknown may contribute in raising or lowering susceptibility of diabetics to macrovascular disease. Several are listed on page 354. Some of these have received little attention in epidemiologic studies.

Factors other than atherosclerosis that increase risk of heart disease in diabetes will be discussed in the section below on heart disease.

Interrelationships of Risk Factors

For reasons outlined above, it has been difficult to determine in macrovascular disease the causal importance of the various factors associated with diabetes. Epstein (1973) has reviewed these problems. Some of the analytic instruments developed earlier in the epidemiologic study of vascular disease have been helpful in the analysis of diabetes-related data. These have been reviewed by Moss (1975), Susser (1973), and Feinstein (1973). Multivariate analysis of the type described by Truett, et al (1967) is sometimes applicable. Methods of this kind showed, for example, that the association between diabetes and increased risk of macrovascular disease was to a considerable degree independent of the other principal risk factors (Garcia, et al, 1974). Other techniques of this type include multiple linear regression, multiple logistic regression, and discriminant function analysis. On the whole, however, the need for more and better data is greater than the need for more powerful analytic instruments. Better application of existing analytic tools is of course desirable.

Geographic and Racial Differences

It is now apparent that the geographic differences in diabetic macrovascular disease are real, substantial in degree, and not primarily attributable to race. Thus these geographic variations provide important and exciting clues to the prevention and mitigation of one of the world's worst health problems. It will be appropriate, therefore, to discuss these differences in some detail.

EARLY OBSERVATIONS

In 1895 Bose described rather vaguely some geographic differences in the manifestations of diabetes. Similar observations were made by many other clinicians of the East in the early part of the 20th century, but as indicated above the association of atherosclerosis and diabetes was little appreciated before the discovery of insulin (1921). Even before he recognized the connection between atherosclerosis and gangrene, Joslin (1923) placed great emphasis on the significance of the rarity of gangrene in Japan as communicated to him by Muryama and Yamaguchi. But many years were to pass before clinicians and scientists of the West recognized the significance of these early observations. In 1937 Wang published an outstanding study of a large group of 405 diabetics in China. Manifestations of coronary and leg-vessel disease were rare. Only a few Western clinicians (eg, Snapper in 1941) seemed to appreciate the significance of this kind of information. The interesting publication of DeZoysa (1951) wasn't much noticed either. He cited very impressive data on the low incidence of peripheral vascular disease in diabetics of Ceylon.

MODERN OBSERVATIONS

The main stimulus for the eventual recognition of the significance and importance of geographic differences was the international work of cardiologists and pathologists studying the geography of atherosclerosis. Systematic study of the geographic aspects of diabetic vascular disease by epidemiologic methods began in the 1960s. These geographic variations will be discussed by race. One reason for this will be to minimize the problem of ascertaining whether observed geographic differences in vascular disease are due to genetic or to environmental factors.

Japanese

In 1962, Rudnick and Anderson reported results of observations on diabetics and nondiabetics of Hiroshima, Japan. Even in diabetics, coronary and peripheral vascular disease were rare. Serum cholesterol levels were low in diabetics, although higher in diabetics than in the general population. Levels of serum triglyceride were not significantly different in diabetics and nondiabetics.

These observations have been extended by many subsequent studies in Japan. Wada, et al (1964) reported clinical studies in diabetes documenting the low rates of coronary and peripheral vascular disease. In 1968 Goto and Fukuhara reported on 933 autopsies of diabetics in Japan as gathered from the records of the Japanese Pathologic Society (1958–1965). Death from ischemic heart disease was quite uncommon (6%). The percentage in decedent Joslin Clinic diabetics was roughly eight times as high (Bradley, 1971). Sasaki, et al (1976) found vascular disease to be a very common cause of death in Osaka diabetics, but cerebrovascular disease was a much more important cause of death than coronary disease. On death certificates on which diabetes was mentioned as a contributing cause, atherosclerotic heart disease was the underlying cause in only 9.2%. In the United States this figure was 42.7% (Marks and Krall, 1971). In Japan a particularly high proportion of deaths from vascular disease in diabetics are caused by glomerulosclerosis. This is probably because rates of large-vessel disease are relatively low. In Japan 88% of autopsied diabetics died of vascular disease (Goto and Fukuhara, 1968), a fraction similar to that usually observed in the West (Bradley, 1971; Schliack, et al 1974). This may be in part the result of a balance in certain parts of Japan of low serum lipid levels and high blood pressure levels. The relatively modest frequency of stroke in Western diabetics is in part the result of the high rates of death from heart disease. Adult-onset diabetics don't survive long enough to die of stroke or glomerulosclerosis.

Other studies in Japan have confirmed the observations cited above. These data have been well summarized in the publications of Mimura (1970) and in the highly informative volumes edited by Tsuji and Wada (1970) and by Baba, et al (1975). Several observers in Japan, including Hashimoto (1974), found coronary disease more common in diabetics than in nondiabetics. Kosaka, et al (1975) reviewed data from several studies in Japan, suggesting that in diabetics coronary disease was increased at least twofold.

The relative immunity to atherosclerosis enjoyed by diabetics in Japan is probably not attributable to social or genetic factors, or to the type of diabetes. Microvascular disease is rife. Rates of coronary disease rise as they adopt Western ways (Bassett, et al, 1969; Kawate, et al, 1975). Kawate, et al (1975) found that diabetic Japanese of Hawaii had rates of ischemic heart disease comparable to those in local whites, and far higher than those of diabetics in Japan. More studies are needed, however, in American diabetics of Japanese descent. As indicated in the section on hyperlipidemia, serum lipids are low in diabetics of Japan. Fukui, et al (1970) found serum lipids higher in diabetics than in nondiabetics, and among diabetics lipids were higher in those with macrovascular disease. The main reason for the paucity of atherosclerosis in diabetics of Japan is probably their low serum lipid levels.

Among the more informative clinical studies in Japan were those of Horiuchi, et al (1970) in 2,014 diabetics of a Tokyo clinic. Coronary disease was found in only 2.4%. Only one patient of the 2,014 had had a "leg lesion"! It does appear, however, that rates of macrovascular disease are rising in diabetics of Japan. In 1970 Okamoto, et al reported myocardial infarction in 17.5% of autopsies of diabetics of Kyoto. Hirata and Mihara (1975) reported an increase in rates of coronary disease in a cooperative autopsy study. This increase is not surprising in view of the recent dramatic changes in way of life in Japan. Hyperlipidemia is no longer rare (Okuno, et al, 1975). Between 1951 and 1967, fat consumption per capita in Japan increased from 18.0 gm to 42.5 gm daily (Oiso, 1970).

Reviews on vascular disease in Japanese diabetics are in press (Goto, 1977; Kawate, et al, 1977).

There have been many clinical and pathologic studies on large-vessel disease in Japanese diabetics but few epidemiologic investigations. More are needed.

Chinese

Wang (1937) and Snapper (1941) observed that rates of macrovascular disease were low in diabetics of China. Even in modern China rates of atherosclerosis have remained low in diabetics. In 1962 Chung reported observations in a series of 922 diabetics in a Shanghai clinic. Only 3.4% had "coronary sclerosis or infarction". Gangrene was seen in only 0.09%. Atherosclerosis was also uncommon in Chinese diabetics of Hong Kong. McFadzean and Yeung (1968) found "myocardial ischemia" in only 4.7% and peripheral vascular disease in only 1.4%. Rates of macrovascular disease have increased substantially in diabetics of Taiwan. Tsai (1971) reported that at autopsy 50.9% of diabetics had some evidence of cardiovascular disease. Peripheral vascular disease is less common than in the West but no longer rare (Tsai, 1970). Tsai (1971) observed that fat consumption had increased almost threefold between 1955 and 1968.

It does not seem likely that the previous immunity of Chinese diabetics to vascular disease is a racial peculiarity. Ischemic heart disease is rife in Chinese of Hawaii, particularly in diabetics (Bassett and Schroffner, 1970).

Africans

In Africa, clinical studies revealed low rates of large-vessel disease in blacks of Johannesburg (Seftel, 1961), Leopoldville (Bourgoignie, et al, 1962), Durban (Hathorn, et al, 1961; Campbell, 1963), Uganda (Shaper, 1962), Nigeria (Kinnear, 1963), Rhodesia (Gelfand and Forbes, 1963), and Dar Es Salaam (Haddock, 1964). Low rates of macrovascular disease in African diabetics were also described by Wicks and Jones in Rhodesia (1974); and in excellent reports of a very large Nigerian clinic series by Greenwood and Taylor (1968) and Osuntokun (1969).

These observations in Africans were reviewed and extended by Jackson (1970, 1972) and his colleagues, who studied blacks and other races in the Capetown area. These clinical and epidemiologic observations in African blacks indicated that rates of macrovascular disease were very low despite diabetes, but they also suggested that rates of diabetic macrovascular disease were beginning to increase in certain urbanized elements of the population

377

(Jackson, 1970). Although macrovascular disease was very uncommon in black diabetics, it did not appear to be quite as rare as in nondiabetics. Dodu (1958) reported from Ghana that only two cases of myocardial infarction had ever been observed in black women of his locality; both of these were diabetic. Weinstein (1962) found macrovascular disease rare in black diabetics of British Guiana. Large-vessel disease was uncommon in Nigerian diabetics; serum cholesterol levels averaged only 140 mg/100 ml in males and 132 in females. (Greenwood and Taylor, 1968). Even so, coronary disease was not quite so rare in diabetic Nigerians as in nondiabetics.

It does not appear that racial factors account for the low rates of macrovascular disease observed in many groups of black diabetics. In American diabetics of African ancestry macrovascular disease is rife. Few systematic epidemiologic observations have been made, but pathologic studies show that amounts of atherosclerosis in urban blacks (New Orleans) have recently reached levels comparable to those in whites, both in diabetics and nondiabetics (Robertson and Strong, 1968). More study is needed but it appears that the incidence of large-vessel disease in urban American black diabetics approximates that in white diabetics. In the general population of Newark, New Jersey no difference was found in coronary disease rates of blacks and whites (Weisse, et al, 1977).

There are many factors that may account for the low rates of macrovascular disease in black diabetics of rural Africa. Prominent among these are low serum cholesterol levels (Shapiro, et al, 1973). Walker (1966) found that mean serum cholesterol levels were 155 mg/100 ml in middle-aged rural Bantus. Other explanations for the low levels of vascular disease may include leanness and relatively high levels of exercise. Walker (1966) found that levels of fibrinolytic activity were higher in Bantu males than in white males. In females no racial differences were found. Serum triglyceride levels in South African Bantu diabetics seem to be similar to those in local white diabetics (Shapiro, et al, 1973). This argues against triglyceridemia as an independent risk factor. Conceivably, however, the effect of triglyceride might depend on factors such as its lipoprotein attachments and the levels of insulinemia present. On the other hand, we find in preliminary studies that large-vessel disease is somewhat less common in Oklahoma Indian diabetics than in whites, despite considerable levels of insulinemia and hyperglycemia, and very high levels of serum triglyceride. Serum cholesterol levels are modest in these diabetics, averaging 215 mg/100 ml, and in nondiabetics about 195.

Serum insulin levels are generally low in African diabetics (Asmal and Leary, 1975). Even in fat Africans, insulinemia is often modest (Joffe, et al, 1975). The low levels of insulin might or might not protect from atherosclerosis. Bantus smoke less than South African whites, and they are also in better physical condition (Walker, 1966).

Asian Indians

The term Indian as used here will refer to individuals whose ancestors lived in the Indian subcontinent of Asia, including what is now Pakistan, Bangladesh, Sri Lanka (Ceylon), and India.

As pointed out above, Bose had described high rates of angina in diabetics of Bengal in 1895. Subsequently, however, most clinicians of India had found rates of macrovascular disease modest in diabetics when compared to rates in Western diabetics. Cosnett reported in 1957, however, that vascular lesions were "extremely common" in Indian diabetics of Durban, South Africa. In 1961 Hathorn, et al also reported high rates of large-vessel diseases in Indian diabetics of Durban, South Africa. On the other hand, Ibrahim (1962) found in a clinic of West Pakistan that coronary disease was evident in only 1.6% of a large series of diabetics! Other manifestations of macrovascular disease were also rare in this group. DeZoysa (1951) had found macrovascular disease rare in Ceylon. Campbell (1963) reported further from Durban that both large- and small-vessel disease were rife in diabetic Indians. This included disease of vessels of the heart, brain, and legs. Shaper (1962) found high rates of coronary disease at autopsy in Indians of East Africa. Shaper and Jones (1959) had reported previously that Indians of Kampala had high levels of serum cholesterol, high-fat diets, and high rates of atherosclerosis. Pathology studies of Strong and Robertson (1968) showed that amounts of atherosclerosis in Indians of Durban were comparable to those in New Orleans whites, both in nondiabetics and diabetics.

In modern India rates of macrovascular disease have been measured in many groups of diabetics (Seftel, 1964a; Patel and Talwalker, 1966; Lal, et al, 1968; Sathe, 1973; Raychaudhuri, 1973). Rates have been highly variable, generally ranging from low to moderate in frequency. Much of this variation is due to marked differences of criteria and of methods of data collection. Some of these intergroup differences are probably real. It would be highly desirable to collect more data in the various regions and ethnic groups of India using well-defined standardized conventions and methods.

In British Guiana, coronary disease had been found in 7 of 70 Indian diabetics, a rate lower than is usually seen in whites of Europe and America, but higher than in local black diabetics (Weinstein, 1962). Results of Cassidy (1967) in Fiji were similar. In a clinic series large-vessel disease was rare in diabetic natives but moderately common in local diabetic Indians. Bakani (1975) found in Fiji that fat consumption was two to three times greater in the Indians. Hypercholesterolemia was regularly observed in Indians with myocardial infarction; a majority had values above 300 mg/100 ml. In Indians myocardial infarction was about 30 times more frequent than in natives of Fiji. Bakini thought that the high rates of diabetes in the Indians was a major contributing factor to their high rate of coronary disease. Twenty-eight percent of Indian cases with acute myocardial infarction had known diabetes.

In the Capetown area of South Africa vascular disease has been studied by Jackson (1972) and associates in Indians and other races. Rates of coronary disease were about equally high in Indian and white diabetics. Rates of peripheral vascular disease seemed to be somewhat less common in Indians. The evidence gathered by Jackson and his group was strengthened by observations in screenee groups drawn from general populations, as well as studies in clinics. These data from clinics often provide important clues, but must be interpreted with caution because of many potential sources of bias. Other data on vascular disease, diet, and diabetes in Indians of South Africa were summarized by Walker (1966).

According to Walker (1966), fat typically constitutes about 30% to 40% of calories in diets of South African Indians. There are, however, significant differences in this respect among the different ethnic subgroups of the Indian population in both India and South Africa (Seftel, 1964a). In Uganda, Shaper (1959) estimated that fat consumption in Indians ranged from 30% to 45% of calories. In Indian diabetics of Durban levels of serum cholesterol and triglyceride are high (Asmal and Leary, 1975). In general, levels of serum insulin are high in Indians of South Africa (Asmal and Leary, 1975). Hathorn, et al (1961) found decreased levels of fibrinolysis in Indian diabetics of Durban. Fibrinolysis in Indians of the Johannesburg area was slightly less than in whites (Walker, 1966); serum cholesterol levels were similar in the two races. Cholesterol values were higher in Indians with diabetes than in nondiabetic Indians. According to Walker (1966) serum cholesterol levels of South African Indians were substantially higher than in "privileged" Indians of India (Walker and Seftel, 1962). Seftel (1964a) and Ahuja (1976) reviewed the differences and apparent differences among various ethnic and social groups of Indians of India and South Africa with respect to diabetes and its vascular manifestations.

In some groups of Indian diabetics large-vessel disease is uncommon (Ibrahim, 1962; Patel and Talwalker, 1966). The reasons for these variations are not clear, but differences in saturated fat consumption are probably a major factor. Among many other possibilities are differences in exercise levels, adiposity, and insulinemia. In general, the South African Indians with coronary disease are fat (Walker and Seftel, 1962). There are great differences among "Indians" in genetic and anthropologic characteristics. The possibility cannot now be excluded that these "racial" and genetic differences among Indian subpopulations have influence in this respect, even though environmental factors are clearly important. The marked variations among Indian populations in diet and way of life present excellent potentialities for productive epidemiologic investigations.

American Indians

Table 33 (West, 1974) summarizes variations among North American tribes in rates of diabetic vascular disease. Precise intertribal comparisons have not been possible because of incomplete data and incomplete standardization of methods and criteria. We (West, 1977) have found coronary disease less common in Oklahoma Indians than in local whites. In Indian diabetics coronary disease is common, but not so frequent as in white diabetics. Serum triglyceride levels are quite high in these Indian diabetics, but cholesterol values are lower than in white diabetics (West, 1977). The most detailed observations on coronary disease in Indian tribes are those of Inglefinger, et al (1976) in Pimas. Coronary disease is more common in diabetics than in nondiabetics, although less common than in white diabetics. In nondiabetics coronary disease is less

TABLE 33 Vascular Lesions of American Indian Diabetics: Summary of Studies and Clinical Impressions

Authors, Years and Tribes	Retinopathy	Nephropathy	Coronary Disease	Other Observations and Comments
Cohen (1954). Mixed group (Arizona, Utah, Nevada)†	Common	Common	Less common than in white diabetics	
Parks and Waskow (1961) Pimas*	Common	Common	Less common than in white diabetics	Autopsy studies in diabetics at Phoenix Indian Hospital
Reichenbach (1967). Mixed group (78% either Pima, Papago, or Apache)†		Common	Less common than in white diabetics; 7 out of 60 had myocardial infarct at autopsy	
Bennett, Miller, Kamenetzky, et al (1971–1976). Pimas‡	Common	Very common	Less common than in white diabetics	Very detailed studies
Richey (1966). Mojaves of Arizona and California*			Rare	"Secondary complications of diabetes were minimal".
Sochet (1958). Kiowas and Comanches of Oklahoma*		Not significantly different from whites	Less common than in whites	
Drevets (1965). Choctaws of Oklahoma*	Probably uncommon		Probably less common than in whites	
Johnson and McNutt (1964) Alabama-Coushatta*	Uncommon (2 of 41 had retinopathy)			
Waring (1970). Winnebagos and Omahas of Nebraska†	Common	Very common		
Westfall and Rosenbloom (1971). Seminoles of Florida*				"Patients with diabetes had serious vascular disease".
Petersen (1969). Sioux and Assiniboine*				"Few complications in spite of relatively high blood sugars".
Prosnitz and Mandell (1967). Navajos, Hopis of Arizona†	Rare	Common	Very rare	
Saiki and Rimoin, 1968 Navajos†	Rare	Common	Very rare	

Source: West (1974).
*Clinical impression only or based on limited number of systematic observations.
†Systematic informative studies that were necessarily limited in character by local resources or circumstances.
‡Highly systematic and detailed studies.

381

frequent than in North American whites. Serum cholesterol levels are lower in these Indians than in US whites. Fat consumption was probably less in Pimas than in US whites (Reid, et al, 1971).

Oklahoma Indians consume moderate amounts of cholesterol but high levels of fat, about 45% of total calories. Caloric intake is high, and obesity rife (West, 1974). In both diabetic and nondiabetic adults diastolic blood pressure values in the range of 90 to 100 are very common, but severe hypertension is uncommon. Smoking is common, but moderate to heavy smoking is probably less common than in local whites. Peripheral vascular disease is common in elderly diabetics, but present data in both American whites and Oklahoma Indians are inadequate to permit comparisons of frequency or severity. Peripheral vascular disease was common in diabetics of the Pima, Chactaw, Winnebago, and Omaha tribes, and rare in Navajos and Mojaves (West, 1974).

Very low rates of macrovascular disease have been observed in diabetics of some tribes. In each instance coronary disease has been rare in the general populations from which they were derived. This was the case, for example, in Navajos (Sievers, 1967). Autopsy studies in Guatemalan diabetics (a population with a considerable proportion of Indian blood) showed little atherosclerosis, but more than in local nondiabetics (Strong and Robertson, 1968). Levels of serum cholesterol in Navajos seemed to be only slightly lower than in American whites, even though macrovascular disease was rare in diabetics and nondiabetics (Sievers, 1968). Serum insulin levels in nondiabetics were relatively high, even in lean Indians (Rimoin, 1969). But diabetes of long duration is still rare in Navajos. More data are needed. Sievers (1967, 1968) has reviewed the subject of coronary disease in Southwestern Indians.

These marked intertribal differences in degree of macrovascular disease present excellent epidemiologic opportunities for determining the relative importance of various etiologic factors.

Whites and other races

Rates of macrovascular disease have been high in diabetic Polynesians in New Zealand and Hawaii (West, 1974). In diabetics Jackson (1972) found rates of macrovascular diseases in Malays of Capetown to be intermediate between those of local blacks and whites. In an Indonesian diabetes clinic 34 of 407 (8%) had coronary disease (Sujono and Sukaton, 1970). The rarity of macrovascular disease in diabetic natives of Fiji has been cited above (Cassidy, 1967). It should be kept in mind that mean age in diabetic populations of poor societies tends to be much younger than in affluent societies.

Differences have been observed in the frequency of macrovascular disease among various Jewish groups. In Israel, Brunner, et al (1964) found macrovascular disease rare in a group of diabetic Yemenites. They had consumed diets low in fat and high in starch. On the other hand, large-vessel disease is rife in Jews of South Africa (Walker, 1966) and in diabetic Jews of the United States (Joslin, 1927; Joslin, et al, 1959). Diabetic macrovascular disease is also common in certain elements of the Israeli population (Goldbourt, et al, 1975).

In whites the geographic differences have, in general, not been as dramatic as those in Chinese, Indians, or blacks. This may only reflect the lesser degrees of environmental differences in whites. On the other hand, very significant differences have been demonstrated among white populations (eg, in the autopsy data of Robertson and Strong, 1968).

Results of Mulcahy, et al (1969) in Ireland suggest that hyperglycemia may be a risk factor for macrovascular disease of lesser importance than in the United States. Gordon, et al (1974) found little effect of hyperglycemia on rates of coronary disease in Puerto Rico. In a Copenhagen hospital, rates of diabetes were not excessive in a group of 597 patients with acute myocardial infarction (Kretny, 1976). Grönberg, et al (1967) observed that rates of large-vessel disease were only slightly higher in Swedish diabetics than in nondiabetics. Other studies in Sweden, however, have shown a substantial effect of diabetes (Sievers, et al, 1961), as have studies in Norway (Westlund, 1969) and Finland (Pyorala, et al, 1976). The huge (3,254) autopsy series of Schliack (1974) in East Berlin indicates that atherosclerosis is about as common in these diabetics as in those of Boston (Bradley, 1971).

In New Zealand Bailey and Beaven (1968) found that among patients with myocardial infarction 6% of men and 12% of women were diabetic. These rates were more than twice those for diabetes in the general population at the same age levels. Yefimov (1972) found macrovascular disease very common in diabetics of Kiev. Very low rates of macrovascular disease were reported in Algerian diabetics by Lebon, et al (1953). In Warsaw mortality rates in diabetics were excessive by a factor of 1.3, and most of this excess was attributable to macrovascular disease (Krolewski, et al, 1977).

Many other observations on macrovascular disease in white populations have been cited in preceding sections of this chapter.

Methodologic Problems in Geographic Comparisons

Many of the citations above have been intentionally worded in only general terms. When one clinic reports that 21% have "coronary disease" and another reports that 13% have "ischemic heart disease", it is typically quite difficult to interpret and compare because of differences or incomplete information with respect to methods, criteria, age distribution, etc. Among the useful data that are frequently missing are distributions by age, sex, duration of known diabetes, degree of glycemia, cholesterolemia, and triglyceridemia, adiposity, blood pressure, definition of "diabetes", and descriptions of criteria and methods for identifying macrovascular disease.

Rabb-Smith (1967) has reviewed the difficulties in interpreting mortality data on coronary disease. Gillum, et al (1976) have reported on their rich experience in Framingham concerning methodologic problems in community studies of cardiovascular disease. Higgins, et al (1965) discussed problems of gathering and comparing electrocardiographic data. Walker (1970) and Moss (1975) have reviewed some of the problems in the epidemiologic study of coronary disease. Risk factors have been reviewed by Dawber (1975). An excellent summary on cardiovascular survey methods was prepared under sponsorship of the World Health Organization by Rose and Blackburn (1968). As indicated below, epidemiologic methods of measuring and comparing rates and amounts of vascular disease in the brain and legs are in a rather primitive state. Kagan (1970) has discussed cardiovascular studies in migrants.

A common problem in interpreting electrocardiographic data is that endemic diseases other than coronary atherosclerosis may have appreciable effects on rates of certain electrocardiographic abnormalities (Florey, et al, 1973). Some electrocardiographic changes are highly specific for coronary atherosclerosis, but they are usually infrequent. Restriction of analyses to these highly specific changes usually requires that very large samples be tested. Another problem is that certain kinds of electrocardiographic effects are often produced by the ingestion of glucose or meals. This phenomenon has been reviewed by Riley, et al (1972). In the course of surveys it is often convenient to perform electrocardiography between the ingestion of glucose and a subsequent determination of blood glucose. But, whenever possible, electrocardiography should not be done for at least ninety minutes after eating or glucose ingestion. If this cannot be avoided, the temporal relationship should be noted and taken into account in interpreting the results.

Other Aspects of Heart Disease

Certain epidemiologic observations concerning the association of diabetes and coronary atherosclerosis have been reviewed above. This section has four additional purposes. One is to summarize the magnitude of the excess morbidity from diabetes-related heart disease. Another is to describe some factors other than atherosclerosis that may contribute to this occlusive disease. A third purpose will be to review the factors other than occlusive coronary disease that are responsible for excessive heart disease in diabetics. Finally, some special features of ischemic heart disease in diabetes will be reviewed, including the especially pronounced effect of diabetes in women, the high rates of silent infarcts, and the poor prognosis when ischemic heart disease is associated with diabetes.

Blackburn (1974), Kuller (1976) and Stamler (1973) have published excellent reviews on the epidemiology of coronary disease. Methods and methodologic problems in ascertaining and comparing rates of heart disease have been discussed above in this chapter, both in the general discussion on methods and in the section on geographic variations. Jarrett (1977) recently published a good review on coronary disease and diabetes.

Toll

Many observations indicating the importance of coronary disease have been cited above in this chapter and in Chapter 6 on mortality. Before the advent of modern epidemiologic studies, the very high rate of ischemic heart disease had been established by clinical studies. These have been well summarized by Bradley (1971). Typical were the observations of Lewis and Symons (1958) in Britain, who found abnormal electrocardiograms in 42.5% of their diabetic patients, and stigmata of heart disease in 59.5%. A recent report of an expert group in Britain concluded that in Western societies coronary heart disease was two to three times more common in diabetic men than in nondiabetic men (Royal College of Physicians and British Cardiac Society, 1976). They estimated that rates of coronary disease were five to six times greater in diabetic women than in nondiabetics. In a well-controlled study, Pell and D'Alonzo (1963) found risk of myocardial infarction increased by a factor of 2.5 in diabetics. As indicated above, these excesses are not entirely due to diabetes itself. Some are the result of the high frequency of other risk factors in diabetics. Other evidence cited above suggests that only about half of the coronary disease in diabetics is attributable to diabetes. Even so, the toll from this excess of ischemic heart disease is now vast. In the US National Survey 21% of all diabetic respondents said they had a "heart condition" (Bauer, 1967). Roughly 20% more have occult heart disease (Bradley, 1971; West, et al, 1976). Testing with especially sensitive methods, such as electrocardiography after exercise, would probably raise the total portion with heart disease to almost half of all American diabetics. Chapter 6 on mortality reviews evidence that in Western countries most of the excessive mortality in diabetes is attributable to the excess of heart disease.

Several factors prevent a precise estimate of the contribution of diabetes to rates of morbidity and mortality from heart disease. These include uncertainties concerning both rates of occult diabetes and the effects of very mild hyperglycemia on the enhancement of vascular disease.

Aarseth (1953) found that more than half of Oslo diabetics had electrocardiographic abnormalities. Lundbaeck (1953) studied long-duration diabetics in the population of Aarhus, Denmark. About half had evidence of heart disease. He also studied the records of dead diabetics in the same cohort. About three quarters had developed evidence of heart disease before death. Of diabetics with diagnosed heart disease, 80% had had symptoms of heart disease, and about one quarter had been "disabled". Of the long-duration diabetics over 59 years of age, about two thirds had diagnosed coronary disease.

In affluent populations, about one third of middle-aged persons with manifestations of atherosclerosis have "abnormal" tolerance. Falsetti, et al (1970) found in a series of American patients with an angiographically proven coronary disease, 63% had abnormal glucose tolerance by conventional criteria. The relationship between mild glucose intolerance and atherosclerosis has been discussed above in detail. The discussion below indicates that the enhancement of heart disease by diabetes is not limited to acceleration of coronary atherosclerosis.

One of the important challenges for epidemiologists is the development of a more precise estimate of the toll from diabetes-related heart disease. One could argue from present data that in the United States as much as 20% of the mortality from heart disease is caused by diabetes. On the other hand, it could be argued that this figure is as low as 2%. The high figure is based on the assumption that even those with normal fasting glucose levels and "abnormal" glucose tolerance have an increased risk of ischemic heart disease relating directly and independently to the "hyperglycemia". Moreover, as indicated below, there are factors other than enhanced atherosclerosis that make diabetics particularly susceptible to heart disease. The low estimate is based on the arguments that only those with unequivocal fasting hyperglycemia have an increased risk relating directly to hyperglycemia, and that much of the risk of heart disease in those with unequivocal diabetes is independent of diabetes itself.

Probably the actual contribution of diabetes is about halfway between these high and low estimates. Assuming that 20% of Americans with fatal heart disease have significant hyperglycemia, and that this "diabetes" accounts for half of this morbidity and mortality, then about 10% of heart disease deaths could be attributed to diabetes. This number (about 70,000 per year) would slightly exceed the number of deaths from any single type of cancer or from auto accidents. Among persons under 70 years of age the number of deaths from all causes of cancer combined would be greater, and the number from all other causes of ischemic heart disease combined would be much greater. But ischemic heart disease has many causes. Of these hyperlipidemia is probably the most important, but in many societies diabetes appears to rank with hypertension as an inciting factor of heart disease. Moreover, hyperlipidemia has many causes, as does diabetes. Thus, relative ranking of various etiologic factors depends greatly on semantics, criteria, and definitions. It is clear, however, that heart disease incited by diabetes is one of the leading causes of morbidity and mortality in the more affluent half of the world, and an increasingly significant problem in the less privileged societies.

OTHER CAUSES OF OCCLUSIVE CORONARY DISEASE

The main occlusive factor appears to be intensification by diabetes of the usual type of atherosclerosis. A few observations have suggested the possibility that there may be some qualitative differences in the biochemical characteristics of the atherosclerotic lesions of the coronary vessels in diabetics and nondiabetics (Lundbaeck and Petersen, 1953; Goodale, et al, 1962). But the similarities of the lesions in diabetics and nondiabetics are more striking than the differences. Nor is it clear whether the qualitative differences observed were the direct effect of diabetes or of other differences in the groups compared (eg, levels of blood lipids, blood pressure, adiposity).

Several factors other than atherosclerosis have been proposed as contributing agents in the excessive occlusive disease in diabetics. Some are listed on page 354. These include various aberrations of coagulation that might enhance propensity to thrombosis (Colwell, et al, 1977; Coller, et al, 1978). But Goodale, et al (1962) observed no evidence on pathologic examination that propensity to thrombosis was greater in diabetes when degree of atherosclerotic occlusion was matched in diabetics and nondiabetics.

It has been suggested by many that microvascular lesions of coronary vasculature may contribute to impairment of blood flow. These changes in capillaries are clearly present, but it isn't certain whether they interfere with rates or amounts of flow (Ledet, 1968). Conceivably, such lesions might interfere with the function of the myocardium or impair nutrition or metabolism of walls of large vessels. Evidence to this effect is not very impressive at present (Barner, et al, 1975).

FACTORS OTHER THAN OCCLUSIVE CORONARY DISEASE

It is now rather well established that the excessive rates of heart disease in diabetics are not entirely attributable to increased atherosclerosis. This was suggested by Lundbaeck as early as 1953. Other factors considered as possible contributors to the high rates of heart disease in diabetes include enhanced blood viscosity (McMillan, 1975) and aberrations of neurologic function (Fekete, et al, 1976; Watkins, et al, 1976; Lloyd-Mostyn and Watkins, 1976; Neubauer and Gunderson, 1976). Among the mechanisms by which neurologic pathology may impair cardiac functions are inhibition of adjustments of rhythm and rates to challenges such as postural changes and exercise. Aarseth found neuropathy in 7% of a group of diabetics (25 of 371). All of those with neuropathy had symptoms of cardiovascular disease.

Hemochromatosis produces cardiac lesions; and the renal complications of diabetes induce cardiac manifestations in several ways. Fibrosis of the myocardium is more frequent and extensive in diabetes (Pearce, 1973). Probably not all of this is secondary to coronary atherosclerosis. Lundbaeck (1973) described observations of Ledet establishing that myocardial fibrosis was especially common and extensive in diabetes, and that the degree was strongly related to duration of diabetes. The papillary heart muscles of diabetes contain excessive amounts of lipids (Alavaiko, et al, 1975).

Rubler, et al (1972) reported severe heart disease in diabetics with patent coronary vessels. Ahmed, et al (1975) have described diabetes-related aberrations of myocardial function (in man and animals) that were not attributable to occlusive coronary disease. Neubauer and Christensen (1976) found depletion of norepinephrine in heart muscle of diabetics. Hamby, et al (1974) and Dash, et al (1974) described a type of cardiomyopathy that was especially common in diabetics. In a patient with congestive heart failure Axelrod (1975) reported marked improvement that seemed to be attributable to mitigation of hyperglycemia. In Framingham Kannel, et al (1974) observed that rates of congestive heart failure were much more frequent in diabetics. This excess did not appear to be accounted for entirely by the higher rates of ischemic heart disease in the diabetics. Congestive failure was about five times more frequent in diabetic women than in nondiabetic women. Harlan, et al (1977) have suggested some criteria of definition for congestive failure.

The University Group (1970, 1971) found that death from cardiovascular disease was more common in patients taking tolbutamide than in controls. Rates of death from heart disease here also thought to be excessive in those taking phenformin. Certain other controlled studies have not found any evidence of increased cardiac morbidity or mortality with these drugs (Carlstrom 1976; Keen, 1975; Jarrett, et al, 1976; Feldman, et al, 1976 and 1977). Lichtstein, et al (1976) studied 265 diabetics who were under intensive coronary care. In those receiving oral antidiabetic drugs, there was no significant increase in death rate or ventricular fibrillation. The conflicting evidence concerning the cardiac effects of these drugs has been well reviewed by Keen (1975) and the University Group (1976). Goodkin (1975) and Krolewski (1977) found excess of mortality greater in diabetics on insulin than in diabetics on oral agents.

Some Special Features of Ischemic Heart Disease in Diabetes

Bradley (1971) summarized evidence indicating that occult ischemic heart disease is more frequent in diabetics. This includes painless myocardial infarction. More recent epidemiologic evidence confirms this. Margolis, et al (1973) found in Framingham that 39% of electrocardiographically documented infarcts in diabetics had not been diagnosed previously. In nondiabetics this proportion was only 22%. In Tecumseh results were similar in this respect (Ostrander, et al, 1967). In Israel, however, occult heart disease was not more common in hyperglycemic subjects (Medalie, et al, 1976).

Certain of the results described above show the especially strong effect of diabetes in increasing rates of ischemic heart disease in women. This was strongly evident, for example, in the data of Lundbaeck (1953) and Aarseth (1953). In some circumstances the protection conferred by female sex has been completely obliterated by diabetes, even in premenopausal women. In other circumstances the loss of immunity has been only partial. For example, Westlund (1969) found in Oslo that deleterious effects of diabetes were greater in women, but rates of death from coronary disease remained greater in diabetic men than in diabetic women. Diabetes narrowed the gap but not completely. Correction for levels of smoking would probably have narrowed the gap further. In Warsaw results were unusual. Excess mortality from coronary disease was at least as great in male diabetics as in female diabetics (Krolewski, et al, 1977). In Cape Town, Tansey, et al (1977) found that, among patients hospitalized for myocardial infarction, excessive mortality in diabetics was attributable to a very high death rate in obese diabetic women.

Dawber (1975) found in Framingham that the incidence of coronary disease was increased fivefold in diabetic women 30 to 39 years of age. A recent analysis of Framingham data by Gordon, et al (1977) showed no clear *independent* effect of diabetes on risk of coronary disease in men; but in women the independent effect of diabetes was even stronger than the effect of low-density lipoprotein cholesterol. What is there about the pathophysiologic effects of diabetes and of status of sex that accounts for the failure of female sex to protect diabetic women?

Most, but not all, studies have shown higher death rates in ischemic heart disease (eg, acute myocardial infarction) when diabetes is present (Henning, et al, 1975; Bradley, 1971; Modan, et al, 1975). Some of this difference is probably attributable to more advanced degrees of atherosclerosis in diabetics. But Brusche, et al (1973) found mortality higher in diabetics than in nondiabetics with the same degree of occlusion of the coronary vessels as determined angiographically. In Framingham (Garcia, et al, 1974), and in the studies of Goodkin, et al (1975), excessive risks of morbidity and mortality were much greater in patients taking insulin than in those taking oral agents. But blood glucose levels were probably higher in those taking insulin.

Acute myocardial infarction often causes hyperglycemia, and frequency of hyperglycemia seems to be greater when infarction is severe (Ravid, et al, 1975). Fasting blood glucose levels and glucose tolerance tend to return to normal during convalescence but, as indicated above, a rather substantial portion of those with myocardial infarctions have hyperglycemia prior to and long after infarction.

In a prospective study in Israel, Herman, et al (1977) found subsequent rates of acute myocardial infarction to be excessive in both newly diagnosed and established diabetics, but rates of sudden death and of angina were excessive only in those who had established diabetes at entry into the study.

Cerebrovascular Disease

FREQUENCY

The epidemiology of stroke has not been so extensively studied in diabetes as has coronary disease. One reason for this is that it has seemed to be a less important problem for diabetics.

Bauer (1967) reported on rates of stroke in diabetics included in the National Health Survey sample of American interviewees. In a group of about 2,000 diabetics, 2.2% had had "paralysis", and 3.3% were thought to have had "vascular disease of the central nervous system". Age-matched data for nondiabetics were not presented. This technique of sampling excludes persons living in institutions. This would substantially reduce stroke rates. Prevalence is also greatly limited by the typically short survival of stroke patients.

Autopsy studies in Boston (Bradley, 1971) and East Berlin (Schliak, 1974) revealed rates of cerebrovascular disease in diabetics that were not much different than usually observed in nondiabetics. In decedent Joslin Clinic patients studied by Kessler (1970) the frequency of death from cerebrovascular disease was only slightly excessive in diabetics (mortality ratio of 1.2). The experience of Grönberg, et al in Sweden was similar.

On the other hand, stroke rates have been quite excessive in some groups of diabetics. In Framingham Garcia found the incidence of strokes quite excessive in diabetics (about twofold). In Birmingham, Alabama (Peacock, et al, 1972), previously diagnosed diabetes was three times as common in stroke patients than in a control group matched for age and other characteristics. Stroke rates were not elevated, however, in persons found to have previously undiagnosed hyperglycemia.

389

In Israel rates of stroke appear to be much higher in diabetics (Lavy, et al, 1973; Najenson, et al, 1976, 1973). Librach, et al (1977) studied a population of retired Israelis. The incidence of stroke was 37.8 per 1000 per year in diabetics and 22.4 in nondiabetics. In persons born in Asia or Africa the rates of stroke were 54.7 in diabetics and 15.8 in nondiabetics. Westlund found that death from stroke was four times more frequent in Oslo diabetics under 70 years of age than in age-matched persons from the general population. In older diabetics, stroke rates were twice as high as in nondiabetics. In a series of 240 patients with transient attacks of brain ischemia, Toole, et al (1974) found 28% had diagnosed diabetes.

Shafer, et al (1974) summarized the results of eleven clinical series from several countries of patients with nonembolic cerebral infarction. These included groups of patients that were exclusively or predominantly blacks and groups that were mainly whites. Rates of diagnosed diabetes in these groups ranged from 2% to 28%. In North Carolina 13.9% of hospitalized stroke patients were known to have diabetes, in Michigan 18.3% (Wylie and Carpenter, 1976). In a case-control study of Abu-Zeid, et al (1977) in Missouri, relative risk of cerebral hemorrhage was not significantly excessive in diabetics but brain infarction was excessive by a factor of 2.5.

In some Japanese groups of diabetics, stroke has been the leading cause of death (Mimura, 1970). But rates of stroke have varied greatly in reports from Japan (Tsuji and Wada, 1970). One of the reasons for this is probably the great variability in frequency of hypertension in different parts of Japan. In some communities salt consumption and rates of hypertension are very high (Meneely and Dahl, 1961). Probably rates of stroke are higher in Japanese diabetics than in nondiabetics (Wade, et al, 1964), but few well-collected data are available concerning this matter. In Osaka diabetics cerebrovascular disease was a much more important cause of death than coronary disease (Sasaki, et al, 1976).

It seems quite likely that much of the association sometimes observed between diabetes and stroke may be incidental to the higher rates of other stroke risk factors in diabetes, particularly hypertension. Very few data are available on the degree of independence of diabetes as a risk factor in stroke. It appears that hypertension is a much stronger risk factor for stroke than diabetes. In diabetics, as in nondiabetics, hypertension greatly increases risk of stroke (Vernet, et al, 1975).

In a small autopsy series of 107 diabetics Grunnet (1963) studied the cerebral vessels, comparing their status to that of a control group. Atherosclerosis was greater in the diabetics, and as great in diabetic females as in diabetic males. No effect of hypertension or duration of diabetes was demonstrated. Atherosclerosis was greater in those with hypercholesterolemia or history of ketosis.

Considerable differences have been found by geography and race in rates of cerebrovascular disease in diabetics (Ahuja and Tandon, 1966). The reasons for these differences are not entirely clear, but no direct effects of race have been demonstrated independent of well-known risk factors such as hypertension. In diabetics of Fiji (Cassidy, 1967) cerebrovascular disease was more common in

Indians than the aboriginal people. In British Guiana, East Indian diabetics had less cerebrovascular disease than local blacks (Weinstein, 1962), while in Durban the opposite was observed (Campbell, 1963).

QUALITATIVE FEATURES

These have been well reviewed by Christlieb (1974). Malignant hypertension and its cerebrovascular manifestations are especially rare in diabetics (Christlieb, 1974; Osuntokun, 1972). Aronson (1973) reported an especially informative study of cerebral vessels in 5,479 autopsies of which 677 were on diabetics. There was no excess in the diabetics of major cerebral infarction. Brain weight was less and encephalomalacia more common in diabetics. In diabetics there was an increase in frequency and severity of lesions of certain small vessels of the paramedian perforating arteries serving the pons, thalamus, and basal ganglia. Diminished brain size was particularly evident in the infratentorial region. Both cerebral hemorrhage and arteriolar necrosis were less frequent in diabetics. In the huge autopsy series of Bell (1952) it was also found that encephalomalacia was more common in diabetes. In diabetics under 60 years of age major hemorrhage was less frequent than in nondiabetics.

During the acute phase of stroke, transient hyperglycemia is common, but rarely persists. Also, immobility after severe stroke probably tends to impair glucose tolerance; but these effects of stroke on glucose tolerance do not explain the high rates of fasting hyperglycemia seen in some series of stroke patients. However, stroke patients are probably more likely to be tested for diabetes under some circumstances.

Much more study is needed on the effects of diabetes on cerebrovascular disease and of the factors that affect this relationship.

Peripheral Vascular Disease

GENERAL NATURE OF THE PROBLEM

Gangrene is one of the most important and distressing manifestations of diabetes. It is not generally appreciated that among populations of diabetics there are very great differences in susceptibility to this dreaded complication. These circumstances suggest excellent opportunities for elucidation and prevention, through epidemiologic approaches. But rather little has been learned previously concerning the epidemiology of gangrene and other disorders secondary to diabetes-related peripheral vascular disease. Indeed, the present status of data in this field is an epidemiologist's nightmare! Methods and standardization are poorly developed. Except in Scandinavia, few studies have been performed in representative samples of diabetics or nondiabetics. Controls have been few and suboptimal in character. The relationship between diabetes and peripheral vascular disease is so strong that little need has been perceived for investigation. To most Western clinicians this suggested an inevitability of association, and tended to stifle incentives to look for preventive measures.

391

The most prominent and important of these manifestations of excessive leg-vessel disease in diabetes is gangrene, but there are other morbid effects. These include intermittent claudication, and pain at rest in the legs or feet. Ulcerations of the toes and feet are often disabling. There are no counterparts of these lesions in the upper extremities. Probably "leg-artery disease" would be more appropriate than peripheral vascular disease, but the latter term has become customary and is, therefore, employed here.

Some of the history of the development of concepts concerning diabetic gangrene were reviewed by Lundbaeck (1953). The pathophysiology and clinical aspects of this problem are covered in the excellent book of Levin and O'Neal (1977). The main cause of the morbidity is occlusive disease of large vessels of the leg and foot. There are, however, several other contributing factors. The most important of these is impairment of sensation secondary to diabetic neuropathy. In populations in which atherosclerosis is rare, gangrene is rare in diabetics even though neuropathy appears to be common in all these populations. Some observers have concluded that occlusive capillary lesions (diabetic microangiopathy) may contribute substantially in impairing circulation to the feet (Pederson and Olsen, 1962; Blumenthal, et al, 1966). Present data do not exclude a significant contribution, but most evidence now suggests that the role of microvascular disease is not of substantial importance in this respect (Strandness, 1964; Barner, 1976).

Both Monckeburg sclerosis and atherosclerosis are intensified in the leg vessels of diabetics. There is some uncertainty concerning the degree to which the concomitants of Monckeburg sclerosis, such as calcification and fibrosis of the media, interfere with blood flow. It now appears that they do contribute to the impairment of flow along with the major culprit atherosclerosis (Neubauer, 1971; Christensen, 1968a; Ferrier, 1967). Intimal fibrosis usually attends Monckeburg sclerosis; this may be functionally significant (Christensen, 1973).

The main problem, however, is that diabetics are especially prone to atherosclerosis of the leg vessels. In diabetics this atherosclerosis occurs more extensively, at an earlier age, and spares the female sex to a lesser degree, than in nondiabetics. There is some conflict of evidence and opinion about the extent to which the anatomic distribution of atherosclerosis in diabetics is peculiar. Most studies have found that the atherosclerotic process in diabetics is more generalized throughout the leg, and that it is particularly excessive below the knee (Gensler, et al, 1961; Vogelberg, et al, 1975; Ferrier, 1967; Strandness, 1964). Strandness (1964) and Ferrier (1967) called attention to the peculiarly extensive occlusion in foot vessels of diabetics. Linear calcification of leg vessels is especially common in diabetics (Ferrier, 1964; Neubauer, 1971).

Toll

The toll from diabetic leg-vessel disease is huge. Dry and Hines reported in 1941 that leg-vessel disease was about 30 times more common in diabetics than in nondiabetics. In nondiabetics disease was about six or seven times more common in men than in women, but in diabetics leg-vessel disease was only about twice as common in men. Rabkin and Field (1962) found that 7% of diabetics admitted to the Massachusetts General Hospital had amputation or vascular surgery. These admissions are typically long in both amputees and in those with severe leg-vessel disease who escape amputation. For this reason leg-vessel disease accounts for a very substantial portion of diabetes-related hospitalization in the affluent West, perhaps as much as one quarter. Viskum (1969) studied length of hospitalization in diabetics with gangrene treated conservatively. Hospital stay averaged seventy-seven days.

In the United States roughly half of leg amputations are secondary to diabetes. In the very large autopsy series of Bell (1950) about half of gangrene in men and approximately two thirds in women was diabetes related. Of patients with major amputations in the series of Kramer and Perilstein (1958), 58.6% were diagnosed diabetics; in that of Silverstein and Kadish (1973), 65%. But this portion varies greatly depending on the sources of the patients in whom amputations are performed and other factors. Even in certain institutions of communities in which diabetes is rather common, diagnosed diabetes has been present in a much lesser portion of gangrene cases. Only one third of the American cases of Ottoman and Stahlgren had had diagnosed diabetes. In several series from Western clinics cited by Selvaag (1962) the portion with diagnosed diabetes ranged from 8% to 50%. Hansson (1964) found in Gothenburg that 43% of leg amputees were known to have diabetes, but more than half were diagnosed diabetics after exclusion of those in whom amputation was caused by tumors or trauma. In the Australian series of Little, only 23% of amputees were diagnosed diabetics. More detailed data on the prominence of diabetes as a cause of gangrene are provided below, mainly from the excellent epidemiologic surveys conducted in Scandinavia. Extrapolations from data of Hierton and James (1973) suggest that in Uppsala County, Sweden, the annual rate of diabetes-related amputation was about 10 per 100,000 population. Assuming similar rates in the United States the annual number of diabetes-related amputations would be about 22,000.

Death rates are high with gangrene requiring amputation. Silverstein and Kadish (1973) reported a death rate of 34% in diabetics undergoing major surgery for leg-vessel disease. Most series report mortality rates that are not quite so high (Warren and Record, 1967), but in all large series mortality is common, typically 20%. Mainly this is the result of the very extensive amounts of coronary disease in this group of patients.

The monetary cost of this disability from leg-vessel disease is great. In the United States a typical cost of a period of hospitalization for amputation is $4,000. The annual costs of medical care for diabetes-related leg-vessel disease in this country probably exceeds $100 million. The yearly number of amputations in the United States is not known. Based on data cited above and below it is probably at least 20,000 and perhaps as high as 30,000. In the large group of diabetics studied by Kramer and Perilstein (1958), 7% had had gangrene and 6% more "threatened gangrene". Probably about one third of American diabetics will ultimately have some degree of disability or discomfort from leg-vessel disease. In many populations this toll is decidedly less. In the populations of Asia, diabetic peripheral vascular disease is a significant problem, but rates of morbidity are generally much lower.

About one third of patients with intermittent claudication have diabetes or occult hyperglycemia (Wahlberg, 1966).

Diabetic peripheral vascular disease tends to be relentless. Of American diabetics who required amputation, about half of the survivors required an amputation of the second leg within five years (Silberg, 1952). In the study of Hansson (1964) in Sweden, 25% of diabetic amputees were bilateral amputees. Goldner (1969) and Whitehouse, et al (1968) have shown that bilateral amputation would be exceedingly common were it not for the short life expectancy in these amputees.

EPIDEMIOLOGIC OBSERVATIONS

Many studies have been cited above in the sections on the general aspects of atherosclerosis, its history, geography, risk factors, etc. The following section will review some additional observations.

Methods

Among the indexes used in the study of leg-vessel disease are the following: counts of deaths attributed to gangrene, counts of amputees, indexes that identify disease by history (eg, intermittent claudication), physical examination for indexes of leg-vessel disease (eg, absent pulses, ulcers or low blood pressure at the ankles), and laboratory procedures such as roentgenography for calcification of vessels, thermography, and oscillographic tests.

Few of these tests have been sufficiently standardized for use in carrying out comparative interpopulation studies, but some recent developments are encouraging. Rose and Blackburn (1968) described a standardized questionnaire for determining the presence or absence of intermittent claudication. They also discuss some of the other methods applicable in the study of leg-artery disease, as well as their state of development. The University Diabetes Group (1970a) have also developed some standardized methods applicable to the study of leg-vessel disease.

More information is needed on most of these methods with respect to sensitivity, specificity, inter- and intraobserver variation, etc. Peripheral pulses are a case in point. Nilsson, et al (1967) did publish the prevalence of absent pulses by age and sex in a control series with no apparent diabetes. More data of these kinds are needed. Even with very primitive methods much could be accomplished. For example, it would be desirable simply to know the incidence of major amputation in the United States, and the factors to which amputation relates such as age and sex, and the major risk factors. To a considerable extent the risk factors for atherosclerosis of leg vessels may be expected to reflect those found in more detailed previous studies of atherosclerosis in other anatomic regions such as the coronary arteries. It is already evident, however, that very significant peculiarities exist by anatomic region.

Smoking is an especially strong risk factor for leg disease, while hypertension seems to be relatively less important etiologically than in coronary or cerebrovascular disease. More data are needed.

Studies designed to measure the interrelationships of risk factors in diabetic leg-vessel disease have been rare. The extent to which observed associations have been independent or dependent has seldom been clear. Analyses of this kind usually require numbers of cases greater than in previous studies. Because death rates are very high in persons with leg-vessel disease, studies of incidence offer considerably more potential than the cross-sectional studies of prevalence, but they are more expensive to conduct. Large numbers are needed to procure some of the types of information that are required (thousands, not hundreds). There are, however, other potentialities in studies on a smaller scale. Indexes should be used for which the interobserver differences are known and of modest degree, so that populations can be compared. These indexes should also be well standardized and defined. Interpretation of previous data has been difficult or impossible because of lack of standardization and convention. Even if the prevalence of "peripheral vascular disease" is said to be 5% in one group and 25% in another, one cannot be certain of a real difference without knowing details. Typically, about one third of diabetics will have some evidence of disease of the leg arteries, but as few as 3% may be amputees at any given time. Among the simple indexes that may be considered are the following: age, sex, duration of known diabetes, type of antidiabetic medication (if any), height (or former height of amputee), weight, lifetime maximum weight, present fasting blood glucose, serum cholesterol and triglyceride, presence or absence of dorsalis pedis pulsation, blood pressure at the ankle, level of amputation if present and year of amputation, presence of ulceration on feet, history of intermittent claudication (Rose and Blackburn, 1968), history of smoking (Rose and Blackburn, 1968), x-ray of legs or feet for calcification (Neubauer, 1971), electrocardiography (Rose and Blackburn, 1968), and presence or absence of diagnosed ischemic heart disease.

Many other indexes could be used, some of which may be found to be epidemiologic instruments superior to those cited above. Oscillometry, for example, deserves further study as an epidemiologic tool. Loss of pain sensation is an important etiologic factor, but simple reproducible field methods for measuring this have not yet been promulgated. Other indexes of neurologic function may reflect the degree of deficit in pain sensation, but the degree of this correspondence is not known. These other measurable parameters include sense of vibration and deep-tendon reflexes. In the study of Nilsson, et al (1967) the correlation coefficient in diabetics between the latter two indexes was not very strong (.36).

Observations

Some of the important studies have been cited above in the sections on the epidemiology of atherosclerotic lesions and their geographic variations. These profound geographic differences are of greatest importance. Their degree and causes require much more study, but even the present evidence is quite impressive. In the American diabetics of Kramer and Perilstein (1958) gangrene was roughly 100 times as frequent as in the Japanese diabetics of Horiuchi, et al (1970). These geographic and racial differences do not appear to correspond precisely with differences in coronary disease. In diabetic Indians of South Africa Jackson, et al (1970) observed that, relative to whites, rates of leg-vessel disease did not seem to be quite so high as rates of coronary disease. Even in localities where rates of peripheral vascular disease are modest, diabetes appears to have a substantially deleterious effect. In India Tandon, et al (1973) found peripheral vascular disease in only 9% of their diabetics, but this was more than ten times as frequent as in their nondiabetic patients (0.8%).

Among the more informative studies were those of Nilsson, et al (1967) who compared the status of a large (598) representative group of diabetics with a control group of persons with no apparent diabetes. There was a strong effect of diabetes and duration of diabetes on vessel calcification as determined by x-ray. Severe calcification was present in 4.8% of controls, 8.7% of short-duration diabetics, and 17.9% of long-duration diabetics. Calcification was not observed at all in nondiabetic women under 40 years of age, nor in young diabetics of short duration; while in women under 40 with diabetes of long duration it was common (23.1%). These data are unusual in that they correct for age and duration of diabetes. Many other studies on diabetic peripheral vascular disease have failed to show an effect of degree and duration of hyperglycemia, but these have seldom been analyzed or collected in a manner capable of excluding this relationship. Confounding variables frequently pose formidable problems. A major difficulty has been that age has a profound effect on risk and degree of leg-vessel disease. Effects of other variables cannot be examined satisfactorily when age is not controlled for or taken into account.

Christensen (1973) showed an effect of duration of diabetes on impairment of blood flow to the feet. The data of Nilsson, et al (1967) also showed a strongly deleterious effect of both age and diabetes, but the effect of duration of diabetes on foot pulses was less pronounced and consistent than on calcification. Even so, there was an impressive effect of duration on occlusion of foot pulses in some subgroups. In women from 40 to 59 years of age, absent pulsations were not observed when diabetes was absent or of short duration, but 5.3% of long-duration diabetics in this age group had absent pulses. The correlation coefficient between status of pulses and calcification was -0.31.

Nilsson's group examined the correlations between indexes of leg-vessel disease and several other variables. By the methods employed, no significant effect of blood glucose level was observed, but it was not clear whether an effect was obscured by the greater age of those with lower blood glucose levels. Even in this large exemplary study (598 diabetics), the numbers of subjects in the various cells and subcells was too small for certain kinds of evaluations.

The results of Christensen (1969) in Denmark were similar to those of Nilsson, et al, in showing a strong effect of diabetes and of duration of diabetes on calcification. In this study there was also a strong association of calcification and morbidity of the leg. Christensen (1973) also showed a relationship of calcification to impairment of blood flow. Ferrier (1963) found a strong relationship of diabetes to medial calcification. Data of Dr. Priscilla White (1972) have shown a high degree of association between calcification of arteries and duration of diabetes. It is interesting that calcification of the musculatures of the vas deferens occurs occasionally in long-duration diabetics. A substantial majority of men in whom this has been observed have had diabetes, usually of long duration.

There have been very few studies of leg-artery disease in general populations. In Tecumseh it was found that foot pulses were absent twice as frequently in those whose blood glucose levels were in the top quintile. In Framingham intermittent claudication was studied (Garcia, et al, 1974). Its incidence was quite excessive in diabetics, by a factor of 4.5.

Hansson (1964) studied the epidemiology of leg amputation in Gothenburg, Sweden. There were 93 with amputation from arteriosclerotic disease and no evident diabetes, while 143 amputees had diabetes. Only one of the diabetics was less than 50 years of age; 73 were men and 70 were women. Because of the excess of diabetes in Swedish women, the number of diabetic women at risk was probably considerably greater. In 11% of cases of diabetic gangrene, diabetes was discovered at the time of the gangrene. In only one female did diabetic gangrene occur before age 60. Average age of onset of diabetes in all diabetic amputees was 62 years. Of the 143 diabetic amputees, 36 (25%) had had bilateral amputation. In 14 instances this second amputation had occurred within one year of the first. Of 125 who died, death was due to circulatory diseases in 112. Mean age at amputation for the diabetics was 69 years, and for the 93 nondiabetics, 72 years. Only 14% of the diabetics were free of other physical handicaps at time of amputation.

Another good comprehensive community survey of amputation was conducted in Aalborg, Denmark, by Christensen (1976). Amputations were studied through the period 1961–1971 in this country with 260,000 residents. Of 372 amputations, 175 (41%) were in diabetics. Of amputations not due to trauma or tumors, about half were in diabetics. The rate of amputation for diabetic gangrene was approximately 7 per 100,000 per year. Of 151 amputations in diabetics, 95 were above the knee, 56 below the knee, and 3 were reamputations at unspecified sites. Healing time and rate of complications at the surgical site were similar in diabetics and nondiabetics with occlusive vascular disease. Survival rate was slightly less in diabetics, even though they were three years younger at the time of amputation. Only one fifth of the diabetics survived for four years. Twenty-five percent of the diabetics were bilateral amputees. The rate of amputation for diabetic gangrene was constant during this period. In some Scandinavian studies rates appeared to increase in the years immediately following World War II, but recent studies have shown a plateau in incidence. This was shown, for example, by Hierton and James (1973) in Uppsala County, Sweden. In this informative study in a whole community, it was found that 60% of amputations were in diabetics. The annual rate of diabetes-related

397

amputation was about 10 per 100,000. Among the segment of the population over 60 years of age the rate of amputation from all causes was 85 per 100,000, and the rate from diabetic gangrene about 53 per 100,000.

Tibell (1971) performed an excellent study in Malmo, Sweden. His publication includes an outstanding review of the literature. Records of virtually all medical facilities in the community were examined on admissions during a period between 1949 and 1965. There were 967 cases of peripheral vascular insufficiency identified, of whom 373 were persons with known diabetes. Only 8 of these 373 were less than 50 years of age and only 7 had been found to be diabetic before age 40. In interpreting the very low number of youth-onset cases it is important to keep in mind the very low number of youth-onset diabetics at risk. In most affluent populations less than 10% of all diabetics have had onset in childhood and only a small fraction of these survive to age 50. There is no evidence that youth-onset diabetics are any less susceptible to peripheral vascular disease than maturity-onset cases. Indeed, they are probably more susceptible, but they usually die of other causes before reaching the age of susceptibility to severe leg-vessel disease.

There were 209 females and 164 males in the group studied by Tibell. Average age at first admission for leg-vessel disease was 68. In these diabetics rates of hospital admission were about 50% higher in the autumn than during other seasons. First admission for leg-vessel disease occurred an average of 9.6 years after diagnosis of diabetes. In 20% the diagnosis of diabetes was made during this first admission. About half these diabetics survived three years after their first admission for peripheral vascular disease. The average duration of hospitalization per admission was fifty-seven days. Moreover, about one third of those who survived were discharged to chronic care facilities. The average duration of stay in the chronic disease hospitals for this condition was one hundred forty-three days. Tibell estimated that the annual incidence of hospitalization for leg-vessel disease was about 1% for diabetics in the sixth decade, 2% in the seventh decade, 3% in the eighth, and 4%–5% in the ninth. He estimated that in octogenerians risk of severe peripheral vascular disease was excessive in diabetics by a factor of about 8. In younger diabetics the degree of excess was considerably greater. During the seventeen-year course of these studies the incidence of diabetes-related leg-vessel disease increased slightly, but this change was not clearly significant. It is probable, for example, that the frequency and sensitivity of testing for diabetes increased during this period between 1949 and 1965.

The data of Nilsson, et al (1967) described above are among the few on the status of the leg vessels in representative samples of the general population. More control data of this type are needed. Widmer, et al (1964) reported results of physical examinations of 6,400 employees of a drug industry, all of whom were under 65 years of age. Arterial occlusion in the leg was found in 1.3% of the men and 0.7% of the women.

A number of studies of prevalence of peripheral vascular disease have been performed in clinic populations. Poor standardization of methods, criteria, and definitions make comparisons difficult. Redisch, et al (1974) examined a series of 684 diabetics (mainly Puerto Ricans) in their New York City clinic. These investigators found that 37% of their diabetics had peripheral vascular disease, but they included persons with minimal stigmata. They estimated on the basis of indirect evidence that prevalence of leg-artery disease was increased by a factor of more than 7 in their diabetic men, and by more than 30 in their diabetic women. In the very large series (3,788) from a London clinic studied by Oakley, et al (1957), only 3.9% of all diabetics were deemed to have had occlusive disease of the leg arteries. This rate rose to 10.5% in diabetics over 69 years of age. In long-duration juvenile diabetics studied by Deckert, et al (1975) in Denmark, 12% had had amputation.

The high rate of death in patients with severe leg-vessel disease tends to hide the high incidence of this important cause of disability. Lundbaeck (1953) studied rates of leg-vessel disease in all patients in his series who had died and on whom data were available. Forty-four percent (22 of 50) had had occlusive vascular disease. None of the patients under 40 years of age had been affected, but half of those over 60 had had leg-vessel disease. In 60 dead patients on whom information was available, 17 (28%) had had gangrene. In Lundbaeck's living patients with diabetes of fifteen to twenty-five years' duration, occlusive vascular disease was present in 39% and gangrene had occurred in 14%. This group was an almost complete sample of all diabetics of this duration in the community of Aarhus, Denmark.

The frequency of diagnosed and occult diabetes has been highly variable in groups of patients with disease of the leg arteries. In general, prevalence of diabetes has been higher in patients with severe leg-vessel disease. Very high rates of diabetes in amputees have been cited above; in the United States rates of 50% in amputees have been typical. Where prevalence of diabetes is less, the proportion who are diabetic is less, but rates of diagnosed diabetes in patients with severe peripheral vascular disease are typically about ten times as high as in age-matched elements of these general populations. Rates of occult diabetes have varied greatly in groups of patients with arterial disease in the legs. Results depend on many factors, including age distribution and the definition of diabetes.

Risk factors

Studies of Wahlberg (1966) showed that rates of impaired glucose tolerance were quite excessive in patients with peripheral vascular disease, even after control for the effects of age on glucose tolerance. These studies did not reveal whether the association was incidental or causal. It is not yet established whether persons with normal fasting blood glucose levels and "abnormal" tolerance have excessive risk of leg-vessel disease after correction for other known risk factors. No consistent relationship, positive or negative, has been shown between smoking and diabetes (Jarrett and Keen, 1975). In Poland diabetics smoked less than nondiabetics (Czyzyk and Krolewski, 1976). But compared to nondiabetic groups, diabetics usually have greater adiposity, higher blood pressure, and greater concentrations of serum lipids. Level of physical conditioning is probably less.

Gordon and Kannel (1972) found in Framingham that the strongest risk factor for the incidence of intermittent claudication was smoking. This was followed, in order of strength, by hyperglycemia, hypercholesterolemia, and hypertension. Others have also found that blood pressure levels have only modest effects on risk of leg-vessel disease. Indian subjects of Jackson (1972) in South Africa had higher blood pressure than whites, but lower rates of peripheral vascular disease. In the Australian cases of Little, et al (1973) with peripheral vascular disease, only 6% had hypertension.

The frequency of hyperlipoproteinemia has been high in most clinical studies of diabetic peripheral vascular disease in Western populations. In the series of Greenhalgh, et al (1971), 39% had abnormal lipoprotein patterns; in the series of Newall and Bliss (1973) the rate was 60%. The latter workers thought risk was probably highest in patients with both hypercholesterolemia and hypertriglyceridemia. In the series of Greenhalgh, hypertriglyceridemia was more common than hypercholesterolemia. In diabetics with peripheral vascular disease Vogelberg, et al (1975) found prognosis worse in those with Type II lipoprotein abnormalities than in those with Type IV. On the other hand, Sorge, et al (1976) found a positive relationship between triglyceride levels and diabetic peripheral vascular disease. Cholesterol levels were, however, similar to those in a nondiabetic control group. In the series of Selvaag (1962), cholesterol values in diabetics with peripheral vascular disease were not (1962), cholesterol values in diabetics with peripheral vascular disease were not higher than those of nondiabetics with this disorder; and Lundbaeck (1953) found no difference in serum cholesterol levels of diabetics with and without leg-vessel disease. Rosen and Depalma (1973) showed, however, that in patients with leg-vessel disease, serum cholesterol levels often fall substantially over time, so that present values do not necessarily reflect previous levels.

Although the effects of "hypercholesterolemia" on leg-vessel disease appear to be modest when traditional Western definitions of this term are used, a different perspective emerges if most Westerners are deemed to have "hypercholesterolemia". Rates of leg-artery disease have been extremely low in diabetics of populations in which cholesterol values below 170 mg/100 ml are typical. This paucity of leg-vessel disease is probably not entirely attributable to the low serum cholesterol values, but it is likely that cholesterol values are a very important etiologic factor.

Data on the effects of hypertriglyceridemia on leg-vessel disease are quite insufficient to determine whether it has a causal role, and of what degree, in either diabetics of nondiabetics. The same uncertainty applies with respect to the effects of insulinemia and of adiposity. Sorge, et al (1976) found in 65 diabetics with peripheral vascular disease that serum triglycerides and insulin levels were much higher than in nondiabetics with peripheral vascular disease.

These differences were not attributable to obesity. But Ghilchik and Morris (1971) found that both hypoinsulinemia and hyperinsulinemia were common in diabetic patients with atherosclerotic leg-vessel disease. Normal insulin levels were common in nondiabetics with leg-vessel disease. In the United States a very high percentage of diabetic amputees have formerly been decidedly overweight, but data are insufficient to determine whether obesity itself is an important independent risk factor. Lean childhood-onset cases of long duration have high rates of peripheral vascular disease (Lundbaeck, 1953). Gangrene is also common in older patients with low levels of endogenous insulin who have never received insulin therapy. Thus, obesity and hyperinsulinemia are not critical factors. Present data do not, however, exclude the possibility that these factors contribute to some extent. Adiposity and hyperinsulinemia as risk factors in atherosclerosis are discussed in detail above.

The high degree of male predominance in peripheral vascular disease is substantially reduced when diabetes is present, but not entirely obliterated. The higher rates of smoking in men contribute to this male predominance. Few data are available on diabetics in which data on smoking were collected systematically. In the series of Selvaag (1962) the male:female ratio was 3.2:1 in all cases of occlusive vascular disease of the legs, and 2:1 in the diabetics. In the diabetics of Oakley, et al (1957) it was 3:1 in those with leg-vessel disease. In nondiabetics sex ratios in leg-vessel disease have ranged, typically, from 2:1 to 11:1. In general, the disparity between sexes declines with age. The same phenomenon is seen in diabetics. In the autopsy series of Bell there were as many females as males with diabetic gangrene, but there were no diabetic females under 50 with gangrene. Among the diabetics there were, however, five males under 50 with gangrene (4% of male cases). In interpreting these ratios it should be kept in mind that in many populations the number of diabetics at risk differs by sex. In the series of Bell the number of females with gangrene was the same as the number of males, but the number of female diabetics was about twice as great as the number of male diabetics. Thus the percentage of diabetic males who had gangrene was substantially higher. In the series of diabetics of Redisch, et al (1974) that included all degrees of peripheral vascular disease, rates were not significantly different in the sexes. In Taiwan and Indonesia gangrene is not common, but in both countries it had been observed somewhat more frequently in females (Tsuji and Wada, 1970). The effect of diabetes on sex predominance is also well illustrated in the studies of Nilsson, et al (1967) on calcification of vessels. In nondiabetics 40 to 59 years of age, calcification of vessels was six times as frequent in males. In long-duration diabetics of this age, calcification was only twice as common in males.

Age is a powerful risk factor. In the autopsy series of Bell (1950) only 1 of 244 cases of diabetic gangrene was less than 40 years of age. Peripheral vascular disease was very rare prior to age 50 in the groups of Oakley, et al (1957) and Selvaag (1962). Among cases of diabetic gangrene observed by Kramer and

401

Perilstein (1958) none was less than 40 years of age. In that series of 100 there were 10 in the fifth decade, 34 in the sixth, 43 in the seventh, 12 in the eighth, and one over 79 years of age. In general, rates of peripheral vascular disease are low in juvenile-onset diabetics, but only because few survive to the age of susceptibility. In a subgroup of childhood-onset patients who had survived forty years or more of diabetes, Paz-Guevara, et al (1975) found that 40% had peripheral vascular disease. This rate is probably higher than would be expected in adult-onset cases of similar age.

The possible role of degree and duration of glycemia has been discussed above. Although in many studies no effect of duration has been apparent, an effect has been shown in several investigations (cited above) in which it was possible to control for age or take it into account. An effect of degree of glycemia has not been well demonstrated. Present data neither establish or exclude an effect of degree of glycemia. Because of the profound effects of other factors, particularly age, very large numbers of well-collected data will be required to confirm or disprove an effect of degree of glycemia. This effect, if present, could be direct or it could relate to the effect of degree of glycemia on blood lipids or other factors. Observations cited above on geographic differences indicate that degree of glycemia has little importance in the enhancement of leg-artery disease when serum lipids are very low (as in Japan), but this does not exclude the possibility of a deleterious effect of glycemia in the presence of higher serum lipid levels.

The possible roles of genetic factors and of microvascular disease as etiologic agents have been discussed above in the section on atherosclerosis. Lundbaeck and his associates (1973) found no evidence that blood flow to the leg was particularly impaired in patients with retinopathy. In diabetics studied by Nilsson, et al (1967), there was no relationship between proteinuria and calcification of leg vessels. In diabetics over 40 there was little relationship of retinopathy to calcification of leg vessels. These latter results were not, however, adjusted for factors such as degree of glycemia, blood lipids, or duration of diabetes.

Observations of Barndt, et al (1977) indicate that under certain circumstances the atherosclerotic lesions in the legs are to some extent reversible.

MICROANGIOPATHY

Introduction

Diabetes causes several kinds of microscopic lesions of the arterioles and capillaries. Microangiopathy has been observed in muscle, skin, gingiva, heart, kidney, eye, and other tissues. Because of certain common characteristics, these different microlesions are often lumped in a manner suggesting they are manifestations of the same etiologic processes. But among these lesions there are important differences that deserve more emphasis than they have received.

It is not rare, for example, to see patients without evident glomerulosclerosis who have severe retinopathy. And the histologic features of arteriolonephros-clerosis differ considerably from those in the capillaries of the retinae. Among the challenges for epidemiology, as well as for clinical and basic investiga-tions, is a determination of the degree to which etiologic factors are common to the various pathologic expressions of microangiopathy.

Only the two main aspects of microangiopathy will receive detailed attention here. They are visual impairment from retinopathy, and kidney failure from glomerulosclerosis. McMillan (1975) has recently published an excellent review of diabetic microangiopathy. Other good general sources of information include Joslin's book (Marble, et al, 1971), that of Ellenberg and Rifkin (1970), and that of Keen and Jarrett (1975). The report of the United States National Commission on Diabetes also has a detailed section on this subject (Prout, et al, 1976). Other sources of general and specific information on retinopathy and on glomerulosclerosis will be listed below.

In recent years much attention has been given to microscopic examination of capillary basement membrane as an index of microangiopathy. Work of Siper-stein, et al (1973) had suggested the possibility that a slight but significant broadening of the basement membranes of muscle capillaries might be detecta-ble before the onset of hyperglycemia in prediabetics. But most evidence now suggests that these lesions do not develop until hyperglycemia has been present for months or years (Lundbaeck, 1974; Williams, et al, 1976). Parving, et al (1976) have presented and reviewed evidence suggesting that hypergly-cemia produces a functional permeability of the capillaries.

Among populations of diabetics geographic variations in microangiopathy are not nearly so great as in atherosclerosis. But present data are decidedly suboptimal. As indicated below, geographic differences in rates of retinopathy of considerable magnitude have been reported. These differences are to some extent related to factors such as intergroup variations in duration of diabetes and in methods of identifying microangiopathy. But it seems probable that some of these interpopulation differences are to some extent real. There is a need for more systematic study to determine the degree and character of environmental influences on susceptibility to microangiopathy.

Retinopathy

General Description

Excellent general reviews have been published by Caird, et al (1969), Bradley and Ramos (1971), Kohner and Oakley (1975), Kohner and Dollery (1975), and Palmberg (1977). Most diabetics eventually develop clinically detectable lesions of the retinae. In many cases they are of small degree and do not interfere with vision. But in about half of long-duration diabetics they impair vision to varying degrees. Diabetic retinopathy is one of the leading causes of blindness. In some countries it is the leading cause of new cases of blindness in adults under the age of 70.

The first lesions detected by routine ophthalmoscopic examination are usually tiny red dots that represent microaneurysms. Hemorrhages and exudates usually appear later in the course of the disease. These intraretinal hemorrhages and exudates seldom produce substantial impairment of vision unless they are in the macula or unless they are unusually large. These less virulent pathologic changes are often referred to as "background retinopathy". The lesion most often associated with visual impairment is the development of new retinal vessels (neovascularization). This is frequently attended by large retinal and vitreous hemorrhages, retinal and vitreous fibrosis, and retinal detachment. The most frequent final causes of blindness include large hemorrhages and fibrosis darkening the vitreous, destruction of the maculae, and retinal detachment.

Applicability of Epidemiologic Study

The nature and importance of these lesions require further basic and clinical studies employing several disciplines. Epidemiologic study also has potential here. Why is it that one person develops malignant retinopathy and complete blindness after a few years of diabetes, while another has good retinae after forty years of severe diabetes? In groups of diabetics from various parts of the world, rates of retinopathy have ranged from 1% to 50%. To what extent are these differences real? To what are they attributable? The risk factor most firmly established is duration of diabetes. The risk factor for which further investigation is most needed is probably degree of glycemia. There is also need for more descriptive data on the scope, character, and magnitude of the problem and of the factors that affect them. It is not known, for example, to what extent the current registries on blindness understate the problem. Studies of Kahn and Hiller (1974) suggest that American nonwhite women may have very high rates of blindness from diabetic retinopathy. About 90% of these "nonwhites" are black. It is not clear to what extent this high rate of blindness is the result of a special propensity of black women to develop the severe lesions when they have diabetes, or whether it is attributable to a great excess in the frequency of diabetes in black women. Since black women are especially fat there is need to determine whether this adiposity contributes directly or indirectly to the high rate of blindness. Amos (1974) reviewed some aspects of the epidemiology of diabetes-related blindness.

Previous studies on risk factors in retinopathy are described below. Often they have been inconclusive. A frequent problem has been that there is a considerable degree of interdependence among these factors. An association observed between retinopathy and age may, for example, be partly attributable to an association of age and duration of diabetes. Associations may also be obscured unless data are appropriately gathered and analyzed. For example, a relationship between degree of glycemia and retinopathy may be obscured by a longer duration of undiagnosed diabetes in those with mild hyperglycemia, , or by a greater susceptibility of old retinae to damage at the same level of glycemia. The effect of duration is so strong that it often obscures other associations or makes them seem stronger than they are. Another problem is that the other characteristics of long- and short-duration diabetics usually do not match well. Even when adjustments are made to take duration into account, there are often other confounding variables. Other factors having a possible relationship to retinopathy are themselves interrelated (eg, age, blood pressure, and fatness). For these reasons most studies have not contained numbers sufficient to determine the extent to which these associations with retinopathy are dependent, independent, or casual; or whether such associations have been obscured or intensified by confounding associations.

More information is also needed on the sensitivity, specificity, and predictive value for subsequent visual impairment of the various indexes of retinopathy. To what extent, for example, is the presence or degree of retinal exudate attended by an increased risk of subsequent neovascularization? To what extent is this association independent of other retinoscopic findings or risk factors? To what extent, if any, are adiposity and hypertension independent risk factors?

Here are listed some of the etiologic factors that affect or may affect risk or degree of retinopathy.

1. Hyperglycemia:

    Duration (actual duration does not coincide with known duration);

    Degree;

    Degree of lability of blood glucose;

2. Ketonemia

3. Blood pressure

4. Adiposity

5. Sex

6. Age

7. Serum insulin

8. Serum lipids

9. Race and genetic factors

10. Ocular tension (negative relationship?)

11. Diet and nutritional status

12. Type of therapy

13. Pregnancy and oral contraceptives

14. Neuropathy and glomerulosclerosis

15. Smoking

16. Aberrations of:

    Capillary permeability (functional or anatomic);

    Capillary fragility;

405

Serum proteins and glycoproteins

Growth hormone

Other hormones

Blood pH

Serum phosphate

Serum enzymes

Retinal blood flow

Coagulability (fibrinogen, fibrinolysis, platelet aggregation, etc)

Blood viscosity

Immunopathy (eg, autoimmunity, immune reaction to injected insulin)

Serum lactic acid

Ascorbic acid metabolism

Retinal oxygenation

Methods and Methodologic Problems

Among the indexes and measurements commonly employed in the study of retinopathy are the following: presence or absence of any evidence of retinopathy; degree of visual impairment; duration of diabetes prior to onset of retinopathy; presence or absence of retinal hemorrhages, exudates, neovascularization, fibrosis; and the number, size, characteristics, and location of these lesions.

Results in studies of retinopathy are greatly affected by the methods employed in ascertaining the presence of both retinopathy and diabetes. Rates of retinopathy are much lower in populations of diabetics containing high proportions with early diabetes. Typically, "duration" of diabetes is computed using the time of diagnosis as a starting point. In populations where screening and detection activities are few, the disparity between duration and known duration tends to be greater, provided that circumstances are otherwise the same. But there are other factors that influence this important disparity between known and actual duration. In general, diabetes is occult for longer periods in the obese. In moderately fat people, mild hyperglycemia is often present for decades without producing symptoms. Any kind of mild hyperglycemia tends to remain longer in the occult stage. These factors make it difficult to evaluate the effect of degree of hyperglycemia. If, for example, after five years of *known* diabetes, rates and degrees of retinopathy are the same in those with moderate hyperglycemia and in those with severe hyperglycemia, the failure to find a difference could be due to the longer *actual* duration in the cases with moderate hyperglycemia. One alternative is to date onset of diabetes from onset of symptoms of diabetes rather than from date of diagnosis. Generally, this is difficult and subject to many problems of definition. Also, truly characteristic symptoms usually do not begin until blood glucose levels are two to three times normal. Correspondence between time of onset of symptoms and time of onset of disease is poor; time of onset is usually impossible to estimate reliably either in individuals or groups. The single exception is a circumstance in which populations or samples thereof are followed prospectively with frequent blood glucose determinations, as in the studies of the Pima Indians (Dorf, et al, 1976).

A frequent problem in interpreting previous clinical studies is caused by circumstances of data collection that create bias in selection of patients. For example, patients with poor vision or retinopathy are more likely to be sent to ophthalmologists for examination, and they tend to be examined more often. Patients who are concerned about their condition are more likely to go or be referred to famous clinics or specialists.

In previous studies methods of ascertainment of retinopathy have often been poorly standardized and incompletely defined. Methods have varied greatly in sensitivity. In some clinics rates of retinopathy are much higher than rates of diagnosed retinopathy. Koerner, et al (1977) have reviewed some methodologic problems in the study of retinopathy. Among the factors affecting sensitivity of ascertainment are the care and skill with which ophthalmoscopic examination is done, the methods used, and the frequency of examination. Waltman, et al (1977) have recently described a quantitative method for measuring photometrically the leakage into the vitreous of injected fluroescein. Kahn, et al (1975) have reviewed needs and methods for standardization of diagnostic procedures in ophthalmology.

Many systems of classification have been offered. Some of these have been cited by Burditt, et al (1968). But no widely accepted standards exist for describing the severity or characteristics of retinopathy. There are, however, a few classification systems that could form the basis of useful epidemiologic conventions. One is the O'Hare Classification (Davis, et al, 1968); another is the Hammersmith system. Both of these are well summarized by Kohner and Dollery (1975). A highly simplified system is being used by the collaborators in the WHO multinational study on the vascular lesions of diabetes. In this system the retinae are examined with an ophthalmoscope after dilating the pupils. Each retina is searched for two minutes to determine the presence or absence of microaneurysms, of hemorrhages, of exudates, or of new vessels (or other evidence of proliferation such as fibrosis). Microaneurysms are defined as red dots having a diameter less than that of the largest retinal artery. The system also provides for crude quantitation. For example, it is determined whether there is one small red dot, a few (two to five) or many (more than five). Hemorrhages with diameters larger than the optic disc are identified as "large" and categorized separately.

Another problem has been the lack of a standard definition of "blindness". Such definitions exist, but data collection in diabetes-related blindness has not been well standardized in this respect. The number who cannot read large print is, for example, much greater than the number who cannot perceive light.

Usually, crude estimates of visual acuity suffice, but standardization and definition are highly desirable. When facilities are available, the standard and more precise methods of assessing visual acuity may be used. Evaluation of data on visual acuity requires information on the status of the lens in all with impaired vision. This is because cataract is common in diabetics and impairment of visions is often secondary to lens opacity rather than retinopathy. Lens opacity also affects the sensitivity of the retinal exam, and sometimes precludes examination altogether. Recently, the popularity of photocoagulation has complicated the grading of retinopathy. But most of these retinae have or have had proliferative lesions, so that the therapy may not affect the category to which they are assigned when severity is graded.

Among the more sensitive methods employed in detecting retinopathy is examination after fluorescein injection. Examination or photography is carried out immediately after injection of this dye, as it is passing through the retinal vessels. Often small lesions are seen that are not appreciated by the standard procedures of examination. Kinnear, et al (1972) have described loss of acuity for color vision as a very early manifestation of retinopathy. Retinal photography is now being used rather widely as an epidemiologic tool (Oakley, et al, 1967). Its employment adds considerably to expense, but offers several advantages, including opportunity for independent and objective measurements, and evaluations of data collected from multiple geographic sites. This approach tends to increase standardization, and also makes possible reevaluation and revision of methods and criteria during the course of a study, if this proves desirable. Another advantage is the opportunity to make subsequent measurements and assessments not requiring the presence of the subject.

Some other methodologic problems relating to the epidemiologic study of retinopathy have been reviewed by Carpenter and Taylor (1963) and by Kahn and Hiller (1974).

NATURAL HISTORY AND TOLL

These have been well summarized in the publications cited above under general description. At the time of discovery of diabetes some diabetics have already developed detectable retinopathy. In groups this portion has ranged from zero to 10% depending on many factors, the most important of which is probably the duration of occult diabetes. For example, in the study of Jackson, et al (1970) of 200 new diabetics in whom diabetes was discovered in the course of screening surveys, none had retinopathy, although this lesion was very common in established diabetics of this same population. After ten years of known diabetes, about half of all diabetics have clinically detectable retinopathy; at twenty years the portion is usually about three quarters. Roughly 5% to 10% escape retinopathy even after thirty to fifty years of diabetes. The incidence of retinopathy declines after fifteen to twenty years of diabetes (details below). In some circumstances even the prevalence may decline after twenty years of duration, because the rate of death is particularly great in those with retinopathy. In groups of diabetics that have included all ages and durations of diabetes, when standard examining methods are employed, it has usually been found that one quarter to one half have retinopathy. Visual impairment ultimately occurs in a substantial portion of persons in whom duration of diabetes exceeds fifteen years. In some groups blindness has occurred eventually in as many as one third of all long-duration cases. However, the prevalence of blindness at any one time in long-duration diabetes tends to be considerably less than one third because of the high death rates of blind diabetics.

In a series of 92 diabetics of more than thirty-nine years' duration studied by Oakley, et al (1974), only 6 were blind, although 10 others had proliferative retinopathy. Thirty-six of these 92 were free of retinopathy. Why? Khurana and White (1976) reported on 153 Joslin Clinic patients who had survived more than forty years of diabetes. Seventy-four percent had retinopathy, but only 31% had impairment of vision, and only 12% were blind.

Fortunately, rates of impaired vision are far lower than rates of retinopathy. In the study in Pima Indians, for example, only 7% of those with retinopathy had proliferative or neovascular changes (Dorf, et al, 1976). Knowles (1971) estimated that about one third of juvenile diabetics developed blindness in the first three decades of diabetes. Blindness in the first decade of diabetes is very rare in juvenile-onset cases. Severe retinopathy in the first decade of known diabetes is less rare in maturity-onset diabetes, but diabetes is often present for years or decades before its discovery in maturity-onset diabetes.

Although retinopathy tends to increase with time, spontaneous improvement is rather common (Gerritzen, 1973). Natural history is discussed further below in the section on descriptive studies.

The toll from diabetes-related blindness in populations has been well summarized by Caird, et al (1969), Keen (1972), Amos (1974), Sorsby (1973), and by Kahn and Hiller (1974). In some countries, including the United States and Britain, diabetes is the leading cause of blindness in middle-aged persons. It is widely believed that in America this toll has been increasing in recent years, but there is little evidence to support this belief (Kahn and Hiller, 1974). It is clear, however, that retinopathy is much more common than heretofore in certain populations and subpopulations in which epidemics of diabetes have recently occurred. This includes American Indians and American black women.

Data reviewed by Kahn and Hiller (1974) suggest that diabetes accounts for roughly 10% of new cases of blindness in the United States. This proportion is substantially higher in persons under 70 years of age. In persons 45-74, diabetes accounts for about 20%. The present reporting systems tend to understate the frequency of diabetes-related blindness in the United States, but based on data that are reported, the prevalence rate of diabetes-related blindness has been about 24 per 100,000 population (Amos, 1974). A small portion of these cases are due to diabetes-related conditions other than retinopathy, but probably more than 80% are the result of retinopathy. The incidence of diabetes-related blindness in 1969–1970, based on registry data in states with reporting systems, was about 1.5 cases per 100,000 per year (Kahn and Hiller, 1974). Kahn and Hiller concluded that, because of under-reporting, the actual incidence rates may be as much as twice this high. In the general population of

Framingham, Massachusetts the prevalence of diabetic retinopathy in those greater than 51 years of age was 3.1% (Kahn, et al, 1977).

Similar data on rates of diabetes-related blindness in Britain have been reviewed by Caird, et al (1969). There were about 8,000–9,000 blind diabetics in the British Isles. Approximately one fifth of this blindness was the result of cataracts, and almost all the rest were caused by retinopathy. According to Keen (1972) blindness occurred in about 5% to 10% of British diabetics after twenty years of diabetes, and an additional portion had a lesser degree of visual impairment. Keen concluded than in Britain diabetes was probably the leading cause of blindness in middle-aged persons. The British Diabetes Association has estimated that about 2% of British diabetics are blind (Kohner and Dollery, 1975). In Britain the annual incidence of diabetes related blindness appears to exceed 1.5 cases per 100,000 (Kohner and Dollery, 1975).

The British Diabetes Association crudely evaluated the sensitivity of the present registry system. Of 44 blind diabetics, only 25 had been registered (Kohner and Dollery, 1975). More studies of this type are needed. The excellent review of Palmberg (1977) summarizes the social costs of diabetic retinopathy in the United States.

Descriptive Studies

Detailed studies have been made for many years in the patients of the Joslin Clinic by Beetham, Waite, Root, Marble, White, Bradley, and others. These have been summarized by Bradley and Ramos (1971). While these data have been quite useful, they must be interpreted in the light of the fact that the patients who come to this famous clinic are not a representative sample of the general population of diabetics. The problem of bias in this situation can be mitigated by studies in which cohorts of newly discovered cases are studied prospectively or retrospectively, excluding cases referred or self-referred during the later course of the disease. Kahn and Bradley (1975) have described some strategies of this kind for epidemiologic studies in this very large group of diabetics. In their study of a sample of 914 Joslin Clinic patients followed from onset of diabetes, retinopathy was rare (2%) in young diabetics when duration was less than ten years. In middle-aged diabetics with less than ten years of known duration, retinopathy was present in 7%, and in elderly diabetics 12%. After fifteen years of known diabetes, retinopathy was equally common in older and younger diabetics (about two thirds of both groups had retinopathy). Among several possible interpretations of these results, one likely explanation is that the disparity between known duration and actual duration is much greater in adult-onset diabetes. It is also possible that old retinae are more susceptible to damage than young retinae.

Caird, et al (1968) performed longitudinal studies in a large group of diabetics residing in the area of Oxford, England. Some of these results will be cited below. One interesting observation was that mortality rates were similar in those with no retinopathy and those who had only microaneurysms. When exudate was present life expectancy was much shorter, almost as short as in those with proliferative retinopathy.

Among the pioneering descriptive studies in large groups were those of Lundbaeck in Denmark (1953) and Kornerup (1955) in Sweden. The nature of the recruitment process in these two studies was such that the findings probably reflected rather well the status of the entire population of diabetics in those communities. Kornerup performed retinal examinations in a consecutive series of 1,000 diabetics, and found that 46.8% had retinopathy. Lundbaeck (1953) studied retinopathy in a cohort of diabetics from the population of Aarhus, Denmark, in whom diabetes had been known for fifteen to twenty-five years. About three quarters of the living patients had retinopathy. No effect of age was observed on prevalence of retinopathy. Six percent of living patients had proliferative retinopathy. The rate of proliferative retinopathy was probably higher in the patients of this cohort who had died, but the latter data were incomplete. Only 3% of the living patients were blind, while 7% of the dead patients had been blind from diabetes.

Knowles (1975) recently summarized 21 different studies on the prevalence of diabetic vascular lesions, including retinopathy. Results of these clinic groups of the Occident and Japan were similar to those described above when account is taken of duration of diabetes.

One of the better studies was that of Nilsson, et al (1967). Favorable attributes included fairly large numbers and systematic measurement of many other variables. The sample included a very high percentage of all diabetics in the population under study. These results will be discussed further below under risk factors and analytic studies. In 483 diabetics incidence of retinopathy was constant and prevalence progressively greater during the first fifteen years of known diabetes. In those with durations of less than eight years, only 7.3% had retinopathy; in those with durations of eight to fifteen years prevalence was 35.1%, while 81.3% of those with longer durations had retinopathy. A further rise in incidence occurred between the 15th and 18th year of diabetes, followed by a decline. This decline in incidence resulted in a plateau in prevalence between the 20th and 30th year. These same phenomena have been observed by other investigators (Szabo, et al, 1967; Inoue, et al, 1970; Miki, et al, 1969). The plateau or decline in prevalence observed after the 20th year is attributable both to a decline in incidence and the high death rates in those with retinopathy. Probably death rates are peculiarly low in long-duration diabetics without retinopathy. More study is needed to determine the degree to which each of these factors contribute. Rogot, et al (1966) found that survival of newly-blind diabetics averaged only about five years.

Nilsson also studied the degree of retinopathy and its relationship to several factors, including duration of diabetes. Although 34.7% of all diabetics had retinopathy, proliferative lesions were present in only 1.0% of all diabetics and in 2.9% of those with retinopathy. But it should be kept in mind that death rates are very high in patients with proliferative retinopathy. Fukuda (1972) in a

411

study of 1,393 Japanese diabetics found that all patients who had died of uremia had also had proliferative retinopathy. For these reasons data on prevalence of proliferative retinopathy tend to greatly understate its importance. One method that has been used to express more satisfactorily the frequency of proliferative disease is to measure and state the rate over time as a cumulative percentage. This has been done by Knowles (1971) and White (1972). Such counts include dead subjects. Data of these kind analyzed by Knowles suggest that almost half of juvenile-onset diabetics have eventually developed proliferative retinopathy at some time during the course of thirty years of diabetes or prior to death (Figure 1, chapter 3).

Although incidence of retinopathy and of proliferative retinopathy decline after twenty years of diabetes, it was shown by Oakley, et al (1974) that onset of retinopathy or severe retinopathy is not rare even in the fourth and fifth decades of diabetes.

One of the few studies on retinopathy over time in a population was that in Bedford (Keen, 1972). Diabetics (116) discovered in a 1962 survey were examined in 1962 and 1967. No microaneurysms were observed initially in 26 persons with two-hour blood glucose levels from 200 to 239 mg/100 ml, but 3 had microaneurysms five years later. In those with still higher blood glucose levels about one quarter had microaneurysms after five years. Examination of Keen's graph suggests that about 8% of the newly discovered diabetics with two-hour glucose levels greater than 239mg/100 ml had microaneurysms at the time of discovery of diabetes. In the entire group of 116, 3 developed impairment of vision from retinopathy during the first five years of known diabetes.

Among the most informative studies were those of Dorf, et al (1976) in a whole population of adult Pima Indians. One of the several accomplishments of this study was the measurement of indexes of retinopathy in those with clearly normal glucose tolerance. In those with two-hour glucose values of less than 100 mg/100 ml, microaneurysms were found in 0.5% and exudates in 0.5%. In those with two-hour values from 100 to 199 mg/100 ml, microaneurysms were also quite rare (0.7%), but exudates were observed in 2.0%. It seems likely, however, that this subgroup was older than the subgroup with two-hour values below 100 mg/100 ml. Proliferative changes were not observed in any of 1,274 persons with two-hour values below 200. In 366 persons with higher glucose values, 76 (21%) had some evidence of retinopathy. Of those with retinopathy, 5 of 76 (7%) had proliferative changes. Thus only 5 of 366 diabetics (1.4%) had proliferative retinopathy. Of 62 diabetics who had diabetes ten years or more, 47% had retinopathy. Proliferative retinopathy was not observed in any subject with diabetes of less than ten years duration.

Kojima, et al (1970) reported the results of a cooperative study of 4,875 diabetics from 37 university hospitals in Japan. Retinopathy was found in 33.9%. Visual acuity of less than 0.1 was seen in 10% of those with less than ten years of diabetes and in 30% of those with diabetes of longer duration. In this group (which may or may not be representative of the general population of

diabetics) there was in relation to age an interesting bimodality in the prevalence of retinopathy. This was seen in both sexes but was particularly marked
in women. Rates were highest in the seventh decade, relatively low in the fifth
decade, and intermediate in the third decade. About half of female diabetics in
the third decade had retinopathy, while only one quarter of those in the fifth
decade had retinopathy. The most likely explanation is that a large portion of
the Japanese diabetics in the third decade are long-duration childhood-onset
diabetics, while in the fifth decade a large fraction are adult-onset cases of short
duration.

The observations of Goto, et al (1975) in Japan are among the better descriptive studies on the relationship of incidence of retinopathy to duration and age
of onset of diabetes. They studied 2,771 cases. Results were similar to those of
other investigators described above. Persons with onset of diabetes in the
fourth decade seemed to have a more favorable prognosis.

In Oxford, England, Burditt, et al (1968) studied in 2,184 diabetics both the
prevalence and incidence of retinopathy over a fifteen-year period. This group
was probably a rather good representation of the entire universe of diabetics of
the Oxford area. When diabetes had been known for less than five years,
retinopathy was present in only 4% of young diabetics (less than 30 years of
age), 22% of those 30–59 years of age, and 34% of those over 59. With long
duration of known diabetes, rates of retinopathy were about the same in older-
and younger-onset patients. In patients with background retinopathy, progression to malignant retinopathy was more common in young patients. Malignant
retinopathy was observed in 85 patients during the fifteen-year period (about
4% of all diabetics examined). Other informative data from this group in
Oxford are provided in the excellent book of Caird, et al (1969).

It is difficult to know how to interpret these and other data on incidence of
retinopathy and malignant retinopathy in youth-onset and maturity-onset diabetics. When known duration is short, prevalence of malignant retinopathy is
much greater in maturity-onset cases. At least in part this is probably the result
of the longer duration of undiscovered diabetes in the maturity-onset cases. But
perhaps older retinae are more easily damaged. The higher subsequent incidence of severe retinopathy in youth-onset cases might be due to their higher
glucose levels. It also may be due to the fact that a greater portion of susceptible
diabetics in the older group have already developed severe retinopathy in the
first few years of discovered diabetes, leaving a relatively small portion at risk
of new retinopathy. Data-gathering and interpretation are complicated by the
high death rates in patients with severe retinopathy, both old and young.
Malignant retinopathy appears to be less common when diabetes begins after
age 60 (Burditt, et al, 1968), but more data are needed. Hyperglucemia tends to
be particularly mild in this group.

There are also important differences in the distribution of specific causes of
retinopathy blindness in old and young diabetics. In older cases maculopathy
is relatively more common, while proliferative retinopathy is a more common

cause of blindness in youth-onset cases. It is not yet clear whether this difference is mainly or entirely the result of differences in the ages of the retinae, or whether the type and degree of diabetes are of importance in this respect.

One of the largest of the clinical studies was that of Cullen (1974) in Edinburgh. He reported on retinal examinations in 5,147 diabetics. The prevalence of retinopathy was 41% in males and 58% in females. In an excellent longitudinal study of 1,323 selected cases in Tokyo, Fukuda (1975) found that 47.5% of diabetics had retinopathy. Eleven percent had proliferative retinopathy. His data suggest that about one quarter of diabetics eventually develop proliferative retinopathy. He showed that, if they occur, proliferative lesions usually appear within a few years after the onset of clinically detectable retinopathy. In only 5% of his cases of proliferative retinopathy had background retinopathy been present more than six years! The main cause of blindness was tabulated for 158 eyes. In 34% blindness was due to retinal detachment; in 20%, vitreous opacity; in 15%, macular lesions; in 14%, fibrous tissue; and in 13%, glaucoma.

It appears that persons with typical retinal hemorrhages of moderate degree are more likely to develop proliferative retinopathy than are diabetics without retinopathy. This is consistent with the concept that proliferative retinopathy is simply an advanced stage of "background" retinopathy, but the relationship between the two is decidedly inconsistent. Persons with little background retinopathy may develop proliferative lesions and those with severe background retinopathy may not develop proliferation. This suggests the need for study of each of the various expressions of retinopathy to elucidate the strength and significance of their relationships. Particularly, this includes microaneurysms, exudates, intraretinal hemorrhages, neovascularizations, vitreous hemorrhages, fibrosis, and retinal detachments.

More and better data are needed, particularly on the incidence of severe blinding retinopathy and the factors to which it relates. Data of Caird, et al (1968) suggest, for example, the possibility that risk of proliferative retinopathy may be relatively modest even in youth-onset diabetes of long duration, perhaps as small as 20%. As indicated above, other investigators have found very high rates of cumulative incidence, as high as 50% (Knowles, 1975). There is an urgent need to determine the extent to which these differences are real and, if so, the reasons for the differences.

Analytic Studies and Risk Factors

Most of the factors that have been considered as causes or possible causes of retinopathy in diabetics have been listed on pages 405–406.

Duration of diabetes
This is by far the most powerful of the known etiologic factors. Studies cited above and many other observations have consistently shown a stronger effect of duration than of any other factor. Also reviewed above is evidence that inci-

dence of severe retinopathy tends to decline after two decades of diabetes. This phenomenon deserves further study, since it suggests that the majority who are susceptible will usually develop retinopathy after ten to twenty-five years of diabetes, leaving in the surviving group a very high proportion who are unusually resistant. The frequent presence of retinopathy in the first ten years of known maturity-onset diabetes is probably mainly the result of the lengthy duration of undiscovered diabetes in such cases.

Degree of hyperglycemia

The extent to which level of hyperglycemia determines risk of retinopathy is not at all clear. This is the most important issue at hand and deserves high priority in epidemiologic research.

Because duration of diabetes has such a strong effect, it seems quite probable that degree of hyperglycemia would also have an effect. But there are alternate possibilities. For example, it might be that the strong relationship between duration of hyperglycemia and retinopathy is not causal. A common factor might be at the root of both. Most recent research in animals and in man tends to preclude this possibility. Retinopathy has been produced by several investigators in animals with no evident genetic propensity to diabetes by making them hyperglycemic (Bloodworth, 1973; Kohner and Dollery,1975; Engerman, 1977). On the other hand, *proliferative* retinopathy has rarely been observed in animals with either spontaneous or induced diabetes. Evidence cited above suggests that diabetic retinopathy is extremely rare in euglycemic persons with prediabetes. As indicated below, retinopathy is very common in long-duration diabetes secondary to pancreatitis and hemochromatosis (Balodimos, 1971; Verdonk, et al, 1975). Fraser (1973) has pointed out that retinopathy is common in acromegalics with hyperglycemia, but has not been reported in acromegalics without hyperglycemia. Even so, the present epidemiologic evidence does not yet, in itself, establish that degree of glycemia is an important risk factor. Neither does existing evidence exclude that possibility. Knowles (1971,1975) analyzed results on a large number of clinical studies on this subject, and concluded that the available evidence was indecisive with respect to this issue.

As pointed out by Kaplan and Feinstein (1973), none of these clinical studies was designed in a manner that could be expected to yield a conclusive result. This issue appeared to be a rather simple one not requiring a design of great scope and sophistication. But we are finally learning that the requirements of such a design are quite considerable, for many reasons. One is that the characteristics of subjects with mild and severe hyperglycemia are quite different. Persons with mild hyperglycemia typically have a longer duration of occult hyperglycemia and as a group they are older. In general, study groups have been too small to determine whether the association between retinopathy and degree of hyperglycemia is hidden or enhanced by these other confounding variables.

Dramatic reversal of retinopathy has occasionally been observed after sharp reductions of blood glucose (Dollery and Oakley, 1965; Kohner and Dollery,

1975), but this experience is uncommon. Another problem in interpreting remissions of modest degree is that they often occur spontaneously (Gerritzen, 1973). Results of the University Group studies (1970) suggest that under ordinary conditions traditional attempts at therapy often have rather little influence on blood glucose levels in patients with mild maturity-onset diabetes. Very substantial mitigation of hyperglycemia is possible, but not very commonly achieved in actual practice. It is also clear that in typical juvenile-onset cases blood glucose levels are quite unphysiologic even when well-conceived therapy is employed. Thus, comparisons of "good" and "poor" control in patients without endogenous insulin are usually comparisons between poor control and very poor control. Knowles (1971) found rates of morbidity and mortality about the same in juvenile diabetics who consumed unmeasured diets as in groups of patients that received more conventional dietary prescriptions. But there is no evidence to indicate whether or not patients of Knowles had glucose levels that were, in general, higher than in those advised to consume traditional diabetic diets. It is quite clear that glycemic levels of some childhood-onset cases are considerably lower or higher than the average of the group. Even if those with lower glucose levels are found to have less retinopathy, it will not be certain that the favorable outcome is a direct result of the lower glucose levels.

A majority of clinical studies addressed to this issue have found some degree of positive relationship between degree of glycemia and risk of retinopathy, but a substantial number have not (Colwell, 1966; Knowles, 1971). Only a few of these clinical studies will be reviewed. This discussion will be confined mainly to studies in groups of cases that appear to be substantially representative of the populations of diabetics in the communities from which they were drawn, or very large clinical studies. Among the more impressive of the clinical studies suggesting a relationship between degree of hyperglycemia and risk or severity of retinopathy are those conducted at the Joslin Clinic (Bradley and Ramos, 1971), and those of Miki, et al (1969), Fukuda (1975), Pirart (1977), Szabo, et al (1967), Burditt, et al (1968), Job, et al (1976), and Hunter, et al (1977). The study of Hardin, et al (1956) was one of the first to suggest that mitigation of hyperglycemia protected against retinopathy. In 1913 Frederick Allen presented arguments pro and con on the issue of whether hyperglycemia was directly deleterious. Forty years later (1953) he argued eloquently that risk of vascular disease could be reduced by mitigation of hyperglycemia. Arguments against this notion have been presented by Hutton, et al (1972). They observed microaneurysms commonly in patients without hyperglycemia. Some of these had a family history of diabetes. But visual impairment from diabetic retinopathy has not been reported in the absence of hyperglycemia. There are no data establishing that normoglycemic subjects with a strong family history of diabetes have microaneurysms more frequently than well-matched controls.

The University Group (1971) found no relationship of level of glycemia to incidence of retinopathy over a period of several years. In this study the spectrum of blood glucose values was relatively narrow. These results do suggest that differences in blood glucose levels of modest degree (eg, 50 mg/ 100 ml) are not associated with great differences in the incidence of retinopathy. They do not exclude the possibility that modest differences over a long period of time might be significant in this respect. Data have not yet been reported by the University Group on the extent to which the relationship between glycemia and retinopathy was affected by factors such as age, duration of diabetes, sex, adiposity, and blood pressure.

Results were similar in the studies of Pima Indians. No significant association was observed between retinopathy and level of glucose in 366 with unequivocal diabetes, despite a broad spectrum of blood glucose levels. Here again, however, possibility was not excluded that an association was hidden by differences of other characteristics in those with minimal, moderate, and severe hyperglycemia. Those with slight hyperglycemia may have been older, and they may have had had occult diabetes longer than those with greater hyperglycemia. Even with these rather substantial numbers (366 diabetics and 76 with retinopathy) of well-collected data, it is not possible to confirm or refute the possibility that a significant causal association exists between degree of glycemia and retinopathy.

In the study of Nilsson, et al (1967) the association between retinopathy and blood glucose was examined in 483 diabetics, of whom 168 had retinopathy. This group included a very high percentage of all diabetics in this geographic area. The correlation coefficient was .28 in men and .14 in women. There is a strong possibility that the strength of this association could have been enhanced or reduced by the confounding variables discussed above.

Bradley and Ramos (1971) found that 97.5% of all their patients with proliferative retinopathy required insulin. This could be the result of any one of several factors, but this observation fits well the possibility that risk of proliferative retinopathy is higher in persons who have higher blood glucose levels. Most observers, including Bradley and Ramos, have found the incidence of proliferative retinopathy higher in insulin-dependent diabetes except during the first few years of known diabetes, at which time the actual duration is less in insulin-dependent cases. As indicated above, Knowles (1971) concluded from his analysis of data from several sources that about half of juvenile diabetics eventually develop proliferative retinopathy. Few comparable data are available on very long-duration maturity-onset cases, but risk of proliferative retinopathy would appear to be lower (even though it is higher in the first few years of known diabetes in these older diabetics). More data are needed, however, to confirm or refute this. The number of persons blinded is far greater among older adults, but in affluent societies the number of maturity-onset diabetics at risk is typically more than ten times greater than the number of juvenile-onset patients. In Edinburgh, for example, 7% of those with known diabetes had been diagnosed in the first two decades of life (Falconer, et al, 1971).

The high rates of death in youth-onset and maturity-onset cases with severe retinopathy make it difficult to interpret data on the relative prevalence of

417

malignant retinopathy in these two groups, even when corrections are made for apparent duration of diabetes. Other confounding variables include the longer duration of undiagnosed diabetes and the greater age of the maturity-onset cases. Among the 1,393 diabetics studied in Japan by Fukuda (1972), there were 120 with proliferative retinopathy. Fukuda thought it significant that 80% of the 120 had had "indifferent" control of diabetes during the first year it was known to be present. In 1975 Fukuda presented additional evidence in a large series strongly suggesting a favorable effect of early aggressive control of the blood glucose. In a group of 744 diabetics in Geneva studied by Vernet, et al (1975), retinopathy was significantly more common in insulin-dependent diabetics. Observations of this kind suggest a causal relationship between degree of hyperglycemia but are not conclusive for several reasons, including uncertainties concerning a possible dependence on other factors of this relationship between type of therapy and retinopathy.

Caird, et al (1969) reviewed evidence from many sources, including their own data, and concluded that degree of hyperglycemia was probably etiologically important, particularly in the early stages of diabetes. They could discern little evidence of a favorable effect of mitigation of hyperglycemia after retinopathy was well established. Szabo, et al (1967) studied 324 diabetics in whom the disease had been known for at least ten years. They found severe retinopathy more common in those who had had higher blood glucose levels.

Several investigators have shown a strong association between retinopathy and capillary permeability (Lundbaeck, 1953; Hart and Cohen, 1968; Christensen, 1968; Hunter, et al, 1969). Parving, et al (1976) have demonstrated that capillary permeability is increased when metabolic control is less satisfactory and hyperglycemia greater.

Low rates of both microvascular and macrovascular disease are notable in the group of patients with mild hyperglycemia having its onset in youth (Tattersall, 1973; Fajans, et al, 1975). This evidence supports the notion of a causal relationship between degree of hyperglycemia and risk of retinopathy. These persons seem to have less microvascular disease than those with mild hyperglycemia beginning later in life. One possible interpretation of this is that young capillaries are less susceptible to damage than old capillaries.

Balodimos (1971) reviewed a large number of reports on the prevalence of microangiopathy in patients with diabetes of secondary types such as pancreatitis, pancreatectomy, and acromegaly. Retinopathy has been common, particularly in cases having diabetes more than ten years. This was true, for example; in the studies of Lyra de Lacerda, et al (1977). In the series of Verdonk, et al (1975) of cases with "pancreatic diabetes" there were 24 patients who had had known diabetes more than thirteen years of whom 12 (50%) had microangiopathy. Of 26 cases with a duration of diabetes of ten years or more, 7 had retinopathy. In this group there was no significant difference in frequency of retinopathy in those with a family history of diabetes (3 of 12) and those without such histories (4 of 14). Frequency of microangiopathy was much greater in patients who required insulin (19 of 20) than in those who did not (2 of 56), but these latter data were not corrected for duration of diabetes. These latter results suggest, however, either that degree of glycemia is etiologically important or that insulin therapy causes retinopathy. The former seems more likely. Soeldner, et al (1976) found that "prediabetics" had shorter retinal circulation times than controls. This could reflect a prediabetic lesion, but the small differences might have been the result of other differences in the characteristics of the two groups.

As shown by Peterson, et al (1977), several of the hematologic aberrations observed in diabetes are dependent on hyperglycemia and proportional to its degree.

Khurana and White (1976) found in 153 juvenile diabetics who had survived more than forty years that all had experienced hypoglycemic reactions, but only 14% had had ketosis.

Engerman, et al (1977) produced retinopathy in dogs. The degree of pathology seemed to be related to the degree of hyperglycemia.

The degree of hyperglycemia probably influences susceptibility to retinopathy, but more and better studies are needed on this important issue.

At what level of glycemia does increased risk of retinopathy begin? Few directly relevant data are available; this writer is not aware of any report of impairment of vision from diabetic retinopathy in a person who has never exhibited fasting hyperglycemia. Microaneurysms and exudates have been observed frequently in persons with normal glucose tolerance. This has led some to conclude that these lesions are not the direct effect of hyperglycemia (Hutton, et al, 1972). But these cases have regularly exhibited a degree of retinal change that is functionally quite trivial. It has been shown above that in many poor societies, for every diabetic there are several with the genetic potential for developing diabetes. Yet, clinically significant glomerulosclerosis and retinopathy have not been reported in euglycemic persons in these countries. The degree of rarity of such cases even in affluent societies is consistent with the possibility that these very rare cases formerly had mild occult hyperglycemia.

The most relevant data are those of Dorf, et al (1976) in a whole population of Pima Indians, and of Keen (1972) and his associates in Bedford, England. In 1,274 Pimas with two-hour glucose values less than 200 mg/100 ml, only 0.7% had microaneurysms and 1.5% exudates. None had a degree of retinal pathology that threatened vision. Such minor lesions may or may not be diabetes-related. Results of Keen (1972) in Bedford were very similar. Microaneurysms were occasionally observed in persons with normal or borderline glucose tolerance. None with borderline glucose tolerance had more than three microaneurysms at either the baseline examination or at a subsequent examination five years later. The extent to which such minor lesions are diabetes-related cannot be discerned on the basis of present evidence. At five years, rates of these minimal retinal abnormalities were slightly higher in the small group with borderline glucose tolerance than in those with clearly normal tolerance, but numbers were not adequate to determine precisely the level of glycemia at which increased risk begins. Another problem in interpreting the data from

419

both Arizona and Bedford is that those with normal tolerance were younger than those with borderline tolerance. The available data do suggest that risk of retinopathy is quite small in those with two-hour blood glucose values below 200 mg/100 ml (Jarrett and Keen, 1976).

More data of this type are needed, with larger numbers. Among the potentialities of such data would be their bearing on the urgent need for determining the normal limits of glucose tolerance. There are apparently no data establishing that risk of clinically significant retinopathy (eg, retinal hemorrhage) is increased prior to the development of fasting hyperglycemia. *The disparity is particularly striking between the millions of old people with "abnormal" glucose tolerance and the extreme rarity of visual impairment from retinopathy in these elderly persons when fasting glucose levels are normal.*

Geography and race

Geographic differences in retinopathy have not been nearly so impressive as the geographic differences in atherosclerosis. Rates of retinopathy in diabetics of Japan, for example, seem to be similar to those found in Europe or North America. There are, however, several reports of particularly low rates of retinopathy that suggest a need for further study of the possible importance of environmental or racial factors.

Campbell (1963) found rates of retinopathy much higher in his Indian diabetics of Natal, South Africa than in local black diabetics. Shaper (1958) had reported low rates of retinopathy in his Kenyan black diabetics. Even though duration of adults was relatively brief in this group, the low rates were impressive. Only 5% of his Type II (insulin-independent) cases had retinopathy. Campbell did not think that the interracial differences in his diabetics were explained by interracial differences in either duration or diabetes or levels of glycemia. On the other hand, Steel, et al (1977) observed retinopathy rather commonly in black diabetics of Nairobi. Seftel and Walker (1966) found retinopathy in 45% of their black South Africans when duration of diabetes exceeded seven years. Jackson, et al (1966) did not find much difference in rates of retinopathy between Indians and blacks of Capetown. It seems probable that in certain circumstances the interval between onset of diabetes and its discovery might differ in ethnic groups. This might account for some of the differences described above and below. The effect of duration is so critical that data on rates of retinopathy are often difficult to interpret unless there are adequate numbers of cases with diabetes of at least ten years duration.

Bourgoignie, et al (1962) examined 34 black diabetics in the Congo. None had retinal hemorrhages or exudates, but only one had had diagnosed diabetes for more than ten years. Gelfand and Forbes (1963) found retinopathy in only 4% of their black Rhodesian diabetics. In general, duration of diabetes was short in this group. Sujano and Sukaton (1970) observed retinopathy rather infrequently in Indonesian diabetics (8%), but average duration of diabetes was also short in this clinic. Retinopathy had been diagnosed in only 1% of the Pakistani diabetics of Ibrahim (1962). Details were not given on methods of ascertainment or rates of retinopathy by duration. In India Lal, et al (1968) found retinopathy about equally common in the various types of diabetes. After correction for duration of diabetes, retinopathy did not seem especially uncommon in any of these subgroups. Another frequent problem in interpreting many of the reports of clinical studies of this type is that circumstances of selection and methods of examination are not well described.

Osuntokun (1969) reported in some detail the results of retinal examinations in 758 Nigerian diabetics. This represented almost all the patients in a clinic for diabetics. Rates of retinopathy were low even after correction for known duration of diabetes. Only 4.6% of all diabetics had retinopathy. In those with known duration of ten to fifteen years, 11.7% (7 of 60) had retinopathy. Of ten patients with diabetes of sixteen to twenty years duration, three had retinopathy. Otim (1975) studied retinal status in 105 black Ugandan diabetics. Only nine had retinopathy and one proliferative retinopathy. Only three had retinal hemorrhages. In 18 with known diabetes for eleven to twenty years, 4 had retinopathy. Edwards, et al (1976) have reported low rates of retinopathy in diabetic Australian aborigines, some of whom had been diabetic as long as fifteen years.

Precise information is lacking, but it appears that US black diabetics have at least as much retinopathy as whites (Kahn and Hiller, 1975). Among the possible explanations for the apparently disparate results in various groups of blacks residing in Africa is that risk may be related to factors associated with "urbanization". In general, rates of retinopathy appear to be less in very lean blacks than in fat blacks, but the relationship to adiposity may or may not have causal significance. In Haiti Charles and Medard (1969) reported the complete absence of retinopathy in a group of 90 black diabetics who were very poor and extremely lean. Information on duration of diabetes was not provided. In more affluent Haitian diabetics retinopathy was not rare.

A paucity of retinopathy has also been reported in other racial groups. Lebon, et al (1953) examined the retinae of 67 Algerian diabetics. None had retinopathy! Mekkawi and Aswad (1972) reported low rates in 137 Libyan diabetics. When diabetes had been known for five to ten years retinopathy was present in 14%; in those of longer duration 17% had retinopathy. Retinopathy was apparently uncommon in Navajo Indian diabetics (Prosnitz and Mandell, 1967; Saiki and Rimoin, 1968), and in certain other tribes of American Indians (Table 33).

Chung (1962) reported very low rates of retinopathy in the Chinese diabetics of Shanghai. In a clinic with more than 900 diabetics proliferative retinopathy had not been observed, and only 7.4% were reported to have had retinopathy. In other groups of Chinese diabetics higher rates have been observed. In Hong Kong McFadzean and Yeung (1968) found that retinopathy was present in 26% of Chinese diabetics who had a known duration of diabetes of ten years or more. In diabetics of Taiwan retinopathy is rather common (Tsai, 1971).

Considered in the aggregate these and other data on racial and geographic variations do not suggest very strongly an effect of race itself. Both high and low rates of retinopathy have been reported in each of several races. Low rates have not been reported in any racial group living under relatively affluent circumstances. It appears that environmental circumstances may influence risk of retinopathy to a moderate degree. Some of the factors that may be responsible will be discussed below.

Age

This has been discussed above. There are many problems in determining the extent to which age has an independent effect on susceptibility to retinopathy. One problem is that age is related to duration of diabetes and, in general, negatively related to degree of hyperglycemia. Present evidence does not establish or refute the possibility that susceptibility to retinopathy is increased with age. This possibility deserves investigation, but very large numbers of well-collected data will be required to evaluate this hypothesis by epidemiologic means.

Dorf, et al (1976) concluded that age was probably not of substantial importance in determining susceptibility to retinopathy, but they acknowledged that present evidence was indecisive. Studies of Burditt, et al (1968) suggested that severe retinopathy was less frequent when diabetes was discovered in old age than when it appeared in middle age. This does not support the notion that old retinae are more susceptible to damage. But another possibility is that the lesser pathology in the elderly is the result of a lesser degree of hyperglycemia. Typically, the elderly are not as fat as persons of middle age. This suggests other possibilities; it may be, for example, that duration of undiscovered diabetes is longest in those found to be diabetic in middle age.

Sex

In many clinical studies rates of retinopathy have been similar in the sexes. Typical results include those of Kahn and Bradley (1975). In a group of 914 they found retinopathy in 24% of men and 27% of women. In several studies, rates have been somewhat higher in females. A greater risk in females seems to be rather generally acknowledged in Japan (Tsuji and Wada, 1970). Nilsson, et al (1967) observed a particularly low frequency and severity of retinopathy in diabetic males over 59 years of age. In black diabetics of South Africa, Seftel and Walker (1966) found retinopathy more common in women. Blindness from diabetes is far more frequent in US black women than in black men, but much or all of this difference may be due to the much higher rate of diabetes in American black women as compared to black men. In Libya retinal exudates appeared to be rare except in fat women (Mekkawi and Aswad, 1972).

These differences between the sexes do not, of course establish an independent relationship between female sex and retinopathy. It is possible for example, that in certain circumstances the duration of occult diabetes is longer in women. Females are often fatter and have a higher renal threshold for glucose (Gordon, et al, 1964; Butterfield, et al, 1967).

In Indonesia Sukaton found retinopathy somewhat more prevalent in males (Tsuji and Wada, 1970). Yuen and Kahn (1976) studied incidence of blindness by sex and age in certain US states with registry systems. They found new blindness more common in diabetic males than in diabetic females in persons under 45 years of age. In older diabetics, new blindness was slightly more common in females. Among several possible explanations for the observed differences is that female hormones are protective. As pointed out by these latter investigators, these data should be interpreted with caution because the methods for ascertaining blindness and the frequency of blindness in these circumstances were necessarily crude. For example, it is possible that blindness is more frequently reported when present in young men, and it is possible that the number of diabetics at risk may have been underestimated to a greater degree in one sex than another. In 4,875 diabetics of Japan, Kojima, et al (1970) found the prevalence of retinopathy higher in females at all age levels.

Adiposity and insulinemia

Diabetic retinopathy and blindness seemed to be much less common before the discovery of insulin. Patients who take insulin probably have generally higher blood insulin levels than do normal persons. Fat diabetics who do not take insulin also have relatively generous levels of blood insulin. These considerations prompted the suggestion that excessive insulin levels might cause retinopathy. Several other considerations militate against this possibility. Obese nondiabetics have very high levels of serum insulin and no retinopathy. Although the frequency of retinopathy has not been well measured in insulinopenic diabetics who do not take insulin, retinopathy appears to be common in this subgroup. Conceivably, however, insulinemia could enhance the effects of some other more fundamental agent such as hyperglycemia. In lean primitive populations in which retinopathy has been uncommon, the percentage of diabetics who are insulinopenic, but not on insulin, is probably higher than that of groups of diabetics in affluent societies. Retinopathy is, however, rather common when diabetes is secondary to pancreatic disease, after ten years of diabetes (Verdonk, et al, 1975). But more data are needed in this group, including the subgroup on insulin therapy and without insulin treatment.

In the much larger group of diabetics with no evident disease of the exocrine pancreas, it has been very difficult to evaluate comparisons of those who take or do not take insulin. These groups differ substantially in many important characteristics, such as age, degree of glycemia, levels of endogenous insulin, and duration of undiscovered diabetes. It would be possible to match for or correct for most of those variables, but very large numbers of well-collected data would be required to determine in an epidemiologic study whether there was an independent effect of insulin therapy or of blood insulin level on risk of retinopathy. In the University Group study (1970) no evidence could be found that insulin therapy enhanced retinopathy or protected against it.

Kohner and Oakley (1975) studied levels of endogenous insulin in 220 diabetics not being treated with insulin. After oral glucose, rises in serum insulin were less in patients with retinopathy than in those without retinopathy.

In the 1,000 diabetics studied by Kornerup (1955) there was a relationship between fatness and retinopathy. It was not discerned whether the association was independent of other variables. It may be, for example, that duration of undiscovered diabetes was longer in the fatter patients. Fat people tend to have higher serum lipids and higher blood pressures. Nilsson, et al (1967) also found an association of fatness and retinopathy, but Szabo, et al (1967) did not.

In their studies of 146 patients with diabetes and chronic pancreatitis, Verdonk, et al (1975) found that the frequency of microangiopathy was substantially higher in patients taking insulin (18 of 70) than in those not taking insulin (2 of 56). These latter data were not, however, adjusted for duration and degree of hyperglycemia. Hunter, et al (1977) found that in long-duration diabetics with most severe retinopathy were heavier than those with least severe retinopathy.

Serum lipids

It does not seem likely that levels of serum lipids are an important determinant in retinopathy, but present evidence does not exclude a causal role of modest degree for lipidemia. Although serum lipid levels are much lower in Japan, Japanese diabetics seem to have about as much retinopathy as North American or European diabetics. Kojima, et al (1970) could not demonstrate a consistent relationship between retinopathy and serum cholesterol in a very large study of 4,875 Japanese diabetics. But in certain subgroups of the entire diabetic population there was some evidence of a positive association between retinopathy and cholesterolemia. Osuntokun (1969) found that Nigerian diabetics with retinopathy had higher serum cholesterol values than diabetics without retinopathy. This of course does not establish a causal relationship. Lebon, et al (1953) thought that the low rates of retinopathy in Algerians might be due to their low blood lipid levels. The diabetics of Balodimos, et al (1969) who had no retinopathy also had lower serum cholesterol levels than those who had retinopathy. This relationship was also observed by Job, et al (1973) and by Kuzuya and Kosaka (1970) and Kohner and Oakley (1975). This was not seen in the patients of Szabo, et al (1967). In the study of Nilsson (1967) the association between retinopathy and serum cholesterol was quite weak. The correlation coefficient was .2 in males and .05 in females.

In the study of Deckert, et al (1967) of patients with proliferative lesions, prognosis for vision was worse in those with high serum cholesterol values. It was not possible to discern whether this had causal significance. In some circumstances a significant confounding variable is that cholesterol levels are elevated by severe glomerulosclerosis.

Several studies summarized by Kohner and Dollery (1975) suggest that lowering the serum cholesterol level has a clearing effect on retinal exudates. But there has been no evidence of improvement in vision with such clearing. Exudates usually do not interfere with vision, but when they occur in the macular area they may do so. Few data are available on the frequency and severity of exudates that would make possible interpopulation comparisons. The multinational study of the World Health Organization is gathering such data.

Caird, et al (1968) reviewed some of the earlier clinical studies linking serum lipid levels to retinopathy. They concluded that these data were indecisive with respect to the causal effect of lipidemia.

Verdonk, et al (1975) measured levels of serum cholesterol in diabetics with chronic pancreatitis. In 15 with microangiopathy mean serum cholesterol was 201 mg/100 ml. In 68 without microangiopathy the mean was 215.

Blood pressure

Blood pressure may be an independent risk factor for diabetic retinopathy. Present evidence is not decisive. In several studies there has been an association between blood pressure and retinopathy, but nephropathy causes elevation of blood pressure, and persons that have retinopathy are more likely to have nephropathy. Blood pressure is also, usually, associated with several other of the possible risk factors for retinopathy, including age, duration of diabetes, and adiposity. Clinical studies linking blood pressure and risk of retinopathy include those of Kornerup (1958), Kojima, et al (1970), Job, et al (1973), Szabo, et al (1967), Harrold (1971), and Adler, et al (1975). Oakley, et al (1974) noted that blood pressure levels were low in diabetics who survived forty years or longer. A substantial portion of these had escaped severe retinopathy.

This relationship of blood pressure and retinopathy has also been observed in epidemiologic studies, including those of Bennett, et al (1976a) and Nilsson, et al (1967). In the study of Nilsson the association between blood pressure and retinopathy was very weak. The correlation coefficient between systolic blood pressure and retinopathy was .18 in males and .10 in females. This degree of association may have been attributable to the association in this group between retinopathy and nephropathy (which causes higher blood pressure).

In a clinical study Keen (1972) found a very weak relationship between blood pressure and retinopathy. He concluded that a causal role of blood pressure was neither established or excluded.

In Pima Indians risk of retinopathy is impressively related to blood pressure, even after corrections for duration of diabetes and presence of nephropathy (Bennett, et al, 1976a). In newly discovered diabetics with baseline systolic blood pressures above 139 mm Hg, 32% had subsequently developed retinopathy, while only 8% of those with lower blood pressure had developed retinopathy.

Systematically collected data on blood pressure are few in the populations that seem to have low rates of retinopathy. In such lean poor people, blood pressure levels have usually been relatively low. In Nigerians, however, hypertension was very common in diabetics without retinopathy (Osuntokun, 1969). According to Osuntokun, hypertensive retinopathy is also uncommon in non-diabetic Nigerians with hypertension.

Genetic factors

Several types of genetic influence are possible. The genetic traits that lead to hyperglycemia could produce retinopathy by mechanisms independent of hyperglycemia. This possibility still has adherents, mainly because an independent effect of degree of hyperglycemia on retinopathy has not yet been well demonstrated in the production of retinopathy. But there is strong evidence against this "genetic retinopathy" hypothesis. This negative evidence is also reviewed in other sections of this book and by Caird, et al (1968), Lundbaeck (1974), and Kohner and Oakley (1975). But there are other possibilities that genetic factors could influence either susceptibility or resistance to retinopathy, even if the basic etiologic factor is hyperglycemia (see below).

Bradley and Ramos (1971) reviewed some observations from Joslin Clinic studies on the presence and severity of retinopathy in diabetics and other diabetics from the same family. Little evidence was found of a genetic influence. The experience of Caird, et al (1968) was also generally negative in this respect. Kojima, et al (1970) in their study of 4,875 diabetics found "no clear relation" between retinopathy and family history of diabetes. On the other hand, Tattersall and Pyke (1972) demonstrated rather striking similarities in identical twins in susceptibility to retinopathy. All too frequently it is assumed that the genetic factor to look for is one that enhances retinopathy. More attention is warranted for genetic influences on resistance. Both positive and negative genetic effects could be mediated by any of many mechanisms or by combinations thereof. These include blood pressure, capillary permeability, enzymatic responses to injury of retinal vasculature.

In a small series it was found by Shin, et al (1977) that diabetics without retinopathy had the HLA-A1 antigen more frequently than diabetics with retinopathy. Anderson, et al (1975) found that proliferative retinopathy was more common in juvenile-onset diabetes in those patients with histocompatibility antigens HLA-B8 and W15. Neither Barbosa, et al (1977) nor Chuck, et al (1977) found a relationship between HLA antigen status and diabetic complications. Becker, et al (1977) observed no such association in youth-onset cases, but in diabetics with later onset those without retinopathy had an excessive frequency of HLA-A1 and B8. In a group of prediabetics Soeldner, et al (1976) found retinal circulation time slightly shorter than in controls. In identical twins Pyke (1977) found more retinopathy in twins concordant for diabetes than in diabetics with a nondiabetic twin.

Nutritional factors

Adiposity and lipedemia have been discussed above. Nutritional factors are a major cause of retinopathy in that they strongly affect susceptibility to diabetes. In established diabetes, however, there is little evidence that qualitative features of diet are important in determining risk of retinopathy. This does deserve further investigation. Kempner, et al (1958) found impressive evidence of improvement of retinopathy in patients who consumed rice diets. Fat diabetic patients of the Occident who observe such diets usually lose substantial amounts of weight; and blood pressure and plasma glucose decline. There is other evidence that favorable effects of rice diet seen under certain conditions are probably not a direct effect of the qualitative features of this diet.

Retinopathy is common in many populations in which rice consumption is very high (eg, in Japan).

The effects of extreme leanness deserve further study. "Nonobese" subjects in affluent societies have, on the average, about three times as much body fat as the people of certain primitive societies in whom retinopathy appears to be uncommon (eg, Pakistan and rural Africa). In cross-sectional studies, an effect of degree of adiposity might be hidden by a decline in weight that frequently occurs after the development of complications such as glomerulosclerosis. In diabetics who are particularly thin at onset of diabetes, the period between onset of diabetes and onset of symptoms is probably shorter than in fatter diabetics.

Other factors

Several other factors that deserve further study are listed under the section (above) on Applicability of Epidemiologic Study (page 405). Most, but not all, are secondary to hyperglycemia. These latter factors have been well reviewed by Caird, et al (1969), Bradley and Ramos (1971), Kohner and Oakley (1975), McMillan (1975) and Palmberg (1977). As indicated above, capillary permeability is increased in patients with retinopathy. Permeability is decreased with hypophysectomy (Christensen, 1968a) and with mitigation of hyperglycemia (Parving, et al, 1976).

In some circumstances a negative relationship has been observed between ocular tension and retinopathy; in other conditions the reverse obtained. It has been suggested that raising ocular tension might increase resistance to retinopathy. It seems more likely that changes in ocular tension are the result rather than the cause of retinopathy. These relationships do deserve more investigation. Some of the work relating to these associations between ocular tension and retinopathy has been reviewed by Keen (1972), and Kohner and Dollery (1975), and by Shin, et al (1977). Smoking may be a risk factor for proliferative diabetic retinopathy (Paetkau, et al, 1977), but present data are not conclusive.

Relationship to other manifestations of diabetes

Beginning with its original description in 1936 by Kimmelstiel and Wilson, glomerulosclerosis has been thought to be closely related to retinopathy. Both are strongly related to duration of diabetes. Both are the result of morbid changes in capillaries. But there are impressive differences in the character of pathologic changes. Severe retinopathy is not infrequent in patients without evident glomerulosclerosis. More data are needed on the strength and character of this relationship.

In the study of Lundbaeck (1953) associations were also observed between retinopathy and heart disease, leg-vessel disease, and kidney disease. It was not clear whether these associations were independent of factors other than degree and duration of hyperglycemia.

Clinicians have long been impressed with a general association of neuropathy and retinopathy (Fagerberg, 1959; Pirart, 1965), but exceptions to this association are also common. In the study of Nilsson, et al (1967) there was a negative association between retinopathy and both vibratory sense and Achilles reflexes. Neuropathy has been very common, however, in some populations of diabetics in which retinopathy has been uncommon (Osuntokun, 1969; Levin and Gelfand, 1973).

Data on the strength and character of these associations between the various manifestations are a potentially rich source of clues concerning the factors that enhance or inhibit the different lesions. Particularly deserving of special study are the characteristics of patients who have severe retinopathy and no proteinuria, or severe glomerulosclerosis and little retinopathy. In the study of Nilsson the association of proteinuria and retinopathy was of only modest strength. The coefficient of correlation was .37. Deckert, et al (1967) demonstrated in patients with proliferative lesions that prognosis for vision was much worse in those with proteinuria. In the study of Fukuda (1972) all patients who died of uremia had proliferative retinopathy. In the long-duration diabetics of Lundbaeck (1953) who were studied in collaboration with Jensen, 92% of those with clinical evidence of nephropathy also had retinopathy. Root, et al (1959) found that of 331 deaths in patients with proliferative retinopathy almost half (147) were from renal failure. But about one third of Root's cases of proliferative retinopathy did not have proteinuria at the time proliferative retinopathy was found. Watkins, et al (1972) showed that glomerulosclerosis was commonly present on renal biopsies of such patients despite absence of proteinuria.

In the group of long-duration diabetics over 59 years of age studied by Lundbaeck (1953), retinopathy was significantly more common in patients with heart disease (88%) than in those without heart disease (56%). In younger diabetics no significant relationship between these two complications was observed. In the study of Szabo, et al (1967) no relationship was found between retinopathy and any of the manifestations of arteriosclerosis. The frequent disparities between microvascular and macrovascular manifestations are quite striking both in individual patients and among populations. In Japan, for example, gangrene is rare and retinopathy is very common.

Much of the strength of the relationship of retinopathy to other morbid effects of diabetes, such as neuropathy and glomerulosclerosis, may be dependent on duration of diabetes.

Glomerulosclerosis

Introduction

Although it is a very important cause of morbidity and mortality, this kidney lesion has received considerably less epidemiologic study than coronary disease and retinopathy, for several reasons. Probably the major one is that there has been little evidence of interpopulation differences in the incidence and character of this lesion. Mitigation of hyperglycemia appears to have a favorable influence, but no other striking clues have emerged concerning its etiology or prevention in established diabetes. Glomerulosclerosis does, however, deserve further epidemiologic study. It is not known why some persons develop severe kidney lesions after a few years of diabetes, while others maintain excellent kidney function for decades despite severe diabetes. Although interpopulation differences have not been established, differences of modest degree have not been excluded. There is need, therefore, for both intrapopulation and interpopulation studies to determine the factors responsible for the substantial intraindividual differences in susceptibility to glomerulosclerosis.

The most important issue is the extent to which degree of hyperglycemia influences the risk of glomerulosclerosis and the rate at which this lesion develops. Data from animal experiments and from some clinical studies suggest that degree of glycemia may be important, but previous clinical and epidemiologic evidence has not been decisive. The difficulties in gathering conclusive evidence are several. Duration of glycemia has a powerful effect and, in general, the duration of undiscovered diabetes is greater in patients with mild hyperglycemia than in those with marked hyperglycemia. It is difficult to measure degree of glycemia over time with precision. No generally accepted standards and conventions exist for expressing degree of glycemia over time. For example, there are no standard definitions for terms such as *good control, mild diabetes,* or *severe hyperglycemia.* Nor are there standardized methods of ascertaining the presence or severity of renal morbidity. Because renal biopsy is not feasible under most circumstances, the major index of the presence of glomerulosclerosis has been proteinuria. Although a very useful index, proteinuria is neither highly sensitive nor highly specific in identifying glomerulosclerosis, or in measuring its degree. None of these problems presents an unsurmountable obstacle to the development of effective epidemiologic designs. Levels of hemoglobin A1$_c$ (glycosylated hemoglobin) seem to reflect fairly well the levels of blood glucose over the previous few weeks. This may provide a method for evaluating the effects of blood glucose levels on other variables.

Diabetics often have other kidney lesions, particularly pyelonephritis. The importance of other causes of nephropathy are conceded, but this discussion will concentrate on the most frequent and serious lesion, glomerulosclerosis.

HISTORY AND GENERAL NATURE

Even in the 19th century it was known that kidney pathology was common in diabetes. But progress in the understanding of the renal lesions was quite limited prior to the clear description of glomerulosclerosis in 1936 by Kimmelstiel and Wilson. In both the British symposium on diabetes in the tropics (Havelock Charles, 1907) and in Allen's book (1913) there is evidence of controversy on whether hyperglycemia itself damaged the kidney. Lundbaeck's excellent publication (1953) contains a good summary of the history of the development of an understanding of glomerulosclerosis.

Retrospective review of mortality data in the early 20th century for both the United States and New York City shows that rates of death from kidney disease were decidedly excessive in diabetes. The fatal cases of nephropathy in diabetes were usually labeled Bright's disease. In New York City, death was attributed to Bright's disease or "nephritis" in about 5%, while in diabetics these causes of death were cited in about 14%. This highly significant evidence was little noticed. Systematic follow-up of these clues would have shortened the long delay in the appreciation of the importance of kidney pathology in diabetes.

By 1949 Mann, et al had shown that nephropathy was the leading cause of death in youth-onset diabetes. In childhood-onset diabetes, proteinuria appears frequently in the second decade of diabetes. The kidney disease typically progresses relentlessly. Often patients with proteinuria are asymptomatic for a few years before the onset of edema and then uremia. Death usually occurs four to ten years after the onset of proteinuria, but a shorter or longer course sometimes obtains.

Details of this disorder have been well set forth by Cameron, et al (1975) and by Balodimos (1971). Others contributing to an understanding of diabetic nephropathy have included Root (1954), Marble (1976), and White (1956) at the Joslin Clinic; Bell (1953); Lundbaeck (1953, 1974); and Thomsen (1955). Other recent contributors will be credited below.

Knowles (1974) has reviewed the toll exacted by diabetic nephropathy. About 40% of juvenile-onset diabetics are killed by these lesions (Marks and Krall, 1971). A small portion of these fatal cases are the result of renal pathologic changes other than glomerulosclerosis, especially pyelonephritis, but more than 90% are caused primarily by glomerulosclerosis. The nodular and diffuse hyaline lesions of the glomeruli are often accompanied by other lesions that some would consider an integral part of "glomerulosclerosis" while others would classify them as separate lesions. These other aberrations include arteriolonephrosclerosis of the afferent and efferent glomerular arterioles. The degree of renal disability is rather closely associated with the diffuse lesions in the glomeruli (Gellman, et al, 1959), but it is not known to what extent the various elements of these pathologic changes (eg, nodular glomerular lesions, thickening of mesangium and basement membrane, arteriolar occlusion) contribute to impaired function. These matters have been well reviewed by Cameron, et al (1975).

Death from nephropathy is not nearly so common in adult-onset diabetes as in the childhood-onset cases. In the Joslin Clinic patients, kidney disease accounted for only 2% of deaths when onset of diabetes was between ages 40 and 59 (Marks and Krall, 1971). Only 1% with later onset were killed by kidney disease. When onset of diabetes occurred between ages of 20 and 39 years, 10% of deaths were from kidney disease. One reason for the infrequency of renal disease as a cause of death in older diabetics of the affluent Occident is that they tend to die from manifestations of atherosclerosis before severe glomerulosclerosis has developed. Data of FitzGerald presented in the book of Malins (1968) show very well that onset of proteinuria occurs with shorter known duration of diabetes in patients with later onset of diabetes. It seems likely that this is mainly the result of the longer interval between onset and discovery of diabetes in older patients. Death registration data have usually been difficult to interpret with respect to rates of death from glomerulosclerosis. In many circumstances these cases are reported as death from "diabetes". In groups of adult-onset cases that have been studied in other ways, diabetic nephropathy has typically accounted for about 8% of all deaths. In Japan the proportion has been higher, probably because death from coronary disease is relatively uncommon. In the autopsy study reported by Goto and Fukuhara (1968) 15% of deaths of diabetics were attributed to kidney disease. Childhood-onset cases were included, but they constitute a very small portion of diabetics in Japan.

The natural history of diabetic renal disease has been well described by Caird (1961), Watkins, et al (1972 and 1977), Cameron, et al (1975), and Miki, et al (1972). Aarseth (1953) found that one fourth of his Oslo diabetics had persistent proteinuria. At autopsy "distinct glomerulosclerosis" was observed in 14% of all cases. Lundbaeck (1953) studied nephropathy in a whole population of diabetics. While this series was modest in size, it was unusually informative because the sample was to a high degree representative of all long-duration diabetics in a community (Aarhus, Denmark), and because the observations were very detailed. Data were gathered concerning both living and dead diabetics. About one quarter of living patients, who had had known diabetes from fifteen to twenty-five years, had albuminuria. But among patients who had died, kidney disease had been found before death in about half of the patients.

Techniques of electron microscopy developed subsequently have greatly increased the sensitivity of ascertainment on autopsy or biopsy specimens. In a large series of juvenile-onset diabetics studied by White (1956), about two thirds of those who had survived more than thirty years had proteinuria. It is clear, however, from these data and those of Oakley that even after forty years of diabetes a significant portion of diabetics are free of proteinuria. Why? This unusual immunity to renal pathology is relative and not absolute. Ruth Osterby (1972) has pointed out that with modern electron microscopic techniques some degree of pathologic abnormality is almost invariable with long-duration diabetes. Further studies on the natural history of diabetic nephropathy in Joslin Clinic patients have been reported recently by Kussman, et al (1976).

GEOGRAPHIC AND RACIAL DIFFERENCES

Highly variable rates of prevalence of kidney disease have been reported in groups of diabetics from the same and from different countries. This is not surprising in view of the profound effect of duration of diabetes and the lack of standardization of criteria and methods. When especially sensitive criteria and methods (eg, renal biopsy) are used, a substantial majority are sometimes found to have kidney lesions, while rates of diagnosed kidney disease in other circumstances are frequently less than 15%. It seems quite likely that the differences observed in prevalence are more apparent than real, but the possibility of modest differences among populations cannot now be excluded.

In Algeria, Lebon, et al (1953) observed that kidney disease was rare in natives with diabetes, but few details were given on duration of diabetes or methods of ascertainment of kidney disease. In 1958 Shaper reported that glomerulosclerosis had not yet been observed in African diabetics of Uganda. But only a few of these patients had had long-duration diabetes.

Hathorn, et al (1961) and Campbell (1963) reported that in Natal, South Africa, kidney disease seemed to be considerably more common in Indian diabetics than in African diabetics. They could not account for this difference on the basis of duration of known diabetes or blood glucose levels. Several subsequent reports on Indians of India, South Africa, and elsewhere do not, however, suggest an especially high rate of nephropathy. When duration of diabetes is taken into account nephropathy was not rare in other diabetic Africans residing in Africa (Seftel and Schultz, 1961; Haddock, 1964; Greenwood and Taylor, 1968; Jackson, et al, 1970). Rates of glomerulosclerosis have also been highly variable in groups of diabetics in various communities of India (Ahuja and Tandon, 1966). In Ceylon, Ramachandrum, et al (1973) found glomerulosclerosis was common. They thought nodular lesions were less common than in diabetics of the West. It seems possible that these variations and those in Africa are mainly or entirely the result of differences in duration of diabetes and methods of ascertainment, but more detailed investigation is warranted.

EPIDEMIOLOGIC STUDIES

Only a few epidemiologic studies in whole populations have been centered on diabetic nephropathy. The pioneering observations of Lundbaeck (1953) have been described above. Ahlmen (1975) studied chronic renal insufficiency in Gothenburg, Sweden, during a six-year period. Diabetic glomerulosclerosis was the third leading cause of renal failure in persons 16 to 65 years of age. Pyelonephritis was about twice as common, but glomerulonephritis was only slightly more frequent than glomerulosclerosis. Glomerulosclerosis accounted for about one sixth of all severe renal insufficiency. The annual incidence of azotemia from glomerulosclerosis in this age group was estimated to be about 22 cases per million population. The annual incidence of fatal uremia from glomerulosclerosis was estimated at 20 per million in this age group. Among 38 cases with glomerulosclerosis and terminal uremia, death was caused by another complicating illness in 12. In seven, the primary cause of death was judged to be heart disease and in two, stroke. In 24 patients with glomerulosclerosis, progress was followed from onset of azotemia. Only three survived more than a year. Watkins, et al (1972) observed coronary disease very commonly in patients with severe glomerulosclerosis.

Ueda, et al (1976) studied prospectively a cohort of an entire community in Japan (Hisayama). Of 1,621 subjects over 40 years of age, 330 died in a ten-year period and autopsies were performed on 270 (81% !). Initially, 131 of the 1,621 (8%) were known or found to be diabetic. Of these 131, 41 died during the study period of ten years. Autopsies were performed in 33. Diabetic glomerulosclerosis was found in 3.7% of all autopsies (known diabetics and others) and in 29% of diabetics. None of these patients died of glomerulosclerosis, and the lesions were, for the most part, minimal or moderate. No relationship was demonstrated between degree of hyperglycemia and presence or severity of glomerular lesions in this series, but the number with marked hyperglycemia was extremely small. Only four patients had fasting blood glucose levels over 130 mg/100 ml. All of these had glomerular lesions. Of 14 with two-hour or fasting levels greater than 200 mg/100 ml, two had no glomerular lesions, five had equivocal lesions, and seven had more definite pathologic changes. It is quite possible that an appreciable portion of these "diabetics" were elderly subjects whose glucose tolerance was not really abnormal after taking their age into account. The rarity of severe lesions was noteworthy in this group with very mild hyperglycemia.

Nilsson, et al (1967) studied glomerulosclerosis in a much larger population. Almost all diabetics of Kristianstad, Sweden, in the age group of 20 to 79 years were studied. The observations included 598 diabetics and a control group. All these diabetics had unequivocal fasting hyperglycemia. Slight proteinuria (0.1 to 0.3 gm/liter) was found in 10% of diabetics and 2.4% of controls. Proteinuria of 0.4 gm/liter or more was observed in only 0.4% of controls and in only 0.6% of short-duration diabetics (less than four years), while 6.2% of long-duration diabetics (more than six years) had this degree of proteinuria. In the diabetics the correlation coefficient between presence of proteinuria of any degree and presence of retinopathy was 0.40 in males and 0.24 in females. The correlations between presence of proteinuria and indexes of other complications of diabetes were quite weak (r values were -0.1 for foot pulsations, 0.1 for calcification of leg vessels, 0.1 for Achilles reflex, and 0.04 for cataract).

One of the early studies of nephropathy was that of Bjerkelund (1951) in 1,335 Oslo diabetics. Proteinuria was found in 22% but in about half of these the proteinuria was thought to be unrelated to diabetes. The frequency of diabetic renal disease was judged to be 32% in those with diabetes of more than fifteen years duration. Retinopathy was present in 7% of those without diabetic nephropathy and in 80% of those with diabetic nephropathy. Risk of nephropathy seemed unrelated to serum cholesterol or weight. Hypertension was common only in the late phase of nephropathy. Lundbaeck (1953) whose results are described elsewhere in this section, also found no evidence that risk of nephropathy was related to levels of serum cholesterol. Cholesterol levels were elevated late in the course of nephropathy but not before.

One of the most informative of the epidemiologic studies was that of Kamentzky, et al (1973) in a whole population of Pima Indians. This group included 1,716 subjects over 14 years of age of whom 404 were diabetic. Severe proteinuria was 15 times more common in the diabetics than in the nondiabetics. These data are unusual in that status of glucose tolerance was known in all subjects. Autopsies were performed in 62 diabetics of whom 65% had diffuse glomerulosclerosis. Nodular sclerosis was not observed in nondiabetics but was present in 59% of diabetics. In this population in which rates of diabetes are quite high, glomerulosclerosis is the most common cause of kidney disease. It is of interest that diabetes is uncommon in some tribes of American Indians living in more primitive conditions who are related to more affluent groups in whom diabetes is rife (West, 1974). Glomerulosclerosis has not been described in any of these euglycemic Indians who have been protected from hyperglycemia by their primitive way of life. This evidence fits poorly the notion that glomerulosclerosis is a genetically-induced lesion independent of hyperglycemia.

In the Pimas proteinuria was strongly related to duration of diabetes. In patients which characteristic glomerular lesions at autopsy, 80% had had proteinuria. In those in whom diabetes had been discovered recently, proteinuria was decidedly more common in older persons. Even these excellent data are not decisive in establishing the degree to which age and level of glycemia influence susceptibility to glomerulosclerosis. However, further prospective studies with larger numbers over a longer period in this and other populations have potentialities in this respect.

Pell and D'Alonzo (1967) studied the occurrence of proteinuria over time in 660 diabetics and 660 controls in a large population of employees. Of the controls 4.8% had proteinuria on one or more occasions while 14.8% of diabetics had proteinuria at least once. They also studied the frequency of persistent proteinuria (three or more tests positive) in subjects with various characteristics. In patients with hypertension, proteinuria was present in 7% while only 2.3% of those with normal blood pressure had proteinuria. In diabetics who did not take insulin proteinuria was present in 2.0%. In those who took less than 50 units daily the rate was 6.7% and in those on dosages of 50 units or more the rate of persistent proteinuria was 12.5%. The rate of persistent proteinuria was also related negatively to age of onset and positively to frequency of glycosuria during the course of repeated health examinations over a ten-year period. All of the differences cited in this paragraph were statistically significant, but none of these data were adjusted for duration of diabetes. These results are of particular interest because of the large number of diabetics, the parallel observations in controls with similar characteristics, and the relatively long period (ten years) over which observations were made.

ANIMAL AND CLINICAL RESEARCH

The section on retinopathy lists (page 405) a large number of factors that are of possible etiologic importance in retinopathy. Almost all of these have also been considered in glomerulosclerosis, but only a few have been measured in epidemiologic studies of glomerulosclerosis. The etiologic factor of greatest current interest is degree of glycemia. Several clinical studies and the epidemiology study of Pell and D'Alonzo (1970) have suggested that mitigation of hyperglycemia in the early stages of diabetes may reduce risk of glomerulosclerosis. But many other studies have been inconclusive or negative in this respect. This positive and negative evidence has been reviewed by Balodimos (1971), Knowles (1971), and by Cameron, et al (1975). The methods used in previous clinical studies have been roundly criticized by Kaplan and Feinstein (1973).

In Bedford, England, Jarrett, et al (1969) studied the occurrence of protein-uria in three matched groups. One was made up of those recently discovered to be diabetic, another had clearly normal glucose tolerance, and the third group had "borderline" glucose tolerance (two-hour capillary glucose values between 120 and 199 mg/100 ml after 50 gm of oral glucose). Using an especially sensitive method for the ascertainment of very small amounts of albumin, they found that slight albuminuria was more common in those with "borderline" status of glycemia than in those with good glucose tolerance. They suggested that there might be a causal association between slight elevations of blood glucose and the proteinuria. Recent work of Parving, et al (1976) also suggests that hyperglycemia may produce a functional leakage from capillaries.

Takazakura, et al (1975) found a relationship between rate of progression of glomerulosclerosis and degree of hyperglycemia when serial biopsies were performed. These results were impressive but the numbers of cases and obser-vations were too small to be entirely decisive.

Glomerulosclerosis is common in "secondary" diabetics (eg, pancreatitis, hemachromatosis), provided that duration of diabetes is sufficiently long (Balo-dimos, 1971; Verdonk, et al, 1975).

Recent work in animals is very encouraging. Glomerulosclerosis has been observed by Gibbs, et al (1966) in monkeys made diabetic by administration of alloxan. Other reports of glomerulosclerosis in artificially-induced diabetes in animals have been summarized by Cameron, et al (1975) and Vaisrub (1976). Regression of the glomerular lesions has been observed by Mauer, et al (1975) and by Koesters, et al (1977) in diabetic rats after correction of hyperglycemia by transplantation of beta cells. Skepticism about the importance of degree of glycemia arose for several reasons. One was that glomerulosclerosis has been observed a few times in patients with no apparent hyperglycemia. These cases have been well reviewed by Harrington, et al (1973). Because remission of diabetes occurs occasionally and because improvement of the diabetic state frequently follows renal decompensation (Hatch, et al, 1961), it is quite possi-ble that these persons had mild hyperglycemia for months or years at some time prior to the discovery of glomerulosclerosis. Even with severe diabetes in patients with a family history of diabetes, glomerulosclerosis is quite rare in the first months of diabetes (Osterby, 1972). When transplanted kidneys from nondiabetic donors are implanted in diabetics, they tend to develop glomeru-losclerosis (Najarian, et al 1976).

Berkman and Rifkin (1973) have described a case of unilateral glomerulos-clerosis. The blood supply of the kidney without glomerulosclerosis had been reduced by an arteriosclerotic occlusion of the main renal artery.

FUTURE STUDIES

Thus, there is strong evidence that hyperglycemia itself produces glomeru-losclerosis and that its mitigation reduces the rate at which glomerulosclerosis develops. But more evidence is needed on the extent to which degree of glycemia is critical. Even assuming that duration and degree of glycemia are very important, it is quite clear that still other factors are at work. These require study using several approaches.

The considerations cited above indicate that epidemiologic studies will require rather large numbers of well-collected data in order to elucidate these matters further. For example, numbers must be large enough to permit a determination of whether the associations between various possible risk factors and glomerulosclerosis are independent of duration of diabetes, and whether associations are hidden by failure to correct for duration or degree of hyperglycemia. Among the factors that deserve further study are age, age of onset, diet, blood pressure, capillary permeability, serum glycoproteins, and genetic factors.

NEUROPATHY

Introduction

In 1953 Lundbaeck described the status of observations on diabetic neuropathy as "bewildering". Seventeen years later little progress was evident with respect to clinical and epidemiologic data. Bruyn and Garland (1970) described the subject as one of "total confusion". Few well-collected data are available. Methods are still poorly standardized, control observations rare (Danowski, et al, 1966). Considerable progress has, however, been made through approaches other than epidemiologic study. Good reviews have been published by Locke (1971), Ellenberg (1976), and by Thomas and Ward (1975).

It is now clear that detectable neuropathic changes are present in most diabetics. Frequently, these are trivial in their effects, but disabling neuropathic lesions are also common. These include pain, weakness, paralysis, diarrhea, bladder dysfunction, and in males, sexual impotence. Bruyn and Garland (1970) have observed that in clinical reports the prevalence of neuropathy in groups of diabetics has ranged from zero to 93%! For the most part these differences seem to be more apparent than real. On the other hand, the available evidence does not preclude the possibility that factors other than glycemia may influence susceptibility to neuropathy. Many types of functional and histologic lesions occur. One challenge in this field is ignorance concerning whether these various neurologic manifestations have a common cause or difference causes.

The most important issue is the extent to which degree of hyperglycemia determines risk and extent of the various types of neuropathy. It has now been well established that some of the aberrations of neurologic function (eg, motor conduction velocity) can be improved by mitigation of hyperglycemia (Christensen, 1973; Thomas and Ward, 1975). It is also clear that many typical pathological changes can be produced by artificially inducing diabetes (eg, with streptozotocin in animals). On the other hand, the association between degree of hyperglycemia and neuropathy is decidedly imperfect. Severe neuropathy is often seen in patients with mild hyperglycemia of short duration (Ellenberg, 1963; Chochinov, et al, 1972), and persons with severe hypergly-cemia of long duration sometimes have little neuropathy. Studies of Pirart (1965) did, however, show an impressive general association between neuropa-thy and degree of hyperglycemia. A major problem here has been that large numbers of subjects needed to correct for the profound effects of age on certain indexes of neuropathy. In the observations of Nilsson, et al (1967), for example, absence of the Achilles reflex was not observed in nondiabetics under 60 years of age, but 25% of older nondiabetic subjects had no Achilles reflex.

Among the least sensitive indicators of neuropathy are data on paralysis and severe pain. These are not rare but are much less frequent than the more subtle evidences of neuropathy. With sophisticated multifaceted testing, some degree of dysfunction can be demonstrated in almost all diabetics. These methods include measurement of motor conduction velocity and electromyography. The prevalence of neuropathy is also increased by increasing the scope and intensity of the medical history and of standard clinical procedures for examin-ing the neurologic system. For example, sexual impotence resulting from neuropathy is very frequent in diabetic men, as are mild degrees of bladder dysfunction. Medical records of persons with these disorders frequently fail to mention the presence of these problems. In a group with recent onset of diabetes, Christensen (1973) found that neurologic impairments were demon-strable frequently, but at this stage no autonomic dysfunctions were evident. In diabetics, Abbasi, et al (1977) found impairment of taste (for salt, sugar, urea, and acid). The degree of this impairment seemed to be related to duration of diabetes and to the extent of neuropathy as determined by other tests.

Little is known about the degree of interobserver difference in results with commonly employed tests of neurologic function such as tendon reflexes and evaluations of sensory function. Nor is much known about the degree of correlation between deficits in these more easily measurable dysfunctions and the risk of gross disability (eg, pain, weakness, sexual impotence, gangrene). There is urgent need for some standard methods, criteria, conventions, and definitions.

Epidemiologic Studies

Only a few investigations have been performed in whole populations or representative samples thereof.

Nilsson, et al (1967) studied vibratory sensation and Achilles reflexes in 598 diabetics of Kristianstad, Sweden, and compared these observations to those in a control group. Achilles reflexes were absent in 8.5% of the controls, 10.5% of the diabetics of short duration, and 15.2% of the diabetics of long duration. As indicated above, response was strongly related to age, indicating a need to take this factor into account in any such studies. Vibratory sense was absent at the ankle malleoli in 2.9% of controls, 7.6% of short-duration diabetics, and 11.7% of long-duration diabetics. These investigators also presented data, by age and duration of diabetes, on prevalence of partial impairment of these neurologic functions. Under these conditions, neurologic function was not significantly related in diabetics to blood glucose level, but this association may have been hidden by the negative association between age and blood glucose level. There was no correlation between these impairments and family history of diabetes.

The association between Achilles jerk and vibratory sense was of only modest strength. The correlation coefficient was .36. There was an association of moderate degree between these neurologic impairments and indexes of leg-vessel disease, but this appeared to be mainly the result of the association of both with age. The relationship of retinopathy to the neurologic impairments was weak. It was not possible to determine from these data whether this latter relationship would have been significantly strengthened or weakened by correction for other factors such as age and blood pressure.

The University Group (1970a) has described some standardized methods by which neurologic status may be evaluated. One of these was a measurement of vibratory sensation using the "biothesiometer". This instrument was also used by Bennett (1973a) in evaluating vibratory sensation in Pima Indians. Bennett and his associates tested vibratory sensation in the toes of 703 subjects, and in the fingers of 816 subjects. Data were analyzed in four subgroups. These were subjects with known diabetes, with newly-discovered diabetes, with clearly normal glucose tolerance, and with borderline tolerance (two-hour plasma glucose values between 140 and 199 mg/100 ml). Vibratory sensation in the toes was the same in all groups except the overt diabetics in whom sensation was significantly less. In the fingers vibratory sensation was somewhat diminished in those with newly-diagnosed diabetes in the age group of 35 to 54 years. There was considerable overlap of acuity of vibratory sensation in normals and diabetics. Multiple regression analysis on vibration in the toes showed that only 35% of variation was predictable on the basis of known or suspected variables such as age, duration of diabetes, degree of glycemia. Age accounted for 30% of the fraction that was predictable, and blood glucose level accounted for only 12% of this predictable fraction. In the fingers only 12% of variability was accounted for by all these factors; almost all of this 12% was related to age. Keen (1973) and his group also used this method to test neurologic function. In the group of older women with newly-discovered diabetes, vibration sensation was less than in those with clearly normal tolerance. No deficits were identified in any other subgroups with newly-discovered diabetes or borderline glucose tolerance.

Some of the studies in large diabetic clinics were performed under circumstances that suggest that results were crudely representative of those that might be expected in the general population of diabetics. But it should be kept in mind that bias of referral or self-referral to specialty clinics in diabetes or neurology may considerably affect the experiences in such clinics. Some of these clinical studies have been reviewed by Bruyn and Garland (1970) and by Thomas and Ward (1975). Of these clinical studies those of Fagerberg (1959) and Pirart (1965) were among the more informative.

There is a need to examine independently the various types of neuropathy. The factors that cause or protect against impairment of sensory function may not be the same as those relevant to motor function or to the autonomic system. Certain features of palsies of ocular muscles suggest a pathogenesis different than that in other diabetes-related neurologic disease. Microvascular disease may contribute in certain types of neuropathy. But there is little epidemiologic data that can be applied in answering these questions.

Because neuropathy is sometimes present before the discovery of diabetes and imperfectly related to degree of hyperglycemia, the possibility has been considered that genetic factors might operate directly in producing neuropathy by mechanisms independent of hyperglycemia. Evidence against this is not entirely conclusive but rather strong. It includes the demonstration that neuropathy occurs commonly in "secondary" diabetes and in animals made hyperglycemic by destroying beta-cell function.

Differences among populations in apparent rates of neuropathy have been reported. But for reasons set forth above it is not possible to discern whether racial or environmental differences have any effects independent of degree and duration of hyperglycemia. Neurologic manifestations have been common in all groups of diabetics in whom intensive searches have been made. Osuntokun, et al (1971) found neuropathy very common in Nigeria. Chuttani and Chawala (1974) have reported on neuropathy in India. If they could be properly standardized, interpopulation studies might provide some useful clues and insights concerning the influence of factors such as degree of hyperglycemia, diet, race, genetics, microvascular diseases, type of diabetes.

OTHER MANIFESTATIONS

In this book only the most important of the morbid effects of diabetes are reviewed. There are, however, several other manifestations that deserve further epidemiologic study. These include cataract, certain diabetes-related infections (eg, tuberculosis), and ketoacidosis.

In some societies diabetic coma is a more important manifestation than macrovascular disease. Because it is a complex metabolic disorder the primary causes of which are well understood, ketoacidosis has rarely been the subject of epidemiologic study. Yet its cost has not been well measured. To a very high degree, ketoacidosis is a preventable disorder for which several interrelated factors are responsible, including social, economic, administrative, and medical determinants. It seems likely that systematic epidemiologic study would be helpful in developing a more effective program of preventive measures. Ganda and Marble (1976) recently reviewed some epidemiologic aspects of ketoacidosis.

Some of the effects of maternal diabetes on the fetus have been discussed in Chapters 7 and 9. Other aspects deserve further study. These problems have been reviewed by O'Sullivan, et al (1976), Pedersen (1977), and Pehrson (1974).

Gabbe (1977) has published a good review on congenital malformations in infants of diabetic mothers. This problem has also been studied by Goodman (1976). It is generally believed that periodontal disease is excessive in diabetics, but present evidence is not conclusive in this respect (Pennel and Keagle, 1977). Better data are needed.

Bibliography

Aarseth S: Cardiovascular-renal disease in diabetes mellitus: A clinical study. *Acta Med Scand* 281:218–244, 1953.

Abbasi A, King D, Dykes M, et al: Hypogeusia in diabetes mellitus. *Diabetes* 26(suppl 1):385, 1977.

Abernethy MH, Andre C, Beaven DW, et al: A random blood sugar diabetes detection survey. *N Zea Med J* 86:123–126, 1977.

Abou-Daoud KT: Diabetes mellitus in a Lebanese population group. *Am J Epidemiol* 89:644–650, 1969.

Abramovich DR: Glucose tolerance tests in pregnancy. *J Obstet Gynaecol Br Commonw* 73:105–112, 1966.

Abrams NE: Oral glucose tolerance and related factors in a normal population sample: II. Interrelationship of glycerides, cholesterol, and other factors with the glucose and insulin response. *Br Med J* 1:599–602, 1969.

Abu-Zeid HA, Choi NW, Maini KK, Nelson NA: Relative role of factors associated with cerebral infarction and cerebral hemorrhage. *Stroke* 8(No. 11):106–112, 1977.

Ackerman RF, Williams EF Jr, Packer J, et al: Comparison of Benedict's solution, Clinitest, TesTape, and Clinistix. *Diabetes* 7:398–402, 1958.

Adams SF: Seasonal variation in the onset of acute diabetes: Age and sex factors in 1,000 diabetic patients. *Arch Intern Med* 37:861–864, 1926.

Adams SF: Obesity as a precursor of diabetes. *J Nutr* 1:339–342, 1929

Adelstein AM: National statistics. *Postgrad Med J* 51(suppl 2):57–67, 1975.

Author's Note: With few exceptions the publications listed here are cited in the text. A few recent publications are cited in the text but not listed here.

Adi FC: Diabetes mellitus associated with epidemic of infectious hepatitis in Nigeria. *Br Med J* 1:183–185, 1974.

Adler R, Freedman J, Kukar N: Various parameters of diabetic retinopathy among clinic populations. *Ann Ophthalmol* 7:1447–1454, 1975.

Agar JMB: Silent myocardial infarction in diabetes mellitus. *Med J Aust* 3:284, 1962.

Ahlmen J: Incidence of chronic renal insufficiency. *Acta Med Scand* 582:1–50, 1975.

Ahlvin RC: Biochemical screening—a critique. *N Engl J Med* 283:1084–1086, 1970.

Ahmed SS, Jaferi GA, Narang RM, Regan TJ: Preclinical abnormality of left ventricular function in diabetes mellitus. *Am Heart J* 39(No. 2):153–158, 1975.

Ahrens RA, Welsh SS, Adams YL, et al: Effect of source of carbohydrate as influenced by dietary fat: carbohydrate ratio and forced exercise in rats. *J Nutr* 95:303–310, 1968.

Ahuja MMS: Vicissitudes of epidemiological studies of diabetes mellitus. *J All India Inst Med Sci* 2:5–13, 1976.

Ahuja MMS, Chhetri MK, Gupta OP, Mutallik GS, et al: National collaborative study on epidemiology of diabetes in India, in Bajaj JS (ed): *Current Topics in Diabetes Research*, Proceedings of 9th Congress of the International Diabetes Federation, India. Amsterdam, Excerpta Medica, Series 400, 1976, p. 183.

Ahuja MMS, Talwar GP, Varma VM, et al: Diabetes mellitus in young Indians. *Indian J Med Res* 53:1138–1147, 1965.

Ahuja MMS, Tandor HD: Diabetic vascular disease in North Indian diabetics. *Indian J Med Sci* 20:172–180. 1966.

Ahuja MMS, Varma VM, Shankar U: A Pilot study to determine the prevalence of diabetes mellitus in Delhi. *J Indian Med Assoc* 46:415–418, 1966.

Ahuja MMS, Viswanadham K: Differential mobilization of non-esterified fatty acids and insulin reserve in various clinical types of diabetes mellitus in India. *Indian J Med Res* 55:870, 1967.

Aikawa T: World War and diabetes mellitus. *Nippon Jishinpo* 1295:321, 1949.

Ajgaonker SS: References in Indian literature on diabetes mellitus, in Patel JC, Talwalker NG (eds): *Diabetes in the Tropics* Bombay, Diab Assoc of India, 1966, p 641–661.

Ajgaonkar SS: The problem of treatment of diabetes in the tropics (with special reference to developing countries, in Rodriguez RR, Vallance-Owen J (eds): *Diabetes*. Proc 7th Congr of Int Diab Fed, Buenos Aires, Series 209, 1970 p. 833–842. 1972.

Akanuma Y, Miki E, Hayashi M, et al: Importance of weight control for prevention of retinopathy, in Bajaj JS (ed): *Current Topics in Diabetes Research*, Proc 9th Congr of Int Diab Fed, India, Series 400, 1976, p. 121.

Aksoy M: Carbohydrate metabolism in severe and longstanding iron-deficiency anemia due to dietary and zinc deficiencies. *Am J Clin Nutr* 25:262–264, 1972.

Alapat JL, Anathachari MD: A preliminary study of the structure and function of enlarged parotid glands in chronic relapsing pancreatitis by sialography and biopsy methods. *Gut* 8:42, 1967.

Alavaikko M, Elfving R, Hirvonen J, Jarvi J: Triglycerides, cholesterol and phospholipids in normal heart papillary muscle and in patients suffering from diabetes, cholelithiasis, hypertension and coronary atheroma. *J Clin Pathol* 26:285–293, 1973.

Albanese AA, Lorenze EJ, Orto LA: Effect of strokes on carbohydrate tolerance. *Geriatrics* 23:142–150, 1968.

Alberti KG, Caird FL: The accuracy of Dextrostix in the estimation of blood sugar. *Lancet* 2:319–321, 1965.

Alberti KG, Hockaday TD: Biochemistry of the complications of diabetes mellitus, in Keen H, Jarrett RJ (eds): *Complications of Diabetes.* London, Edward Arnold Publishing Co, 1975, p. 221–264.

Albertsson V: Diabetes in Iceland. *Diabetes* 2:184–186, 1952.

Albrink MJ: Triglyceridemia. *J Am Dietetic Assoc* 62:626–630, 1973.

Albrink MJ: Diabetes as a risk factor for arteriosclerotic vascular disease. *Adv Exp Med Biol* 63:279–285, 1975.

Albrink MJ, Davidson PC: Imparied glucose tolerance in patients with hypertriglyceridemia. *J Lab Clin Med* 67:573, 1966.

Albrink MJ, Lavietes PH, Man AB: Vascular disease and serum lipids in diabetes mellitus: Observation of 30 years (1931–1961). *Ann Intern Med* 58:305, 1963.

Albrink MJ, Meigs JW: Interrelationships between skinfold thickness, serum lipids and blood sugar in normal men. *Am J Clin Nutr* 15:255–261, 1964.

Alex M, Baron EK, Goldenberg S, Blumenthal HT: An autopsy study of cerebrovascular accident in diabetes mellitus. *Circulation* 35:663–673, 1962.

Alezzandrini AA: Fluorescein angiography in diabetic retinopathy. *Acta Diabetol Lat* 10:1325, 1973.

Alford FP, Kiss ZS, Martin FIR, et al: "Type J" diabetes in New Guinea: Studies of insulin release and insulin sensitivity. *Aust Ann Med* 2:111–117, 1970.

Alford FP, Martin FIR, Pearson MJ: The significance and interpretation of mildly abnormal oral glucose tolerance. *Diabetologia* 7:173–180, 1971.

Allan FN, Georgeson LW: A candy tolerance test in the detection of early diabetes. *Med Clin North Am* 44:429–432, 1960.

Allen E: The glucosuria of pregnancy. *Am J Obstet Gynecol* 38:982, 1939.

Allen FM: *Glycosuria and Diabetes.* Cambridge, Harvard University Press, 1913.

Allen FM: Experimental studies in diabetes, Series IV Lipemia: II. The production of diabetic lipemia in animals and observations in some possible etiologic factors. *J Metabol Res* 2:219–298, 1922.

Allen FM: The dietetic management of diabetes. *Am J Med Sci* 167:554–570, 1924.

Allen FM: Current judgments on metabolic control and complications in diabetes. *N Engl J Med* 248:133–136, 1953.

Allen FM, Stillman E, Fitz R: Total dietary regulation in the treatment of diabetes, monograph No. 11, Rockefeller Institute for Medical Research, 1919.

Allen OP: Symptoms suggesting prodromal stage of diabetes mellitus. *Ohio Med J* 49:213–215, 1953.

Allen RJ, Brook M, Lister RE, et al: Metabolic differences between dietary liquid glucose and sucrose. *Nature* 211:1104, 1966.

443

Allison RS: Carbohydrate tolerance in overweight and obesity. *Lancet* 1:537–540, 1927.

Almer L- O: Effect of obesity on endogenous fibrinolytic activity in diabetes mellitus. *J Med* 6:351–367, 1975.

Almer L- O, Nilsson IM: On fibrinolysis in diabetes mellitus. *Acta Med Scand* 198:101–106, 1975.

Alpert S: Imparied glucose tolerance, a consequence of excessive carbohydrate consumption. *Ann Intern Med* 42:927–931, 1955.

Altman DF, Baker SD, McCally M, et al: Carbohydrate and lipid metabolism in man during prolonged bed rest. *Clin Res* 17:543, 1969.

Altschul A, Nathan A: Diabetes mellitus in Harlem Hospital outpatient department in New York. A comparison of certain etiologic factors in negro and white patients. *JAMA* 119:248–252, 1942.

Altshuler CW: Diabetes mortality: A statistical analysis. *J Am Statistics Assoc* 35:341–345, 1940.

Alvavaikko M, Elfving R, Hirvonen J, Jarvi J: Triglycerides, cholesterol. and phospholipids in normal heart papillary muscle and in patients suffering from diabetes, cholelithiasis, hypertension, and coronary atheroma. *J Clin Pathol* 26:285–293, 1973.

Amatuzio DS, Rames ED, Nesbitt S: Practical application of the rapid intravenous glucose tolerance test. *J Lab Clin Med* 48:714, 1956.

Amatuzio DS, Stutzman FL, Vanderbilt MJ, Nesbitt S: Interpretation of the rapid intravenous glucose tolerance test in normal individuals and in mild diabetes mellitus. *J Clin Invest* 32:428, 1953.

American Diabetes Association, special rep of Committee on Professional Education (Hanwi GJ, Fajans SA, Cahill GF, et al). Classification of genetic diabetes mellitus. *Diabetes* 16:540, 1967.

Amer Diab Assoc, report of Committee on Statistics (Klimt CR, et al): Standardization of the oral glucose tolerance test. *Diabetes* 18:299–310, 1969.

American Diabetes Association (Meinert CL, et al): Standardization of the oral glucose tolerance test. December 1972.

American Diabetes Association, The Endocrine Society, and American Medical Association. Statement on hypoglycemia. *JAMA* 223:682, 1973.

American Diabetes Association: Detection and diagnosis of diabetes: Plasma glucose procedures (brochure). Detection and Education Program. New York, 1974.

American Diabetes Association, policy statement (Cahill GF, Etzwiler DD, Freinkel N): Blood glucose control in diabetes. *Diabetes* 25 (organizational section), 1976.

American Heart Association Committee on Reduction of Risk of Heart Attack and Stroke, *Coronary Risk Handbook*, 1973.

Amos JF: The epidemiology of diabetes mellitus and blindness due to diabetes. *Am J Optom Physiol Opt* 51:676–679, 1974.

Anders JM, Jameson HL: Adiposity and other etiologic factors in diabetes mellitus. *Am J Med Sci* 170:313–324, 1925.

Andersen J, Lauritzen E: Blood groups and diabetes mellitus. *Diabetes* 9:20–24, 1960.

Anderson JW, Herman RH: Effect of fasting, caloric restrictions and refeeding on glucose intolerance of normal men. *Am J Clin Nutr* 25:41–52, 1972.

Anderson JW, Herman RH: Effects of carbohydrate restriction on glucose tolerance of normal men and reactive hypoglycemic patients. *Am J Clin Nutr* 28:748–755, 1975.

Anderson NV, Strafuss AC: Pancreatic disease in dogs and cats. *J Am Vet Med Assoc* 159:885–891, 1971.

Anderson O, Vejtorp L, Christy M, Platz R, et al: HL-A factors in insulin dependent diabetes mellitus. Clinical significance. *Diabetologia* 11:329, 1975.

Anderson RS, Ellington A, Gunter LN: The incidence of arteriosclerotic heart disease in Negro diabetic patients. *Diabetes* 10:114, 1961.

Anderson TW: The duration of unrecognized diabetes mellitus. *Diabetes* 15:160–163, 1966.

Andres R: Diabetes and aging. *Hospital Practice,* October 1967, p 63–67.

Andres R: Aging and diabetes. *Med Clin North Amer* 55:835–846, 1971.

Andres R: Effect of age in interpretation of glucose and tolbutamide tolerance tests, in Fajans SS, Sussman KE (eds): *Diabetes Mellitus: Diagnosis and Treatment,* vol 3. New York, American Diabetes Association, 1971a, p 115–119.

Andres R: *Aging and Glucose Tolerance.* vol 3, part I. Report of National Commission on Diabetes to the Congress of the US. US National institutes of Health and Dept of HEW Publ (NIH) 76-1021, 1976, p 105–111.

Andres R, Tobin J: Aging, carbohydrate metabolism and diabetes. 9th Int. Congress of Gerontology, Kiev, 1972, p 276–280.

Andrews CT: A survey of diabetes in West Cornwall. *Br Med J* 1:427–433, 1957.

Armstrong B, Doll R: Bladder cancer mortality in diabetics in relation to saccharin consumption and smoking habits. *Br J Prev Soc Med* 29:73–81, 1975.

Armstrong B, Lea AJ, Adelstein AM, et al: Cancer mortality and saccharin consumption in diabetes. *Br J Prev Soc Med* 30:151–157, 1976.

Armstrong ML: Regression of atherosclerosis, in Paoletti R, Gotto AM Jr: *Atherosclerosis Review,* vol 1. New York, Raven Press, 1976, p 137–182.

Arney GK, Pearson E, Sutherland AB: Burn stress pseudo-diabetes, *Ann Surg* 152:77–99, 1960.

Aronoff SL, Bennett PH, Gorden P: Early phase insulin release to IV glucose in prediabetic and normal Pima Indians and normal caucasians. *Diabetes* 24:402, 1975.

Aronoff SL, Bennett PH, Gorden P, et al: Unexplained hyperinsulinemia in normal and "prediabetic" Pima Indians compared with normal caucasians. An example of racial differences in insulin secretion. *Diabetes* 26:827–840, 1977.

Aronoff SL, Bennett PH, Rushforth, NB, Miller M, Unger RH: Normal glucagon response to arginine infusion in "prediabetic" Pima Indian. *J Clin Endocrinol Metab* 43:279–286, 1976.

Aronson SM: Intracranial vascular lesions in patients with diabetes mellitus. *J Neuropathol Exp Neurol* 32:103–106, 1973.

Aschner B: Beziehungen der Fettsucht zu arteriolleon Hochdruck. Diabetes mellitus and cholelithiasis. *Z F Klin Med* 116:669–679, 1931.

Ashley DJB: Diabetes in Wales. *J Med Genet* 4:274–276, 1967.

Asmal AC, Leary WP: Carbohydrate tolerance, plasma insulin, growth hormone and lipid levels in Indian and black diabetics. *S Afr Med J* 49:810–812, 1975.

Aspevik E, Jorde R, Raeder S: The diabetes survey in Bergen, Norway 1956. *Acta Med Scand* 196:161–169, 1974.

Astwood EB, Glynn M, Krayer O: Effect of continuous intravenous infusion of glucose in normal dogs. *J Clin Invest* 21:621, 1942.

Auerbach E: Die Sterblichkeit der Juden in Budapest 1901–1905. *Z Demog Statist* 4:164–168, 1908.

Aurell E: Hjortzberg-Nordlund H, Tibblin G: Obesity in 50-year old men: somatic aspects. *Sven Tandlak Tidskr* 63:520–525, 1966.

Axelrod L: Response of congestive heart failure to correction of hyperglycemia in the presence of diabetic neuropathy. *N Engl J Med* 293:1243–1245, 1975.

Ayad H: The incidence of diabetes mellitus in Egypt (UAR), in Ostman J, Milner RDG (eds): *Diabetes.* Proc 6th Congr of Int Diab Fed, Stockholm, Series 140, 1967, p 25.

Aykroyd WR: Sweet malefactor: sugar, slavery and human society, in *Sugar in the Modern World.* London, Heinemann, 1967, p 102–129, chap 12.

Baba S: Diabetes mellitus from the ecological viewpoint. in Baba S, Goto Y, Fukui I (eds): *Diabetes Mellitus in Asia.* Proc. 2nd Symposium of Int Diab Fed, Kyoto. Series 390, 1975, p 3–11.

Baba S, Matsuoka A, Takaishi T, et al: Clinical significance of double-loading glucose tolerance test and immunoreactive insulin response in diabetics, in Tsuji S, Wada M (eds): *Diabetes Mellitus in Asia.* Proceedings of a Symposium in Kobe, Japan. May 1970, p. 120–129.

Bacque M: Quelques reflexions sur le diabete en Afrique. Comparison entre une consultation du diabete a Durban (Natal) et a Casablanca (Maroc). *J Med Bordeauz* 5:733–746, 1964.

Bagriacik N, Onen K, Ipbuker A, Erek E, et al: The results of diabetes detection in Turkey and comments on renal glycosurias, in Hoet, JJ, Lefebre, P, Butterfield, WJH, et al (eds): Proc 8th Congr of Int Diab Fed, Belgium, *Series 280,* 1973, p 159–160.

Bailey RR, Beavan DW: Diabetes mellitus and myocardial infarction. *Aust NZ J Med* 17:312, 1968.

Baird JD: Diet and development of clinical diabetes. *Acta Diabetol Lat* (suppl 1)9:621–637, 1972.

Baird JD: Diabetes mellitus and obesity. *Proc Nutr Soc* 32:199–204, 1973.

Bakani IR: Acute myocardial infarction in Suva, Fiji. *NZ Med J* 81:288–292, 1975.

Balazs N, Bradshaw R, Welborn T: Use of test strips with colour meter to measure blood-glucose. *Lancet* 1:1232, 1970.

Balcerzak SP, Peternal WW, Heinle EW: Iron absorption in chronic pancreatitis. *Gastroenterology* 53:257, 1967.

Balcerzak SP, Mintz DH, Westerman MP: Diabetes mellitus and idiopathic hemochromatosis. *Am J Med Sci* 255:53–62, 1968.

Bale GS, Entmacher PS: Estimated life expectancy of diabetics. *Diabetes* 26:434–438, 1977.

Bale JF Jr: John Harvey Kellogg MD and the American diet. *U Mich Med Center J* 41:56–58, 1975.

Balodimos MD: Diabetic nephropathy, in Marble A, White P, (eds): *Joslin's Diabetes Mellitus.* ed 11. Philadelphia, Lea & Febiger, 1971, p 526–561.

Bang I: *Der Blutzucker.* Wiesbaden, 1913.

Banting F: The history of insulin. *Edin Med J* 36:1–2, 1929.

Banwell JG, Campbell J, Blackman V, Hutt MV, Leonard P: Studies of intestinal function in Ugandan diabetic patients. *East Afr Med J* 40:277–287, 1963.

Banwell JG, Hutt MR, Leonard PJ, et al: Exocrine pancreatic disease and the malabsorption syndrome in tropical Africa. *Gut* 8:388, 1967.

Barbosa J: HLA and diabetes mellitus. *Lancet* 1:906–907, 1977.

Barbosa J: Chromium and diabetes. *Br Med J* 2:266, 1977a.

Barbosa J, King R, Noreen H, Yunis EJ: The histocompatibility system in juvenile, insulin-dependent diabetic multiplex kindreds. *J Clin Invest* 60:989–998, 1977.

Barbosa J, Noreen H, Goetz F, Simmons R, et al: Juvenile diabetes and viruses. *Lancet* 1:371, 1976.

Barndt R Jr, Blankenhorn DH, Crawford DW, Books SH: Regression and progression of early femoral atherosclerosis in treated hyperlipoproteinemic patients. *Ann Intern Med* 86:139–146, 1977.

Barner HB: Vasculitis in maturity-onset diabetes mellitus. *JAMA* 235:2495, 1976.

Barner HB, Kaiser GC, Codd JE, Willman VI: Coronary graft flow and glucose tolerance: Evidence against the existence of myocardial microvascular disease. *Vasc Surg* 9:220–227, 1975.

Barner HB, Kaiser GC, Willman VL: Blood flow in the diabetic leg. *Circulation* 43:391–394, 1971.

Barnes AJ, Bloom A, Crowley MF, et al: Is glucagon important in stable insulin-dependent diabetics? *Lancet* 2:734–737, 1975.

Barnes RJ: Sugar, heart disease and diabetes. *Lancet* 1:355–356, 1974.

Barringer TB Jr: The incidence of glycosuria and diabetes in New York City between 1902 and 1907. *Arch Intern Med* 3:295–298, 1909.

Barta L: Frequency of chemical diabetes in the parents of diabetic children. *Acta Paediatr Acad Sci Hung* 15:275–280, 1974.

Barta L, Kammerer L, Regoly-Merci A: Examination of heterogeneity in diabetics. *Diabetologia* 12:379, 1976.

Barta L, Simon S: Role of HLA B8 and Bw15 antigens in diabetic children. *N Engl J Med* 296:397, 1977.

Bassett DR, Moellering RD, Rosenblatt G, et al: Coronary heart disease in Hawaii, serum lipids and cardiovascular, anthropometric and related findings in Japanese and Hawaiian men. *J Chron Dis* 21:565–583, 1969.

Bassett DR, Rosenblatt G, Moellering RC, Hartwell AS: Cardiovascular disease, diabetes mellitus and anthropometric evaluation of Polynesian males on the Island of Niihau 1963. *Circulation* 34:1088–1097, 1966.

447

Bassett DR, Schroffner VB: Blood lipids and lipoproteins, glucose tolerance and plasma insulin response in Chinese men with and without coronary heart disease in Hawaii. *Isr J Med Sci* 5:666–670, 1969.

Bassett DR, Schroffner WG: Coronary heart disease in Chinese men in Hawaii. Serum lipids, plasma glucose and cardiovascular, anthropometric and related findings. Comparisons and findings with Japanese men. *Arch Intern Med* 125:476–487, 1970.

Bastenie PA, Conard V, Franckson JR: Effect of cortisone on carbohydrate metabolism measured by the "glucose assimilation coefficient". *Diabetes* 3:285, 1954.

Bastenie PA, Gepta J (eds): *Immunity and Autoimmunity in Diabetes Mellitus.* Proceedings of Francqui Fdn Colloq, Brussels. Amsterdam, Excerpta Medica, 1974.

Bauer ML: Characteristics of persons with diabetes. National Center for Health Statistics, Series 10, 1967, p 1–44.

Baumslag N, Yodaiken RE, Varady JC: Standardization of terminology in diabetes. Types and family histories. *Diabetes* 19:664–669, 1970.

Beardmore M, Reid JJA: Diabetic children. *Br Med J* 2:1383–1384, 1966.

Beardwood JT: Report of diabetes surveys in Philadelphia, in Proceedings of the New York Diabetes Association, February 1944. *Am J Dig Dis* 11:345–355, 1944.

Beaser SB: The clinical characteristics of early diabetes mellitus. *N Engl J Med* 239:765–769, 1948.

Beaumont P, Hollows FC: Classification of diabetic retinopathy with therapeutic implications. *Lancet* 1:419, 1972.

Beaven DW, Arcus AC, Bell JP, et al: Epidemiology of diabetes mellitus. *NZ Med J* 80:291–299, 1974.

Becker D, Rabin B, Villalpando S, Foley T, et al: Juvenile diabetes mellitus (JDM) as part of an autoimmune endocrinopathy, abstract. *Diabetes* 26(suppl 1):387, 1977.

Becker B, Shin DH, Burgess D, et al: Histocompatibility antigens and diabetic retinopathy. *Diabetes* 26:997–999, 1977.

Beck-Nielsen H: The diurnal variation in insulin receptors. Insulin receptors in glucose metabolism. *Diabetologia* 12:380, 1976.

Bednarzewski J, Kutarski A: Analysis of hospital mortality in patients with myocardial infarction and diabetes (in Polish with English summary at end). *Pol Tyg Lek* 31:279–281, 1976.

Beetham WP: Visual prognosis of proliferating diabetic retinopathy. *Br J Ophthalmol* 47:611, 1963.

Belcher DW: Diabetes mellitus in Northern Ethiopia. *Ethiop Med J* 8:73–84, 1970.

Bell ET: Incidence of gangrene of the extremities in nondiabetic and in diabetic persons. *Arch Pathol Lab Med* 49:469–473, 1950.

Bell ET: A postmortem study of vascular disease in diabetics. *Arch Pathol Lab Med* 53:444–455, 1952.

Bell ET: Renal vascular disease in diabetes mellitus. *Diabetes* 2:376–389, 1953.

Bell ET: *Diabetes Mellitus.* Springfield, Ill, Charles C Thomas, 1960.

Belsky JL, Tachikawa K, Jablon S: The health of atomic bomb survivors: A decade of examinations in a fixed population. *Yale J Biol Med* 46:294–296, 1973.

Benarroch IS, deSalama AR: Beeinflussung der Triglyzeridamie des Diabetikers: Wirkung einer kohlenhydratreichen Diät mit starkem Fruktose-Anteil. *Munch Med Wochenschr* 113:1197, 1971.

Benedict AL: Is the ingestion of sugar a cause of diabetes? *Dietet Hyg Gaz NY* 25:459–462, 1909.

Bengtsson C: A survey to trace previously unknown diabetes mellitus. Results from part of the Health Survey in the County of Varmland. *Acta Med Scand* 181:129–141, 1967.

Bengtsson C: Ischaemic heart diease in women. *Acta Med Scand* (suppl 549):5–20, 1973.

Bengtsson C, Blohme G, Waldenstrom J: Diabetes mellitus, carbohydrate tolerance and early insulin response to an intravenous glucose injection in a population sample of women and in women with ischaemic heart diease. *Acta Med Scand* (suppl 549) 1973, p 65–74.

Bennett C, Tokuyama GH, Bruyers PT: Health of Japanese Americans in Hawaii. *Public Health Rep* 78(No. 9):753–762, 1973.

Bennett MJ, Coon E: Mellituria and postprandial blood sugar curves in dogs after the ingestion of various carbohydrates in the diet. *Nutrition* 88:163–170, 1966.

Bennett PH: Discussion on tests of neurological function in Pima Indians, in Camerini-Davalos RA, Cole HS (eds): *Vascular and Neurological Changes in Early Diabetes.* New York, Academic Press, 1973, p 273–275.

Bennett PH, Burch TA, Miller M; Diabetes mellitus in American (Pima) Indians. *Lancet* 2:125–128, 1971.

Bennett PH, Miller M, Burch TA: Diabetes mellitus in American Indians: The Pima of Arizona, in Ostman J, Milner RDG (eds): *Diabetes.* Proc 6th Congr of Int Diab Fed, Stockholm, Series 140, 1967, p 26.

Bennett PH, Rushforth NB, Miller M, LeCompte PM: Epidemiologic studies in diabetes in the Pima Indians. *Recent Prog Horm Res* 32:333–376, 1976a.

Bennett PH, Rushforth NB, Steinberg AG, Burch TA, Miller M: Diabetes in the Pima Indians: Evidence of bimodality in glucose tolerance distributions. *Diabetes* 18:333, 1969.

Bennett PH, et al: *Report of Workgroup on Epidemiology.* National Commission on Diabetes, vol 3, part 2. US Department of Health, Education, and Welfare Publication (NIH) 76-1022, 1976, p 65–135.

Bennion LJ, Grundy SM: Effects of diabetes mellitus of cholesterol metabolism in man. *N Engl J Med* 296:1365–1371, 1977.

Berger H: Method of increasing sensitivity of glucose tolerance test. *JAMA* 148:364, 1952.

Berger M, Baumhoff E, Gries FA: Gewichtereduktion and glucose intoleranz bei adipositas. (Weight reduction and glucose intolerance in obese patients). *Dtsch Med Wochenschr* 9:307–311, 1976.

Berger M, Berchtold P, Drost H, et al: Metabolic effects of muscular exercise in diabetics, in Bajaj JS (ed): *Current Topics in Diabetes Research.* Proc 9th Int Diab Fed, India, Series 400, 1976a, p. 70.

Berk ME, Page LE, Herbst VCO: An analysis of the Queen's Hospital diabetic clinic: 1. The physician's data. *Hawaii Med J* 6:22–25, 1946.

Berkman J, Rifkin H: Unilateral modular diabetic glomerulosclerosis (Kimmelstiel-Wilson): Report of a case. *Metabolism* 22:715–722, 1973.

Berkow JW, Patz A, Fine S: A followup of blind diabetic patients. *Ann Ophthalmol* 7:79–82, 1975.

Berkowitz D: Serum lipid and fat tolerance determinations in controlled diabetics. *Diabetes* (suppl 2)11:56–61, 1962.

Berris RF, Huttner WA, LeRogers R: Routine postprandial blood glucose determinations in a general hospital. *JAMA* 198:135, 1966.

Berry JH, Chakravarty RN, Gupta HD, Malik K: Prevalence of diabetes mellitus in a North Indian town. *Ind J Med Res* 54:1025–1047, 1966.

Bertillion J: *Transactions of the Fifteenth International Congress on Hygiene and Demography,* 1, part 2, 1912, p 364–366.

Beygui HE: Epidemiology of diabetes in Iran, in Bajaj JS (ed): *Current Topics in Diabetes Research.* Proc 9th Congr of Int Diab Fed, India, Series 400, 1976, p 176.

Bhoola KD: A necropsy study of diabetes mellitus in Natal blacks. *S Afr Med J* 50:1364–1366, 1976.

Bierens deHann B, Scherrer JR, Stauffacher W, Pometta D: Iron excess, early glucose intolerance and impaired insulin secretion in idiopathic haemochromatosis. *Eur J Clin Invest* 3:179–187, 1973.

Bierman EL, Nelson R: Carbohydrates, diabetes, and blood lipids. *World Rev Nutr Diet* 22:280–287, 1975.

Billis A, Rastogi GK: Studies in methods of investigating carbohydrate. *Diabetologia* 2:169–177, 1966.

Binazzi M, Calandra P, Lisi P: Statistical association between psoriasis and diabetes: Further results. *Arch Dermatol Res* 254:43–48, 1975.

Bing FC: Dietary fiber—in historical perspective. *J Am Diet Assoc* 69:498–505, 1976.

Birkbeck JA: Growth in juvenile diabetes mellitus. *Diabetologia* 8:221–224, 1972.

Birkenstock WE, Louw JH, Terblanche J: Smoking and other factors affecting the conservative management of peripheral vascular disease. *S Afr Med J* 49:1129–1132, 1975.

Birmingham Diabetes Working Party. Glucose tolerance and glycosuria in the general population. *Br Med J* 2:655–659, 1963.

Birmingham Diabetes Working Party (Crombie DL, et al): Five year followup report on the Birmingham diabetes survey of 1962. *Br Med J* 3:301–305, 1970.

Birmingham Diabetes Survey Working Party: Ten year followup report on Birmingham Diabetes Survey of 1961. *Br Med J* 2:35–37, 1976.

Bisht DB, Krishnamurthy M, Rangaswamy R: Gustatory threshold for sugar in diabetics and their sibs utilizing sucrose. *Assoc Phys India* 19:431–433, 1971.

Bjerkelund CJ: Diabetic renal disease: Clinical studies of 1,335 diabetics treated in Med Dept A of the University Hospital, Oslo, 1930–1950. *Acta Med Scand* 139:133–145, 1951.

Bjorntorp P, deJounge K, Sjostrom K, Sullivan L: The effect of physical training on insulin production in obesity. *Metabolism* 19:631–638, 1970.

Bjorntorp P, Berchtold P, Tibblin G: Insulin secretion in relation to adipose tissue in men. *Diabetes* 20:65–70, 1971.

Bjorntorp P, Fahlen M, Grimby G, Gustafson A, Holm J, et al: Carbohydrate and lipid metabolism in middle-aged, physically well-trained men. *Metabolism* 21:1027–1044, 1972.

Bjorntorp P, Holm G, Jacobsson B, Schillder-deJounge K, Lundberg PA, et al: Physical training in human hyperplastic obesity: 4. Effects on the hormonal status. *Metabolism* 26:319–320, 1977.

Bjorntorp P, Sjostrom L: Number and size of adipose tissue fat cells in relation to metabolism in human obesity. *Metabolism* 20:703–713, 1971a.

Bjurulf P: Atherosclerosis and body-build with special reference to size and number of subcutaneous fat cells. *Acta Med Scand* (suppl 349), 1959.

Blackard WG, Omori Y, Freedman L: Epidemiology of diabetes mellitus in Japan. *J Chron Dis* 18:415–427, 1965.

Blackburn H: Progress in the epidemiology and prevention of coronary heart disease. *Progress in Cardiology* 3:1–36, 1974.

Blackburn H: Coronary disease prevention. Controversy and professional attitudes. *Adv Cardiol* 20:10–26, 1977.

Blackburn H, Keys A, Simonson E, et al: The electrocardiogram in population studies: A classification system. *Circulation* 21:1160, 1960.

Block MB, Berk JE, Fridhandler LS, et al: Diabetic ketoacidosis associated with mumps virus infection. Occurrence in a patient with macromylasemia. *Ann Intern Med* 78:663–667, 1973.

Bloodworth JMB Jr, Engerman RL, Anderson PJ: Microangiopathy in the experimentally diabetic animal, in Camerini-Davalos RA, Cole HS (eds): *Vascular and Neurological Changes in Early Diabetes.* New York, Academic Press, 1973, p 245–250.

Bloom A: Relation of the complications of diabetes to the clinical state. *Proc R Soc Med* 60:149–152, 1967.

Bloom A, Hayes TM, Gamble DR: A register of newly diagnosed diabetic children. *Br Med J* 3:580–583, 1975.

Bloom A, Hayes TM, Gamble DR: A register of newly diagnosed diabetic children. *Int Diab Fed Bull,* October 1975a, p 20–23.

Blotner H: Studies in glycosuria and diabetes mellitus in selectees. *JAMA* 131:1109–1114, 1946.

Blotner H, Hyde RW: Studies in diabetes mellitus and transient glycosuria in selectees and volunteers. *N Engl J Med* 229:885–892, 1943.

Blotner H, Marble A: Diabetes control: Detection, public education and community aspects. *N Engl J Med* 245:567–575, 1951.

Blumenthal HT, Alex M, Goldenberg S: A study of lesions of the intramural coronary artery branches in diabetes mellitus. *Arch Pathol Lab Med* 70:13, 1960.

Blumenthal HT, Berns AW, Goldenberg S, Lowenstein PW: Etiologic considerations in peripheral vascular disease of the lower extremities with special reference to diabetes mellitus. *Circulation* 33:98, 1966.

Blumenthal HT, Probstein JG, Berns AW: Inter-relationships of diabetes mellitus and pancreatitis. *Surgery* 87:844, 1963.

Bock OAA, Bank S, Marks IN, Jackson WPU: Exocrine pancreatic function in diabetes mellitus. *S Afr Med J* 41:756–758, 1967.

Bodmer J, Bodmer WF: Population genetics of the HL-A system. A summary of data from the fifth International Histocompatibility Testing Workshop. *Isr J Med Sci* 9: 1257–1268, 1973.

Boedhi-Darmojo RA: Some features of myocardial infarction as a complication of diabetes mellitus (a hospital study). Second symposium on Diabetes Mellitus in Asia, Kyoto, 1975, p 24.

Bojanowiez K: Remarks on the incidence of diabetes in Poland. *Int Diab Fed Rep*, 1968, p 82–84.

Booen S, Balitskaya LL, Barovik LN, et al: The incidence and the characteristics of complications and concomitant diseases in patients with diabetes Mellitus. *Probl Endokrinol* 20:20–24, 1974.

Booyens J, DeWaal VM: The level of sucrose intake by three groups of Indian Subjects. *S Afr Med J* 44:1415–1417, 1970.

Booyens J, Frank M, deWaal V: The food intake and activity patterns of offspring of connubial Indian diabetics. *S Afr Med J* 44:278–281, 1970a.

Boozer CN, Mayer J: Effects of long-term restricted insulin production in obese-hyper-glycemic (Genotype ob/ob) mice. *Diabetologia* 12:181–187, 1976.

Bose KC: Diabetes mellitus and its prevention. *Ind Med Gaz* 30:135–144, 1895.

Bose RKC: Comments on diabetes in the tropics. *Br Med J*, October 1907, p 1053.

Boshell BR, Wilsensky AS, Wayland J, Carr JH Jr: A new oral diagnostic test for diabetes mellitus. *Metabolism* 12:108–116, 1963.

Botella-Llusia J, Pereion A: Diabetes, latent diabetes and prediabetes complicating pregnancy: A clinical study of 500 patients. *Int J Gynecol Obstet* 7:56, 1969.

Botros M: Skin glucose tests for screening diabetes mellitus. *J Egypt Med Assoc* 49:231–235, 1966.

Bouchardat A: *De la glycosurie ou diabete sucre,* vol 2. Paris, Germer-Bailliere, 1875.

Boulay A: Un cas de diabete sucre h chez un noir d'Afrique. *Bull Soc Pathol Exot* 21:701–708, 1928.

Bourgoignie J, Sonnet J, Dechef G: Clinical study of diabetes mellitus in the Bantu in the region of Leopoldville. *Ann Soc Belg Med Trop* 3:261–294, 1962.

Bowcock HM: Diabetes mellitus in the negro race: A study of one hundred consecutive cases. *South Med J* 21:994–999, 1928.

Bowen AJ, Reeves RL: Diurnal variation in glucose tolerance. *Arch Intern Med* 119:261–264, 1967.

Bowyer RC, Curnow DH, Stenhouse NS: The second Busselton adult population survey (1969). Twelve biochemical variables. *Pathology* 5:197–208, 1973.

Bowyer RC, Curnow DH, Stenhouse NS: The second Busselton adult population survey (1969): Serum cholesterol. *Pathology* 6:147–152, 1974.

Boyns DR, Crossley JN, Abrams ME: Oral glucose tolerance and related factors in a normal population sample. *Br Med J* 1:595–598, 1969.

Brach VD: Prevalence of diabetes mellitus among the population of Kharkov. (In Russian). *Vrach Delo* 4:8–11, 1975.

Bradley RF: Cardiovascular disease, in Marble A, White P, et al (eds): *Joslin's Diabetes Mellitus,* ed 11. Philadelphia, Lea & Febiger, 1971.

Bradley RF, Ramos E: The eyes and diabetes, in Marble A, White P, et al (eds): *Joslin's Diabetes Mellitus,* ed 11. Philadelphia, Lea & Febiger, 1971, p 478–525.

Brandman O, Redisch W: Incidence of peripheral vascular change in diabetes mellitus: A survey of 264 cases. *Diabetes* 2:194–198, 1953.

Brandt L, Norden A, Schersten B, et al: A diabetes detection campaign in Southern Sweden. Results of 69,000 examinations. *Acta Med Scand* 176:555–561, 1964.

Bray G, et al (eds): *Obesity in Perspective.* US Dept of HEW (NIH) 75-708, 1975.

Breitbach A: The determination by a nomogram of the coefficient of assimilation, K, of Conard for an intravenous glucose load. *Diabetologia* 4:167–168, 1968.

Briethaupt DJ: Discussion of a mortality study of insured diabetics. Medical Section of American Life Convention, 1961.

Breslow L: Multiphasic screening examinations: An extension of the mass screening technique. *Am J Public Health* 40:274, 1950.

Bridges JM, Dalby AM, Millar JHD, Weaver A: An effect of d-glucose on platelet stickiness. *Lancet* 1:75–77, 1965.

Brigham CB: *An Essay upon Diabetes Mellitus.* Boston, Press of Abner A Kingman, 1868.

Brill IC: The effect of a normal meal upon the blood sugar level in health and in certain conditions of disease. *Am J Med Sci* 185:717–731, 1923.

British Diabetic Association Committee on Blindness: *Diabetic Blindness in the United Kindgom, 1967–1969.*

British Medical Journal. Heritability of diabetes, editorial. *Br Med J* 4:127–128, 1975.

British Medical Journal: Diabetes in Madras. Diabetes among the educated classes, anonymous correspondent. *Br Med J:* October 1914, p 604.

Brook CGD: Evidence for a sensitive period in adipose-cell replication in man. *Lancet* 2:624–627, 1972.

Brook CGD, Lloyd JK: Adipose cell size and glucose tolerance in obese children and effects of diet. *Arch Dis Child* 48:301–304, 1973.

Brook CGD, Lloyd JK, Wold OH: Relation between age of onset of obesity and size and number of adipose cells. *Br Med J* 2:25–27, 1972.

Brown GD, Thompson WH: The diabetic child: An analytic study of his development. *Am J Dis Child* 59:238–254, 1940.

Brown WC: Discussion on diabetes in the Tropics. *Br Med J* 2:1062, 1907.

Brozek J: Interaction of human and animal research on body composition. Symposium 1967 (Columbia, Missouri), National Academy of Science Publ 1598, 1968, p 3–15.

Bruhn JG, Wolf S: Studies reporting "Low Rates" of ischemic heart disease: A critica review. *Am J Public Health* 60:1477–1495, 1970.

Brunner D, Altman S, Nelken L, Reider J: The relative absence of vascular disease in diabetic Yemenite Jews: 1. A study of clinical findings. *Diabetes* 13:268–272, 1964.

Brunzell JD, Bierman EL: Plasma triglyceride and insulin levels in familial hypertriglyceridemia, brief report. *Ann Intern Med* 87:198–199, 1977.

Brunzell JD, Hazzard WR, Matulsky AG, Bierman EL: Evidence for diabetes mellitus and genetic forms of hypertriglyceridemia as independent entities. *Metabolism* 24:1115–1121, 1975.

Brunzell JD, Lerner RL, Hazzard WR, et al: Improved glucose tolerance with high carbohydrate feeding in mild diabetes. *N Engl J Med* 284:521, 1971.

Brunzell JD, Schrott HG, Motulsky AG, Bierman EL: Myocardial infarction in the familial forms of hypertriglyceridemia. *Metabolism* 25:313–320, 1976.

Bruschke AVG, Proudfit WL, Sones FM: Progress study of 590 consecutive nonsurgical cases of coronary disease followed 5–9 years. *Circulation* 68:1154–1163, 1973.

Brusis OA, McGandy RB: Nutrition and man's heart and blood vessels. *Fed Proc* 30:1417–1420, 1971.

Bruyn GW, Garland H: Neuropathies of endocrine origin, in Vinken PJ, Bruyn GW (eds): *Handbook of Clinical Neurology: 2. Diseases of Nerves*. New York, North Holland-Elsivier Publishing Co., 1970, p 29–71.

Buchanan WM: Bantu siderosis: A review. *Cent Afr J Med* 15:105–113, 1969.

Buckley RE: Induction of hyperglycemia as treatment for peptic ulcers. *Lancet* 2:497, 1967.

Burch GE, O'Meallie LP: Senile diabetes. *Am J Med Sci* 254:601–607, 1967.

Burch PRJ, Rowell NR: Hepatic cirrhosis and diabetes mellitus. *Lancet* 1:275–276, 1967.

Burditt AF, Caird FI, Draper GJ: The natural history of diabetic retinopathy. *Q J Med* 37:303–317, 1968.

Burgi W: Oral glucose tolerance test: Significant differences between capillary and venous tolerance curves. *Schweiz Med Wochenschr* 104:1698–1699, 1974.

Burkeholder JN, Pickens JM, Womach WN: Oral glucose tolerance test in siblings of children with diabetes mellitus. *Diabetes* 16:156–160, 1967.

Burkitt DP, Trowell HC: *Refined Carbohydrate Foods and Disease: Some Implications of Dietary Fiber*. New York, Academic Press, 1975.

Burkitt DP, Walker ARP, Painter NS: Dietary fiber and disease. *JAMA* 229:1068–1074, 1974.

Burn JL: A diabetic survey. *Med Officer* 96:5, 1956.

Burns TW, Bregant R, Van Peenan HJ, Hood TE: Observations on blood glucose concentration of human subjects during continuous sampling. *Diabetes* 14:186–193, 1965.

Burns TW, Terry BE, Langley PE, Robison GA: In-vitro observations on isolated adipose tissue cells from hyperobese subjects. *Diabetes* 26:657–662, 1977.

Buschard K, Andersen OO, Christau B, et al: Islet-cell antibodies—a marker of subclinical diabetes? A pathogenic factor? *Diabetologia* 13:386, 1977.

Bush OB Jr: Prevalence of diabetes in Japan, in Patel JC, Talwalker NG (eds): *Diabetes in the Tropics*. Bombay, Diab Assoc of India, 1966, p 8–16.

Bush OB Jr, Moriwaki T: Diet and diabetes mellitus, in Patel JC, Talwalker NG (eds): *Diabetes in the Tropics.* Bombay, Diab Assoc of India, 1966, p 553–539.

Butterfield WJH: Summary of results of the Bedford Diabetes Survey. *Proc R Soc Med* 57:196–200, 1964.

Butterfield WJH: Diabetes mellitus: A definition of the problem, in McKeown T (ed): *Screening in Medical Care: Reviewing the Evidence.* New York, Oxford University Press, 1968, p 54–80.

Butterfield WJH, Abrams ME, St John DJB, Whichelow MJ: The intravenous glucose tolerance test: Peripheral disposal of the glucose load in controls and diabetics. *Metabolism* 16:19, 1967.

Butterfield WJH, Abrams ME, Whichelow MJ: The 25 cm intravenous glucose tolerance test; a critical appraisal. *Metabolism* 20:255–265, 1971.

Butterfield WJH, Hanley T, Whichelow MH: Peripheral metabolism of glucose and free fatty acids during oral glucose tolerance tests. *Metabolism* 14:851–866, 1965.

Butterfield WJH, Keen H, Whichelow M: Renal glucose threshold variations with age. *Br Med J* 4:505–507, 1967.

Cabanac M, Duclaux R: Obesity: Absence of satiety, aversion to sucrose. *Science* 168:496–497, 1970.

Cahill GF, Soeldner JS: A noneditorial on non-hypoglycemia. *N Engl J Med* 291:905–906, 1974.

Caird FI: Survival of diabetics with proteinuria. *Diabetes* 10:178–181, 1961.

Caird FI, Burditt AF, Draper GJ: Diabetic retinopathy: A further study of prognosis for vision. *Diabetes* 17:121–123, 1968.

Caird FI, Garrett CJ: Prognosis for vision in diabetic retinopathy. *Diabetes* 44:389, 1963.

Caird FI, Pirie A, Ramsell TG: *Diabetes and The Eye.* Oxford, Blackwell Scientific Publications, 1969.

Calderon R, Llerena LA, Munive L, Kruger F: Intravenous glucose tolerance test in pregnancy in women living in chronic hypoxia. *Diabetes* 15:130–132, 1966.

Camerini-Davalos RA, Cole HS: Vascular and neurological changes in early diabetes, in *Advances in Metabolic Disorders* (suppl 2 to 1973). New York, Academic Press, 1973.

Cameron DP, Poon TKY, Smith GC: Effects of monosodium glutamate administration in the neonatal period on the diabetic syndrome in KK mice. *Diabetologia* 12:621–626, 1976.

Cameron JS, Ireland JT, Watkins PJ: The kidney and renal tract, in Keen H, Jarrett RJ (eds): *Complications of Diabetes.* London, Edward Arnold Pub Co, 1975, p 99–150.

Cammidge PJ: Diabetes mellitus and heredity. *Br Med J* 2:738, 1928.

Campbell CH: Diabetes mellitus in the territory of Papua and New Guinea. *Med J Aust* 2:607–610, 1963.

Campbell GD: Insulin-independent young diabetics in Natal. *Br Med J* 2:537–538, 1960.

Campbell GD: Diabetes in Asians and Africans in and around Durban. *S Afr Med J* 37:1195, 1963.

Campbell GD: Some observations upon 4,000 African and Asiatic diabetics collected in Durban between 1958 and 1962. *East Afr Med J* 5:267–276, 1963a.

455

Campbell GD: Some thoughts on the syndrome of diabetes in Indian people in Natal. *Leech* 34:125, 1964.

Campbell GD: The epidemiology of diabetes in Africa, in Ostman J, Milner RDG (eds): *Diabetes.* Proc 6th Congr of Int Diab Fed, Stockholm, 1967. Excerpta Medica Fdn, 1969, p 693–695.

Campbell GD: The distribution of diabetes mellitus. Frequency in Africa, Asia, Australasia and the Pacific Islands, in *Handbook of Diabetes Mellitus*, vol 2. Munchen, JF Lehmanns Verlag, 1970.

Campbell GD: Frequency of diabetes with special respect to diet, in Rodriguez RR, Vallance-Owen J (eds): *Diabetes.* Proc 7th Congr of Int Diab Fed, Buenos Aires, 1970a, p 325–330.

Campbell GD: The epidemiology of diabetes in mammals (comments from Tongast Sugar Survey Company). *Horm Metab Res* (suppl 4, 1974), pp 128–134.

Campbell GD, Batchelor EL, Goldberg MD: Sugar intake and diabetes, letter to the editor. *Diabetes* 16:62–63, 1967.

Campbell GD, Goldberg MD: The sugar orgy. *S Afr Med J* 2:365–397, 1966.

Campbell GD, McNeil WG: Initial experiences in a biracial subtropical diabetic clinic. Annual report, City Medical Officer of Health, Durban, 1958.

Canelo CK, Bissell DM, Abrams H: A multiphasic screening survey in San Jose. *Calif Med* 71:409–413, 1949.

Cannon WB, Sholib AT, Wright WS: Emotional glycosuria. *Am J Physiol* 29:280, 1911.

Capani F, Sensi S: Circadian rhythm of hypoglycemic effect of insulin in healthy and obese subjects, in Bajaj JS (ed): *Current Topics in Diabetes Research.* Proc 9th Congr of Int Diab Fed, India, Series 400, 1976, p 163–164.

Caplash VK, Khattri HN, Bidwai PS, Rastogi GK: Frequency of ischemic heart disease in patients with overt diabetes mellitus. *J Assoc Physicians India* 23:373–376, 1975.

Cardonnet LJ, Nusimovich B: On the epidemiology of diabetes: Prevalence rate in the urban population of Argentina. *Int Diab Fed Rep,* 60–68, 1968.

Carlson LA, Bottiger LE: Ischaemic heart disease in relation to fasting values of plasma triglycerides and cholesterol. *Lancet* 1:865 1972.

Carlson LA, Wahlberg F: Serum lipids, intravenous glucose tolerance and their interrelation studied in ischemic cardiovascular disease. *Acta Med Scand* 180:307–315, 1966.

Carlstrom S, Lundquist A, Lundquist I, Norden A, et al: Borderline glucose tolerance not followed by overt diabetes. *Acta Med Scand* 189:415, 1971.

Carlstrom S, Persson G, Lundquist I, et al: A followup study of patients with borderline glucose tolerance. *Diabetologia* 8:365, 1972.

Carlstrom S, Persson G, Schersten B: Antidiabetic treatment in the prevention of cardiovascular disease of subjects with borderline glucose tolerance. *Diabetes* 24:414, 1975.

Carpenter AM, Goetz FC, Najarian JS, Lazarow A: Juvenile onset idabetes: Quantitation of glomerular basement membrane thickness after renal transplantation *Diabetes* 25(suppl 1):357, 1976.

Carpenter CCJ, Solomon N, Silverberg SG, et al: Schmidt's syndrome (thyroid and adrenal insufficiency): A review of the literature and a report of 15 new cases including ten instances of coexistent diabetes mellitus. *Medicine* 43:153–180, 1964.

Carpenter RG, Taylor KW: Statistical methods for examining retinopathy in relation to the control of diabetes and other factors. *Br J Ophthalmol* 47:590–595, 1963.

Carr WR, Gelfand M: The incidence of diabetes mellitus in the African: A survey in Highfield, Salisbury, Southern Rhodesia. *Cent Afr J Med* 7:332–335, 1961.

Carroll KF, Nestel PJ: Diurnal variation in glucose tolerance and in insulin secretion in man. *Diabetes* 22:333–348, 1973.

Caspary WE, Creutzfeldt W: Gastrointestinal manifestations of diabetes, in Sussman KE, Metz RJS (eds): *Diabetes Mellitus*, ed 4. New York, American Diabetes Assoc, 1975.

Cassidy J: Diabetes in Fiji. *NZ Med J* 66:167–172, 1967.

Castells S, Avruskin T, Reddy CM, Hashemi SE: Maximum stimulation of insulin secretion in children with chemical diabetes and obesity. *Am J Med Sci* 271:25–30, 1976.

Castren O, Kallio V, Ruponen S: Screened glucosuria during pregnancy. Correlation with intravenous glucose tolerance test and serum lipids. *Acta Obstet Gynecol Scand* 53:323–327, 1974.

Castro A, Scott JP, Grettie DP, et al: Plasma insulin and glucose responses of healthy subjects of varying glucose loads during 3-hour glucose tolerance tests. *Diabetes* 19:842–851, 1970.

Cathelineau G: HLA system and diabetes mellitus. *Int Diab Fed Bull* 21:24–25, 1976.

Cattaneo R, Saibene V, Pozza G: Peripheral T-lymphocytes in juvenile-onset diabetics (JOD) and in maternity-onset diabetics (MOD). *Diabetes* 25:223–226, 1976.

Cawley T: A singular case of diabetes consisting entirely in the quality of the urine with an inquiry into the different theories of that disease. *London Med J* 9:286–308, 1788.

Cerasi E, Efendie S, Luft R: Dose response relation between plasma-insulin and blood-glucose levels during oral glucose loads in prediabetic and diabetic subjects. *Lancet* 1:794–797, 1973.

Chakravarty A: A study on diabetes and its treatment with special reference to the Bengalees and their diet. *India Med Record* 58:65–80, 1938.

Chakravarty S: Comments on diabetes in India. *Br Med J*, October 1907, p 1056.

Chance GW: Control of hyperlipidaemia in juvenile diabetes: Standard and corn-oil diets compared over a period of 10 years. *Br Med J* 3:616–618, 1969.

Chance GW, Albutt EC, Edkins SM: Serum lipids and lipoproteins in untreated diabetic children. *Lancet* 1:1126, 1969.

Chandalia HB, Boshell BR: Diagnosis of diabetes. The size and nature of carbohydrate load. *Diabetes* 19:863–869, 1970.

Chandraprasert S, Samranvej P, Arthaschinta S, Isarsena S: Diabetes mellitus and tropical form of chronic calcific pancreatitis in Thailand. *Aust NZ J Med* 6:316–320, 1976.

Chapman JM, Coulson AH, Clark VA, Borun ER: The differential effect of serum cholesterol, blood pressure and weight on the incidence of myocardial infarction and angina pectoris. *J Chron Dis* 23:631–645, 1971.

Charbonnel B, Chupin M, Guillon J: Glucose tolerance in viral hepatitis, in Bajaj JS (ed): *Current Topics in Diabetes Research.* Proc 9th Congr of Int Diab Fed, India, Series 400, 1976, p 67–68.

Charles RW, Medard F: Relation of diabetes mellitus to nutrition in Haiti, abstract. *Diabetes* 18(suppl 1):349, 1969.

Chase HP, Glasgow AM: Juvenile diabetes mellitus and serum lipids and lipoprotein levels. *Am J Dis Child* 130:1113–1117, 1976.

Chavez A, Balam G, Zubiran S: Estudio epidemiologico dela diabetes en tres communicados de la zona Henequenata del Estado de Yucatan. *Rev Invest Clin* (Span.) 15:333, 1963.

Cheah JS, Tambyah JA, Mitra NR: Prevalence of diabetes mellitus among the ethnic groups in Singapore. *Trop Geogr Med* 27:14–16, 1975.

Chertack MM, Sherrick JC: Screening for diabetes by the glucose oxidase method. *JAMA* 169:1059–1061, 1959.

Chesrow EJ, Bleyer JM: Diabetes case finding among 1000 patients over 60. *Geriatrics* 10:479–486, 1955.

Chevers N: A commentary on the diseases of India. London, J and A Churchill, 1886, p 371–372.

Chey WY, Shay H, Shuman CR: External pancreatic secretion in diabetes mellitus. *Ann Intern Med* 59:812–821, 1963.

Chiang BN, Perlman LV, Epstein FH: Overweight and hypertension: A review. *Circulation* 39:403–421, 1969.

Childs P: Dietary fat, dyspepsia, diarrhoea, and diabetes. *Br J Surg* 59:669–691, 1972.

Chinn H, Broday H, Silverman S Jr, DiRaimondo V: Glucose tolerance in patients with oral symptoms. *J Oral Ther Pharmacol* 2:261–269, 1966.

Chiumello G, delGuercio MJ, Carnelutti M, Bidone G: Relationship between obesity, chemical diabetes and beta pancreatic function in children. *Diabetes* 18:238–243, 1969.

Chlouverakis C, Jarrett RJ, Keen H: Glucose tolerance, age, and circulating insulin. *Lancet* 1:806–807, 1967.

Chochinov RH, Ullyot LE, Moorhouse JA: Sensory perception thresholds in patients with juvenile diabetes and their close relatives. *N Engl J Med* 286:1233–1236, 1972.

Christacopoulos P, Karamanos B, Papadimitrious P, Tountas C: The prevalence of diabetes mellitus in males and females in the Greek rural population by decade. *Diabetes* 25(suppl 1):358, 1976.

Christau B, Kromann H, Andersen OO, et al: Incidence, seasonal and geographical patterns of juvenile-onset insulin-dependent diabetes mellitus in Denmark. *Diabetologia* 13:281–284, 1977.

Christau B, Kromann H, Kristensen H, Steinrud J, Nerup J: Incidence, sex and seasonal patterns of juvenile diabetes mellitus. *Diabetologia* 12:384, 1976.

Christensen NJ: Muscle blood flow measured by xenon and vascular calcifications in diabetics. *Acta Med Scand* 183:449, 1968.

Christensen NJ: Increased skin capillary resistance after hypophysectomy in long-term diabetics. *Lancet* 2:1280–1291, 1968a.

Christensen NJ: Diabetic macroangiopathy blood flow and radiological studies, in Camerini-Davalos RA, Cole HS (eds): *Vascular and Neurological Changes in Early Diabetes.* New York, Academic Press, 1973, p 129–134.

Christensen S: Lower extremity amputations in the county of Aalborg, 1961–1971: Population study and followup. *Acta Orthop Scand* 47:329–334, 1976.

Christiansen I, Deckert T. Kjerulf K, Midtgaard K, Worning H: Glucose tolerance, plasma lipids and serum insulin in patients with ischaemic heart diseases. *Acta Med Scand* 184:283–287, 1968.

Christie T: Notes on diabetes mellitus as it occurs in Ceylon. *Edinburgh Med and Surg J* 7:285–299, 1811.

Christlieb AR: Diabetes and hypertensive vascular disease: Mechanisms and treatment. *Am J Cardiol* 32:592–606, 1973.

Christophe J, Mayer J: Effect of exercise on glucose uptake in rats and men. *J Appl Physiol* 13:269–272, 1958.

Christopherson JB: Comments on diabetes in the Sudan. *Br Med J,* October 1907, p 1962.

Christy M, Deckert T, Nerup J: Immunity and autoimmunity in diabetes mellitus. *Clin Endocrinol Metab* 6:305–332, 1977.

Christy M, Nerup J, Bottazzo GF, Doniach D, Platz P, Svejgaard A, Ryder LP, Thomsen M: Association between HLA B8 and autoimmunity in juvenile diabetes mellitus. *Lancet* 2:142–143, 1976.

Chuck AL, Cudworth AG: Plasma fibrinogen, plasma viscosity, lipoproteins and HLA phenotypes in relation to the complications of diabetes. *Diabetologia* 13:387, 1977.

Chukwuemeks AC, Fulton WFM, M'Ngola EN: Ischaemic heart disease among African diabetics in Nairobi. *East Afr Med J* 49:11, 1972.

Chun JWH: Remarks on the incidence of certain diseases in Chinese and Europeans. *Natl Med J China* 10:145–152, 1923–1924.

Chun JWH: The influence of the Chinese diet on disease. *Chin Med J* 39:1046–1049, 1925.

Chung CS, Bassett DR, Moellering RC Jr, Rosenblatt G, Stokes J, Yoshizaki H: Risk factors for coronary heart disease in Hawaiian and Japanese males in Hawaii. *J Med Genet* 6:59–66, 1969.

Chung HL, Tah JH, Lin YS, Chiu PJ, et al: Diabetes mellitus, a clinical analysis of 922 cases. *Chin Med J* 82:511, 1962.

Chutorian AM, Nicholson JF, Killian P: Reactive hypoglycemia in children. *Trans Am Neurol Assoc* 98:188–192, 1973.

Chuttahi PN, Chawla LS: Diabetic neuropathy in India. *Indian J Med Res* 62:99, 1974.

Cleave TL: The neglect of natural principles in current medical practice. *J R Nav Med Serv* 42:55–83, 1956.

Cleave TL: *The Saccharine Disease.* Bristol, Wright, 1974.

Cleave TL: The saccharine disease, letter. *Lancet* 1:1124, 1974a.

Cleave RL, Campbell GD: *Diabetes, Coronary Thrombosis and the Saccharine Disease,* ed 2. Bristol, John Wright and Sons Ltd, 1969.

Clements RS Jr, Morrison AD, Winegrad AI: Polyol pathway in aorta: Regulation by hormones. *Science* 166:1007–1008, 1969.

459

Cochran HA, Buck NF: A mortality study of an insured diabetic population. *Proc Med Sect Am Life Insur Assoc* 49:145–178, 1961.

Coelingh-Bennink HJT, Schreurs WH: Improvement of oral glucose tolerance in gestational diabetes by pyridoxine. *Br Med J* 3:13–14, 1975.

Cohen AM: Prevalence of diabetes among different ethnic Jewish groups in Israel. *Metabolism* 10:50, 1961.

Cohen AM: Fats and carbohydrates as factors in atherosclerosis and diabetes in Yemenite Jews. *Am Heart J* 65:291–293, 1963.

Cohen AM: Effect of dietary carbohydrate on the glucose tolerance curve in the normal and the carbohydrate-induced hyperlipemic subject. *Am J Clin Nutr* 20:126–130, 1967.

Cohen AM: Environmental aspects of diabetes. *Isr J Med Sci* 8:358–363, 1972.

Cohen AM, Bavly S, Poznanski R: Change of diet of Yemenite Jews in relation to diabetes and ischaemic heart-disease. *Lancet* 2:1399–1401, 1961.

Cohen AM, Canaani ZZ, Landau J, Braun K: Diabetes and arteriosclerosis: A study on sixty diabetic Yemenites. *Diabetes* 12:46–49, 1963.

Cohen AM, Shafrir E: Carbohydrate metabolism in myocardial infarction, behavior of blood glucose and free fatty acids after glucose loading. *Diabetes* 14:84, 1965.

Cohen AM, Teitelbaum A: Effect of different levels of protein in "sucrose" and "starch" diets on the glucose tolerance and growth. *Metabolism* 15:1034–1038, 1966.

Cohen AM, Teitelbaum A, Rosenman E: Diabetes induced by a high fructose diet. *Metabolism* 26:17–22, 1977.

Cohen AM, Teitelbaum A, Salternik R: Genetics and diet as factors in development of diabetes mellitus. *Metabolism* 21:235–240, 1972.

Cohen SL, Legg S, Bird RA: Bedside method of blood glucose estimation. *Lancet* 2:883–884, 1964.

Cohen SM: Diabetes mellitus among Indians of the American Southwest: Its prevalence and clinical characteristics in a hospitalized population. *Ann Intern Med* 40:588–599, 1954.

Cohen T: Trends in frequency of juvenile diabetes mellitus in Israel. *Isr J Med Sci* 8:844–845, 1972.

Cohen T: Diabetes mellitus among children in Israel. *Isr J Med Sci* 9:1404–1405, 1973.

Cohen T, Nelken L, Wolfsohn H: Juvenile diabetes mellitus in immigrant populations in Israel. *Diabetes* 19:585–590, 1970.

Cohn C, Joseph D, Bell L, Allweiss D: Studies on the effects of feeding frequency and dietary composition on fat deposition. *Ann NY Acad Sci* 131:507–518, 1965.

Cohn PF, Gabbay SI, Weglicki WB: Serum lipid levels in angiographically defined coronary artery disease. *Ann Intern Med* 84:241–245, 1976.

Colby AO: Neurologic disorder of diabetes mellitus. *Diabetes* 14:424–429, 516–525, 1965.

Cole HS, Bilder JH: Capillary blood sugar values in infants and children during oral glucose tolerance tests. *Diabetes* 19:176–181, 1970.

Collen MF, Kidd PH, Feldman R, Cutler JL: Cost analysis of a multiphasic screening program. *N Engl J Med* 280:1043–1045, 1969.

Collins IA: Medicine in the Torres Straits. *Med J Aust,* November 1968, p 863.

Collins SD: Economic status and health. *Public Health Bull* 165:1–74, 1927.

Coltart TM, Crossley JN: Influence of dietary sucrose on glucose and fructose tolerance and triglyceride synthesis in the baboon. *Clin Sci Mol Med* 38:427–437, 1970.

Colwell AR, Meyer K: Small blood vessel involvement in diabetes mellitus. *Am Inst of Biol Sci,* 1964.

Colwell JA: Effect of diabetic control on retinopathy. *Diabetes* 15:497, 1966.

Colwell JA, Lein A: Diminished insulin response to hyperglycemia in prediabetes and diabetes. *Diabetes* 16:560–565, 1967.

Colwell JA, Sagel J, Crook L, Chambers A, et al: Correlation of platelet aggregation, plasma factor activity, and megathrombocytes in diabetic subjects with and without vascular disease. *Metabolism* 26:279–285, 1977.

Comessatti G: Über die Änderung der assimilations grenze fur Zucker durch Muskelarbeit. *Beitr Z Chem Phys u Path Brnschwg* 60:67–73, 1906.

Comstock GW, Kendrick MA, Livesay VT: Subcutaneous fatness and mortality. *Am J Epidemiol* 83:548–563, 1966.

Conant RG, Perkins JA, Ainley AB: Stroke morbidity, mortality and rehabilitative potential. *J Chron Dis* 18:397–403, 1958.

Conard V, Franckson JRM, Bastenie PA, et al: Étude critique du triangle D'hyperglycemie intraveineux chez l'homme normal et determination d'un coefficient d'assimilation glycidique. *Arch Int Pharmacodyn Ther* 93:277–292, 1953.

Concepcion I: Incidence of diabetes mellitus among Filipinos. *J Philippine Island Med Assoc* 2:57, 1922.

Conn HO, Schreiber W, Elkington SG, Johnson TR: Cirrhosis and diabetes: I. Increased incidence of diabetes in patients with Laennec's cirrhosis. *Am J Dig Dis* 14:837–852, 1969.

Conn JW: Interpretation of the glucose tolerance test: The necessity of a standard preparatory diet. *Am J Med Sci* 199:555–564, 1940.

Conn JW: Hypertension, the potassium ion, and impaired carbohydrate tolerance. *N Engl J Med* 273:1135–1143, 1965.

Conn JW, Fajans SS: The prediabetic state. *Am J Med* 31:839–850, 1961.

Connell AM: Dietary fiber and diverticular disease. Hosp Prac, March 1976, p 119–123.

Cook AR: Notes on the disease met with in Uganda. *Cent Afr J Trop Med* 4:178, 1901.

Cooke AM, FitzGerald MG, Malins JM, et al: Diabetes in children of diabetic couples. *Br Med J* 2:674–676, 1966.

Cooper GR: Methods for determining the amount of glucose in blood. *CRC Crit Rev Clin Lab Sci,* August 1973, 101–145.

Cooper KH, Pollock ML, Martin RP, et al: Physical fitness levels vs. selected coronary risk factors: A cross-sectional study. *JAMA* 236:116–119, 1976.

Cornblath H, Schwartz R: Transient diabetes in early infancy, in *Disorders of Carbohydrate Metabolism in Infancy,* vol 3. Philadelphia, WB Saunders Co, 1956, p 105–112.

Cosnett JE: Illness among Natal Indians. *S Afr Med J* 31:1109, 1957.

Cosnett JE: Diabetes among Natal Indians. *Br Med J* 1:137, 1959.

Costill DL: Physiology of marathon running. *JAMA* 221:1024, 1972.

Costin G, Kogut MD, Hyman C, Ortega JA: Carbohydrate metabolism and pancreatic islet-cell function in thalassemia major. *Diabetes* 26:230–240, 1977.

Cotton LT, Higton DIR, Berry HE: Diabetes and vascular surgery. *Postgrad Med J* 47:84, 1971.

Cotton RB, Cornelius LM, Therna P: Diabetes mellitus in the dog: A clinicopathologic study. *J Am Vet Med Assoc* 159:863–870, 1971.

Craighead JE, Steinke J: Diabetes mellitus-like syndrome in mice infected with encephalomyocarditis virus. *Am J Pathol* 63:119, 1971.

Crane RK: Intestinal absorption of sugars. *Physiol Rev* 40:789–825, 1960.

Crapo PA, Reaven G, Olefsky J: Plasma glucose and insulin responses to orally administered simple and complex carbohydrates. *Diabetes* 25:741–747, 1976.

Crapo PA, Reaven G, Olefsky J: Postprandial plasma-glucose and -insulin responses to different complex carbohydrates. *Diabetes* 26:1178–1183, 1977.

Crawford T: A standard intravenous glucose tolerance test: *Arch Dis Child* 13:69–78, 1938.

Creutzfeldt W, Kobberling J, Neel JV (eds): *The Genetics of Diabetes Mellitus*. New York, Springer-Verlag, 1976.

Cristol R, Cottet J, Cloaric M: Study of glucose regulation by an intravenous tolbutamide test in coronary insufficiency. *Presse Med* 78:739–742, 1970.

Cudworth AG: Recent advances in the genetics of diabetes. *J Hum Nutr* 30:113–116, 1976.

Cudworth AG, Gamble DR, Landrum R, Bloom A, White GBB, Woodrow JC: Aetiology of juvenile onset diabetes: A prospective study. *Lancet* 1:385–388, 1977.

Cudworth AG, Woodrow JC: HL-A system and diabetes mellitus. *Diabetes* 24:345–349, 1975.

Cudworth AG, Woodrow JC: Genetic susceptibility in diabetes mellitus: Analysis of the HLA association. *Br Med J* 2:846–848, 1976.

Cudworth AG, Woodrow JC: Classification of diabetes. *Lancet* 1:949–950, 1977.

Cullen JF, Town SM, Campbell CJ: Double-blind trial of Atromid-S in exudative diabetic retinopathy. *Trans Ophthalmol Soc UK* 94:554–562, 1974.

Curnow DH, Cullen KJ, McCall MG, Stenhouse NS, Welborn TA: Health and disease in a rural community: A western Australian study. *Aust J Biol Sci* 31:281–285, 1969.

Czyzyk A, Brzezinski ZJ, Krolewski AS, et al: Fate of diabetic patients: I. Plan of the study, methods, and study group. (In Polish with English Summary on last page.) *Przegl Epidemiol* 29:449–460, 1975.

Czyzyk A, Krolewski AS: Is cigarette smoking more frequent among insulin-treated diabetics? *Diabetes* 25:717–718, 1976.

Dahlberg G, Jorpes E (eds): Diabetes mellitus in Sweden. *Acta Med Scand* (suppl)188:1–67, 1947.

Dalderup LM, Van Haard WB: Er is geen reden om aan te nemen dat suiker een primaire rol speelt bij het ontstaan van atherosclerotisch hart-en vaat aandoeningen, even-min bij het onstaan von obesitas of ten aanzien van de levensduur. *Voeding* 32: 569, 1971.

Dales LG, Siegelaub AB, Feldman R, et al: Racial differences in serum and urine glucose after glucose challenge. *Diabetes* 23:327–332, 1974.

Danaraj TJ, Acker MS, Danaraj W, et al: Ethnic group differences in coronary heart disease in Singapore: An analysis of necropsy records. *Am Heart J* 58:516–526, 1959.

Dandrow R, O'Sullivan JG: Obstetrical hazards of gestational diabetes. *Am J Obstet Gynecol* 96:1144, 1966.

Danowski TS: *Diabetes Mellitus: With Emphasis on Children and Young Adults.* Baltimore, Williams and Wilkins Co, 1957.

Danowski TS: Emotional stress as a cause of diabetes mellitus, editorial. *Diabetes* 12:183, 1963.

Danowski TS: Classifications of diabetes mellitus, in Kryston LJ, Shaw RA (eds): *Endocrinology and Diabetes.* New York, Grune and Stratton, 1975, p 321–328.

Danowski TS, Aarons JH, Hydovitz JD, Wingert JP: Utility of equivocal glucose tolerances. *Diabetes* 19:524–526, 1970.

Danowski TS, Fisher ER, Khurana RC, Nolan S, Stephan T: Muscle capillary basement membrane in juvenile diabetes mellitus. *Metabolism* 21:1125–1132, 1972.

Danowski TS, Khurana RC, Gonzalez AR, Fisher ER: Capillary basement membrane thickness and the pseudo-diabetes of myopathy. *Am J Med* 51:757–766, 1971.

Danowski TS, Khurana RC, Nolan S, et al: Insulin patterns in equivocal glucose tolerance tests (chemical diabetes). *Diabetes* 22:808–812, 1973.

Danowski TS, Limaye NR, Cohn RE, Grimes BJ, et al: Sex distribution and frequency of diabetic concomitants of complications. *Diabetes* 15:507–510, 1966.

Danowski TS, Moses C, Weir TF, Wingert JP, et al: Diabetes detection in hospitalized patients, in Diabetes in Pennsylvania. *Pa Med* 69:1–7, 29–36, 1966a.

Darlow JM, Smith C, Duncan LJP: A statistical and genetical study of diabetes: III. Empiric risks to relatives. *Ann Hum Genet* 37:157–174, 1973.

Darragh JH, Hutchinson AR, Mangola EN: The diabetic clinic, Kenyatta National Hospital: Review of results of treatment and recommendations. *East Afr Med J* 48:327–335, 1971.

Dash H, Johnson RA, Dinsmore RE, et al: Syndromes of coronary artery disease: In diabetics and nondiabetics. *Circulation* 49, 50 (suppl 3):109, 1974.

Datey KK, Nanda NC: Hyperglycemia after acute myocardial infarction: Its relation to diabetes mellitus. *N Engl J Med* 276:262, 1967.

Datta SN, Prasad BG, Jain SP: An epidemiological study of diabetes mellitus in a defence population in Lucknow cantonment. *J Indian Med Assoc* 61:23–27, 1973.

Datta SP, Sing Verma NP, Gopalkreshnan R, Ghosh BN: Survey of diabetes in Pondicherry, in Patel JC, Talwalker NG (eds): *Diabetes in the Tropics.* Bombay, Diab Assoc of India, 1966, p 33–39.

Daubs JG: Diabetes screening with the corneal aesthesiometer. *Am J Optom Physiol Opt* 52:31–35, 1975.

463

Davidson JK: Plasma glucose lowering effect of caloric restriction in obesity-induced insulin-treated diabetes mellitus, abstract. *Diabetes* 26(suppl 1):355, 1977.

Davidson JK, Reuben D, Sternberg J: Diabetes screening using a quantitative urine glucose method, abstract. *Diabetes* 24(suppl 2):430, 1975.

Davidson PC: Effect of activity on glucose tolerance. *Diabetes* 16:521–522, 1967.

Davies LEC, Hanson S: Eskimos of the Northwest Passage. *Can Med Assoc J* 92:205, 1965.

Davis AE, Badenoch J: Iron absorption in pancreatic disease. *Lancet* 2:6–8, 1962.

Davis MD: Natural course of diabetic retinopathy, in Kimura SJ, Caygill WM (eds): *Vascular Complications of Diabetes Mellitus.* St Louis, CV Mosby Company, 1967.

Davis MD, Norton EWD, Myers FL: The Arlie classification of diabetic retinopathy, *Symposium on Treatment of Diabetic Retinopathy.* Public Hlth Serv Publication 1890, 1968.

Dawber TR: Risk factors for atherosclerotic disease, in *Current Concepts,* a Scope Publication. Kalamazoo, Mich, Upjohn Co, 1975.

Dawber TR, Kannel WB, Friedman GD: Vital capacity, physical activity and coronary heart disease, in Rabb W (ed): *Prevention of Ischemic Heart Disease: Principles and Practice.* Springfield, Ill, Charles C Thomas Co, 1966, p 254–265.

Day AJ, Nestel PJ, Reeder JR, Turtle JR, White HM: Dietary fat and coronary heart disease: A review (prepared by a standing subcommittee appointed by the Natl Heart Fed of Australia to maintain a continuing review of research developments in the field of diet as related to heart disease). *Med J Aust,* May 1971, p 1155–1160.

Day JL, Tattersall RB: Glucagon secretion in unaffected monozygotic twins of juvenile diabetics. *Metabolism* 24:145–151, 1975.

Dayal B, Moshal MG, Asmal AC: Pancreatic (exocrine) function in calcific pancreatitis with and without diabetes, in Bajaj JS (ed): *Current Topics in Diabetes Research.* Proc 9th Congr of Int Diab Fed, India, Series 400, 1976, p 168–169.

Dean G: The causes of death among the South African-born and immigrants to South Africa. *S Afr Med J* (suppl)39:1–20, 1965.

Deckert T, Poulsen JE: Prognosis for juvenile diabetics with late diabetic manifestations. *Acta Med Scand* 183:351–356, 1968.

Deckert T, Poulsen JE, Larsen M: Prognosis in juvenile diabetes mellitus. *Diabetologia* 11:329–385, 1975.

Deckert T, Simonsen SJE, Poulsen JE: Prognosis of proliferative retionopathy in juvenile diabetes. *Diabetes* 16:728, 1967.

DeCoek NM: The interpretation of the results of oral glucose tolerance tests in older subjects. *Aust NZ J Med* 16:132–138, 1967.

deHertogh R, Vanderheyden I, deGasparo M: Glucose tolerance in a Saharan Nomad population: The Broayas, from the Toubou ethnic group. *Diabetes* 24:983–987, 1975.

DeJong RN: The neurologic manifestations of diabetes mellitus, in Vinken PJ, Bruyn GW (eds): *Handbook of Clinical Neurology, Part 1: Metabolic Deficiency Diseases of the Nervous System,* vol 27. New York, North Holland-Elsevier Publishing Co, 1976, p 99–142.

DeLangen CD, Schut H: Medilingen Borgelijken Genees, Diente in Nederland. *Indie* 3:65–88, 1919.

Del Greco F, Scapellato L: Transient diabetes with coma following short term excessive consumption of carbohydrate. *Diabetes* 2:457–561, 1953.

Del Prete GF, Betterle C, Padovan D, et al: Incidence and significance of islet-cell autoantibodies in different types of diabetes mellitus. *Diabetes* 26:909–915, 1977.

DeMoor P, Meulepas E: Factors related to the age at discovery of diabetes mellitus. *J Clin Endocrinol Metab* 28(part 2):1487, 1968.

DePorte JV: Sickness in Essex County: Survey of morbidity during 52 weeks October 2, 1927–September 29, 1928. *NY State J Med* 29:1310–1316, 1929.

Deren MD: Dextrose tolerance in the aged. *J Lab Clin Med* 22:1138–1141, 1936.

Desai HG, Antia EP: Effect of posture on glucose tolerance curve, in Patel JC, Talwalker NG (eds): *Diabetes in the Tropics*. Bombay, Diab Assoc of India, 1966, p 191–193.

Deschamps I, Giron BJ, Lestradet H: Blood glucose, insulin and free fatty acid levels during oral glucose tolerance tests in 158 obese children. *Diabetes* 26:89–93, 1977.

deSilva WH: Comments on diabetes in Ceylon. *Br Med J*, October 1907, p 1060.

Dewees EJ, Langer PH Jr: Study of glucose tolerance tests and significance of glycosuria. *Trans Assoc Life Insur Med Dir Am* 29:105–134, 1943.

DeZoysa VP: Clinical variations of the diabetic syndrome in a tropical country (Ceylon). *Arch Intern Med* 88:812–818, 1951.

Dickie MM: Genetics of animals with spontaneous diabetes. *Adv Metab Disord* (suppl 1):23–31, 1970.

Dippe SE, Bennett PH, Savage PJ: How the fasting glucose relates to the two-hour post-load glucose level. *Diabetes* 23:350, 1974.

Disease Detection Information Bureau: State Health Department programs find 3,000 new diabetics in 1976. *DDIB Newsletter* 8(no. 10):1, 1977.

Ditschuneit H: Obesity and diabetes mellitus. Proc 7th Congr of Int Diab Fed, Buenos Aires 1970. Stockholm, Excerpta Medica, 1971, p 526–543.

Djokomoeljanto R, Soetardjo H, Boedhi-Darmojo R: A community study of diabetes mellitus in an urban population in Semarang, Indonesia, in Baba S, Goto Y, Fukui I (eds): *Diabetes Mellitus in Asia*. Proc 2nd symp Kyoto, 1975. Amsterdam, Excerpta Medica, 1976.

Dobbs R, Faloona G, Unger RH: Effects of intravenously administered glucose on glucagon and insulin secretion during fat absorption. *Metabolism* 24:69–75, 1975.

Dobson HL, Shaffer R, Burns R: Accuracy of urine testing for sugar and acetone by hospital ward personnel. *Diabetes* 17:281–285, 1968.

Dodu SRA: The incidence of diabetes mellitus in Accra (Ghana), a study of 4,000 patients. *West Afr Med J* 7:129–134, 1958.

Dodu SRA: Diabetes and haemosiderosis—haemochromatosis—in Ghana. *Trans R Soc Trop Med Hyg* 52:425–430, 1958a.

Dodu SRA: Diabetes in the tropics. *Br Med J*, June 1967, p 747–750.

Dohan FC, Lukens FDW: Experimental diabetes produced by the administration of glucose. *Endocrinology* 42:244–262, 1948.

Dolder MA, Oliver MF: Myocardial infarction in young men: Study of risk factors in nine countries. *Br Heart J* 37:493–503, 1975.

Dolger H: Clinical evaluation of vascular damage in diabetes mellitus. *JAMA* 134:1289–1291, 1947.

Dollery CT, Oakley NW: Reversal of retinal vascular changes in diabetes. *Diabetes* 14:121–127, 1965.

Donowitz M, Hendler R, Spiro HM, Binder HJ, Felig P: Glucagon secretion in acute and chronic pancreatitis. *Ann Intern Med* 83:778–781, 1975.

Dorf A, Ballintine EJ, Bennett PH, Miller MN: Retinopathy in Pima Indians: Relationships to glucose level, duration of diabetes, age at diagnosis of diabetes and age at examination in a population with a high prevalence of diabetes mellitus. *Diabetes* 25:554–560, 1976.

Dornhorst A, Ouyang A: Effect of alcohol on glucose tolerance. *Lancet* 2:957–959, 1971.

Drash A: Diabetes mellitus in childhood: A review. *J Pediatr* 78:919–941, 1971.

Drash A: Chemical diabetes mellitus in the child. *Metabolism* 22:295, 1973.

Drash A: Relationship between diabetes mellitus and obesity in the child. *Metabolism* 22:337–344, 1973a.

Drash A: Diabetes mellitus, in Vaughan VC, McKay RJ (eds): *Nelson's Textbook of Pediatrics*. Philadelphia, WB Saunders Co, 1975, p 1259–1270.

Dreiling DA, Janowitz HD, Ferrier CV: *Pancreatic Inflammatory Disease: A Physiologic Approach*. New York, Harper & Row, 1964.

Drenick EJ, Johnson D: Evolution of diabetic ketoacidosis in gross obesity. *Am J Clin Nutr* 28:264–272, 1975.

Dreyer K, Hey A: Forekomst og fordeling af diabetes mellitus i Danmark. *Ugeskr Laeger* 115:27, 1069–1073, 1953.

Dreyer K, Hey A: Dodelighedsforhold blandt diabetikere. *Ugeskr Laeger* 116:273–276, 1954.

Dreyfuss F, Abramov A, Peritz E: A comparison of the number of pregnancies up to the age of 45 in diabetic and nondiabetic women. *Isr J Med Sci* 8:1953–1955, 1972.

Drossel MR: Kaiser plan automates multiphasic testing. *Mod Hosp* 106:113–116, 1966.

Drury MI, Timoney FJ: Changing sex ratios in diabetes. *Br Med J* 1:181, 1972.

Drury MI, Timoney FJ: Mortality in diabetes mellitus. *Ir Med J* 66:484, 486, 1973.

Dublin and Marks: The influence of weight on certain causes of death. *Hum Biol* 2:159, 1930.

Dubois A: La Pathologic du Congolais. *Ann Soc Belg Med Trop* 24:13–28, 1944.

Duffy T, Phillips N, Pelligrin F: Review of glucose tolerance: A proglem in methodology. *Am J Med Sci* 265:117–133, 1973.

Duncan LJP: Cortisone induced impairment of glucose tolerance in the detection of the diabetic diathesis. *Q J Exp Physiol* 41:453–461, 1956.

Duncan LJP: The intravenous glucose tolerance test. *Q J Exp Physiol* 41:85, 1956a.

Dunlop DM, Lyon RMM: A study of 523 cases of obesity. *Edinburgh Medical Journal* 38:561–577, 1931.

Dunn JP, Ipsen J, Elsom KO, Ohtani M: Risk factors in coronary artery disease, hypertension and diabetes. *Am J Med Sci* 259:309–322, 1970.

Dunn LJ, Merchant JA, Bradbury JT, Stone DB: Glucose tolerance and endometrial carcinoma: A controlled study. *Arch Intern Med* 121:246–254, 1968.

Dunnigan MG, Fyfe T, McKiddie MT, Crosbie SM: The effects of isocaloric exchange of dietary starch and sucrose on glucose tolerance, plasma insulin and serum lipids in man. *Clin Sci Mol Med* 38:1–9, 1970.

Dunstone MW: Diabetes mellitus: A report from the Australian General Practitioner Morbidity and Prescribing survey, 1969–1974. *Aust Fam Phys* 584:479–480, 1976.

Dupre J, Chisholm DJ: Gastrointestinal factors and insulin release, in Fajans SS, Sussman KE (eds): *Diabetes Mellitus: Diagnosis and Treatment,* vol 3. New York, Amer Diab Assoc, 1971, p 47–50.

Dutt MM: Diabetes in Bengal. Trans 7th Congr of Far East Association on Tropical Medicine, 1:179–189, 1927.

Dyer AR, Stamler J, Berkson DM, et al: Relationship of relative weight and body mass index to 14 year mortality in the Chicago Peoples' Gas Company study. *J Chron Dis* 28:109–123, 1975.

Dymock IW, Cassar J, Pyke DA, Oakley WG, Williams R: Observations on the pathogenesis, complications and treatment of diabetes in 115 cases of hemochromatosis. *Am J Med* 52:203–210, 1972.

Eastwood MA, Fisher N, Greenwood GT, Hutchinson JB: Perspectives on the bran hypothesis. *Lancet* 1:1029–1032, 1974.

Eaton RP, Kipnis DM: Effects of high-carbohydrate diets on lipid and carbohydrate metabolism in the rat. *Am J Physiol* 217:1160–1168, 1969.

Eaton RP, Nye WHR: The relationship between insulin secretion and triglyceride concentration in endogenous lipemia. *J Lab Clin Med* 81:682–695, 1973.

Eddington GM, Gilles HM: *Pathology in the Tropics.* Baltimore, Williams and Wilkins Co, 1969.

Edginton ME, Hodkinson J, Seftel HC: Disease patterns in a South African rural Bantu population, with a commentary on comparisons with the pattern in urbanized Johannesburg Bantu. *S Afr Med J* 46:968–976, 1972.

Edwards FM, Wise PH, Craig RJ, et al: Visual acuity and retinal changes in South Australian Aborigines. *Aust NZ J Med* 6:205–209, 1976.

Elizabeth T, Stephen PM: Pancreatic calculi. *J Indian Med Assoc* 24:126, 1954.

Elkeles RS, Lowry D, Wyllie ADH, Young JL, Fraser TR: Serum insulin, glucose and lipid levels among mild diabetics in relation to incidence of vascular complications. *Lancet* 1:880–883, 1971.

Ellenberg M: Diabetic complications without manifest diabetes: Complications as presenting clinical symptoms. *JAMA* 183:916–980, 1963.

Ellenberg M: Diabetic neuropathy in Sussman KE, Metz RJS (eds): *Diabetes Mellitus,* ed 4. New York, Comm on Prof Educ, Amer Diab Assoc, 1975.

Ellenberg M: Diabetic neuropathy: Clinical aspects. *Metabolism* 25:1627–1655, 1976.

Ellenberg M, Rifkin H (eds): *Diabetes Mellitus: Theory and Practice.* New York, McGraw-Hill, 1970.

467

Elmfeldt D, Vedin A, Wilhelmsson C, et al: Morbidity in representative male survivors of myocardial infarction compared to representative population samples. *J Chron Dis* 29:221–231, 1976.

Embleton D: Glucose tolerance curves in 500 obese cases. *Br Med J* 2:739–742, 1938.

Emerson H, Larimore LD: Diabetes mellitus: A contribution to its epidemiology based chiefly on mortality statistics. *Arch Intern Med* 34:585–630, 1924.

Emmer M, Gorden P, Roth J: Diabetes in association with other endocrine disorders. *Med Clin North Am* 55:1057–1064, 1971.

Endocrine and Metabolic Division of Peking Union Hospital: Endocrinology in New China. *Chin Med J* 79:304–325, 1959.

Engerman RA: Panel on diabetic retinopathy. 33rd annual meeting, Amer Diab Assoc, June 15, 1975.

Engel A: Late complications of diabetes. (Summary in English.) *Nord Med* 43:902–908, 1950.

Engle HJ, Page HL, Campbell WB: Coronary artery disease in young women. *JAMA* 230:1531–1534, 1974.

Entmacher PS: An insurance-clinical dialogue on diabetes. *Trans Assoc Life Ins Med Dir Am* 55:205–217, 1972.

Entmacher PS: Long-term prognosis in diabetes mellitus, in Sussman KE, Metz RJS (eds): *Diabetes Mellitus*, ed 4. New York, Comm on Prof Educ, Amer Diab Assoc, 1975, p 191–196.

Entmacher PS: Report of economic impact, in Report of the National Commission on Diabetes: *Scope and Impact of Diabetes*, vol 3, part 2. US Dept of HEW Publ (NIH) 76-1022, p 305–351, 1976.

Entmacher PS, Marks HH: Diabetes in 1964: A world survey. *Diabetes* 14:212–223, 1965.

Entmacher PS, Marks HH: Socioeconomic considerations in the life of a diabetic, in Marble A, et al (eds): *Joslin's Diabetes Mellitus*, ed 11. Philadelphia, Lea & Febiger, 1971, p 783–796.

Entmacher PS, Root HF, Marks HH: Longevity of diabetic patients in recent years. *Diabetes* 13:373–377, 1964.

Epstein FH: Glucose intolerance and cardiovascular disease. *Triangle* 12:3–8, 1973.

Epstein FH, Francis T Jr, Hayner NS, et al: Prevalence of chronic diseases on distribution of selected physiologic variables in a total community, Tecumseh, Michigan. *Am J Epidemiol* 81:307–322, 1965.

Epstein FH, Ostrander LD, Johnson BC, Payne MW, et al: Epidemiological studies of cardiovascular disease in a total community-Tecumseh, Michigan. *Ann Intern Med* 62:1170–1187, 1965a.

Erhardt CI, Weiner L: Changes in mortality statistics through the use of the new international statistical classification. *Am J Public Health* 40:6–16, 1950.

Ernest I, Linner E, Svanborg A: Carbohydrate-rich, fat-poor diet in diabetes. *Am J Med* 39:594–600, 1965.

Esmann V, et al: Types of exudates in diabetic retinopathy. *Acta Med Scand* 174:375, 1963.

Eswaraiah G, Bali RS: Palmar flexion creases and dermatoglyphics among diabetic patients. *Am J Phys Anthrop* 47:11–14, 1977.

Ettinger PO, Oldewurtel HA, Sethi V, Regan TJ: Glucose intolerance in cardiac patients without myocardial ischemia and its relation to cardiac output. *Trans Assoc Am Physicians* 84:262–271, 1971.

Ettinger PO, Oldewurtel HA, Weisse AB, Regan TJ: Diminished glucose tolerance and immunoreactive insulin response in patients with nonischemic cardiac disease. *Circulation* 38:559–567, 1968.

European Diabetes Epidemiology Study Group: A brief account of the European Diabetes Epidemiology Study Group and its activities. *Diabetologia* 6:453–454, 1970.

Evans JG, Ostrander LD: Fasting serum-triglycerides concentration and distribution of subcutaneous fat. *Lancet* 1:761–762, 1957.

Exton WG, Rose AR: The one-hour, two-dose dextrose tolerance test. *Am J Clin Pathol* 4:381, 1934.

Ezcurra Cebreiro, JM, Sancez Plaza N, Pirta E: Epidemiology of diabetes in 40,438 inhabitants of the Province of Vizcaya, Spain. Proc 6th Congr Int Diab Fed, Stockholm, Series 140, 1967, p 27.

Fabry P, Fodor J, Hejl Z, et al: The frequency of meals: Its relation to overweight, hypercholesterolaemia, and decreased glucose-tolerance. *Lancet* 2:614, 1964.

Fabrykant M: Clinical versus laboratory hypoglycemia: An analysis of 81 oral glucose tolerance tests with arterial and venous blood glucose measurements. *Metabolism* 4:153–159, 1955.

Fabrykant M, Gelfand ML: Symptom-free diabetes in angina pectoris. *Am J Med Sci* 247:665–668, 1964.

Faerman I, Faccio E, Miliei J, et al: Autonomic neuropathy and painless myocardial infarction in diabetic patients. Histologic evidence of their relationship. *Diabetes* 26:1147–1158, 1977.

Fagerberg SE: Diabetic neuropathy: A clinical and histological study on the significance of vascular affections. *Acta Med Scand* 164:1, 1959.

Fahlen M, Oden A, Bjorntorp P, Tibblin G: Seasonal influence on insulin secretion in man. *Clin Sci* 41:453–458, 1971.

Fain A: L'hypertrophie parotidienne chronique chez les indigenes du Congo Belge. *Receuil de Truvaux Sciences Medicales au Congo Belge* 6:75–80, 1947.

Fajans SS: Classification and natural history of genetic diabetes mellitus, in Fajans SS, Sussman KE (eds): *Diabetes Mellitus: Diagnosis and Treatment,* vol 3. New York, Amer Diab Assoc, 1971, p 89–94.

Fajans SS (ed): *Diabetes Mellitus.* Dept of HEW Publication (NIH) 76-854, 1976.

Fajans SS, Conn JW: An approach to the prediction of diabetes mellitus by modification of the glucose tolerance test with cortisone. *Diabetes* 3:296–304, 1954.

Fajans SS, Conn JW: The early recogniation of diabetes mellitus. *Ann NY Acad Sci* 82:208–218, 1959.

469

Fajans SS, Conn JW: Tolbutamide-induced improvement in carbohydrate intolerance of young people with mild diabetes mellitus. *Diabetes* 9:83, 1960.

Fajans SS, Conn JW: Comments on the cortisone-glucose tolerance test. *Diabetes* 10:63, 1961.

Fajans SS, Floyd JC Jr, Pek S, Conn JW: The course of asymptomatic diabetes in young people as determined by levels of blood glucose and plasma insulin. *Trans Assoc Am Physicians* 82:213, 1969

Fajans SS, Floyd JC, Tattersall RB, et al: The various faces of diabetes in the young. *Arch Intern Med* 136:194–202, 1976.

Fajans SS, Weissman PN, Willis PW III, Floyd JC Jr, et al: Search for macroangiopathy in patients with latent diabetes, in Camerini-Davalos RA, Cole HS (eds): *Vascular and Neurologic Changes in Early Diabetes*. New York, Academic Press, 1973, p 19–28.

Falconer DS: The inheritance of liability to diseases with variable age of onset with particular reference to diabetes mellitus. *Ann Hum Genet* 31:1–20, 1967.

Falconer DS, Duncan LJP, Smith C: A statistical and genetical study of diabetes: 1. Prevalence and morbidity. *Ann Hum Genet* 34:347–369, 1971.

Falsetti HL, Schnatz JD: Heart disease and diabetes mellitus, in Ellenberg M, Rifkin H (eds): *Diabetes Mellitus: Theory and Practice*. New York, McGraw-Hill Book Co, 1970, p 870–889.

Falsetti HL, Schnatz JD, Greene DG, Bunnell IL: Serum lipids and glucose tolerance in angiographically proved coronary artery disease. *Chest* 58:111, 1970.

Falta M, Boller R: Insularer und resistenter diabetes. *Klin Wochnschr* 10:438–443, 1931.

Faludi G, Bendersky G, Gerber P: Functional hypoglycemia in early latent diabetes. *Ann NY Acad Sci* 148:868–874, 1968.

Fariss BL: Prevalence of post-glucose-load glycosuria and hypoglycemia in a group of healthy young men. *Diabetes* 23:189–191, 1974.

Farnam LW: Pancreatitis following mumps: Report of a case with operation. *Am J Med Sci* 153:859–870, 1922.

Farquhar JW: Prognosis for babies born to diabetic mothers in Edinburgh. *Arch Dis Child* 44:36–47, 1969.

Feinberg LJ, Sandberg H, DeCastro O, Bellett S: Effects of coffee ingestion on oral glucose tolerance curves in normal human subjects. *Metabolism* 17:916–922, 1968.

Feinleib M, Davidson MJ: Coronary heart disease mortality: A community perspective. *JAMA* 222:1129–1134, 1972.

Feinstein AR: Clinical biostatistics 21. A primer of concepts, phrases and procedures in the statistical analysis of multiple variables. *Clin Pharmacol Ther* 14:462–477, 1973.

Fekete T, Rub D, Bogdan E: Absence of respiratory arrhythmia: A possible symptom of cardiac autonomic neuropathy in diabetes mellitus. *Diabetologia* 12:390, 1976.

Feldman R: Oral hypoglycemic agents. *N Eng J Med* 297:394, 1977.

Feldman R, Crawford D, Elashoff R, Glass A: Progress report on the prophylactic use of oral hypoglycemic drugs in asymptomatic diabetes: Neurovascular studies, in Camerini-Davalos RA, Cole HS (eds): *Vascular and Neurological Changes in Early diabetes*. New York, Academic Press, 1973, p 557–573.

Feldman R, Crawford D, Elashoff R, Glass A: Long-term oral hypoglycemic drug prophylaxis in chemical diabetes, in Bajaj JS (ed): *Current Topics in Diabetes Research.* Proc 9th Congr of Int Diab Fed, India, Series 400, 1976, p 88.

Feldman R, Sender AJ, Sieglelaub AB: Difference in diabetic and nondiabetic fat distribution patterns by skinfold measurements. *Diabetes* 18:478–486, 1969.

Felig P: Pathophysiology of diabetes, in Sussman KE, Metz RJS (eds): *Diabetes Mellitus,* ed 4. New York, Committee on Prof Educ, Amer Diab Assoc, 1975, p 1–8.

Felig P, Wahren J: The liver as site of insulin and glucagon action in normal, diabetic and obese humans. *Isr J Med Sci* 11:528–539, 1975.

Fernando HM: Comments on diabetes in Ceylon. *Br Med J,* October 1907, p 1060.

Fernando RE: Diabetics survey among Filipinos: A one-year study involving 3,638 subjects. *J Philipp Med Assoc* 41(suppl):946–953, 1965.

Fernando RE: Frequency and sex distribution of complications among Filipino diabetics. *J Philipp Med Assoc* 43:603, 1967.

Ferrier TM: Radiologically demonstrable arterial calcification in diabetes mellitus. *Aust NZ J Med* 13:222–228, 1964.

Ferrier TM: Comparative study of arterial disease in amputated lower limbs from diabetics and nondiabetics with special reference to feet arteries. *Med J Aust* 1:5–11, 1967.

Fine J: Glucose content of normal urine. *Br Med J* 1:1209–1214, 1965.

Finkelstein S, Zeller E, Walford RL: No relation between HL-A and juvenile diabetes. *Tissue Antigens* 2:74–77, 1972.

Finlay-Jones RA, McComish MJ: Prevalence of diabetes mellitus in Aboriginal lepers: The Derby Survey. *Med J Aust* 2:135–137, 1972.

FitzGerald MG, Keen H: Diagnosis classification of diabetes. *Br Med J* 1:1568, 1964.

FitzGerald MG, Malins MJ, O'Sullivan DJ: The prevalence of diabetes in women 13 years after bearing a big baby. *Lancet* 1:1250–1252, 1961.

FitzGerald MG, Malins JM, O'Sullivan DJ, Wall M: The effect of sex and parity on the incidence of diabetes mellitus. *J Med* 30:57, 1961a.

Fiser RH, Bray GA, Sperling MA, et al: The studies on the mechanisms of insulin resistance in childhood obesity. *Pediatr Res* 8:158, 1974.

Fitz R, Murphy WP: The cause of death in diabetes mellitus. *Am J Med Sci* 168:313–325, 1924.

Fleeson WP, Wenk RE: Pitfalls of mass chemical screening. *Postgrad Med* 48:59–64, 1970.

Flint A: *Principles and Practice of Medicine* ed 2. (revised). Philadelphia, Henry G Lea Publishers, 1867, p 759.

Florence E, Quarterman J: The effectsof age, feeding pattern and sucrose on glucose tolerance, and plasma free fatty acids and insulin concentrations in the rat. *J Nutr* 28:63–74, 1972.

du V Florey C, Lowy C, Uppal S: Serum insulin levels in school children aged 9–12 in Westland, Holland. *Diabetologia* 12:313–317, 1976.

du V Florey C, McDonald H, McDonald J, Miall WEL: The prevalence of diabetes in rural population of Jamaican adults. *Int J Epidemiol* 1:157–166, 1972.

471

du V Florey C, McDonald H, Miall WE, Milner RDG: Serum lipids and their relation to blood glucose and cardiovascular measurements in a rural population of Jamaican adults. *J Chron Dis* 26:85–100, 1973.

Folin O, Wu H: Simplified and improved method for determination of sugar. *J Biol Chem* 41:367–374, 1920.

Ford MJ: Program of diabetes demonstration unit in Jacksonville and DuVal County. *J Fla Med Assoc* 35:416, 1949.

Ford S Jr, Bozian RD, Kowles HC Jr: Interactions of obesity and glucose and insulin levels in hypertriglyceridemia. *Am J Clin Nutr* 21:904–910, 1968.

Forman DT, Grayson SH, Slonicki A: Evaluation of reagent strip reflectance meter serum glucose method. *Lab Med* 3:26–29, 1972.

Forrest JM, Menser MA, Burgess JA: High frequency of diabetes mellitus in young with congenital rubella. *Lancet* 2:332, 1971.

Forster H: Dosage in oral glucose tolerance tests, in Gutsche H, Holler HD (eds): *Diabetes Epidemiology in Europe*. Stuttgart, George Thieme, 1975, p 43–47.

Forster H, Haslbeck M, Geser CA, Mehnert H: Blood glucose and serum insulin after oral administration of glucose and starch syrup in various doses. *Diabetologia* 6:73, 1970.

Forster H, Haslbeck M, Mehnert H: Metabolic studies following the oral ingestion of different doses of glucose. *Diabetes* 21:1102–1108, 1972.

Forsyth CC, Payne WW: Free diets in the treatment of diabetic children. *Arch Dis Child* 31:245–253, 1956.

Foster GL: Studies on carbohydrate metabolism. *J Biol Chem* 55:291–301, 1923.

Foster SJ: Diabetes mellitus—a study of the disease in the cat and dog in Kent. *J Small Anim Pract* 16:295–315, 1975.

Fox JR: The incidence of diabetes mellitus and glycosuria in 19,358 college students. *Lancet* 72:479–481, 500, 1952.

Franckson FRM, Conard V, Bastenie PA: Measurement of the free glucose diffusion space in man by the rapid intravenous glucose tolerance test. *Acta Endocrinol* 32:463, 1959.

Franckson RM, Ooms HA, Bellens R, Conard V, Bastenie PA: Physiologic significance of the intravenous glucose tolerance test. *Metabolism* 11:482, 1962.

François R, Hermier M, Jurlot B, et al: Occurrence of diabetes in infants less than one year old, in *Diabetes in Juveniles*. International Beilinson Symposium on Various Phases of Diabetes in Juveniles, Jerusalem, 1972, p 60–66.

Fraser R: Discussion on retinopathy and acromegaly, in Camerini-Davalos RA, Cole HS (eds): *Vascular and Neurological Changes in Early Diabetes*. New York, Academic Press, 1973, p 265–266.

Fraser R, Lowry C, Elkeles RS, Lewis B, Mancini M: Insulin, glucose and lipid levels in mild diabetics in relation to complications, in Camerini-Davalos RA, Cole HS (eds): *Vascular and Neurological Changes in Early Diabetes*. New York, Academic Press, 1973, p 83.

Fredman H: Somatotypes in a group of Tamil diabetics. *S Afr Med J* 46:1836–1837, 1972.

Fredrickson DS: Hyperlipoproteinemia with carbohydrate intolerance, in Sussman KE, Fajans SS (eds): *Diabetes Mellitus: Diagnosis and Treatment,* vol 3. New York, Comm on Prof Educ, Amer Diab Assoc, 1971, p 377–382.

Freedman LR, Blackard WG, Sagan LA, et al: The epidemiology of diabetes mellitus in Hiroshima and Nagasaki. *Yale J Biol Med* 37:283–299, 1965.

Freeman HJ, Weinstein WM, Shnitka TK, et al: Alpha$_1$-antitrypsin deficiency and pancreatic fibrosis. *Ann Intern Med* 85:73–76, 1976.

Freeman N, Looney JM, Hoskins RG: Spontaneous variability of oral glucose tolerance. *J Clin Endocrinol Metab* 2:431, 1941.

Freis ED: Salt, volume and the prevention of hypertension. *Circulation* 53:589–596, 1976.

Frias JL, Rosenbloom AL: The genetics of diabetes. *Metabolism* 22:355–358, 1973.

Friedman GD: *A Primer of Epidemiology.* New York, McGraw Hill Book Co, 1974.

Friedman JM: Inheritance of susceptibility to histocompatibility-associated disease. *Lancet* 1:49, 1976.

Froesch ER, Renold AE: Specific enzymatic determination of glucose in blood and urine using glucose oxidase. *Diabetes* 5:1–5, 1956.

Frohman LA, Doeblin TD, Emerling FG: Diabetes in the Seneca Indians. *Diabetes* 18:36–43, 1969.

Fromantin M, Beccuau M, Duriez R, Rottembourg J: An appraisal of the diabetic population in 20 year old people: Results of a survey in 100,000 young males. Taille et structures de la population diabetique a 20 ans. *Le Diabete* 19:81–85, 1971.

Fry AJ: The effect of a "sucrose free" diet on oral glucose tolerance in man. *Nutr Metabol* 14:314–323, 1972.

Fukuda M: Prognosis of diabetic retinopathy. *Acta Soc Ophthalmol Jpn* 76:184–193, 1972.

Fukuda M: Natural history of diabetic retinopathy and its treatment in Japan, in Baba S, Goto Y, Fukui I (eds): *Diabetes Mellitus in Asia.* Proc 2nd Symposium Kyoto, Amsterdam, Excerpta Medica, Series 390, 1975, p 225–231.

Fukui I, Masaki K, Fujita Y, Takahata J: Serum lipid levels and fatty acid patterns in Japanese diabetic patients, in Tsuji S, Wada M (eds): *Diabetes Mellitus in Asia.* Proc symp, Kobe, Japan, May 1970, Amsterdam, Excerpta Medica, p 130–135.

Fuller JH, McCartney P, Colwell LM: Blood sugar as a predictor for coronary heart disease. *Diabetologia* 11:343, 1975.

Fung WP, Aw EE, Khoo TT: Chronic pancreatitis in Asian patients in Singapore. *Med J Aust* 1:653, 1970

Furth-Wien E von: Morbiditat und mortalitat bei diabetes. *Munch Med Wochenschr* 83:1259–1261, 1936.

Futcher TB: Diabetes mellitus (Part 9. Constitutional Diseases), in Osler W, (ed): *Modern Medicine—Its Theory and Practice,* vol 1. Philadelphia and New York, Lea Brothers and Co, 1907, p 747–798.

Gabbay KH: The sorbitol pathway and the complications of diabetes. *N Engl J Med* 288:831–836, 1973.

473

Gabbe SG: Congenital malformations in infants of diabetic mothers. *Obstet Gynecol Surv* 32:125–132, 1977.

Gabbe SG, Mestman JH, Freeman RK, et al: Management and outcome of Class A diabetes mellitus. *Am J Obstet Gynecol* 127:465–469, 1977.

Galen RS, Gambino SR: Beyond normality: The predictive value and efficiency of medical diagnosis. New York, John Wiley and Sons, 1975, p 115–119.

Gamble DR: Epidemiological and virological observations on juvenile diabetes. *Postgrad Med J* 50:538–543, 1974.

Gamble DR, Nelson PG, Pyke DA: Diabetes and virus infection. *Lancet* 2:1509, 1974.

Gamble DR, Taylor KW: Seasonal incidence of diabetes mellitus. *Br Med J* 3:631–633, 1969.

Gamble DR, Taylor KW: Epidemiological background to diabetes. *Acta Endocrinol* 83 (suppl):161–166, 1976.

Gamble DR, Taylor KW, Cumming H: Coxsackie viruses and diabetes mellitus. *Br Med J* 4:260–262, 1972.

Ganda OP, Gleason RE: Hypertriglyceridemia: A frequent concomitant of "abnormal" glucose tolerance in non-obese adults. *Diabetes* 26(suppl 1):398, 1977.

Ganda OP, Marble A: Report of workgroup on ketoacidosis or coma of National Commission on Diabetes, vol 3, part 2. Dept of HEW publ (NIH) 76-1022, 1976, p 88–97.

Garcia ML, McNamara PM, Gordon T, Kannel WB: Morbidity and mortality in diabetics in Framingham population: Sixteen year followup study. *Diabetes* 23:105–111, 1974.

Gates EW: Diagnosis of undetected diabetes—report of a study of a group of 1,800 individuals. *Indust Med* 11:387, 1942.

Gebhardt C, Garnett R: Drugs affecting carbohydrate metabolism, in Sussman KE, Metz RJS (eds): *Diabetes Mellitus,* ed 4. Comm on Prof Educ, Am Diab Assoc, 1975, p 271–276.

Geevarghese PJ: *Pancreatic Diabetes.* Bombay, Popular Prakashan, 1968.

Geevarghese PJ: Differentiation of pancreatic and maturity-onset diabetes: A comparative study. *Madhumeh* 9:97, 1969.

Geevarghese PJ: Pathogenesis of tropical pancreatic diabetes, in Bajaj JS (ed): *Current Topics in Diabetes Research.* Proc 9th Congr of Int Diab Fed, India, Series 400, 1976, p 191.

Geevarghese PJ, Pillai VK, Joseph NP, et al: The diagnosis of pancreatogenous diabetes mellitus. *J Assoc Physicians India* 10:173, 1962.

Geevarghese PJ, Pitchumoni CS: Pancreatic diabetes in Kerala, in Patel JC, Talwalker NG (eds): *Diabetes in the Tropics.* Bombay, Diab Assoc of India, 1966, p 223–229.

Geevarghese PJ, Pitchumoni CB, Ramachandren N: Is protein malnutrition an initiating cause of pancreatic calcification? *J Assoc Physicians India* 17:417, 1969.

Geiger E: Nutritional problems connected with diabetes mellitus. *J Am Diet Assoc* 28:905–911, 1952.

Gelfand M: *Diet and Tradition in an African Culture.* Edinburgh and London, E & S Livingstone, 1971.

Gelfand M, Forbes JI: Diabetes mellitus in the Rhodesian African. *S Afr Med J* 97:1208–1213, 1953.

Gellman DD, Pirani CC, Soothill JF, et al: Diabetic nephropathy: A clinical and pathologic study based on renal biopsies. *Medicine* 38:321, 1959.

Gensler SW, Haimovici H, Hoffert P, et al: Study of vascular lesions in diabetic, nondiabetic patients. *Arch Surg* 91:617, 1961.

Genuth SM: Plasma insulin responses to an oral carbohydrate solution. *Diabetes* 18:434–436, 1969.

Genuth SM: Effect of high fat vs. high carbohydrate feeding on the development of obesity in weanling ob/ob mice. *Diabetologia* 12:155–159, 1976.

Genuth SM, Houser HB, Carter JR, et al: Community screening for diabetes by blood glucose measurement: Results of a five-year experience. *Diabetes* 25:1110–1117, 1976.

George PK, Banks PA, Pai KN: Exocrine pancreatic function in calcific pancreatitis in India. *Gastroenterology* 60:858, 1971.

Gepts W: Pathologic anatomy of the pancreas in juvenile diabetes mellitus. *Diabetes* 14:619–633, 1965.

Gepts W, Toussaint D: Spontaneous diabetes in dogs and cats: A pathological study. *Diabetologia* 3:249–265, 1967.

Gerard MJ, Klatsky AL, Siegelaub AB, et al: Serum glucose levels and alcohol-consumption habits in a large population. *Diabetes* 26:780–785, 1977.

German JL: The glucose tolerance test after cortisone administration in obese and nonobese men. *Diabetes* 7:261, 1958.

Gerritsen GC: Experimental prevention of diabetes in prediabetics: Studies of Chinese hamsters. *Compr Ther* 1:25–29, 1975.

Gerritsen GC: The role of nutrition to diabetes in relation to age, in Rockstein M, Sussman ML (eds): *Nutrition, Longevity and Aging*. Proc of a symposium on nutrition, longevity and aging, Miami, 1976. New York, Academic Press Inc, 1976, p 229–252.

Gerritsen GC, Blanks MD, Frankel BJ, Grodsky GM: Amelioration of ketonuria in Chinese hamsters by reduction of dietary fat. *Diabetes* 25(suppl 1):345, 1976.

Gerritsen GC, Blanks MC, Miller RL, et al: Effect of diet limitation on the development of diabetes in prediabetic Chinese hamsters. *Diabetologia* 10:559–565, 1974.

Gerritzen FM: The course of diabetic retinopathy: A longitudinal study. *Diabetes* 22:122–128, 1973.

Gerson CD: Glucose and intestinal absorption in man, in Floch MH (ed): *Comments in Gastroenterology. Am J Clin Nutr* 24:1393–1398, 1971.

Ghilchik MW, Morris AS: Insulin response to glucose in patients with peripheral vascular disease, arteritis and Raynaud's disease phenomenon. *Lancet* 2:1229–1231, 1971.

Gibbs GE, Wilson RB, Gifford H: Glomerulosclerosis in the long-term Alloxan diabetic monkey. *Diabetes* 15:258–261, 1966.

Gibson T, Jarrett RJ: Diurnal variation in insulin sensitivity. *Lancet* 2:947–948, 1972.

475

Gilbert JAL, Dunlop DM: Diabetic fertility, maternal mortality, and foetal loss rate. *Br Med J* 1:48, 1949.

Gillman DD, Pirani CL, Soothill JF, et al: Diabetic nephropathy: A clinical and pathologic study based on renal biopsies. *Medicine* 38:321, 1959.

Gillum RF, Feinleib M, Margolis JR, et al: Community surveillance for cardiovascular disease: The Framingham cardiovascular disease survey. Some methodological problems in the Community study of cardiovascular disease. *J Chron Dis* 29:289–299, 1976.

Gilly R, Dutruge J, Noiret A, Charvet F, et al: Infant diabetes. *Arch Fr Pediatr* 19:995, 1972.

Ginsberg H, Mok H, Grudy S, Zeck L: Increased production of very low density lipoproteintriglyceride (VLDL-TG) in insulin-deficient (ID) diabetics. *Diabetes* 26(suppl 1):399, 1977.

Giza T, Fedecyko D, Pietrzykowa B: Tongue surface test as a screening procedure for diabetes mellitus. *Diabetes* 15:58, 1966.

Glasgow JL, Bonar JR, Tucker TS, Hoskins B: Diabetes induced by Vacor rat-killer. *Diabetes* 25(suppl 1):345, 1976.

Gleason RE, Kahn CB, Funk IB, et al: Seasonal distribution of juvenile diabetes (JD): Onset in Massachusetts, 1964–1973. *Diabetes* 26(suppl 1):399, 1977.

Glogner P, Durr F: Suchaktion auf diabetes und nephropathien. *Dtsch Med Wochenschr* 89:2081, 1964.

Glueck CJ, Tsang R, Fallat R: Familial hypertriglyceridemia: Studies in 130 children and 45 siblings of 36 index cases. *Metabolism* 22:1287–1309, 1973.

Goldberg L, Luft R: A comparison of oral and intravenous dextrose tolerance tests in healthy subjects. *Acta Med Scand* 132:201, 1948.

Goldberg MD, Marine N, Ribiero F, et al: Prevalence of glycosuria and diabetes among Indians and Bantu. *S Afr Med J*, June 1969, p 733–738.

Goldberger J: The etiology of pellagra: The significance of certain epidemiological observations with respect thereto. *Public Health Rep* 29:1683, 1914.

Goldberger J, Wheeler GA: The experimental production of pellagra: A test of diet among institutional inmates. *Public Health Rep* 30:3117, 1915.

Goldbourt U, Medalie JH, Neufeld HN: Clinical myocardial infarction over a five-year period: III. A multivariate analysis of incidence. The Israel ischemic heart disease study. *J Chron Dis* 28:217–237, 1975.

Goldman JA: Glucose tolerance in mothers of offspring with congenital malformation. *Isr J Med Sci* 10:1434–1437, 1974.

Goldman JA, Schechter A: Effect of cigarette smoking on glucose tolerance in pregnant women. *Isr J Med Sci* 3:561–564, 1967.

Goldner MG: The fate of the second leg in the diabetic amputee. *Diabetes* 9:100–103, 1969.

Goldner MG, Knatterud GL, Prout TE: Effects of hypoglycemic agents on vascular complications in patients with adult-onset diabetes: III. Clinical implications of UGDP results. *JAMA* 218:1400–1410, 1971.

476

Goldstein DE, Drash AL, Blizzard RM: Diabetes mellitus: the incidence of circulating antibodies against thyroid, gastric and adrenal tissue. *J Pediatr* 77:304–306, 1970.

Goldstein ME, Schein CJ: Significance of biliary tract disease in the diabetic—its unique features. *Am J Gastroenterol* 39:630–634, 1963.

Gomez F, Jequier E, Chabot V, et al: Carbohydrate and lipid oxidation in normal human subjects: Its influence on glucose tolerance and insulin response to glucose. *Metabolism* 21:381–391, 1972.

Good CS (ed): *The Principles and Practice of Clinical Trials* (symposium, London, 1976). New York, Churchill Livingstone, 1977.

Goodale F, Daoud AS, Florentin R, et al: Chemico-anatomic studies of arteriosclerosis and thrombosis in diabetics: 1. Coronary arterial wall thickness, thrombosis and myocardial infarcts in autopsied North Americans. *Exp Pathol* 1:353–363, 1962.

Goodall JWD, Pilbeam STHH: Diabetes in Nyasaland (Malawi). *Trans R Soc Trop Med Hyg* 58:575–578, 1964.

Goodkin G: How long can a diabetic expect to live? *Nutrition Today* May/June, 1971, 21–29.

Goodkin G: Mortality factors in diabetes. *J Occup Med* 17:716–721, 1975.

Goodkin G, Wolloch LB: Longevity of diabetic. *J Occup Med* 11:522–532, 1969.

Goodkin G, Wolloch L, Gottcent RA, Reich F: Diabetes: A twenty-year mortality study. *Trans Assoc Life Ins Med Dir Am* 58:217–271, 1975.

Goodman MJ: Maternal diabetes and congenital malformations among live births in Hawaii. *Acta Diabetol Lat* 13:99–106, 1976.

Goodman MJ, Chung CS: Diabetes mellitus: Discrimination between single locus and multifactorial models of inheritance. *Clin Genet* 8:66–74, 1974.

Goodman MJ, Chung CS, Gilbert F: Racial variation in diabetes mellitus in Japanese and Caucasians living in Hawaii. *J Med Genet* 11:328–334, 1974.

Gordon T: Further mortality experience among Japanese Americans. *Public Health Rep* 82:973–984, 1967.

Gordon T, Castelli WP, Hjortland MC, et al: Predicting coronary heart disease in middle-aged and older person. *JAMA* 238:497–499, 1977.

Gordon T, Castelli WP, Hjortland MC, Kannel WB, Dawber TR: Diabetes, blood lipids, and the role of obesity in coronary heart disease risk for women. The Framingham study. *Ann Int Med* 87:393–397, 1977.

Gordon T, et al: Glucose tolerance of adults, United States 1960–62, diabetes prevalence and results of glucose tolerance tests by age and sex, vital and health statistics, Series 11, No. 2. US Government Printing Office, 1964.

Gordon T, Garcia-Palmieri MR, Kagan A, Kannel WB, Schiffman J: Differences in coronary heart disease in Framingham, Honolulu and Puerto Rico. *J Chron Dis* 27:329–344, 1974.

Gordon T, Kagan A, Rhoads G: Relative weights in different populations, letters to the editor. *Am J Clin Nutr* 28:304–309, 1975.

Gordon T, Kannel WB: Premature mortality from coronary heart disease: The Framingham study. *JAMA* 215:1617–1625, 1971.

Gordon T, Kannel WB: The Framingham study: Predisposition to atherosclerosis in the head, heart and legs. *JAMA* 221:661–666, 1972.

Gore JK: A world's war against disease. Read before the 21st Annual Convention of the Association of Life Insurance Pres, Statistical Section of Betterment of Life Insurance Service, New York, 1927. p 40.

Gorwitz K, Thompson T, Howen GG: The prevalence of diabetes in school-age children. *Diabetes* 25:122–127, 1976.

Goschke H: Mechanism of glucose intolerance during fasting: differences between lean and obese subjects. *Metabolism* 26:1147–1148, 1977.

Gossain VV, Ahuja MMS: Dietetic analysis and blood lipids, chemical and isotopic studies in vascular disease among Indian diabetics. *Am J Clin Nutr* 20:834, 1967.

Goto Y: Vascular complications in diabetes in Japan, in Bennett PH, Miller M (eds): *Epidemiology of Diabetes.* New York, Academic Press, 1977 (in press).

Goto Y, Fukuhara M: Cause of death in 933 diabetic autopsy cases, abstract. *J Jpn Diabetic Soc* 11:197–206, 1968.

Goto Y, Kato J, Takanami A, Ohneda A: Detection of prediabetes by glucose-tolerance test sensitized by prednisolone. *Lancet* 2:461, 1960.

Goto Y, Maraki T: Statistical observation of diabetic coma in Japan. *Saishin Igaku* 12:118, 1957.

Goto Y, Nakayama Y, Yagi T: Influence of the World War II food shortage on the incidence of diabetes mellitus in Japan. *Diabetes,* March/April 1958, p 133.

Goto Y, Sato SI, Masuda M: Causes of death in 3151 diabetic autopsy cases. *Tohoku J Exp Med* 112:339, 1974.

Goto Y, Toyota T, Masuda M, et al: Vascular complications of diabetic patients in Japan, in Baba S, Goto Y, Fukui I (eds): *Diabetes Mellitus in Asia.* Proc 2nd symp Kyoto, Amsterdam, Excerpta Medica, Series 390, 1975, p 177–192.

Gottlieb MS: Diabetes mellitus in siblings and offspring of matched juvenile and maturity onset probands, abstract. *Diabetes* 22:320, 1973.

Gottlieb MS: The natural history of diabetes: Factors present at time of diagnosis which may be predictive of length of survival. *J Chron Dis* 27:435–445, 1974.

Gottlieb MS, Soeldner JS, Kyner JL, et al: Oral glucose stimulated insulin release in nondiabetic twin siblings of diabetic twins. *Diabetes* 23:684–692, 1974.

Gottstein A, Umber F: Diabetes und drieg. *Dtsch Med Wochenschr* 43:1209, 1916.

Gough WW, Shack MJ, Bennett PH, et al: Evaluation of glucose in the Pima Indians by longitudinal studies. *Diabetes* 19:388, 1970.

Grachev A: Main clinico-pathological data on persons who died of diabetes mellitus in Odessa hospitals from 1945 through 1969. *Vrach Delo* 86:8, 1974.

Grant L, Kyle GC, Teichman A, Mendels J: Recent life events and diabetes in adults. *Psychosom Med* 36:121–127, 1974.

Gray H: Lipoids in 1,000 diabetic bloods with special regard to prognosis. *Am J Med Sci* 168:35–46, 1924.

Greene DA, DeJusus PV, Winegrad AI: Effects of insulin and dietary myoinositol in impaired peripheral motor nerve conduction velocity in acute streptozotocin diabetes. *J Clin Invest* 55:1326–1336, 1975.

Greenhalgh RM, Lewis B, Rosengarten DS, et al: Serum lipids and lipoproteins in peripheral vascular disease. *Lancet* 2:947–950, 1971.

Greenwood BM, Taylor JR: The complications of diabetes in Nigerians. *Trop Geogr Med* 20:1–12, 1968.

Grell GAC: Medical disorders in a small Caribbean island: An analysis of the diseases of adults in Dominica in 1971 and 1973. *Ann Trop Med Parasitol* 70:1–10, 1976.

Greville GD: The intravenous glucose tolerance equation. *Biochem J* 37:17, 1943.

Grey NJ, Goldring S, Kipnis DM: The effect of fasting, diet and actinomycin D on insulin secretion in the rat. *J Clin Invest* 49:881, 1970.

Grey N, Kipnis DM: Effect of diet composition on the hyperinsulinemia of obesity. *N Engl J Med* 285:827–831, 1971.

Griffiths JD, Dymock IW, Davies EW, et al: Occurrence and prevalence of diabetic retinopathy in hemochromatosis. *Diabetes* 20:766–770, 1971.

Griffiths M, Payne PR: Energy expenditure in small children of obese and nonobese parents. *Nature* 260:698–700, 1976.

Grobin W: Progressive deterioration of glucose tolerance in the aged: Mortality in diabetics versus nondiabetics. *Isr J Med Sci* 8:920, 1972.

Grodsky GM, Frankel BJ, Gerich JE, Gerritsen GC: The diabetic Chinese hamster: In vitro insulin and glucagon release, the "chemical diabetic", and the effect of diet on ketonuria. *Diabetologia* 10:521–528, 1974.

Grönberg A: Osteopathia diabetica. *Klinik och terapi Nord Med* 75:10, 283–284, 1966.

Grönberg A: Diabetic osteopathy. *Diabetes* 15:534–535, 1966a.

Grönberg A, Larsson T, Jung J: Diabetes in Sweden: A clinico-statistical epidemiological and genetic study of hospital patients and death certificates. *Acta Med Scand* 477(suppl):1–275, 1967.

Groothof G, Du Plessis JP, Versluis EE, et al: Biochemical aspects of a study of 100 obese white subjects. *S Afr Med J* 49:893–897, 1975.

Grote LR: Public Health provisions for the diabetic. *J State Med* 39:732–737, 1931.

Grunnet ML: Cerebrovascular disease: Diabetes and cerebral atherosclerosis. *Neurology* 13:486–491, 1963.

Gsell O: Epidemiologie des diabetes. *Dtsch Med Wochenschr* 93:2446–2450, 1968.

Guest GM: "Unrestricted Diet" in the treatment of juvenile diabetes. *J Am Diet Assoc* 23:299–303, 1947.

Guest GM: Infantile diabetes mellitus: 3 cases in successive siblings, two with onset at 3 months of age and one at 9 days of age. *J Dis Child* 75:461, 1948.

Guidotti L, Gelfand M: Frequency of diabetes mellitus in Mtoko. *Cent Afr J Med* 22:28–29, 1975.

Gundersen E: Is diabetes of infectious origin? *J Infect Dis* 41:197, 1927.

Gupta DS, Whitehouse FW: Significance of the flat oral glucose tolerance test in Henry JB (ed): *Laboratory Medicine. Postgrad Med* 49, March 1971, 55–59.

Gupta OP, Dave ML, Rawal YM, et al: A study of the prevalence of diabetes mellitus, by means of a house-to-house survey in Ahmedabad (Gujarat), India, in Tsuji S, Wada M: *Diabetes Mellitus in Asia*. Proc Symp of Int Diab Fed, Kobe, 1970. Amsterdam, Excerpta Medica, 1971, p 6–10.

Gupta OP, Dave SK, Gupta PS, Hegde HS, et al: Aetiological factors in the prevalence of diabetes in urban and rural populations in India, in Baba S, Goto Y, Fukui I (eds): *Diabetes Mellitus in Asia.* Kyoto. Amsterdam, Excerpta Medica, Series 390, p 23–24.

Guralnick L: Some problems in the use of multiple causes of death. *J Chron Dis* 19:969, 1966.

Guthrie RA, Guthrie DW, Holland E, Jackson RL: Growth rates in children with diabetes mellitus, in Bajaj JS (ed): *Current Topics in Diabetes Research.* Proc 9th Congr of Int Diab Fed, India, Series 400, 1976, p 83.

Guthrie RA, Guthrie DW, Murthy DYN, et al: Standardization of the oral glucose tolerance test and criteria for diagnosis of chemical diabetes in children. Metabolism 22:275–282, 1973.

Gutsche H, Holler HD (eds): *Diabetes Epidemiology in Europe.* Stuttgart, Georg Thieme, 1975.

Hackel DB, Frohman L, Mikat E, et al: Effect of diet on the glucose tolerance and plasma insulin levels of the sand rat (Psammomys Obesus). *Diabetes* 15:105–114, 1966.

Hadden DR, Harley JMG: Potential diabetes and the foetus: A prospective study of the relation between maternal oral glucose tolerance and foetal result. *Br J Obstet Gynaecol* 74:669–674, 1967.

Hadden DR, Boyle D, Montgomery DA, Weaver JA: Risk factors for myocardial infarction in maturity-onset diabetes mellitus. *Practitioner* 210:655–660, 1973.

Hadden DR, Conley JH, Montgomery DAD, et al: Coxsackie B virus neutralization tests in newly diagnosed diabetic patients: A negative report. *Diabetologia* 9:70–71, 1973.

Hadden DR, Harley JMG, Kajtar TJ, Montgomery DA: A prospective study of three tests of glucose tolerance in pregnant women selected for potential diabetes with reference to the foetal outcome. *Diabetologia* 7:87–93, 1971.

Hadden DR, Montgomery DAD, Weaver JA: Myocardial infarction in maturity-onset diabetics. *Lancet* 1:335–338, 1972.

Haddock DR: Diabetes mellitus and its complications in Dar Es Salaam. *East Afr Med J* 41:145, 1964.

Haddock L, Villavicenio E, Morales P: The oral glucose tolerance test in a normal adult population, in Rodriguez RR, Vallance-Owen J(eds):*Diabetes.* Proc 7th Congr of Int Diab Fed, Buenos Aires, Series 209, 1970, p 58.

Haerer AF, Woosley PC: Prognosis and quality of survival in a hospitalized stroke population from the south. *Stroke* 6:543–548, 1975.

Hagbard L: The prediabetic period and obstetrics. *Acta Obstet Gynecol Scand* 37:497–518, 1958.

Hagbard L, Oslow I, Reinard T: A followup study of 514 children of diabetic mothers. *Acta Paediatr Scand* 48:184, 1959.

Haggard HW, Greenberg LA: The effects of cigarette smoking on blood sugar. *Science* 70:165–166, 1934.

Hagroo AA, Verman NPS, Dalta P, Ajmani NK, Vaishnava H: Observations on lipolysis in ketosis-resistant, growth-onset diabetes. *Diabetes* 23:268, 1974.

Hai VD, Melichar F, Khanh V, Nhu NT: Prevalence of diabetes mellitus in Haiphong (Vietnam Democratic Republic). *Gunma J Med Sci* 14:161–167, 1965.

Haines H, Hackel DB, Schmidt-Nielsen K: Experimental diabetes mellitus induced by diet in the sand rat. *Am J Physiol* 208:297–300, 1965.

Hainline A Jr, Keller DF: An evaluation of the fasting blood-glucose level as an index of abnormal carbohydrate tolerance. *Cleve Clin Q* 31:209–212, 1964.

Haist RE, Campbell J, Best CH: The prevention of diabetes. *N Engl J Med* 223:607–615, 1940.

Hale-White R, Payne WW: The dextrose tolerance curve in health. *Q J Med* 19:393–410, 1926.

Hallpike JF, Claveria LE, Cohen NM: Glucose tolerance and plasma insulin levels in subarachnoid hemorrhage. *Brain* 94:151–164, 1971.

Hambidge KM: Chromium nutrition in man. *Am J Clin Nutr* 27:505–514, 1974.

Hambidge KM, Rodgerson DO: Comparison of hair chromium levels of nulliparous and parous women. *Am J Obstet Gynecol* 103:320, 1969.

Hamby RI, Zoneraich S, Sherman L: Diabetic cardiomyopathy. *JAMA* 229:1749–1754, 1974.

Hamill PVV, Johnston FE, Lameshow S: Height and weight of children: Socioeconomic status. US Dept of HEW Publ (HSM) 73-1601. US National Center for Health Statistics (Series 11, No. 19), October 1972.

Hamilton B, Stein AF: Measurement of intravenous blood sugar curves. *J Lab Clin Med* 27:491, 1942.

Hamman L, Hirschman II: Studies on blood sugar. *Arch Intern Med* 20:761, 1917.

Hamman RF, Bennett PH, Miller M: The effect of menopause on serum cholesterol in American (Pima) Indian women. *Am J Epidemiol* 102:164–169, 1975.

Hamman RF, Miller M: Risk factors in diabetes: An 8-year life table analysis. *Diabetes* 24:434, 1975a.

Hamovici H: Patterns of arteriosclerotic lesions of the lower extremity. *Arch Surg* 95:918, 1967.

Hamwi GJ, Fajans SA, Cahill GF, et al: Classification of genetic diabetes mellitus. Special rep of ADA Comm of Prof Educ. *Diabetes* 16:540, 1967.

Hankin J, et al: Dietary and disease patterns among Micronesians. *Am J Clin Nutr* 23:346–357, 1970.

Hansen AG, Degnbol B: Prevalence of diabetes mellitus among relatives of 187 patients with juvenile diabetes. *Diabetologia* 12:396, 1976.

Hansen KM: The blood sugar in man: Conditions of oscillations, rise and distribution. *Acta Med Scand* 4 (suppl):1–224, 1923.

Hanssen P: Diabetes in Bergen 1925: A study of mortality, causes of death and complications. *Acta Med Scand* 178(suppl):163–179, 1946.

Hansson J: The leg amputee: A clinical followup study. *Acta Orthop Scand* 69(suppl):7–103, 1964.

Harano Y, Shimizu Y, Kim CI, et al: Diabetic exocrine-pancreatopathy: Exocrine pancreatic dysfunction associated with diabetes mellitus, in Bajaj JS (ed): *Current*

Topics in Diabetes Research. Proc 9th Congr of Int Diab Fed, India, Series 400, 1976, 105.

Hardin RC, Jackson RL, Johnston RL, Kelly HG: The development of diabetic retinopathy: Effects of duration and control of diabetes. *Diabetes* 5:397–404, 1956.

Hare PJ: Necrobiosis lipoidica. *Br J Dermatol* 67:365–384, 1955.

Hargreaves ER: The epidemiology of diabetes mellitus. *Public Health* 71:365–370, 1958.

Harkness J: Prevalence of glycosuria and diabetes mellitus: A comprehensive survey in an urban community. *Br Med J* 1:1503–1507, 1962.

Harlan WR, Oberman A, Grimm R, Rosati RA: Chronic congestive heart failure in coronary artery disease: Clinical criteria. *Ann Intern Med* 86:133–138, 1977.

Harrington JT, Garella S, Stilmant MM: Renal failure as the initial manifestation of diabetes mellitus. *Arch Intern Med* 132: 249–251, 1973.

Harris EI: Adverse reactions to oral antidiabetic agents. *Br Med J* 3:29–30, 1971.

Harris HF: A case of diabetes mellitus quickly followed by mumps. *Boston Med Surg J* 140:465–469, 1899.

Harris H, McArthur N: Changes in sex incidence of diabetes mellitus. *Ann Eugen* 16:109, 1951.

Harris S: Hyperinsulinism and dysinsulinism. *JAMA* 83:729–733, 1924.

Harris S: The prevention of diabetes. *Seale Harris Clin Bull* 1:23–24, 1950.

Harrold BP: Diabetic retinopathy and hypertension. *Br J Ophthalmol* 55:225, 1971.

Harrower, ADB: Cardiovascular disease in diabetes mellitus. *Br J of Clin Pract* 31:47–51, 1977.

Harrower ADB, Clarke BF: Experience of coronary care in diabetes. *Br Med J* 1:126–128, 1976.

Hart A, Cohen H: Capillary fragility studies in diabetes. *Br Med J* 2:89–91, 1969.

Harting D, Glenn BB: A comparison of blood sugar and urine sugar determinations for the detection of diabetes. *N Engl J Med* 245:48–54, 1951.

Harvald B, Hauge M: Selection in diabetes in modern society. *Acta Med Scand* 173:459–465, 1963.

Hashimoto T: Clinical prediction of myocardial infarction, Eng. abstract. *Jpn Circ J* 38:683–685, 687–705, 1974.

Hashimoto Y, Okaichi T, Watanabe T, et al: Muscle dystrophy of carp due to oxidized oil and the preventive effect of vitamin E. *Jpn J Smooth Muscle Res* 32:64–69, 1966.

Hatch FE, Watt MF, Kramer NC, et al: Diabetic glomerulosclerosis: A longterm followup study based on renal biopsies. *Am J Med* 31:216–230, 1961.

Hatfield E: Extensified statistics on blindness and vision problems. New York, National Society for Prevention of Blindness, Inc, 1966, p 44–50.

Hathorn M, Gillman T, Campbell GD: Blood lipids, mucoproteins and fibrinolytic activity in diabetic Indians and Africans in Natal: Possible relation to vascular complications. *Lancet* 1:1314–1318, 1961.

Haunz EA, Keranen DC: Clinical interpretation of blood sugar values: A study of Folin-Wu, Somogyi-Nelson, Wilkerson-Heftmann blood sugar determinations in 100 subjects. *Proc Am Diab Assoc* 10:200–216, 1950.

Haunz EA, Keranen DC: Blood sugar methods in clinical medicine. A study of Folin-Wu, Somogyi-Nelson, and Wilkerson-Heftmann blood sugar determinations in 100 subjects. *Lancet* 1:9, 1951.

Havel RJ: Atherosclerosis and diabetes, in Siperstein, et al (eds): *Small Blood Vessel Involvement in Diabetes Mellitus*. Washington, DC, American Institute for Biological Sciences, 1964.

Havelock-Charles R, et al: Discussion on diabetes in the Tropics. *Br Med J*, October 1907, p 1051–1064.

Hawarth JC, Dilling LA: Effect of abnormal glucose tolerance in pregnancy on infant mortality rate and morbidity: A prospective study. *Am J Obstet Gynecol* 122:555–560, 1975.

Hawley TG, Jansen AAJ: Weight, height, body surface and overweight of Fijian adults from coastal areas. *NZ Med J* 74:9–21, 1971.

Hayashi T, Misugi Y, Nagai S: Statistical observations of myocardial infarction in Japanese diabetics, in Baba S, Goto Y, Fukui I (eds): *Diabetes Mellitus in Asia*, Proc 2nd symp Kyoto, Amsterdam, Excerpta Medica, Series 390, 1975, p 208–211.

Hayes TM: Plasma lipoproteins in adult diabetes. *Clin Endocrinol* 1:247–251, 1972.

Hayner NS, Kjelsberg MO, Epstein FH, Francis T Jr: Carbohydrate tolerance and diabetes in a total community, Tecumseh, Michigan: 1. Effect of age, sex, and test conditions on one-hour glucose tolerance in adults. *Diabetes* 14:413–423, 1965.

Hayner NS, Waterhouse AM, Gordon T: The one-hour tolerance test. Vital and Health Statistics series 2, No. 3. Washington, DC, US Govt Printing Office, 1963, p 1–34.

Hayner NS, Waterhouse AM, Gordon T: The one-hour oral glucose tolerance test: Response of middle-aged men to 100 gm and 50 gm doses of glucose given fasting and 1, 2 and 3 hours after a meal. Vital and Health Statistics Series 2, No. 3. Washington, DC, US Govt Printing Office, 1963a.

Hayward RE, Lucena BC: An investigation into the mortality of diabetes. *J Inst Actuaries* 92:286, 1965.

Heaton KW: Food fibre as an obstacle to energy intake. *Lancet* 2:1418–1421, 1973.

Heiberg P, Heiberg KA: Diabetes in Denmark in 1924. *Acta Med Scand* 62:126–130, 1926.

Heimsoth VH, Graffe-Achelis C, Baunach D, et al: Reference values for the urinary glucose concentration of adults, in Bajaj JS (ed): *Current Topics in Diabetes Research*. Proc 9th Congr of Int Diab Fed, India, Series 400, 1976, p 177.

Heinbecker P: Studies on the metabolism of Eskimos. *J Biol Chem* 80:461–475, 1928.

Heinle RA, Levy RI, Frederickson DS, Gorlin R: Lipid and carbohydrate abnormalities in patients with angiographically documented coronary artery disease. *Am J Cardiol* 24:178, 1969.

Heinsalmi P, Heinonen OP: Prevalence of diabetes and results of oral glucose tolerance test (GTT) in the adult population of East Finland. Proc 6th Congr of Int Diab Fed, Stockholm, Series 140, 1967, p 28.

Helmers C: Short and long-term prognostic indices in acute myocardial infarction: A study of 606 patients initially treated in a coronary care unit. *Acta Med Scand* 555(suppl):7–26, 1973.

483

Hendricks DG, Mahoney AW: Glucose tolerance in zinc-deficient rats. *Nutrition* 102:1079–1084, 1972.

Henning R: Swedish co-operative CCU Study: A study of 2008 patients with acute myocardial infarction from 12 Swedish Hospitals with coronary care unit. Part 1. A description of the early stage. Part 2: The short term prognosis. *Acta Med Scand* 586(suppl):7–12, 52–58, 1975; (Part 2, 1–35).

Henningar GR, Cohn RJ, Hartz HD: Nodular glomerulosclerosis: Clinicopathological correlation of 40 advanced cases. *Am J Med Sci* 241:89, 1961.

Herberg L, Coleman DL: Laboratory animals exhibiting obesity and diabetes syndromes. *Metabolism* 26:59–99, 1977.

Herman JB, Medalie JH, Goldbourt U: Diabetes, prediabetes and uricaemia. *Diabetologia* 12:47–52, 1976.

Herman JB, Medalie JH, Goldbourt U: Differences in cardiovascular morbidity and mortality between previously known and newly diagnosed adult diabetics. *Diabetologia* 13:229–234, 1977.

Herman JB, Medalie JH, Kahn HA, et al: Diabetes incidence: A two-year followup of 10,000 men in a survey of ischemic heart disease in Israel. *Diabetes* 19:938–943, 1970.

Herman JB, Mount FW, Medalie JH, et al: Diabetes prevalence and serum uric acid: Observations among 10,000 men in a survey of ischemic heart disease in Israel. *Diabetes* 16:858–868, 1967.

Herzstein J, Dolger H: The fetal mortality in women during the prediabetic period. *Am J Obstet Gynecol* 51:420–422, 1946.

Hesse FGP: Incidence of cholecystitis and other diseases among Pima Indians of Southern Arizona. *JAMA* 170:1789–1790, 1959.

Hierton T, James H: Lower extremity amputation in Uppsala County 1947–1969: Incidence and prosthetic rehabilitation. *Acta Orthop Scand* 44:573–582, 1973.

Higgins ITT, Kannel WB, Dawber TR: The electrocardiogram in epidemiological studies: Reproducibility, validity and international comparison. *Br J Prev Soc Med* 19:53–68, 1965.

Himsworth HP: Diet and the incidence of diabetes mellitus. *Clin Sci Mol Med* 2:117–148, 1935–1936.

Himsworth HP: The influence of diet on the sugar tolerance of healthy men and its reference to certain extrinsic factors. *Clin Sci Mol Med* 2:67, 1935–1936a.

Himsworth HP: Diabetes mellitus: Its differentiation into insulin-sensitive and insulin-insensitive types. *Lancet* 117–120, 1936.

Himsworth HP: The mechanism of diabetes mellitus. *Lancet* 2:171–175, 1939.

Himsworth HP: The syndrome of diabetes mellitus and its causes. *Lancet* 1:465–473, 1949.

Himsworth HP: Diet in the aetiology of human diabetics in the Cause of Diabetes. *Proc Roy Soc Med* 42:323–326, 1949a.

Himsworth HP, Kerr RB: Insulin-sensitive and insulin-insensitive types of diabetes mellitus. *Clin Sci Mol Med* 4:119, 1939.

Himsworth HP, Marshall EM: The diet of diabetics prior to the onset of the disease. *Clin Sci Mol Med* 2:95–115, 1935–36.

Hingston RG, Price AVG: Diabetic surveys in Papua. *Papua New Guinea Med J* 7:33, 1964.

Hinkle LE Jr, Wolf S: The effects of stressful life situations on the concentrations of blood glucose in diabetic and nondiabetic humans. *Diabetes* 1:383, 1952.

Hinkle LE Jr, Wolf S: A summary of experimental evidence relating to life stress to diabetes mellitus. *Mt Sinai J Med NY* 19:537–570, 1952a.

Hirata Y, Mihara T: Principal causes of death among diabetic patients in Japan from 1968–1970, in Baba S, Goto Y, Fukui I (eds): *Diabetes Mellitus in Asia.* Proc 2nd symp Amsterdam, Excerpta Medica, Series 390, 1975, p 91–97.

Hirata Y, Nakamura Y, Kaku M: Characteristics of the treatment of diabetics in Japan, in Tsuji S, Wada M (eds): *Diabetes Mellitus in Asia.* Proc symp May 1970, p 216–220.

Hirohata I: Epidemiologic study of diabetes mellitus: Age distribution at the onset of the disease. *Jpn J Hyg* 24:380–385, 1969.

Hirohata T, MacMahon B, Root HF: The natural history of diabetes: 1. Mortality. *Diabetes* 16:875–881, 1967.

Hirose K: Clinical and pathological features of diabetic nephropathy in Japanese diabetic patients, in Tsuji S, Wada M (eds): *Diabetes Mellitus in Asia.* Proc symp, Amsterdam, Excerpta Medica, 1970, p 177–182.

Hirsch A: Diabetes (vol 2, chronic infective, toxic, parasitic, syptic and constitutional diseases), in *Handbook of Geographical and Historical Pathology* (Creighton, C tr. 2nd German ed). *New Sydenham Soc Pub* 112:642–647, 1885.

Hirsch J: Can we modify the number of adipose cells? *Postgrad Med* 51:83–86, 1972.

Hoet JP: Carbohydrate metabolism during pregnancy. *Diabetes* 3:1, 1954.

Hofeldt FD: Reactive hypoglycemia. *Metabolism* 24:1193–1208, 1975.

Hofeldt FD, Adler RA, Herman RH: Postprandial hypoglycemia. Fact or Fiction? *JAMA* 233:1309, 1975.

Hofeldt FD, Lufkin EG, Hagler L, et al: Are abnormalities in insulin secretion responsible for reactive hypoglycemia? *Diabetes* 23:589–596, 1974.

Hoffer A, Osmond H: *The Chemical Basis of Clinical Psychiatry: 2. Relationship of Schizophrenia to Diabetes Mellitus.* Springfield, Ill, Charles C Thomas Co, 1960, p 238–240.

Hoffman AA, Nelson A, Goss FA: Effects of an exercise program on plasma lipids of senior air force officers. *Am J Cardiol* 20:516–524, 1967.

Hoffman FL: The mortality from diabetes. *Boston Med Surg J* 187:135–137, 1922.

Hofmeister F: Über Resorption und Assimilation der Nahrstoffe. Über den Hugerdiabetes. *Arch Exp Path U Pharm* 26:355, 1889–1890.

Hohe PT: Glucose tolerance testing during gregnancy: Comparison of standard 3-hour glucose tolerance test with a single 2-hr glucose-load test. *Obstet Gynecol* 38:693–696, 1971.

Hollingsworth D: Changing patterns of food consumption in Britain. *Nutr Rev* 32:353–359, 1974.

Hollister LE, Overall JE, Snow HL: Relationship of obesity to serum triglyceride, cholesterol and uric acid, and to plasma-glucose levels. *Am J Clin Nutr* 20:777–782, 1967.

Holme I: Mortality among patients who survived their first myocardial infarction. *J Oslo City Hosp* 26:2–16, 1976.

Holten C, Lundbaek K, Staffeldt I: An investigation of the action of cortisone and prednisone on intravenous glucose tolerance. *Acta Med Scand* 157:257–262, 1957.

Hoogslag W: *Nederlandsch Tijdschr V Geneesk* 2:1934 1922.

Hopkins AH: Studies in the concentration of blood sugar in health and disease as determined by Bang's micromethod. *Am J Med Sci* 149:254–267, 1915.

Horger EC, Miller MC, Conner ED: Relation of large birthweight to maternal diabetes mellitus. *Obstet Gynecol* 45:150–154, 1975.

Horiuchi A, Kitamura S, Tanaka G, et al: Angiopathy of diabetes mellitus in Japan, in Tsuji S, Wada M (eds): *Diabetes Mellitus In Asia*. Proc symp Kobe, 1970, Amsterdam, Excerpta Medica, P 205–212.

Horstmann P: Census of diabetics in Odense County. *Ugeskr Laeger* 112:1437, 1950.

Horstmann P: The annual incidence of diabetes mellitus in a Danish country (Odense). *Diabetologia* 8:364, 1972.

Hoshi M, Kikkawa R, Shigeta Y, Abe H: Estimation of pathological changes from clinico-laboratory data in diabetic nephropathy: Application of canonical correlation analysis in the medical field. *Diabetes* 26(suppl):401, 1977.

Hososake A, Matsuyama T: The incidence of childhood diabetes in the families of Tahata Iron-Manufacturing Company. *J Jpn Diabetic Soc* 9:160–161, 1966.

Houser HB, Mackay W, Verma N, Genuth S: A three-year controlled followup study of persons identified in a mass screening program for diabetes. *Diabetes* 26:619–627 1977.

Houssay BA, Martinez C: Experimental diabetes and diet. *Science* 105:548–549, 1947.

Howard CF Jr: Spontaneous diabetes in Macaca Nigra. *Diabetes* 21:1077–1090, 1972.

Howard CF Jr: Correlations of serum triglyceride and prebetalipoprotein levels to the severity of spontaneous diabetes in Macaca Nigra. *J Clin Endocrinol Metab* 38:856–860, 1974.

Howard CF Jr: Diabetes in Macaca Nigra: Metabolic and histologic changes. *Diabetologia* 10:671–677, 1974a.

Hseueh-Li C, Juei-Hung T, et al: Diabetes mellitus—a clinical analysis of 922 cases. *Chin Med J* 81:511–525, 1962.

Hsu TH, Hsu SH, Chase GA, Bias WB: Intra-HLA recombination frequency in families with juvenile diabetes mellitus. *Diabetes* 26(suppl 1):402, 1977.

Huber AM, Gershoff SN: Effect of zinc deficiency in rats on insulin released from the pancreas. *J Nutr* 103:1739–1744, 1973.

Huff JC, Hierholzer JC, Farris WA: An "outbreak" of juvenile diabetes mellitus: Consideration of a viral etiology. *Am J Epidemiol* 100:277–287, 1974.

Hugh-Jones P: Diabetes in Jamaica. *Lancet* 2:891, 1955.

Hughes RO: Reduced carbohydrate intake in the preparatory diet and the reliability of the oral glucose tolerance test. *Aviat, Space, Environ Med* 46:727–728, 1975.

Humphreys GS, Delvin DG: Insulin and oral therapy in diabetes. *Br Med J* 2:352, 1972.

Hundley JM: Diabetes-overweight: U.S. problem. *J Am Diet Assoc* 32:417–421, 1956.

Hunter PR, Heath H, Bloom A: A clinical comparison between diabetics with no retinopathy after 15 years and severe, deteriorating retinopathy. *Diabetologia* 13:403, 1977.

Hunter PR, Kelsey J, Porter R, et al: The relationship between cutaneous capillary resistance and the severity of hemorrhage in the diabetic retina. *Diabetologia* 5:203, 1960.

Hunziker H: Prevalence of diabetes in Basel. *Schweiz Med Wochenschr* 3:168, 1922.

Hutton WL, Snyder WB, Vaiser A, Siperstein MD: Retinal microangiopathy without associated glucose intolerance. *Trans Am Acad Ophthalmol Otolaryngol* 76:968–980, 1972.

Ibrahim M: Diabetes in East Pakistan. *Br Med J* 1:837–839, 1962.

Ikkos D, Luft R: On the intravenous glucose tolerance test. *Acta Endocrinol* 25:312, 1957.

Imperato PJ, Handelsman MD, Fofana B, Sow O: The prevalence of diabetes mellitus in three population groups in the Republic of Mali. *Trans R Soc Trop Med Hyg* 70:115–158, 1976.

Ingelfinger JA, Bennett MB, Liebow IM, Miller M: Coronary heart disease in the Pima Indians: Electrocardiographic findings and postmortem evidence of myocardial infarction in a population with a high prevalence of diabetes mellitus. *Diabetes* 25:561–565, 1976.

Ingle DJ, Nezamis J: Further study of the specificity of the diabetogenic effect of diethylstilbesterol in the partially depancreatized rat. *Endocrinology* 42:262, 1948.

Inoue M, Sugiyasu K, Moriwaki T: Natural course of diabetic retinopathy estimated by the Theory of Markob process, in Rodriguez RR, Vallance-Owen J (eds): Diabetes. Proc 7th Congr of Int Diab Fed, Buenos Aires, 1970, Series 209, p 132.

Inque S, Frame C, Sperling C, Bray G: Genetic obesity versus experimental obesity: Differences in insulin secretion and sensitivity. *Diabetes* 26(suppl 1):402, 1977.

Ipbuker A, Oker C, Hatemi H, Erkurt R, Biyal F: The epidemiology of diabetes in Turkey. Proc 6th Congr of Int Diab Fed, Stockholm, Series 140, 1967, p 28.

Irsigler K, Veitl V, Ogris E: Body composition, glucose tolerance, serum insulin, and serum lipids in top Austrian sportsmen. *Diabetologia* 12:400, 1976.

Irvine WJ: Classification of idiopathic diabetes. *Lancet* 1:638–642, 1977.

Irvine WJ, Holton DE, Clarke BF: Familial-studies of type-1 and type-II idiopathic diabetes mellitus. *Lancet* 2:325–328, 1977.

Irvine WJ, McCallum CJ, Gray RS, Campbell CJ, et al: Pancreatic islet-cell antibodies in diabetes mellitus correlated with the duration and type of diabetes, coexistent autoimmune disease and HLA type. *Diabetes* 26:138–147, 1977.

Irving EM, Wang I: The effect of previous diet on the glucose tolerance test. *Glasgow Med J* 35: 275–278, 1954.

Ismail, Abdel-aziz: Aetiology of hyperpiesis in Egyptians. *Lancet* 2:275–277, 1928.

Isoda S: Diabetes in children. Nihon Isho Suppan, Kaisha Tokyo 1947. *J Chron Dis* 18:427, 1965.

Israel Journal Medical Science: Apparent rise in mortality from diabetes, editorial in world news section. *Israel J Med Sci* 7:1209–1211, 1971.

487

Iwai T: *Le Diabete Sucre Chez Les Japenais, Tokyo* (tr Le Goff). Paris, Masson et Companie, Editeurs, 1916.

Iwai T: Le Diabete Sucre, tonyo byo, chez les Japanais et son etude comparative avec le diabete observed en Europe et an Amerique. *Arch de Med Exper* 27:1–54, 1916a.

Izumi K, Hoshi M, Shigeta Y, et al: Juvenile unstable diabetes: Its growth and development of vascular complications studies in participants of a summer camp for diabetic children, in Bajaj JS (ed): *Current Topics in Diabetes Research.* Pro 9th Congr of Int Diab Fed, India, Series 400, 1976, p 178.

Jackson RA, Advani V, Perry G: Reproducibility of peripheral metabolism after glucose loading in normal subjects. *Diabetologia* 6:150, 1970.

Jackson RA, Advani U, Perry G, et al: The influence of low-carbohydrate diet on peripheral glucose utilization (dietary diabetes). *Isr J Med Sci* 8:916, 1972.

Jackson RL, Guthrie RA, Murthy DyN, Lang J: The intravenous glucose tolerance test in chemical diabetes. *Metabolism* 22:247–254, 1973.

Jackson WPU: The prediabetic syndrome: Large babies and the prediabetic father. *J Clin Endocrinol* 14:177, 1954.

Jackson WPU: Is pregnancy diabetogenic? *Lancet* 2:1369–1371, 1961.

Jackson WPU: The cortisone glucose tolerance test with special reference to the prediction of diabetes: Diagnosis of prediabetes. *Diabetes* 10:33, 1961a.

Jackson WPU: Effects of pregnancy on glucose tolerance, in *On the Nature and Treatment of Diabetes.* Proc 5th Congr of Int Diab Fed, Series 84, 1965, p 718–721.

Jackson WPU: Diabetes and pregnancy. *Acta Diabetol Lat* 4:1–528, 1967.

Jackson WPU: Diabetes mellitus in different countries and difference races: Prevalence and major features. *Acta Diabetol Lat* 7:361–400, 1970.

Jackson WPU: Diabetes and related variables among the five main racial groups in South Africa: Comparisons from population studies. *Postgrad Med J* 48:391–398, 1972.

Jackson WPU: Epidemiology of diabetes in South Africa, in Bennett PH, Miller M (eds): *Epidemiology of Diabetes.* New York, Academic Press, 1977 (in press).

Jackson WPU, Campbell GD, Goldberg MD, Marine N: Observations on heredity and obesity in the emergence of diabetes. *Diabetologia* 7:405–408, 1971.

Jackson WPU, Campbell GD, Marine N, et al: Triamcinolone-augmented glucose tolerance in offspring of diabetic couples. *Metabolism* 21:807–814, 1972.

Jackson WPU, Goldberg MD, Major V, Campbell GD: Vascular and other diabetes-related disorders among Natal Indian diabetics and nondiabetics. *S Afr Med J* 44:279–285, 1970.

Jackson WPU, Goldberg MD, Marine N, Vinik A: Effectiveness, reproducibility and weight-relation of screening test for diabetes. *Lancet* 2:1101–1105, 1968.

Jackson WPU, Golden C, Marine N: Diabetic-inter-racial comparisons: 2. Retinopathy and heart disease. *S Afr Med J* 40:206–208, 1966.

Jackson WPU, Huskisson JM: Diabetics: Inter-racial comparisons. *S Afr Med J* 39:526–531, 1965.

Jackson WPU, Mieghem W van, Marine N, et al: 1. Diabetes among a Tamilian Indian community in Cape Town: Re-examination after five years. *S Afr Med J* 48:1839–1843, 1974.

Jackson WPU, Vinik AL, Joffe BI, Sacks A, et al: Vicissitudes encountered in a diabetes population study. *S Afr Med J* 44:1283–1287, 1970.

Jacobson TB: Untersuchungen uber den einfluss des Chloralhydrate auf experimentelle Hyperglykamieforemen. *Biochem Z* 51:443–462, 1913.

Jahnke K, Jahnke KA, Reis HE: Regeneration capacity of β-Cell function in obese diabetics after weight reduction. *Dtsch Med Wochenschr* 101:73–76, 1976.

Jaksic Z, Skrabalo Z: Azgreb diabetes survey. Proc 6th Congr of Int Diab Fed, Stockholm, Series 140, 1967.

Jaksic Z, Skrabalo Z: Zagreb diabetes survey. *Diabetologia* 5:366–372, 1969.

James RD, Chase GR: Evaluation of some commonly used semiquantitative methods for urinary glucose and ketone determinations. *Diabetes* 23:474–479, 1974.

James WPT: Food and death-rates from diabetes, letter to the editor. *Lancet* 2:1201–1201, 1974.

James WPT, Cummings JH: Dietary fibre and energy regulation. *Lancet* 1:61–62, 1974.

Janeway TC: The etiology of the diseases of the circulatory system (The Shattuck Lecture). *Boston Med Surg J* 174:925–938, 1916.

Jankelson OM, Beaser SB, Howard FM, et al: Effect of coffee on glucose tolerance and circulating insulin in men with maturity-onset diabetes. *Lancet* 1:527–530, 1967.

Jarrett RJ: Diabetes and the heart: Coronary heart disease. *Clin Endocrinol Metabol* 6:389–402, 1977.

Jarrett RJ, Baker IA, Keen H, Oakley NW: Diurnal variation in oral glucose tolerance: Blood sugar and plasma insulin levels morning, afternoon and evening. *Br Med J* 1:199–201, 1972.

Jarrett RJ, Keen H: Diurnal variation of oral glucose tolerance: A possible pointer to the evolution of diabetes mellitus. *Br Med J* 2:341, 1969.

Jarrett RJ, Keen H: Diurnal variation in oral glucose tolerance: Its degree and significance. *Diabetologia* 6:50, 1970.

Jarrett RJ, Keen H: Cardiovascular disease in diabetes. *Lancet* 1:492–493, 1972.

Jarrett RJ, Keen H: Diabetes and atherosclerosis, in Keen H, Jarrett RJ (eds): *Complications of Diabetes.* London, Edward Arnold Pub Co, 1975, p 179–204.

Jarrett RJ, Keen H: Epidemiology of diabetes, in Sussman KE, Metz RJS (eds): *Diabetes Mellitus* ed 4. Comm on Prof Ed, Amer Diab Assoc, 1975a, p 41–48.

Jarrett RJ, Keen H: Hyperglycaemia and diabetes mellitus. *Lancet* 2:1009–1012, 1976.

Jarrett RJ, Keen H, Boyns DR, Chlouverakis C, Fuller J: The concomitants of raised blood sugar studies in newly-detected hyperglycaemics: 1. A comparative assessment of neurological functions in blood sugar groups. *Guy's Hospital Reports* 118:237–246, 1969.

Jarrett RJ, Keen H. Fuller JH, McCartney M: Controlled trial of phenformin and diet in borderline diabetes, in Bajaj JS: *Current Topics in Diabetes Research.* Proc 9th Congr of Int Diab Fed, India, Series 400, 1976, p 90.

Jarrett RJ, Keen H, Hardwick C: "Instant" blood sugar measurement using dextrostix and a reflectance meter. *Diabetes* 19:724–726, 1970.

Jarrett RJ, Wise PH, Butterfield WJH: The epidemiology of early diabetes, in Camerini-Davalos RA, Cole HS (eds): *Early Diabetes.* New York, Academic Press, 1970, p 359–364.

Jeffrys DB: The effect of dietary fibre on the response to orally administered glucose. *Proc Nutr Soc* 33:11A-12A, 1974.

Jenson WK: The digestive system and diabetes, in Marble A, White P, et al (eds): *Joslin's Diabetes Mellitus,* ed 11. Philadelphia, Lea & Febiger, 1971, p 708–721.

Jivani SKM, Rayner PHW: Does control influence the growth of diabetic children? *Arch Dis Child* 48:109–115, 1973.

Job D, Eschwege E, Guyot-Argento C, Aubry J-P, Tchobroutsky G: Effect of multiple daily insulin injections on the course of diabetic retinopathy. *Diabetes* 25:463–469, 1976.

Job D, Tchobroutsky G, Eschwege E, et al: Relationships between diabetic retinopathy, blood pressure, body weight and serum lipids level. *Diabetologia* 9:74, 1973.

Joffe BI, Goldberg RB, Seftel HC, Distiller LA: Insulin, glucose and triglyceride relationships in obese African subjects. *Am J Clin Nutr* 28:616–620, 1975.

Joffe BI, Jackson WPU, Thomas ME, et al: Metabolic responses to oral glucose in the Kalahari Bushmen. *Br Med J* 4:206–208, 1971.

Johansen K: Different plasma insulin responses to glucose and tolbutamide in young and old people with the same degree of carbohydrate intolerance. *Diabetologia* 6:50, 1970.

Johnsen K: A new principle for the comparison of insulin secretory responses: 2. The effect of obesity on insulin secretion. *Acta Endocrinol* 74:524–541, 1973.

Johansen K: Mild diabetes in young subjects: Clinical aspects and plasma insulin response pattern. *Acta Med Scand* 193:23–33, 1973a.

Johnsen K, Gregersen G: A family with dominantly inherited mild juvenile diabetes. *Acta Med Scand* 210:567–570, 1977.

Johnsen K, Munck O: Correlation between blood glucose/insulin ratio and physical fitness. *Diabetologia* 12:375–428, 1976.

Johansen K, Soeldner JS, Gleason RE: Insulin, growth hormone and glucagon in prediabetes mellitus—a review. *Metabolism* 23:1185–1199, 1974.

Johansen K, Soeldner S, Gleason R, et al: Serum insulin and growth hormone response patterns in monozygotic twin siblings of patients with juvenile-onset diabetes. *N Engl J Med* 293:57–61, 1975.

John HF: A summary of findings in 1100 glucose tolerance estimations. *Endocrinology* 13:388–392, 1929.

John HJ: The diabetic child: Etiologic factors. *Ann Intern Med* 8:198–213, 1934.

John HJ: Statistical study of 6,000 cases of diabetes. *Ann Intern Med* 33:925–940, 1950.

Johnson JE Jr, McNutt CW: Diabetes mellitus in an American Indian population isolate. *Tex Rep Biol Med* 22:110–125, 1964.

Johnson ML, Burke BS, Mayer J: Relative importance of inactivity and over-eating in the energy balance of obese high school girls. *Am J Clin Nutr* 4:37, 1956.

Johnson PC, West KM, Masters F: Albumin binding of chlorpropamide. *Metabolism* 9:1111–1117, 1960.

Johnson TO: Comparative study of screening methods for diabetes mellitus in the elderly Nigerian subject. *West Afr Med J,* June 1971, p 243–246.

Johnson TO: Diabetes mellitus among urban Africans—an epidemiological survey in Lagos, Nigeria. Proc in 8th Congr of Int Diab Fed, Belgium, Series 280, 1973, p 160–161.

Johnston FE, Hamill PVV, Lemeshow S: Skinfold thickness of youths 12–17 years, United States. Dept of HEW Publ (HRA) 74-1614, series 11, No. 132. US Natl Ctr for Hlth Stat, January 1974.

Jolly JG, Sarup BM, Aikat BK: Diabetes mellitus and blood groups. *J Indian Med Assoc* 52:104–107, 1969.

Jonsson A, Wales JK: Blood glycoprotein levels in diabetes mellitus. *Diabetologia* 12:245–250, 1976.

Joplin GF, Wright AD: The detection of diabetes in man, in Dickens F, Randle PJ, Whalen WF (eds): *Carbohydrate Metabolism and Its Disorders,* vol 2. New York, Academic Press, 1968, p 1–24.

Jorde R: *The Diabetes Survey in Bergen, Norway 1956: An Epidemiologic Study of Blood Sugar Values Related to Sex, Age and Weight.* Bergen-Oslo, Norwegian Univ Press, 1962.

Jorde R: The epidemiology of diabetes in Western Europe. in *Diabetes.* Proc 6th Congr of Int Diab Fed, Excerpta Medical 1967, p 669–671.

Jorgensen S: On the differential diagnosis between benign and malignant glycosuria by means of intravenous injections of small quantities of grape sugar. *Acta Med Scand* 58:161–200, 1923.

Jorgensen S, Plum T: Differential diagnosis between benign and malignant glycosuria by means of intravenous injection of small quantities of glucose. *Acta Med Scand* 58:161, 1923.

Joslin EP: *Treatment of Diabetes Mellitus,* ed 1. Philadelphia, Lea & Febiger, 1916.

Joslin EP: *Treatment of Diabetes Mellitus,* ed 2. Philadelphia, Lea & Febiger, 1917, p 17–50.

Joslin EP: The prevention of diabetes mellitus. *JAMA* 76:79–84, 1921.

Joslin EP: *Treatment of Diabetes Mellitus,* ed 3. Philadelphia, Lea & Febiger, 1923.

Joslin EP: Arteriosclerosis and Diabetes. *Ann Clin Med* 5:1061–1079, 1927.

Joslin EP: Discussion of paper of Short JJ, Johnson HJ: Glucose tolerance in relation to weight and age: A study of 541 cases. *Proc of Assoc Life Insur Med Dir Amer* 25:253, 1939.

Joslin EP, Dublin LI, Marks HH: Studies in diabetes mellitus: 1. Characteristics and trends of diabetes mortality throughout the world. *Am J Med Sci* 186:753–773, 1933.

Joslin EP, Dublin LI, Marks HH: Studies in diabetes mellitus: 2. Its incidence and the factors underlying its variations. *Am J Med Sc* 187:433–457, 1934.

Joslin EP, Dublin LI, Marks HH: Studies in diabetes mellitus: 3. Interpretation of the variations in diabetes incidence. *Am J Med Sci* 189:163–192, 1935.

Joslin EP, Dublin LI, Marks HH: Studies in diabetes mellitus: 4. Etiology. *Am J Med Sci* 191:759–775, 1936.

Joslin EP, Dublin LI, Marks HH: Studies in diabetes mellitus: 5. Heredity. *Am J Med Sci* 193:8–23, 1937.

Joslin EP, Lombard HL: Diabetes epidemiology from death records. *N Engl J Med* 214:7–9, 1936.

Joslin EP, Root HF, White P, Marble A: *Treatment of Diabetes Mellitus,* ed 10. Philadelphia, Lea & Febiger, 1959.

Jung Y, Khurana RC, Corredor DG, et al: Reactive hypoglycemia in women: Results of a health survey. *Diabetes* 20:428–434, 1971.

Junker K, Ditzel J: Inaccuracy of test strips with reflectance meter in determination of high blood-sugar. *Lancet* 1:815–817, 1972.

Kadish AH, Sternberg JC: Determination of urine glucose by measurement of oxygen consumption. *Diabetes* 18:467–470, 1969.

Kagan A: Opportunities for studies of cardiorespiratory disease in migrants. *J Chron Dis* 23:335–344, 1970.

Kagan A, Harris BR, Winkelstein W Jr, et al: Epidemiologic studies of coronary heart disease and stroke in Japanese men living in Japan, Hawaii and California: Demographic, physical, dietary and biochemical characteristics. *J Chron Dis* 27:345–364, 1974.

Kagan AR, Sternby NH, Uremura K, et al: Atherosclerosis of the aorta and coronary arteries in 5 towns. *Bull WHO* 53, 1976.

Kageura N: Über den einfluss der Eiweiss-Fettdiat auf den Kohlenhydrastoffwechsel: 1. Mitteilung. *J Biochem* 1:333–389, 1922.

Kahn CB, Soeldner JS, Gleason RE, Royas L, Camerini-davalos RA, Marble A: Clinical and chemical diabetes in offspring of diabetic couples. *N Engl J Med* 281:343, 1969.

Kahn CR, Flier JS, Bar RS, et al: The syndromes of insulin resistance and acanthosis nigricans: Insulin receptor disorders in men. *N Engl J Med* 294:739–745, 1976.

Kahn HA, Bradley RF: Prevalence of diabetic retinopathy. *Br J Ophthalmol* 59:345–349, 1975.

Kahn HA, Herman JB, Medalie JH, et al: Factors related to diabetes incidence: A multivariate analysis of two years observation on 10,000 men. *J Chron Dis* 23:617–629, 1971.

Kahn HA, Leibowitz H, Ganley JP, et al: Standardizing diagnostic procedures. *Am J Ophthalmol* 79:768–775, 1975.

Kahn HA, Leibowitz HM, Ganley JP, et al: The Framingham Eye Study. I. Outline and major prevalence findings. *Am J Epidemiol* 106:17–32, 1977.

Kahn HA, Leibowitz HM, Ganley JP, et al: The Framingham Eye Study. II. Association of ophthalmic pathology with single variables previously measured in the Framingham heart study. *Am J Epidemiol* 106:33–41, 1977.

Kahn HA, Miller R: Blindness caused by diabetic retinopathy. *Am J Ophthalmol* 78:58–67, 1974.

Kahn O: The incidence and significance of gas gangrene in a diabetic population. *Angiology* 25:462–466, 1974.

Kaku M: Dietary effects of the development of diabetes mellitus. *Acta Med* 41:174–191, 1971.

Kalafatic Z: The epidemiology of juvenile diabetes in Croatia, in Gutsche H, Hollen HD (eds): *Diabetes Epidemiology in Europe*. Stuttgart George Thieme, 1975, p 21–26.

Kalant N, Teitelbaum JI, Cooperberg AA: Dietary atheroma in diabetic rats. *Mod Med* 32: 238–242, 1964.

Kalkhoff R, Ferrou C: Metabolic differences between obese overweight and muscular overweight men. *N Engl J Med* 284:1236–1239, 1971.

Kannel WB: Diabetes and cardiovascular disease, the Framingham Study. *Am J Cardiol* 35:147, 1975.

Kannel WB: Coronary risk factors: 1. Recent highlights from the Framingham study. *Aust NZ Med J* 6:373–386, 1976.

Kannel WB, Huortland M, Castelli WP: Role of diabetes in congestive heart failure: The Framingham Study. *Am J Cardiol* 34:29–34, 1974.

Kannel WB, McGee D, Gordon T: A general cardiovascular risk profile: The Framingham Study. *Am J Cardiol* 38:46–51, 1976.

Kaplan MH, Feinstein AR: A critique of methods in reported studies of long-term vascular complications in patients with diabetes mellitus. *Diabetes* 22:160–174, 1973.

Kaplan MH, Feinstein AR: The importance of classifying initial co-morbidity in evaluating the outcome of diabetes mellitus. *J Chron Dis* 27:387–404, 1974.

Kaplan NM: Tolbutamide tolerance test in carbohydrate metabolism. *Arch Intern Med* 107:212, 1961.

Kar BC, Tripathy BB: Clinical observations on a group of young diabetics. *J Assoc Physicians India* 15:9–15, 1967.

Karam JH, Grodsky GM, Forsham PH: Excessive insulin response to glucose in obese subjects as measured by immunochemical assay. *Diabetes* 12:197–204, 1963.

Karam JH, Grodsky GM, Forsham PH: Insulin-resistant diabetes with autoantibodies induced by exogenous insulin. *Diabetes* 18:445, 1969.

Karam JH, Grodsky GM, Forsham PH: Weight gain in infancy and development of juvenile diabetes mellitus. Lancet 1:45, 1976.

Karam JH, Grodsky GM, Pavlatos FC, et al: Critical factors in excessive serum insulin response to glucose: Obesity in maturity-onset diabetes and growth hormone in acromegaly. *Lancet* 1:286–289, 1965.

Karlsson K. Kjellmer I: The outcome of diabetic pregnancies in relation to the mother's blood sugar level. *Am J Obstet Gynecol* 112:213–220, 1972.

Kasi AM: Neonatal diabetes mellitus. *Br Med J* 5417: 1137, 1964.

Kato H, Tillotson J, Nichaman MZ, et al: Epidemiologic studies of coronary heart diseases and stroke in Japanese men living in Japan, Hawaii, and California. *Am J Epidemiol* 97:372–385, 1973.

Kato K: Studies on clinical prediction of myocardial infarction; quantifications of coronary risk factors (author's translation). *Jpn Circ J* 40:1041–1943, 1976.

Kato T, Yasue T, Teshigawara S: Atherosclerotic indices of aortic and coronary arteries in the middle part of Japan (Gifu). English summary of original article written in Japanese. *Jpn Circ J* 38:1013–1031, 1974.

Katsumata K: Studies on the diabetic state of rats fed a high fat diet for 400 days: A postulated mechanism of disturbed carbohydrate metabolism. *Nagoya J Med Sci* 32:261–280, 1970.

Katsumata K: Studies on the dietary factors impairing carbohydrate metabolism of rats. *Nagoya J Med Sci* 33:27–30, 1970a.

Katsumata K, Yamada K: Studies on the relationship between diabetes mellitus and alcohol. Proc 5th Congr Int Diab Fed, Toronto, Series 74, 1964. p 110–111.

Katterman R, Kobberling J: Serum lipids in first degree relatives of diabetes. *Diabetes* 19:952, 1970.

Kaufman BJ, Grant DR, Moorhouse JA: An analysis of blood glucose values in a population screened for diabetes mellitus. *Can Med Assoc J* 100:692, 1969.

Kawa A, Nakazawa M, Sakaguchi S, et al: HLA system in Japanese patients with diabetes mellitus. *Diabetes* 26:591–595, 1977.

Kawate R: Seven-year followup observations on glycosuria and diabetes mellitus in inhabitants of Hiroshima, in Tsuji S, Wada M (eds): *Diabetes Mellitus in Asia*. Proc symp Kobe May 1970, Amsterdam, Excerpta Medica, p 76–82.

Kawate R, Miyanishi M, Nishimoto Y: Prevalence and mortality of diabetes mellitus in Japanese residents on the Island of Hawaii as compared with those in Japan in Baba S, Goto Y, Fukui I (eds): *Diabetes Mellitus in Asia*. Proc 2nd symp Kyoto, Amsterdam, Excerpta Medica, Series 390, p 16.

Kawate R, Miyanishi M, Yamakido M, et al: The prevalence and mortality of diabetes mellitus in Japanese in Japan and on the Island of Hawaii, in Bennett PH, Miller M (eds): *Epidemiology of Diabetes*. New York, Academic Press, 1977 (in press).

Kay RM: Nutrition in the etiology and treatment of diabetes mellitus. *Nutr Rev* 28:97–109, 1974.

Keen H: The Bedford Survey: A critique of methods and findings. *Proc R Soc Med* 57:196–202, 1964.

Keen H: The presymptomatic diagnosis of diabetes. *Proc R Soc Med* 59:1169–1174, 1966.

Keen H: Population screening for diabetes. *Postgrad Med J* (suppl), May 1969, p 49–51.

Keen H: Prevalence of blindness in diabetics. *J R Coll Physicians Lond* 7:53–60, 1972.

Keen H: Glucose tolerance plasma lipids and atherosclerosis. *Proc Nutr Soc* 31:339–345, 1972a.

Keen H: Diabetes and sugar consumption, in Hillebrand SS (ed): *Is the Risk of Becoming Diabetic Affected by Sugar Consumption?* Proc 8th Symp of Int Sugar Res Fed, Bethesda, Maryland, 1974, p 14–17.

Keen H: The incomplete story of diabetes and obesity, in Howard A (ed): *Recent Advances in Obesity Research: 1*. Proceedings of 1st International Congress on Obesity. London, Newman Publishing Ltd, 1974a, p 116–127.

Keen H: Antidiabetic agents and vascular events. *J Clin Pathol* 28(suppl 9):99–105, 1975.

Keen H: Glucose intolerance, diabetes mellitus and atherosclerosis; prospects for prevention. *Postgrad Med J* 52:445–451, 1976.

Keen H, Chlouverakis C, Fuller J, Jarrett RJ: The concomitants of raised blood sugar: Studies in newly-detected hyperglycaemics. 2. Urinary albumin excretion, blood pressure and their relation to blood sugar levels. *Guy's Hosp Rep* 118:247–254, 1969.

Keen H, Jarrett RJ: Modern concepts in the diagnosis of diabetes, in *The New Management of Stable Adult Diabetes*. Springfield, Ill. Charles C Thomas Co, 1969, p 3–30.

Keen H, Jarrett RJ: The effect of carbohydrate tolerance on plasma lipids and atherosclerosis in man, in Jones RJ (ed): *Atherosclerosis. Proc of 2nd Int Symposium*. New York, Springer-Verlag, 1970, p 435–444.

Keen H, Jarrett RJ: Macroangiopathy: Its prevalence in asymptomatic diabetes. *Adv Metab Disord* (suppl 2, 3–9) 1973.

Keen H, Jarrett J: *Complications of Diabetes*. London, Edward Arnold Pub Co, 1975.

Keen H, Jarrett RJ: Complications of diabetes. *Lancet* 2:439, 1975a.

Keen H, Jarrett RJ, Fuller JH: Diet and glucose tolerance in man. *Diabetologia* 10:372, 1974.

Keen H, Jarrett RJ, Thomas B: Sucrose intake and diabetogenesis, in Bajaj JS (ed): *Current Topics in Diabetes Research*. Proc 9th Congr Int Diab Fed, India, Series 400, 1976, p 169.

Keen H, Jarrett RJ, Ward JD, Fuller JH: Borderline diabetics and their response to tolbutamide. *Adv Metab Disord*, suppl 2, 1973, p 521.

Keen H, Rose G, Pyke DA, et al: Blood sugar and arterial disease. *Lancet* 2:505, 1965.

Keen H, Track NS: Age on onset and inheritance of diabetes: The importance of examining relatives. *Diabetologia* 4:317–321, 1968.

Keet JPD, Welborn TA, Stenhouse NS, et al: Evaluation of the "dextrostix" method for estimating blood glucose level in a population survey. *Med J Austr*, 1969, p 973–976.

Keller P, Jackson WPU, Bank S, et al: Plasma-insulin levels in "Pancreatic Diabetes". *Lancet* 2:1211–1213, 1965.

Kellock TD: Birth weight of children of diabetic fathers. *Lancet* 2:1252–1254, 1961.

Kellock TD: Proprietary foods for diabetics. *Nutrition* 20:56–59, 1966.

Kellogg JH: *The Itinerary of a Breakfast*. Battle Creek, Mich, Modern Medicine Publishing Co, 1921.

KEM Hospital Group: Incidence of diabetes, in Patel JC, Talwalker NG (eds): *Diabetes in the Tropics*. Diabetic Assoc of India, Bombay, 1966, p 1 7.

KEM Hospital Group: Vascular complications in 5481 cases of diabetes, in Patel JC, Talwalker NG (eds): *Diabetes in the Tropics*. Bombay, Diab Assoc of India, 1966a, p 352–354.

Kemenetsky SA, Bennett PH, Dippe SE, et al: A clinical and histological study of diabetic nephropathy in the Pima Indians. *Diabetes* 23:61–68, 1974.

Kempner W, Newborg BC, Peschel RL, et al: Treatment of massive obesity with rice/ reduction diet program: An analysis of 106 patients with at least a 45-kg weight loss. *Arch Intern Med* 135:1575–1584, 1975.

Kempner W, Peschel RL, Schlayer C: Effect of rice diet on diabetes mellitus associated with vascular disease. *Postgrad Med* 24:359, 1958.

495

Kenien AG, Hengstenberg FM, Drash A: Lipids in children and adolescents with juvenile diabetes mellitus (JLM). *Diabetes* 26, suppl 1, 1977, p 365.

Kenny AJ, Chute AL: Diabetes in two Ontario communities: Studies in case finding. *Diabetes* 2:187–193, 1953.

Kenny AJ, Chute AL, Best CH: A study of the prevalence of diabetes in an Ontario Community. *Can Med Assoc J* 65:233–241, 1951.

Kent GT, Leonards JR: Mass screening for diabetes in a metropolitan area using finger blood glucose after a carbohydrate load. *Diabetes* 14:295–299, 1965.

Kent GT, Leonards JR: Analysis of tests for diabetes in 250,000 persons screened for diabetes using finger blood after carbohydrate load. *Diabetes* 17:274, 1968.

Kessler II: Cancer mortality among diabetes. *J Natl Cancer Inst* 44:673–686, 1970.

Kessler II: Mortality experience of diabetic patients. *Am J Med* 51:715–724, 1971.

Kessler II, Levin ML: The community as an epidemiologic laboratory: A casebook of Community Studies. Baltimore, Johns Hopkins Univ Press, 1970, p 1–24.

Keys A (ed): Coronary heart disease in seven countries. Circulation (suppl 1)41, 42: 1970.

Keys A, Aravanis C, Blackburn H, et al: Coronary heart disease; overweight and obesity as risk factors. *Ann Intern Med* 77:15, 1972.

Khakpour M, Nikakhtar B: Diabetes mellitus following a mumps epidemic. *J Trop Med Hyg* 78:261–263, 1975.

Khanina EV: Epidemiology of diabetes mellitus in Riga. *Probl Endokrinol (Mosk)*23:17–20, 1977.

Khojandi M, Tsai M, Tyson JE: Gestational diabetes: The dilemma of delivery. *Obstet Gynecol* 48:1–6, 1974.

Khurana RC, White P: Characteristics of patients with more than 40 years of juvenile diabetes: Possible factors for longevity, in Bajaj S (ed): *Current Topics in Diabetes Research.* Proc 9th *Congr* of Int Diab Fed, India, Series 400, 1976, p 105–106.

Kiehm TG, Anderson JW: Reduction in insulin or sulfonylurea requirements in diabetic men treated with high carbohydrate diets. *Diabetes* 25(suppl 1): 345, 1976.

Kikchi S, Shimodaira A, Ito M, Aoyamu S: Study on blood lipids in patients with diabetes in Japan, in Patel JD, Talwalker NG (eds): *Diabetes in the Tropics.* Bombay, Diab Assoc of India, 1966, p 135–137.

Kilo C, Vogler N, Williamson JR: Muscle capillary basement membrane changes related to aging and to diabetes mellitus. *Disease* 21:881, 1972.

Kilpatric JA, Beaven DW, Collins CM, et al: The classification and diagnosis of diabetes mellitus. *NZ Med J* 76:108–110, 1972.

Kim EJ: Diabetes mellitus and its epidemiology in Korea. *J Jpn Diab Soc* 14:25–36, 1971.

Kim EJ: Diabetic retinopathy in Korean diabetics, in Bajaj JS (ed): *Current Topics in Diabetes Research.* Proc 9th Congr of Int Diab Fed, India, Series 400, 1976, p 123.

Kim EJ, Kim KS, Lee TM, Kim DY: Incidence of diabetes mellitus in rural and urban populations in Korea, in Baba S, Goto Y, Fujui I (eds): *Diabetes Mellitus in Asia.* Proc 2nd symp, Kyoto, Amsterdam, Excerpta Medica, Series 390, 1976.

Kimmelstiel P, Wilson G: Intercapillary lesions in the glomeruli of the kidney. *Am J Pathol* 12:83–97, 1936.

Kini MG: Multiple pancreatic calculi with chronic pancreatitis. *Br J Surg* 25:705, 1937–1938.

Kinnear PR, Aspinall PA, Lakowski R: The diabetic eye and colour vision. *Trans Ophthalmol Soc UK* 92:69–78, 1972.

Kinnear TWG: The pattern of diabetes mellitus in a Nigerian teaching hospital. *East Afr Med J* 40:288–294, 1963.

Kipnis DM: Nutrient regulation of insulin secretion in human subjects. Diabetes 21(suppl 2):606–616, 1972.

Kirk RD, Dunn PJ, Smith JR, et al: Abnormal pancreatic alpha-cell function in first-degree relatives of known diabetics. *J Clin Endocrinol Metab* 40:913, 1975.

Kisch EH: Diabetes in the elderly. *JAMA* 44:1038, 1915.

Kitagawa EM, Hauser PM: Education differentials in mortality by cause of death: United States 1960. *Demography* 5:318–353, 1968.

Klatsky AL, Friedman GD, Siegelaub AB, Gerard MJ: Alcohol consumption among white, black, or oriental men and women: Kaiser–Permanente multiphasic health examination data. *Am J Epidemiol* 105:311–323, 1977.

Klimt CR, Canner PL, Jacobs DR, Tominaga S (Coronary Drug Project Research Group): The prognostic importance of plasma glucose levels and of the use of oral hypoglycemic drugs after myocardial infarction in men. *Diabetes* 26:453–465, 1977.

Klimt CR, Meinert CL, Miller M, et al: University Group Diabetes Program (UGDP): A study of the relationships of therapy to vascular and other complications of diabetes. in *Tolbutamide: After Ten Years.* Brook Lodge Symposium of Int Diab Fed. New York, Excerpta Medica Series 149, 1967, p 261–269.

Klimt CR, Wolff FW, Silverman C, Conant J: Calibration of a simplified cortisone glucose tolerance test. *Diabetes* 10:351–356, 1961.

Knowles HC: Prevalence and development of diabetes. *Fed Proc* 27:945–948, 1968.

Knowles HC Jr: Long-term juvenile diabetes treated with unmeasured diet. *Trans Assoc Am Physicians* 84:95–101, 1971.

Knowles HC: Magnitude of the renal failure problem in diabetic patients. *Kidney Int* 1(suppl):2–7, 1974.

Knowles HC Jr: Evaluation of a positive urinary sugar test. *JAMA* 234:961–963, 1975.

Knowles H: Discussion on vascular disease, in Wolf S, Berle BB(eds): *Dilemmas in Diabetes.* New York, Plenum Press, 1975a, p 111–125.

Knowles HC Jr, Guest GM, Lampe J, et al: The course of juvenile diabetes treated with unmeasured diet. *Diabetes* 14:239, 1965.

Knowles HC, Meinert CL, Prout TE: Diabetes mellitus: The overall problem and its impact on the public, in Fajans SS (ed): *Diabetes Mellitus.* Dept of HEW Pub (NIH) 76-854, 1976, p 11–32.

Kobberling J: Studies on the genetic heterogeneity of diabetes mellitus. *Diabetologia* 7:46–49, 1971.

Kobberling J, Creutzfeldt W: Comparison of different methods of the evaluation of the oral glucose tolerance test. *Diabetes* 19:870–877, 1970.

Kobberling J, Kattermann R, Arnold A: Followup of nondiabetic relatives of diabetics by retesting oral glucose tolerance after 5 years. *Diabetologia* 11:451–456, 1975.

Koerner F, Koerner U, Eichenseher N: Diabetic retinopathy study. Data acquisition and its reliability. *Albrecht v. Graefes Arch klin Exp Ophthal* 202:163–173, 1977.

Koesters W, Seelig HP, Strauch M: Reversibility of functional and morphological glomerular lesions by islet transplantation in long-term diabetic rats. *Diabetologia* 13:409, 1977.

Kohner EM: Dynamic changes in the microcirculation of diabetics as related to diabetic microangiopathy. Diabetic microangiopathy *Acta Med Scand* (suppl 578) 1975, p 41–47.

Kohner EM, Dollery CT: Diabetic retinopathy, in Keen H, Jarrett RJ (eds): *Complications of Diabetes*. London, Edward Arnold Pub Co, 1975, p 7–98.

Kohner EM, Oakley NW: Diabetic retinopathy. *Metabolism* 24:1085–1102, 1975.

Kojima K, Nimi K, Watanabe I: Diabetic retinopathy, in Tsuji S, Wada M, et al (eds): *Diabetes Mellitus in Asia*. Proc symp Kobe, Amsterdam, Excerpta Medica, 1971, p 183–192.

Komrower GM: Maternal diabetes and congenital malformation (a letter). *Arch Dis Child* 52:519–520, 1977.

Koncz L, Soeldner JS, Otto H, Smith TM, Gleason RE: Deranged insulin secretory dynamics in offspring of two diabetic parents after double stimulation with intravenous glucose. *Diabetes* 26:1184–1191, 1977.

Kornerup T: Studies in diabetic retinopathy. *Acta Med Scand* 152:81–101, 1955.

Kornerup T: Retinopathia diabetica proliferans. *Acta Ophthalmol* 36:87, 1958.

Kosaka K, Hagura R, Kuzuya T: Insulin responses in equivocal and definite diabetes, with special reference to subjects who had mild glucose intolerance but later developed definite diabetes. *Diabetes* 26:944–952, 1977.

Kosaka K, Miki E, Kawazu S: Results of 5–18 year follow up of Japanese diabetic patients, with particular reference to vascular complications, in Baba S, Goto Y, Fukui I (eds): *Diabetes Mellitus in Asia*. Proc 2nd symp Kyoto, Amsterdam, Excerpta Medica, Series 390, 1975, p 242–248.

Kosaka K, Mizuna Y, Kuzuya T: Reproducibility of the oral glucose tolerance test and the rice-meal test in mild diabetics. *Diabetes* 15:901–904, 1966.

Kramer DW, Perilstein PK: Peripheral vascular complications in diabetes mellitus: A survey of 3,600 cases. *Diabetes* 7:384–387, 1958.

Kravitz AR, Isenberg PL, Shore MF, Barnett DM: Emotional factors in diabetes mellitus, in Marble A, White P, et al (eds): *Joslin's Diabetes Mellitus*, ed 11. Philadelphia, Lea & Febiger, 1971, p 767–782.

Krikler DM: Diabetes in Rhodesian Sephardic Jews. *S Afr Med J* 43:931–935, 1969.

Krishna Ram B: Atypical behavior of young diabetics: A critical appraisal. *J All India Institute of Med Sci* 2:32–40, 1976.

Krishna Ram B, Kochlar GS, Janah S, et al: The role of various dietary constituents on the serum lipids in diabetics, in Bajaj JS (ed): *Current Topics in Diabetes Research*. Proc 9th Congr of Int Diab Fed, India, Series 400, 1976, p 84.

Kriss B: Zur Kenntnis der Hypoplasie des Pankreas. *Virchows Arch* 263:591–598, 1927.

Krolewski AS, Czyzyk A, Janeczko D, et al: Mortality from cardiovascular diseases among diabetics. *Diabetologia* 13:345–350, 1977.

Krolewski AS, Czyzyk A, Kopczynski J: Prevalence of diabetes mellitus and other diseases among families of persons with juvenile diabetes and adult type diabetes. *Diabetologia* 13:411, 1977a.

Kromann H, Christau B, Kristensen, et al: Incidence, sex, age, and seasonal patterns of juvenile diabetes mellitus, in Bajaj JS (ed): *Current Topics in Diabetes Research.* Proc 9th Congr of Int Diab Fed, India, Series 400, 1976, p 179.

Krook L, Larsson S, Rooney JR: The interrelationship of diabetes mellius, obesity and pyometra in the dog. *Am J Vet Res* 21:120–124, 1960.

Krueger DE: New numerators for old denominators—multiple causes of death. *Natl Cancer Inst Mono* 19:431–443, 1966.

von Kruger HU: Reihenuntersuchungen auf Diabetes mellitus bei Kindern. *Deutsch Gesundh* 20:781–782, 1965.

Kruse-Jarres JD, Werner J: The effect of the intervening variables age, sex and over-weight on the intravenous glucose tolerance test. *J Clin Chem Clin Biochem* 11:114–116, 1973.

Kryston LJ: Diabetes and reactive hypoglycemia, in Kryston LJ, Shaw RA (eds): *Endocrinology and Diabetes.* New York, Grune & Stratton, 1975, p 473–490.

Kuller LM: Epidemiology of cardiovascular diseases: Current perspectives. *Am J Epidemiol* 104:424–456, 1976.

Kurihara M, Matsuyama T, Segi M: Diabetes mellitus mortality in Japan compared with other countries, in Tsuji S, Wada M (eds): *Diabetes Mellitus in Asia.* Amsterdam, Excerpta Medica, 1970, p 25–32.

Kurlander AB, Iskrant AP, Kent ME; Screening tests for diabetes: A study of specificity and sensitivity. *Diabetes* 3:213, 1954.

Kussman MJ, Goldstein HH, Gleason RE: The clinical course of diabetic nephropathy. *JAMA* 236:1861–1863, 1976.

Kuzuya N, Kosaka K: Diabetes in Japan, in Tsuji S, Wada M (eds): *Diabetes Mellitus in Asia.* Proceedings of a symp, Kobe, Amsterdam, Excerpta Medica, 1970, p 11–21.

Kuzuya T, Irie M, Niki Y: Glucose intolerance among Japanese professional sumo wrestlers, in Baba S, Goto Y, Fukui I (eds): *Diabetes Mellitus in Asia.* Proc 2nd symp Kyoto, Amsterdam, Excerpta Medica, Series 390, 1975, p 137–143.

Kvetny J: Diabetes mellitus and acute myocardial infarction. *Acta Med Scand* 200:151–153, 1976.

Kwaan HC, Colwell JA, Cruz S, et al: Increased platelet aggregation in diabetes mellitus. *J Lab Clin Med* 80:236–246, 1972.

Kyner JL, Levy RI, Soeldner JS, et al: Lipid, glucose and insulin interrelationships in normal, prediabetic and chemical diabetic subjects. *J Lab Clin Med* 88:345–367, 1976.

van't Laar A: Comparison of the 50 and 100 gram oral glucose tolerand test in patients with borderline glucose tolerance, abstract. *Diabetologia* 8:71, 1972.

Labbe M, Lenfanten H: Les lesions arterielles des diabetiques decelees par la radiographic. *Bull Mem Soc Med Hop Paris* 48:522–524, 1924.

Lal BH, Bahl AL, Mathur KP, et al: Clinical patterns and complications of diabetes mellitus in India. *Postgrad Med J* 44:223–228, 1968.

Lambert AC: Diabetes mellitus in the Chinese. *Br Med J* 1:19, 1908.

Lambert TH, Johnson RB, Paul GR: Glucose and cortisone glucose tolerance in normal and "prediabetic" humans. *Ann Intern Med* 54:916, 1961.

Lancaster HO: Diabetic prevalence in New South Wales. *Med J Aust* 1:117–119, 1951.

Lancaster HO: Death certification in diabetes. *Lancet* 2:1286–1387, 1962.

Lancaster HO, Maddox JK: Diabetic mortality in Australia. *Aust NZ J Med* 7:145, 1958.

Lancereaux E: Le diabete maigre: Ses symptomes, son evolution, son prognostic et son traitement; ses rapports avec les alterations du pancreas. Etude comparative du diabete maigre et du diabete gras. *Union Med* 29:161–167, 205–211, 1880.

Lancereaux E: Leçons de clinique medicale, review. *Union Med* 14:439–441, 1890.

Lancet: Diabetic neuropathy: A preventable complication, editorial. vol 2, 1972, p 583.

Lancet: Autoimmune diabetes mellitus, editorial. vol 2, 1974, pp 1549–1550.

Lancet: Inheritance of virus-induced diabetes mellitus, editorial. vol 2, 1976, p 28–29.

Langberg R, et al: Diabetes mellitus mortality in the United States 1950–1967, in *Vital and Health Statistics.* Publication of Natl Center for Health Statistics, vol 20, 1971, p 1–39.

Langner PH, Fies HL: Capillary venous differences in blood glucose values during the one-hour, two-dose glucose tolerance test (Exton-Rose procedure). *Am J Clin Pathol* 12:95–102, 1942.

Laron Z (ed): Psychological aspects of balance of diabetes in juveniles. 3rd International Beilinson Symposium, Herzlia 1975, Part II, 1977.

Laron Z, Karp M (eds): Diabetes in Juveniles, medical and rehabilitation aspects, in *Modern Problems in Paediatrics,* vol 12. International Beilinson Symposium on the Various Faces of Diabetes in Juveniles, Jerusalem. New York, S Karger Pub, 1972.

Laron Z, Kauli R: Skinfold measurements in diabetic children and adolescents, in *Diabetes in Juveniles.* International Beilinson Symposium on the Various Faces of Diabetes in Juveniles, Jerusalem. New York, S Karger Pub, 1972, p 121–125.

Larsen HW: Ophthalmoscopic and fluorescein angiographic picture of diabetic retinopathy. Diabetic Microangiopathy. *Acta Med Scand* (suppl 578) 1975, p 31–40.

Larsson T: Mortality from cerebrovascular disease, in Engel A, Larsson T (eds): *Stroke.* Thule Int Symposia, Stockholm. *Nord Med,* 1967, p 15–40.

Larsson T, Sterky G: Long term prognosis in juvenile diabetes *Acta Paediatr* 51(suppl 135):137–143, 1962.

Larsson Y, Lichtenstein A, Ploman KG: Degenerative vascular complications in juvenile diabetes mellitus treated with "free diet". *Diabetes* 1:449–458, 1952.

Lassman MN, Genel M, Wise JK, et al: Carbohydrate homeostasis and pancreatic islet cell function in Talassemia. *Ann Intern Med* 80:65–69, 1974.

Laube H, Schatz H, Nierle C, Fussganger R, Pfeiffer EF: Insulin secretion and biosynthesis in sucrose fed rats. *Diabetologia* 12:441–446, 1976.

Lauvaux JP, Pirart J: Diabetic retinopathy: A statistical study in 4,400 diabetics. Relation to duration and control. Artifactual nature of "early" retinopathy. *Diabetologia* 10:383, 1974.

Lauvaux JP, Pirart J: The course of diabetic retinopathy: A statistical study on its development, progression and regression in 4,400 diabetics. *Diabetologia* 8:358, 1975.

Lauvaux JP, Staguet M: The oral glucose tolerance test: A study of the influence of age on the response to the standard oral 50 g glucose load. *Diabetologia* 6:414–419, 1970.

Lavy S, Melamed E, Cahane E, Carmon A: Hypertension and diabetes as risk factors in stroke patients. *Stroke* 4:751–759, 1973.

Lawrence AM, Kirsteins L, Mitton J: Parotid gland insulin: An extrapancreatic source of insulin in rats. *Diabetes* 25(suppl 1): 328, 1976.

Lawrence RD: Types of human diabetes. *Br Med J* 4703:373–375, 1951.

Lawrence RD: Record incidence of diabetes, foreign letters. *JAMA* 152:624, 1953.

Lawrence RD: Treatment of 90 severe diabetics with soluble insulin for 20–40 years: Effect of diabetic control on complications. *Br Med J* 2:1624, 1963.

Lebon J, Fabregoule M, Choussat H, et al: Aspects cliniques et biologiques du diabete de l'indigen Musulman Algerien. *Sem Hop Paris* 26:2553–2554, 1953.

LeCompte PM: Insulitis in early juvenile diabetes. *Arch Pathol Lab Med* 66:450–457, 1958.

LeCompte PM, Legg MA: Insulitis (lymphocytic infiltration of pancreatic islets) in late-onset diabetes. *Diabetes* 21:762–769, 1972.

LeCompte PM, Steinke J, Soeldner JS, et al: Changes in the islet of Langerhans in cows injected with heterologous and homologous insulin. *Diabetes* 15:586–596, 1966.

Ledet T: Histological and histochemical changes in the coronary arteries of old diabetic patients. *Diabetologia* 4:268–272, 1968.

LeGoff J: De la mortalite chez les diabetiques. A Paris dans le Department de la Seine. *Gaz D Hop* 84:556–558, 1911.

Lehnherr ER: Arteriosclerosis and diabetes mellitus. *N Engl J Med* 208:1307–1313, 1933.

Lehtovirta EO: Comparison of oral and intravenous glucose tolerance in men aged 40–59. *Scand J Clin Lab Invest* 21(suppl 101):25, 1968.

Lehtovirta E: Obesity in relation to glucose tolerance. Proc Institute Occup Health Research Dept Finnish Hlth Assoc, Helsinki, 1973. *Ann Clin Res* 5(suppl 10):7–116, 1973.

Lemann II: Diabetes mellitus among the negroes. *New Orleans Med Surg J* 63:461–467, 1910–1911.

Lemann II: Diabetes mellitus in the Negro Race. *South Med J* 14:522–525, 1921.

Lender M, Menczel J: Characteristics of hospitalizations and death cases of diabetic patients in a general hospital. *Gerontology* 23:23–30, 1977.

Lendrum R, Walker G, Cudworth AG, et al: HLA linked genes and islet-cell antibodies in diabetes mellitus. *Br Med J* 1:1565–1567, 1976.

Lenner RA: Studies of glycemia and glucosuria in diabetics after breakfast meals of different composition. *Am J Clin Nutr* 29:716–725, 1976.

Lennox WG: Repeated blood sugar curves in non-diabetic subjects. *J Clin Invest* 4:331, 1927.

501

Leonards JR, McCullagh EP, Christopher TC: A new carbohydrate solution for testing glucose tolerance. *Diabetes* 14:96–99, 1965.

Leopold EJ: Diabetes in the Negro Race. *Ann Intern Med* 5:285–293, 1931.

Lepine R. *Le Diabete Sucre.* Alcan F (ed): Ancienne Librairie Germer Bailliere et Cie, Paris, 1909.

Lesser GT, Deutsch S, Markofsky J: Use of independent measurement of body fat to evaluate overweight and underweight. *Metabolism* 20:792–793, 1972.

Lester FT, Albulkadir J, Larson D: Quana'a P: Diabetes mellitus: Clinical features in 404 Ethiopians. *Ethiop Med J* 14:185–198, 1976.

Lestradet H, Battistelli F, Combier E, et al: L'heredite du diabete insulino-dependent. *Nouv Presse Med* 3:1077–1080, 1974.

Lestradet H, Besse J: Prevalence and incidence of diabetes mellitus in children and adolescents. (Part II, Proc.). *Acta Paediatr Belg* 30:123–127, 1977.

Lestradet H, Deschamps I, Giron B: Insulin and free fatty acid levels during oral glucose tolerance tests and their relation to age in 70 healthy children. *Diabetes* 25:505–508, 1976.

Levin L, Gelfand M: Diabetic retinopathy in African patients. *S Afr Med J* 47:993–994, 1973.

Levin ME, O'Neal LW (eds): *The Diabetic Foot,* ed. 2. St. Louis, CV Mosby and Co, 1977.

Levine: Comments on effects of feeding meat to poultry. *Horm Metab Res* 4(suppl):152, 1974.

Levine SA: Angina pectoris: Some clinical considerations. *JAMA* 79:928–933, 1922.

Levine SB, Sampliner RE, Bennett PH, et al: Asymptomatic parotid enlargement in Pima Indians: Relationship to age, obesity, and diabetes mellitus. *Ann Intern Med* 73:571–573, 1970.

Levy R: Triglycerides as a risk factor in coronary artery disease. *JAMA* 224:1770, 1973.

Lewis JG, Symons C: Vascular disease in a diabetic clinic. *Lancet* 2:985–988, 1958.

Lewis RA, Said D: Influence of posture on oral glucose tolerance test, in Demole M (ed): *Medicine et Hygiene.* Proc 4th Congr of Int Diab Fed, Geneva, 1961, vol 1, p 231.

Librach G, Schadel M, Seltzer M, et al: Stroke: Incidence and risk factors. *Geriatrics* 32:85–91, 94–96, 1977.

Licenziati M: Diabetes mellitus in the province of Naples: Preliminary notes. *Minerva Med* 59:5057–5058, 1968.

Lichstein E, Kuhn LA, Goldberg E, et al: Diabetic treatment and primary ventricular fibrillation in accute myocardial infarction. *Am J Cardiol* 38:100–102, 1976.

Lickley HLA, Chisholm DJ, Rabinovitch A, et al: Effects of portacaval anastomosis on glucose tolerance in the dog: Evidence of an interaction between the gut and the liver in oral glucose disposal. *Metabolism* 24:1157–1167, 1975.

Like AA, Levine RL, Poffenbarger PL: Studies in the diabetic mutant mouse: 6. Evolution of glomerular lesions and associated proteinuria. *Am J Pathol* 66:193–224, 1972.

Lilienfeld AM: *Foundations of Epidemiology.* New York, Oxford Univ Press, 1976.

Lindhart M: On the frequency fo diabetes mellitus in Denmark. *Dan Med Bull* 1:61–66, 1954.

Lipman RL, Raskin P, Love T, et al: Glucose intolerance during decreased physical activity in man. *Diabetes* 21:101–107, 1972.

Lipman RL, Schnure JJ, Bradley EM, Lecocq FR: Impairment of peripheral glucose utilization in normal subjects by prolonged bed rest *J Lab Clin Med* 8:221–223, 1970.

Little JM, Petritsi-Jones D, Zylstra P, et al: A survey of amputations for degenerative vascular disease. *Med J Aust* 1:329–334, 1973.

Lloyd JK: Diabetes mellitus presenting as spontaneous hypoglycemia in childhood. *Proc R Soc Med* 57:1061–1064, 1964.

Lloyd-Mostyn RH, Watkins PJ: Total cardiac denervation in diabetic autonomic neuropathy. *Diabetes* 25:748–751, 1976.

Locke S: The nervous system and diabetes, in Marble A, White P, et al (eds): *Joslin's Diabetes Mellitus,* ed 11. Philadelphia, Lea & Febiger, 1971, p 562–580.

Logie AW, Stowers JM, Dingwall-Fordyce I: Longitudinal study of untreated chemical diabetes. *Br Med J* 4:630–632, 1974.

Lombard HL, Joslin EP: Certification of death of 1,000 diabetic patients. *Am J Dig Dis* 14:275–278, 1947.

Lopes-Virella MF, Colwell JA: Serum high density lipoproteins in diabetic patients. *Lancet* 1:1291–1292, 1976.

Lopes-Virella MFL, Stone PG, Colwell JA: Serum high density lipoprotein in diabetic patients. *Diabetologia* 13:285–291, 1977.

Lowe CR, McKeown T: Arterial pressure in an industrial population and its bearing on the problem of essential hypertension. *Lancet* 1:1086, 1962.

Lozner EL, Winkler AW, Taylor FHL, Peters JP: The intravenous glucose tolerance test. *J Clin Invest* 20:507–515, 1941.

Lubetzki J, Duprey J, Sambourg CL: Influence of mother's age, parity, obesity and diabetes upon birth weight. *Diabetologia* 9:79, 1973.

Ludwig H, Mayr WR, Schernthaner G: Glucose-tolerance tests in HL-A typed relatives of patients with juvenile onset diabetes mellitus, letter. *Lancet* 2:1152–1153, 1975.

Ludwig H, Schernthaner G, Mayr WR: The importance of HLA genes to susceptibility in the development of juvenile diabetes mellitus. *Diab Metab* 3:43–58, 1977.

Lundbaek K: Metabolic abnormalities in starvation diabetes. *Yale J Biol Med* 20:533–544, 1947.

Lundbaek K: *Long-term diabetes: The clinical picture in diabetes mellitus of 15–25 years duration.* Copenhagen, Ejnar Munksgaard, 1953.

Lundbaek K: Diabetic retinopathy in newly diagnosed diabetes mellitus. *Acta Med Scand* 152:53–60, 1955.

Lundbaek K: Intravenous glucose tolerance as a tool in definition and diagnosis of diabetes mellitus. *Br Med J* 1:1507, 1962.

Lundbaek K: Diabetic angiopathy. *Acta Diabetol Lat* 10:183–207, 1973.

Lundbaek K: Diabetic angiopathy. *Mod Concepts Cardiovasc Dis* 43:103–107, 1974.

Lundbaek K, Keen H (eds): Blood vessel disease in diabetes mellitus: Milano Il Ponte 1971. *Acta Diabetol Lat* 8(suppl 1): 1971.

503

Lundbaek K, Osterby R: Renal disease in diabetes mellitus, in Fajans SS (ed): *Diabetes Mellitus*. US Dept of HEW Publ (NIH) 76-854, 1976, p 227–242.

Lundbaek K, Petersen VP: Lipid composition of diabetic and nondiabetic coronary arteries. *Acta Med Scand* 144:354–359, 1953.

Lunell N-O: Intravenous glucose tolerance in women with previously complicated pregnancies. *Acta Obstet Gynecol Scand* 45(suppl 4):1–89, 75–77, 1965.

Lunnell N-O, Persson B: Potential diabetes in women with large babies: A follow up study. *Acta Obstet Gynecol Scand* 51:293–296, 1972.

Lutjens A, Verleur H, Plooij M: Glucose and insulin levels on loading with different carbohydrates. *Clin Chim Acta* 62:239–243, 1975.

Luyckx AS, Lefebvre PJ: Plasma insulin in reactive hypoglycemia. *Diabetes* 20:435–442, 1971.

Lynn TN, Duncan R, Naughton JP, et al: Prevalence of evidence of prior myocardial infarction, hypertension, diabetes and obesity in three neighboring communities in Pennsylvania. *Am J Med Sci* 254:385–391, 1967.

Lyra de Lacerda SN, Feingold J, Bernades P, et al: Genetic and acquired diabetogenic factors in 262 patients with chronic pancreatitis. *Diabetes* 26(suppl 1):406, 1977.

MacBryde CM: St Louis diabetes detection drive. *Mo Med* 46:776–779,1949.

McConnell RB, Pyke DA, Roberts JAF: Blood groups in diabetes mellitus. *Br Med J* 1:772–775, 1956.

McDonald GW: Diabetes in the Americas, Proc 6th Congr of Int Diab Fed, Stockholm Series 140, 1967, p 657–667.

McDonald GW, et al: *Diabetes Source Book*. US Dept of HEW (PHS), Div Chronic Diseases Publ 1168, 1964 (revised 1968).

McDonald GW, Burnham CE, Lewis WF: Reproducibility of glucose tolerance in 101 nondiabetic women. *Public Health Rep* 84:353–357, 1969.

McDonald GW, Fisher GF: Diabetes prevalence in the United States: Implications for public health programming. *Public Health Rep* 82:334–338, 1967.

McDonald GW, Fisher GF, Burnham CE: Differences in glucose determinations obtained from plasma or whole blood. *Public Health Rep* 79:515–521, 1964.

McDonald GW, Fisher GF, Burnham CE: Reproducibility of the oral glucose tolerance test. *Diabetes* 14:473–480, 1965.

McDonald GW, Hozier JB, Fisher, GF, Ederma AB: Large scale diabetes screening program for Federal employees. *Public Health Rep* 78:553, 1963.

MacDonald I: Diet and human atherosclerosis—carbohydrates. *Adv Exp Med Biol* 60:57–64, 1975.

MacDonald MJ: Equal incidence of adult-onset diabetes among ancestors of juvenile diabetics and nondiabetics. *Diabetologia* 10:767–773, 1974.

MacDonald MJ: Lower frequency of diabetes among hospitalized Negro than white children: Theoretical implications. *Acta Genet Med Gemellol* 24:119–126, 1975.

McFadzean AJS, Yeung R: Diabetes among the Chinese in Hong Kong. *Diabetes* 17:219–228, 1968.

McGavran MH, Unger RH, Recant L: A glucagon-secreting alpha-cell carcinoma of the pancreas. *N Engl J Med* 1408–1413, 1966.

McGlashan ND: Geographical evidence on medical hypothesis. *Trop Geogr Med* 19:333–343, 1967.

MacKay EM, Wick AM, Barnum CP: Ketogenic action of short chain even-numbered carbon fatty-acids in carbohydrate-fed animals. *J Biol Chem* 135:183–187, 1940.

MacKay N, Gordon A, Neilson JM: Observer error in Dextrostix estimation of blood-sugar. *Lancet* 2:269–270, 1965.

Maclaren NK: Viral and immunological bases of beta cell failure in insulin-dependent diabetes. *Am J Dis Child* 131:1149–1154, 1977.

McLaughlin P, Morton B, McLoughlin M, et al: Long term effect of hyperlipidemia, diabetes and smoking on graft patency and progression of disease following aorto-coronary bypass. *Circulation* 49, 50 (suppl 3): 191, 1974.

MacLean AB, Sullivan RC: Dextrose tolerance in infants and in young children. *Am J Dis Child* 37:1146–1160, 1929.

MacLean H, de Wesselow OLV: The estimation of sugar tolerance. *Q J Med* 14:103–119, 1921.

McMahon G, Pugh TF: *Epidemiology: Principles and Methods.* Boston, Little, Brown and Co, 1970.

McMillan DE: Deterioration of microcirculation in diabetes. *Diabetes* 24:944–957, 1975.

MacMillan DR, Kotoyan M, Zeidner D, Hafezi B: Seasonal variation in the onset of diabetes. *Pediatrics* 59:113–115, 1977.

Maempel JVZ: Diabetes in Malta: A pilot survey. *Lancet* 2:1197–1200, 1965.

Magnus-Levy A: *Spez Path u Therap Inn Krank.* Berlin, Kraus und Brugsch, Pub, 1913.

Mahler R: Effect of insulin on lipid metabolism of human arteries, in Camerini-Davalos RA, Cole HS (eds): *Vascular and Neurological Changes in Early Diabetes.* New York, Academic Press, 1973, p 49–54.

Mahler RJ: The pathogenesis of pancreatic islet-cell hyperplasia and insulin insensitivity in obesity. *Adv Metab Disord* 7:213–241, 1974.

Mahler RJ: Diabetes mellitus—distinguishing between patients receiving insulin and those requiring insulin therapy. *West J Med* 120:358–362, 1974a.

Malik TK, Kumar V, Ahuja MMS: Degree of acetonemia following epinephrine infusions to determine biochemical characterization of diabetes mellitus. *Indian J Med Res* 62:80, 1974.

Malins JM: *Clinical Diabetes Mellitus.* London, Eyre and Spottiswoode, 1968.

Malins JM: Diabetes in the population. *Clin Endocrinol Metabol* 1:645–672, 1972.

Malins JM: Food and death rates from diabetes. *Lancet* 2:1201, 1974.

Malins JM: Diabetes. *Lancet* 2:1367–1368, 1974a.

Malins JM: Glucose tolerance and the diabetic population. *Postgrad Med J* 50:529–537, 1974b.

Malins JM, FitzGerald MG: Childbearing prior to recognition of diabetes: Recollected birth weights and stillbirth rate in babies born to parents who developed diabetes. *Diabetes* 14:175–178, 1965.

Malins JM, FitzGerald MG, Wall M: A change in the sex incidence of diabetes. *Diabetologia* 1:121–124, 1965.

Malmros H: A study of glucosuria, with special reference to the interpretation of the incidental finding of a positive reduction test. *Acta Med Scand* 27 (suppl):285–309, 1928.

Mann GV: Hypothesis: The role of vitamin C in diabetic angiopathy. *Perspect Biol Med,* Winter 1974, p 210–217.

Mann I, Potter D: Geographic ophthalmology, a preliminary study of Maoris of New Zealand. *Am J Ophthalmol* 67:358–369, 1969.

Marble A: Diabetes mellitus in the US Army in World War II. *Milit Surg* 105:357–363, 1949.

Marble A: Laboratory procedures useful in diagnosis and treatment, in Marble A, White P, Bradley RF, et al (eds): *Joslin's Diabetes Mellitus,* ed 11. Philadelphia, Lea & Febiger, 1971, p 191–208.

Marble A: The natural history of diabetes. *Horm Metab Res* 4 (suppl):153–158, 1974.

Marble A, Ramos E: Cancer and diabetes, in Marble A, White P, et al (eds): *Joslin's Diabetes Mellitus,* ed 11. Philadelphia, Lea & Febiger, 1971, p 695–700.

Marble A, White P, Bradley RF, Krall LP (eds): *Joslin's Diabetes Mellitus,* ed 11. Philadelphia, Lea & Febiger, 1971.

Margolis JR, et al: Clinical features of unrecognized myocardial infarction—silent and asymptomatic. *Am J Cardiol* 32:1–7, 1973.

Marhuhama Y, Goto Y, Yamagata S: Diabetic treatment and the diurnal plasma triglyceride. *Metabolism* 16:985–995, 1967.

Marigo S, Sachetti G, Benj P, et al: Sex incidence of diabetes: An epidemiological study in the La Spezia area. *Acta Diabetol Lat* 11:9–17, 1974.

Marine N, Vinik EA, Edelstein I, Jackson WPU: Diabetes, hyperglycemia and glucosuria among Indians, Malays, and Africans (Bantus) in Capetown, South Africa. *Diabetes* 18:840–857, 1969.

Marks HH: Longevity and mortality of diabetes. *Am J Public Health* 55:416, 1965.

Marks HH, Krall LP: Onset, course, prognosis and mortality in diabetes mellitus, in Marble A, White P, et al (eds): *Joslin's Diabetes Mellitus,* ed 11. Philadelphia, Lea & Febiger, 1971, p 209–254.

Marks HH, Krall LP, White P: Epidemiology and detection of diabetes, in Marble A, White P, et al (eds): *Joslin's Diabetes Mellitus,* ed 11. Philadelphia, Lea & Febiger, 1971, p 10–34.

Marks V, Dawson A: Rapid stick method for determining blood-glucose concentration. *Br Med J* 1:293, 1965.

Martin FIR, Stocks AE: Insulin sensitivity and vascular disease in insulin-dependent diabetics. *Br Med J* 2:81–82, 1968.

Martin FIR, Warne GL: Factors influencing the prognosis of vascular disease in insulin-deficient diabetics of long duration: Seven-year follow up. *Metabolism* 24:1–9, 1975.

Martin JM, Hartroft WS: Atherogenicity of saturated or unsaturated dietary fats in pancreatectomized diabetic rats, in Liebel BS, Wrenshall GA (eds): *On the Nature and Treatment of Diabetes.* Amsterdam, Excerpta Medica Foundation, 1965, p 410–428.

Martin M: Diabetes mellitus bei Negren der Afrikanischen West-Kuste. *Arch Intern Med* 4:849, 1906.

Martin MM, Martin ALA: Obesity, hyperinsulinism and diabetes mellitus in childhood. *J Pediatr* 82:192–201, 1973.

Martinez C: Experimental diabetes and diet. *Proc Am Diab Assoc* 6:503–510, 1946.

Martinez RA: Diabetes in the Dominican Republic. *Int Diab Fed Rep*, 1968, p 77–81.

Mateo de Acosta O, Amaro S, Diaz O: Diabetes in Cuba. *Acta Diabetol Lat* 10:534–546, 1973.

Mathew TN, David D, Meyer JS: Hyperlipoproteinemia in occlusive cerebrovascular disease. *JAMA* 232:262–266, 1975.

Matsuo T, Shino A, Iwatsuka M, Suzuoki Z: Induction of overt diabetes in KK mice by dietary means. *Endocrinol Jpn* 17:477–488, 1970.

Matsuoka A, Yamaguchi K, Masuyama T, et al: Characteristics of dietary treatment of diabetes mellitus in Japan: Comparison of dietary habits and diabetic pathology in Japanese and American diabetics, in Baba S, Goto Y, Fukui I (eds): *Diabetes Mellitus in Asia*. Proc 2nd symp Kyoto, Amsterdam, Excerpta Medica, Series 390, 1975, p 265–269.

Mauer SM, Steffes MW, Sutherland DER, et al: Studies of the rat of regression of the glomerular lesions in diabetic rats treated with pancreatic-islet transplantation. *Diabetes* 24:280–285, 1975.

Mauer SM, Sutherland ER, Steffes MW, et al: Pancreatic islet transplantation: Effects on the glomerular lesions of experimental diabetes in the rat. *Diabetes* 23:748–753, 1974.

Maugh TH II: Diabetes: Epidemiology suggests a viral connection. *Science* 188:347–351, 1975.

Maugh TH II: Diabetes: Model systems indicate viruses a cause. *Science* 188:436–438, 1975a.

Maxwell JP: Diabetes mellitus in Chinese. *Br Med J* 1:926, 1908.

Mayer J: Inactivity as a major factor in adolescent obesity. *Ann NY Acad Sci* 131:502–506, 1965.

Mayer J, Roy P, Mitra KP: Relation between caloric intake, body weight, and physical work, studies in an industrial male population in West Bengal. *Am J Clin Nutr* 4:169–175, 1956.

Mayer KH, Stamler J, Dyer A, et al: Epidemiologic findings on the relationship of time of day and time since last meal to glucose tolerance. *Diabetes* 25:936–943, 1976.

Mayne EE, Bridges JM, Weaver JA: Platelet adhesiveness, plasma fibrinogen and factor VIII levels in diabetes mellitus. *Diabetologia* 6:436–440, 1970.

Mazovetsky AG, Khachaturov VG, Akmetzyanov AM: Methods of a study of epidemiology. *Probl Endokrinol (Mosk)* 22:19–21, 1976.

Mazzaferri EL, Skillman TG, Lanese RR, Keller MP: Use of test strips with colour meter to measure blood glucose. *Lancet* 1:331–333, 1970.

Medalie JH, Goldbourt U: Angina pectoris among 10,000 men: 2. Psychosocial and other risk factors as evidenced by a multivariate analysis of a five-year incidence study. *Am J Med* 60:910–921, 1976.

Medalie JH, Goldbourt U: Unrecognized myocardial infarction; five-year incidence, mortality, risk factors. *Ann Intern Med* 84:526–531, 1976a.

Medalie JH, Papier C, Herman JB, et al: Diabetes mellitus among 10,000 adult men: 1. Five-year incidence and associated variables. *Isr J Med Sci* 10:681–697, 1974.

Medalie JH, Papier CM, Goldbourt U, Herman JB: Major factors in the development of diabetes mellitus in 10,000 men. *Arch Intern Med* 135:811–818, 1975.

Medalie JH, Snyder M, Groen JJ, et al: Angina pectoris among 10,000 men: 5-year incidence and univariate analysis. *Am J Med* 55:583–594, 1973.

Medley DRK: The relationship between diabetes and obesity: A study of susceptibility to diabetes in obese people. *Q J Med* 34:111–132, 1965.

Megyesi C, Samols E, Marks V: Glucose tolerance and diabetes in chronic liver disease. *Lancet* 2:1051–1056, 1967.

Mehnert H, Forster H: Study of the evacuation mechanism of the stomach after oral administration of different sugars in man and rat. *Diabetologia* 4:26–33, 1968.

Mehnert H, Reichstein W, Sewering H: Clinical and scientific aspect of the Munich campaign for the early detection of diabetes, in Ostman H (ed): Proc 6th Congr of Int Diab Fed, Stockholm Series 172, 1967, 701.

Meier H: Diabetes mellitus in animals: A review. *Diabetes* 9:485–489, 1960.

Meissener WA, Legg MA: The pathology of diabetes, in Marble A, White P, et al (eds): *Joslin's Diabetes Mellitus*, ed 11. Philadelphia, Lea & Febiger, 1971, p 179.

Mekkawi MF, Aswad ME: Diabetic retinopathy in Libyans. *Bull Ophthalmol Soc Egypt* 65:437–440, 1972.

Melani F, Verrillo A, Osorio J, et al: Periodicity in beta-cell responsiveness and diurnal variation of glucose tolerance, in Bajaj S (ed): *Current Topics in Diabetes Research*. Proc 9th Congr of Int Diab Fed, India, Series 400, 1976, p 27–28.

Melin K, Ursing B: Diabetes mellitus son Komplikatin till parotitis epidemica. *Nord Med* 60:1715, 1958.

Meneely GR, Dahl LK: Electrolytes in hypertension: The effects of sodium chloride. The evidence from animal and human studies. *Med Clin North Am* 45:271–283, 1961.

Menser MA, Forrest JM, Honeyman MC, Burgess JA: Diabetes, HL-A antigens, and congenital rubella. *Lancet* 2:1508–1509, 1974.

Menser MA, Forrest JM, Honeyman MC, Burgess JA: Diabetes and asthma in Eskimos. *N Engl J Med* 292:981–982, 1975.

Merikas G, Deliyiannis A, Karamanos B, et al: Unusually low coronary heart disease prevalence in diabetics of Kretan and Corfu, in Bajaj SJ (ed): *Current Topics in Diabetes Research*. Proc 9th Congr of Int Diab Fed, India, Series 400, 1976, p 116.

Merimee TJ, Rimoin DL, Cavalli-Aforza LL: Metabolic studies in the African Pygmy. *J Clin Invest* 51:395–401, 1972.

Merlihot J: Several cases of chronic pancreatitis in Madagascar. *Med Tropicale* 23:52–62, 1963.

Merriman A: Six cases of hyperosmolar non-ketotic diabetic decompensation in a hospital practice in West Africa. *J Trop Med Hyg* 78:94–96, 1975.

Metropolitan Life Ins Co: Girth and death. *Stat Bull Metropol Life Ins Co* 18:2–5, 1937.

Metropolitan Life Ins Co: New weight standards for men and women. *Stat Bull Metropol Life Ins Co* 40:1–4, 1959.

Metropolitan Life Ins Co: Diabetes and socioeconomic level. *Stat Bull Metropol Life Ins Co* 49:3, 1968.

Metropolitan Life Ins Co: Trends in average weights and heights in man: An insurance experience. *Stat Bull Metropol Life Ins Co* 51:6–7, 1970.

Metropolitan Life Ins Co: Diabetes mortality—United States, Canada and Western Europe. *Stat Bull Metropol Life Ins Co* 53 (Sept):5–8,1972.

Metropolitan Life Ins Co: Regional variations in mortality from diabetes. *Stat Bull Metropol Life Ins Co* 54:2–5, 1973.

Metropolitan Life Ins Co: Policyholder mortality declines. *Stat Bull Metropol Life Ins Co* 55:10–12, 1974.

Metropolitan Life Ins Co: Recent trends in mortality from diabetes. *Stat Bull Metropol Life Ins Co* 56:2–5, 1975.

Metz R, Friedenberg R: Effects of repetitive glucose loads on plasma concentrations of glucose, insulin and free fatty acis: Paradoxical insulin responses in subjects with mild glucose intolerance. *J Clin Endocrinol Metabol* 30:602–608, 1970.

Metz R, Surmaczynsja B, Berger S, et al: Glucose tolerance, plasma insulin, and free fatty acids in elderly subjects. *Ann Intern Med* 64:1042–1047, 1966.

Middleton GD, Caird FI: Parity and diabetes mellitus. *Br J Prev Soc Med* 22:100–104, 1968.

Miki E, Fukuda M, Kuzuya T, et al: Relation of the course of retinopathy to control of diabetes, age, and therapeutic agents in diabetic Japanese patients. *Diabetes* 18:773–780, 1969.

Miki E, Kuzuya T, Ide T, et al: Frequency, degree and progression with time of proteinuria in diabetic patients. *Lancet* 1:922–924, 1972.

Miki E, Like AA, Steinke J, Soeldner JS: Diabetic syndrome in sand rats. *Diabetologia* 3:135–139, 1967.

Miki E, Maruyama H: Childhood diabetes mellitus in Japan, in Tsuji, S, Wada M (eds): *Diabetes Mellitus in Asia, 1970,* Amsterdam, Excerpta Medica Fdn, 1970, p 69–75.

Miller DI, Ridolfo AS: The skin surface-glucose test. *Diabetes* 9:48–52, 1960.

Miller HC: The effect of the prediabetic state on the survival of the fetus and the birth weight of the newborn infant. *N Engl J Med* 233:376–378, 1945.

Miller HC, Hurwitz D, Kuder K: Fetal and neonatal mortality in pregnancies complicated by diabetes mellitus. *JAMA* 124:271, 1944.

Miller K, Michael AF: Immunopathology of renal extracellular membranes in diabetes mellitus: Specificity of tubular basement-membrane immunofluorescence. *Diabetes* 25:701–708, 1976.

Miller M, Knatterud GL, Hawkins BS, et al (University Group Diabetes Program): A study of the effects of hypoglycemic agents on vascular complications in patients with adult-onset diabetes: 6. Supplementary report on nonfatal events in patients treated with tolbutamide. *Diabetes* 25:1129–1153, 1976.

Millington JT, Tinsman CA: Diabetes screening in Pennsylvania. *Pa Med* 69:36, 1966.

Mills CA: Diabetes mellitus: Is climate a responsible factor in the etiology? *Arch Intern Med* 46:469–581, 1930.

Mills CA: Diabetes mellitus: Sugar consumption in its etiology. *Arch Intern Med* 46:582–584, 1930a.

Mimura G: Epidemiology of diabetes in Asia, especially in Japan, in Rodriguez RR, Vallance-Owen J (eds): *Diabetes.* Proc 7th Congr of Int Diab Fed, Buenos Aires, Series 209, 1970, p 331–334.

Mimura G, Jinnouchi T, Sakamoto Y, et al: Epidemiology of child diabetes in Kumanoto Perfecture, Japan: Prevalence of glycosuria and child diabetes among 127,451 schoolboys and 123,138 schoolgirls, and their hereditary background, in Baba S, Goto Y, Fukui I (eds): *Diabetes Mellitus in Asia.* Proc 2nd symp, Kyoto, Amsterdam, Excerpta Medica, Series 390, 1975, p 74–81.

Mimura G, Miyaom K, Koganemoro Y, et al: Heredity of diabetes mellitus in Japan, in Tsuji S, Wada M (eds): *Diabetes Mellitus in Asia.* Proc symp 1970, Amsterdam, Excerpta Medica, p 83–97.

Mincu I, Dumitrescu C, Campeanu S, et al.: Epidemiological researches on diabetes mellitus in Roumanian urban and rural population. *Diabetologia* 8:12–18, 1972.

Mincu I, Dumitrescu C, Ionescu-tirgoviste C, et al: Concomitant screening of diabetes mellitus, obesity and hyperlipoproteinemia in large population groups, in Bajaj JS (ed): *Current Topics in Diabetes Research.* Proc 9th Congr of Int Diab Fed, India, Series 400, 1976, p 179–180.

Mintz DH, Chez RA, Hutchinson DL: Subhuman primate pregnancy complicated by streptozotocin (Stz) induced diabetes mellitus. *Clin Res,* January 1971, p 68.

Mirsky JA: Some considerations of the etiology of diabetes mellitus in man. *Proc Am Diab Assoc* 5:119–138, 1945.

Mitchell FL, Pearson J, Strauss WT: Plasma lipids and glucose in normal health, diabetes and cardiovascular disease. *Diabetologia* 4:105–108, 1968.

Mitchell FL, Strauss WT: Relation of postprandial blood glucose level to the oral glucose-tolerance curve. *Lancet* 1:1185–1189, 1964.

Mitra A: Diabetes—the bane of Bengal. *The Indian Lancet* 21:897–898, 1903.

Miyamura K, Mikuni E, Hayashi K: The frequency of diabetes in the hilly districts and a rural town in the Kii Peninsula, in Baba S, Goto Y, Fukui I (eds): *Diabetes Mellitus in Asia.* Proc 2nd symp, Kyoto, Amsterdam, Excerpta Medica, Series 390, 1975, p 118–122.

Modan B, Schor S, Shani M: Acute myocardial infarction prognostic value of white blood cell and blood glucose level. *JAMA* 233:266, 1975.

Molineaux L, Piodc J, Dasnoy J: Analysis of medical admissions to the Gondar Hospital 1963–1965. *Ethiop Med J* 5:47–65, 1966.

Monif GR: Can diabetes mellitus result from an infectious disease? *Hosp Practice,* March 1973, p 124–130.

Montegriffo VME: Height and weight of a United Kingdom adult population with a review of anthropometric literature. *Ann Hum Genet* 31:389–399, 1968.

Montel LR: Etudes de pathologie annemite en Cochinchine. *Bull Soc Pathol Exot* 1:443, 1924.

Montenegro MR, Solberg LA: Obesity, body weight, body length and atherosclerosis. *Lab Invest* 18:594–603, 1968.

Montgomery DAD, Harley JMG, Hadden DR, Kajtar TJ: A prospective study of three tests of glucose tolerance in potential diabetic pregnancy. *Diabetologia* 6:57, 1970.

Montgomery R: The medical significance of cyanogen in plant foodstuffs. *Am J Clin Nutr* 17:103, 1965.

Montoye HJ, Epstein FH, Kjelsberg MO: Relationship between serum cholesterol and body fatness, an epidemiological study. *Am J Clin Nutr* 18:397, 1966.

Moore RH, Buschbom RL: Work absenteeism in diabetics. *Diabetes* 23:957–961, 1976.

Moran JJ, Lewis PL, Reinhold JG, Lukens FDW: Enzymatic tests for glucosuria. *Diabetes* 6:358–362, 1957.

Moriyama IM: Is diabetes mortality increasing? *Public Health Rep* 63:1334–1339, 1948.

Moriyama IM: Use of vital records for epidemiological research. *J Chron Dis* 17:889, 1964.

Moriyama, TM, Dawber TR, et al: Evaluation of diagnostic information supporting medical certification of deaths from cardiovascular disease. *Am J Public Health* 48:1376–1387, 1958.

Moriyama IM, Dawber TR, Kannel WB: Evaluation of diagnostic information supporting medical certification of deaths from cardiovascular disease. *Natl Cancer Inst Monogr* 19:405–419, 1966.

Morrison H: A statistical study of the mortality from diabetes mellitus in Boston from 1896 to 1913 with special reference to its occurrence among Jews. *Boston Med Surg J* 175:54–57, 1916.

Morrison IB, Bogan IK: Calcification of the vessels in diabetes: A roentgenographic study of the legs and feet. *JAMA* 92:1424–1426, 1929.

Morrison LB, Bogan IK: Bone development in diabetic children: A roentgen study. *Am J Med Sci* 174:313–319, 1927.

Morse JL: Diabetes in infancy and childhood. *Boston Med Surg J* 168:530–535, 1913.

Morse WI, Soeldner JS: Adipose and non-adipose body water, sodium space and fat free solid fractions in human obesity. *Clin Res* 9:186, 1961.

Mosenthal HO, Barry E: Evaluation of blood sugar tests: Significance of the nonglucose reducing substances and the arteriovenous blood sugar difference. *Am J Dig Dis* 13:160–170, 1946.

Mosenthal HO, Barry E: Criteria for and interpretation of normal glucose tolerance tests. *Ann Intern Med* 33:1175–1194, 1950.

Mosenthal HO, Bolduan C: Diabetes mellitus—problems of present-day treatment. *Am J Med Sci* 186:605, 1933.

Moses SGP, Gandhi VS: A few aspects of clinical profile and patterns of younger age group diabetics (30 years and below) in Madras, South India. Proc 8th Congr of Int Diab Fed, Belgium, Series 280, 1973, p 161.

Moses SGP, Kannan V: The clinical profile of undernourished diabetics aged 30 or less with associated complications in Madras, India, in Baba S, Goto Y, Fujui I (eds): *Diabetes Mellitus in Asia*. Proc 2nd symp of Kyoto, Amsterdam, Excerpta Medica, Series 390, 1975, p 259–264.

Moss AJ: Profile of high risk in people known to have coronary heart disease: A review. 4. The indicators of risk. *Circulation* 52(suppl 3):147–154, 1975.

Moss JW, Muelholland HB: Diabetes and pregnancy: With special reference to prediabetic state. *Ann Intern Med* 34:678, 1951.

Mouratoff CJ, Carroll NV, Scott EM: Diabetes mellitus in Eskimos. *JAMA* 199:107–112, 1967.

Mouratoff CJ, Carroll NV, Scott EM: Diabetes mellitus in Arthapascan Indians in Alaska. *Diabetes* 18:29–32, 1969.

Mouratoff CJ, Scott EM: Diabetes mellitus in Eskimos after a decade. *JAMA* 226:1345–1346, 1973.

Mouratoff CJ, Scott EM: Diabetes mellitus in the Aleutians of Alaska. *Diabetes* 25 (suppl 1):377, 1976.

Mouriquand G: Obesity in children. *Lyon Med* 129:883, 1920.

Moyer JH, Womack CR: Glucose tolerance: 1. A comparison of four types of diagnostic tests in 103 control subjects and 26 patients with diabetes. *Am J Sci* 219:161–173, 1950.

Mukherjee AB, Pandey GC, Bannerjee N, Gupta MK: Clinical observations on cardiovascular complications of diabetes mellitus, in Patel JC, Talwalker NG (eds): *Diabetes in the Tropics*. Bombay, Diab Assoc of India, 1966, p 329–335.

Mulcahy R, Maurer B, Hickey N: Coronary heart disease: A study of risk factors in 400 patients in 60 years. *Geriatrics* 24:106–114, 1969.

Muller MWA, Faloona GR, Unger RH: The influence of the antecedent diet upon glucagon and insulin secretion. *N Engl J Med* 285:1450–1454, 1971.

Muller R: Diabetic angiopathy and blood viscosity. *Acta Diabetol Lat* 10:1311, 1973.

Munke A: A mass survey to trace previously unknown diabetes mellitus. *Acta Med Scand* 176:169, 1964.

Munro HN, Eaton JC, Glen A: Survey of a Scottish Diabetic Clinic: A study of the etiology of diabetes mellitus. *J Clin Endocrinol* 9:48, 1949.

Murray JT, Hannah EE, Laing JK, et al: Diabetes mellitus in European New Zealanders. *NZ Med J* 69:271–275, 1969.

Murray MJ, Stein N: Does the pancreas influence iron absorption? A critical review of information to date. *Gastroenterology* 51:694, 1966.

Muting D, Kaufmann M: Disorders of glucose tolerance in 2600 histologically confirmed acute and chronic liver patients. *Munch Med Wochenschr* 117:1689–1694, 1975.

Nadon GW, Little JA, Hall WE, et al: A comparison of the oral and intravenous glucose tolerance tests in nondiabetic, possible diabetic, and diabetic subjects. *Can Med Assoc J* 91:1350–1353, 1964.

Nagaratnam N, Gunawardene KRW: Aetiological factors in pancreatic calcification in Ceylon. *Digestion* 5:9–16, 1972.

Najarian JS, Mauer SM, Simmons RG, et al: Rehabilitation and recurrence after 100 kidney transplants to diabetics. *Diabetes* 15(suppl 1):349, 1976.

Najenson T, Mendelson L, Selibiansky H, et al: Diabetes and cerebrovascular accidents. *Isr J Med Sci* 6:598–604, 1970.

Najenson T, Mendelson L, Solzi P, et al: Cerebrovascular accident and diabetes: The pathogenic role of hyperglycemia in diabetic vasculopathy. *Acta Diabetol Lat* 10:1041, 1973.

Nakao Y, Fukunishi T, Koide M, Akasawa K, Ikeda M, Yahata M, et al: HLA antigens in Japanese patients with diabetes mellitus. *Diabetes* 26:736–739, 1977.

National Center for Health Statistics: Comparability of mortality statistics for the 6th and 7th revisions, United States. Vital Health Stat Spec Rep, Vol 51, No. 4. Washington DC, PHS, March 1965.

Natl Center for Health Stat: Blood glucose in adults. Vital Health Stat Pub 1000, Series 11, No. 18. Washington DC, PHS, September 1966.

Natl Center for Health Stat: Characteristics of persons with diabetes, US July 1964–June 1965. Vital Health Stat Publ Health Serv, Publ 1000, Series 10, No. 40, 1967.

Natl Center for Health Stat: Diabetes mellitus mortality in the US, 1950–67. Vital Health Stat Pub 1000, Series 20, No. 10. Rockville, Md, PHS, July 1971.

Natl Center for Health Stat: Mortality trends: Age, color and sex. US 1950–1969. Vital Health Stat, Dept of HEW Publ (HRA) 74-1852, Series 20, No. 15. Washington, DC, Health Resources Admin, November 1973.

Natl Center for Health Stat: Mortality trends for leading causes of death, US 1950–1969. Vital Health Stat, Dept of HEW Publ (HRA) 74-1853, Series 20, No. 16. Washington, DC, Health Resources Admin, March 1974.

Natl Diabetes Commission (United States) Report. Dept of HEW Publ (NIH) 76-1021, 1976.

Natl Heart and Lung Institute (Div of Heart and Vascular Diseases): Clinical applications and prevention. Ref list of Publications 1960–1972, Bethesda, Maryland.

Natl Libr Med: Factors in glucose tolerance in aged humans, January 1964–July 1968: 123 citations. US Dept of HEW Pub Hlth Serv Natl Inst Hlth Literature Search No. 19–68, 1975.

Natl Libr Med: A bibliography on maturity onset diabetes, effect of metabolic control, January 1968–February 1971: 130 citations. Literature Search No. 71-13, 1971.

Natl Libr Med: Dietary fiber, January 1973–October 1975: 105 citations. Pothier PE, Literature Search No. 75-15, 1975.

Naunyn B: *Diabetes Mellitus.* Vienna, Holder, 1898.

Neel JV: Diabetes mellitus: A "thrifty" genotype rendered detrimental by "progress"? *Am J Hum Genet* 14:353–362, 1962.

Neel JV: Diabetes mellitus—a geneticist's nightmare, in Creutzfeldt W, Kobberling J, Neel JV (eds): *The Genetics of Diabetes Mellitus.* New York, Springer-Verlag, 1976, p 1–12.

Neel JV, The genetics of juvenile-onset-type diabetes mellitus. *N Engl J Med* 297:1062–1063, 1977.

Neel JV, Shaw MW, Schull WJ (eds): Genetics and the epidemiology of chronic diseases. *Pub Hlth Serv Pub* 1163, 1965.

Neill MH: Discussion of a mortality study of insured diabetics. *Proc Med Sect Am Life Conv* 49:179–841, 1961.

Nelson PG, Pyke DA: Diabetic complications in concordant identical twins, in Creutz-feldt W, Kobberling J, Neel JV (eds): *The Genetics of Diabetes Mellitus.* New York, Springer-Verlag, 1976, p 215–223.

Nelson PG, Pyke DA: Genetic diabetes not linked to the HLA locus. *Br Med J* 1:196–197, 1976a.

Nelson PG, Pyke DA, Cudworth AG, et al: Histocompatibility antigens in diabetic identical twins. *Lancet* 2:193–194, 1975.

Nelson PG, Pyke DA, Gamble DR. Viruses and the aetiology of diabetes: A study in identical twins. *Br Med J* 4:249–251, 1975.

Nerup J: The inheritance of juvenile diabetes. *Int Diab Fed Bull* 21:6–7, 1976.

Nerup J, Andersen OO, Buschard K, et al: HLA-D typing in insulin-dependent diabetes mellitus (IDDM). *Diabetologia* 13:421, 1977.

Nerup J, Andersen OO, Christy M, et al: HL-A factors, autoimmunity, virus and juvenile diabetes mellitus. *Diabetologia* 8:365–366, 1975.

Nerup J, Andersen OO, Christy M, Platz P, et al: HLA, autoimmunity, virus and the pathogenesis of juvenile diabetes mellitus. *Acta Endocrinol kbh* 83 (suppl):167–175, 1976a.

Nerup J, Platz P, Andersen OO, et al: HL-A antigens and diabetes mellitus. *Lancet* 2:864–866, 1974.

Nerup J, Platz P, Andersen OO, et al: HL-A, autoimmunity and insulin-dependent diabetes mellitus, in Creutzfeldt W, Kobberling J, Neel JV (eds): *Genetics of Diabetes Mellitus.* New York, Springer-Verlag, 1976, p 106–114.

Neubauer B: A quantitative study of peripheral arterial calcification and glucose toler-ance in elderly diabetics and nondiabetics. *Diabetologia* 7:409–413, 1971.

Neubauer B, Christensen NJ: Norepinephrine, epinephrine and dopamine contents of the cardiovascular system in long-term diabetes. *Diabetes* 25:6, 1976.

Neubauer B, Gundersen HJ: Early and progressive loss of autonomic control of the heart in diabetics measured on a standard, resting ECG. *Diabetologia* 12:375–428, 1976.

Newall RG, Bliss BP: Lipoproteins and the relative importance of plasma cholesterol and triglycerides in peripheral arterial disease. *Angiology* 24:297–302, 1973.

Newburgh LH: Control of the hyperglycemia of obese "diabetics" by weight reduction. *Ann Intern Med* 17:935–942, 1942.

Newburgh LH, Conn JW: A new interpretation of hyperglycemia in obese middle-aged persons. *JAMA* 112:7–11, 1939.

Newill VA: Present concepts of incidence and prevalence. *Diabetes* 12:554–559, 1963.

New Zealand Department of Health: Data on high rates of Diabetes in Maoris. Spec Rep No. 1, 1960.

Nichols AB, Ravenscroft C, Lamphier DE, et al: Independence of serum lipid levels and dietary habits: The Tecumseh Study. *JAMA* 236:1948–1953, 1976.

Nicholson WA: Changing sex ratios in diabetes. *Br Med J* 20:465–466, 1971.

Niejadlik DC, Dube AH, Adamko SM: Glucose measurements and clinical correlations. *JAMA* 224:1734–1736, 1973.

Nikkila EA: Triglyceride metabolism in diabetes mellitus. *Prog Biochem Pharmacol* 8:271–299, 1973.

Nikkila EA, Hormila P: Coronary heart disease and its risk factors among chronic insulin-dependent diabetics. *Diabetologia* 12:412, 1976.

Nikkila EA, Miettinen TA, Vesenne MR, et al: Plasma-insulin in coronary heart disease: Response to oral and intravenous glucose and to tolbutamide. *Lancet* 2:508–521, 1965.

Nilsson SE: Genetic and constitutional aspects of diabetes mellitus. *Acta Med Scand* (suppl 375) 1962, p 1–96.

Nilsson SE: On the heredity of diabetes mellitus and its interrelationship with some other diseases. *Acta Genet* 4:97–124, 1964.

Nilsson SE, Lindolm H, Bulow S, et al: The Kristianstad survey 1963–1964. Studies in a normal adult population for variation and correlation in some clinical, anthropometric, and laboratory values, especially the peroral glucose tolerance test. *Acta Med Scand* 177 (suppl 428):1–54, 1964.

Nilsson SE, Nilsson JE, Frostberg E, et al: The Kristianstad Survey II: Studies in a representative adult diabetic population with special reference to comparison with an adequate control group. *Acta Med Scand* (suppl 469) 1967, p 1–42.

Nisell O: The effect of posture and intragastric gas administration on the oral glucose tolerance test. *Acta Med Scand* 157:445–449, 1957.

Nolan S, Stephan T, Chae S, et al: Age related insulin patterns in normal glucose tolerance. *Am Geriatr Soc* 21:106–111, 1973.

Nolan S, Stephan T, Khurana RC, et al: Low profile (flat) glucose tolerances. *Am J Med Sci* 164:33–39, 1972.

Nordsiek FW: The sweet tooth. *Am Sci* 60:41–45, 1972.

Norgaard A: Administrative problems of diabetes. *Br Med J* 2:1, 1933.

North AF, Gorwitz K, Sultz HA: A secular increase in the incidence of juvenile diabetes mellitus. *J Pediatr* 91:706–710, 1977.

Oakley N, Hill DW, Joplin GF, Kohner EM, et al: Diabetic retinopathy: 1. The assessment of severity and progress by comparison with a set of standard fundus photographs. *Diabetologia* 3:402–405, 1967.

Oakley NW, Beard RW, Turner RD: Effect of sustained maternal hyperglycaemia on the foetus in normal and diabetic pregnancies. *Br Med J* 1:466–469, 1972.

Oakley NW, Joplin GF, Kohner EM, et al: Practical experience with a method for grading diabetic retinopathy, in Goldberg MR, Fine SL (eds): *Treatment of Diabetic Retinopathy* US Dept of HEW Public Hlth Serv symposium, 1968, p 3–6.

Oakley W, Catterall RDF, Martin MM: Aetiology and management of lesions of the feet in diabetes. *Br Med J* 2:953, 1968.

Oakley WG, Pyke DA, Tattersall RB, et al: Long term diabetes. *Q J Med* 43:145–156, 1974.

Oakley WG, Pyke DA, Taylor KW: Clinical diabetes and its biochemical basis. Oxford, Blackwell Scientific Publications, 1968a.

Oberdisse K, Jahnke K: *Diabetes Mellitus.* Proc 3rd Congr of Int Diab Fed, Dusseldorf. Stuttgart, Georg Thieme Verlag, 1958.

Ogawa S, quoted in *Sportsmedicine*, World-at-Play Section: "Sumo Wrestlers, Making Gluttony Pay". *Sportsmedicine (The Physician and SportsMedicine)* 2:61, 1974.

515

Ogilvie RF: Sugar tolerance in obese subjects, a review of 65 cases. *Q J Med* 28:345–358, 1935.

Oiso T: Recent annual changes in nutrition in Japan, in Tsuji S, Wada M (eds): *Diabetes Mellitus in Asia,* Proc symp Kobe, Amsterdam, Excerpta Medica, 1970, p 234–242.

Okamoto K, Hazama F, Yamasaki Y: Pathology of diabetes mellitus in Japan, in Tsuji S, Wada M (eds): *Diabetes Mellitus in Asia.* Proc symp, Kobe, Amsterdam, Excerpta Medica, 1970, p 106–119.

Oker C, Ipbuker A, Bagriacik N, et al: The incidence of diabetes mellitus in Turkey. Proc 6th Congr of Int Diab Fed, Stockholm Series 140, 1967, p 31–32.

Okuno G, Tako H, Fukuda K, et al: Vascular complications in diabetic patients with hyperlipemia, in Baba S, Goto Y, Fukui I (eds): *Diabetes Mellitus in Asia.* Proc 2nd symp, Kyoto, Amsterdam, Excerpta Medica, Series 390, 1975, p 183.

Olefsky JM: The insulin receptor: Its role in insulin resistance of obesity and diabetes. *Diabetes* 25:1154–1162, 1976.

Olefsky J, Crapo PA, Ginsberg H, et al: Metabolic effects of increased caloric intake in man. *Metabolism* 24:495, 1975.

Olefsky JM, Farquhar JW, Reaven GM: Do the oral and intravenous glucose tolerance tests provide similar diagnostic information in patients with chemical diabetes mellitus? *Diabetes* 22:202–209, 1973.

Olefsky JM, Reaven GM: Insulin and glucose responses to identical oral glucose tolerance tests performed forty-eight hours apart. *Diabetes* 23:449–453, 1974.

Olefsky J, Reaven GM, Farquhar JW: Effects of weight reduction on obesity: Studies of lipid and carbohydrate metabolism in normal and hyperlipoproteinemic subjects. *J Clin Invest* 53:64–76, 1974.

Olmstead WH, Drey NW, Agress H, Roberts HK: Mass screening for diabetes: The use of a device for the collection of dried urine specimens and testing for sugar (St Louis Dreypak). *Diabetes* 2:37, 1953.

Olurin EO, Olurin O: Pancreatic calcification: A report of 45 cases. *Br Med J* 4:534–539, 1969.

Oppermann W, Iwatsuka H, Reddi AS, et al: Prolonged fasting in mice: A more sensitive approach to genetic diabetes. *Horm Res* 6:150–156, 1975.

Orr JB, Gilks JL: Studies of nutrition: The physique and health of two African tribes, Council special report. *Br Med Res* Series No. 155, 1931.

Orzeck EA, Mooney JH, Owen JA Jr: Diabetes detection with a comparison of screening methods. *Diabetes* 20:109–116, 1971.

Oscarrsson N, Silwer H: Incidence of pulmonary tuberculosis among diabetics: Search among diabetics in the county of Kristianstad. *Acta Med Scand* 1 (suppl):335, 1958.

Osler W: *Diabetes Mellitus in the Principles and Practice of Medicine.* New York, D Appleton and Co, 1894, p 295–305.

Osterby R: Morphometric studies of the peripheral glomerular basement membrane in early juvenile diabetes: 1. Development of initial basement membrane thickening. *Diabetologia* 8:84–92, 1972.

Ostrander LD, Block WB, Lamphiear DE, et al: Altered carbohydrate and lipid metabolism and coronary heart disease among men in Tecumseh, Michigan, in Camerini-

Davalos RA, Cole HS (eds): *Vascular and Neurological Changes in Early Diabetes.* New York, Academic Press, 1973, p 73–82.

Ostrander LD, Epstein FH: Diabetes, hyperglycemia and atherosclerosis: New research directions, in Fajans SS (ed): *Diabetes Mellitus.* US Dept of HEW Publ (NIH) 76-854, 1976, p 194–212.

Ostrander LD Jr, Francis T Jr, Hayner NS, et al: The relationship of cardiovascular disease to hyperglycemia. *Ann Intern Med* 62:1188–1198, 1965.

Ostrander LDJ, Lamphiear DE, Block WD, et al: Biochemical precursors of atherosclerosis, studies in apparently healthy men in a general population, Tecumseh Michigan. *Arch Intern Med* 134:224–230, 1974.

O'Sullivan JB: Problems in comparing population studies of diabetes, in Ostman J, Milner RDG (eds): *Diabetes.* Proc 6th Congr of Int Diab Fed, Stockholm 1967, p 697–700.

O'Sullivan JB: Age gradient in blood glucose levels. *Diabetes* 23:714–715, 1974.

O'Sullivan JB, et al: Report of workgroup on pregnancy of National Commission on Diabetes. US Dept of HEW Publ (NIH) 76-1022, vol 3, part 2, 1976, p 177–277.

O'Sullivan JB, Acheson RM: Comparison of diabetes prevalence rate in Oxford (1946) and Sudbury (1964), in Bennett PH, Miller M (eds): *Epidemiology of Diabetes.* New York, Academic Press, 1977, (in press).

O'Sullivan JB, Charles D, Dandrow R: Treatment of verified prediabetics in pregnancy. *J Reprod Med* 7:21–24, 1971.

O'Sullivan JB, Gellis SS, Dandrow R, et al: The potential diabetic and her treatment in pregnancy. *Obstct Gynccol* 27:683–689, 1966.

O'Sullivan JB, Gordon T: Childbearing and diabetes mellitus: United States 1960–1962. Nat Ctr for Health Stat, Series 11, No. 21, 1966, p 4–5.

O'Sullivan JB, Hurwitz D: Spontaneous remissions in early diabetes mellitus. *Arch Intern Med* 117:769, 1966.

O'Sullivan JB, Kantor N, Wilkerson HC: Comparative value of tests for urinary glucose. *Diabetes* 11:53–55, 1962.

O'Sullivan JB, Mahan CM: Criteria for the oral glucose tolerance test in pregnancy. *Diabetes* 13:278, 1964.

O'Sullivan JB, Mahan CM: Blood sugar levels, glycosuria and body weight related to development of diabetes mellitus: The Oxford epidemiologic study 17 years later. *JAMA* 194:587–592, 1965.

O'Sullivan JB, Mahan CM: Glucose tolerance test: Variability in pregnant and nonpregnant women. *Am J Clin Nutr* 19:345–351, 1966.

O'Sullivan JB, Mahan CM: Prospective study of 352 young patients with chemical diabetes. *N Engl J Med* 278:1038, 1041, 1968.

O'Sullivan JB, Mahan CD, Charles D, et al: Gestational diabetes and perinatal mortality rate. *Am J Obstet Gynecol* 116:901–904, 1973.

O'Sullivan JB, Mahan CM, Charles D, Dandrow RV: Medical treatment of the gestational diabetic. *Obstet Gynecol* 43:817–821, 1974.

O'Sullivan JB, Mahan CM, Friedlander AE, et al: The effect of age on carbohydrate metabolism. *J Clin Endocrinol Metab* 33:619–623, 1971.

O'Sullivan JB, Mahan CM, McCaughan D: Identification of evolving diabetes, in Rodriquez RR, Vallance-Owen J (eds): *Diabetes*. Proc 7th Congr of Int Diab Fed, Buenos Aires, 1970, p 256–260.

O'Sullivan JB, Snyder PJ, Sporer AC, et al: Intravenous glucose tolerance test and its modification by pregnancy. *J Clin Endocrinol Metab* 31:33–37, 1970a.

O'Sullivan JB, Wilkerson HLC, Krall LP: The prevalence of diabetes mellitus in Oxford and related epidemiologic problems. *Am J Public Health* 56:742, 1966.

O'Sullivan JB, Williams RF: Early diabetes mellitus in perspective: A population study in Sudbury Mass. *JAMA* 198:111–114, 1966.

O'Sullivan JB, Williams RF, McDonald GW: The prevalence of diabetes mellitus and related variables—a population study in Sudbury Mass. *J Chron Dis* 20:535–543, 1967.

Osuntokun BO: Diabetic retinopathy in Nigerians: A study of 758 patients. *Br J Ophthalmol* 53:652, 1969.

Osuntokun BO: The neurology of non-alcoholic pancreatic diabetes mellitus in Nigerians. *J Neurol Sci* 11:18–43, 1970.

Osuntokun BO: Cassava diet and cyanide metabolism in Wistar rats. *Br J Nutr* 24:797–800, 1970a.

Osuntokun BO: Hypertension in Nigerian diabetics: A study of 832 patients. *Afr J Med Sci* 3:257–265, 1972.

Osuntokun BO: Diabetes mellitus and infectious hepatitis. *Br Med J* 1:369, 1974.

Osuntokun BO, Akinkugle FM, et al: Diabetes mellitus in Nigerians: A study of 832 patients. *West Afr Med J*, October 1971, p 295–312.

Otim MA: Preliminary observations on diabetic retinopathy in Ugandian African attending Mulago Diabetic Clinic. *East Afr Med J* 52:63–69, 1975.

Otim MA, Kyobe J: Preliminary observations on fasting glucose, triglyceride and cholesterol levels in Mulago Hospital diabetic clinic. *E Afr Med J* 54:96–99, 1977.

Otterman MG, Stahlgren LRH: Evaluation of factors which influence mortality and morbidity following major lower extremity amputations for arteriosclerosis. *Surg Gynecol Obstet* 120:1217–1220, 1965.

Owen JA Jr, Dennis BW, Hollifield G: Pitfalls in diabetes detection during the diagnostic study. *South Med J* 63:161–166, 1970.

Paasikivi J: Long-term treatment of patients with abnormal intravenous glucose tolerance after myocardial infarction, in Camerini-Davalos RA, Cole HS (eds): *Vascular and Neurological Changes in Early Diabetes*. New York, Academic Press, 1973, p 533–538.

Paetkau ME, Boyd TAS, Winship B, Grace M: Cigarette smoking and diabetic retinopathy. *Diabetes* 26:46–49, 1977.

Paffenbarger RS Jr, Wing AL: Chronic disease in former college students: 12. Early precursors of adult onset diabetes mellitus. *Am J Epidemiol* 97:314–323, 1973.

Page L, Friend B: Level of use of sugars in the US, in Sipple HL, McNutt KW (eds): *Sugars in Nutrition*. New York, Academic Press, 1974, p 94–98.

Palmberg PF: Diabetic retinopathy. *Diabetes* 26:703–709, 1977.

Palmer WK, Tipton CM: Effect of training on adipocyte glucose metabolism and insulin responsiveness. *Fed Proc* 33:1964–1968, 1974.

Palumbo PJ: Diabetes mellitus in Rochester Minnesota. *Diabetes* 24:440, 1975.

Palumbo PJ, Connolly DC: Distribution of coronary artery disease in diabetics and nondiabetics. *Diabetes* 25(suppl 1):346, 1976.

Palumbo PJ, Elvebaack LR, Chu CP, et al: Diabetes mellitus: Incidence, prevalence, survivorship and causes of death in Rochester Minnesota 1945–1970. *Diabetes* 25:566–573, 1976.

Park BN, Kahn CB, Gleason RE, Soeldner JS: Insulin-glucose dynamics in nondiabetic reactive hypoglycemia and asymptomatic biochemical hypoglycemia in normals, prediabetics and chemical diabetics. *Diabetes* 2:373, 1972.

Parker AM: Testing skin surface for glucose. *Diabetes* 11:49–52, 1962.

Parson W, MacDonald FW, Shaper AG: African diabetics necropsied at Mulago Hospital, Kampala Uganda 1957–1966. *East Afr Med J* 45:89–99, 1968.

Parving HH, Noer I, Deckert T, et al: The effect of metabolic regulation on microvascular permeability to small and large molecules in short-term juvenile diabetics. *Diabetologia* 12:161–166, 1976.

Patel JC: Epidemiology of diabetes in Asia and Australasia. Proc 6th Congr of Int Diab Fed, 1969, p 673–683.

Patel JC, Dhirawani MK, Doshi JC: Remission in diabetes—study of 24 cases, in Patel JC, Talwalker NG (eds): *Diabetes in the Tropics.* Bombay, Diab Assoc of India, 1966, p 106–109.

Patel JC, Dhirawani MK, Juthami VJ: Incidence of complications in 5481 subjects of diabetes mellitus, in Patel JC, Talwalker NG (eds): *Diabetes in the Tropics.* Bombay, Diab Assoc of India, 1966, p 459–465.

Patel JC, Dhirawani MK, Kabur AN: Juvenile diabetes: A report of 18 cases, in Patel JC, Talwalker NG (eds): *Diabetes in the Tropics.* Bombay, Diab Assoc of India, 1966, p 285–289.

Patel JC, Dhirawani MK, Kadekar SG: Analysis of 5481 subjects of diabetes mellitus, in Patel JC, Talwalker NG (eds): *Diabetes in the Tropics.* Bombay, Diab Assoc of India, 1966, p 94–100.

Patel JC, Talwalker NG (eds): *Diabetes in the Tropics.* Bombay, Diab Assoc of India, 1966.

Patel R, Ansari A, Covarrubias CLP: Leukocyte antigens and disease: 3. Association of HLA-B8 and HLA-BW 15 with insulin-dependent diabetes in three different population groups. *Metabolism* 26:487, 1977.

Patrick A: Acute diabetes following mumps. *Br Med J* 2:802, 1924.

Paullin JE, Sauls HC: A study of the glucose tolerance test in the obese. *South Med J* 15:249–253, 1922.

Paulsen EP, Richenderfer L, Ginsberg-Fellner F: Plasma glucose, free fatty acids, and immunoreactive insulin in 66 obese children: Studies in reference to a family history of diabetes mellitus. *Diabetes* 17:261–269, 1968.

Pavel I, Pieptea R: The prevention of diabetes. *Acta Diabetol Lat* 10:707–724, 1973.

519

Pawliger DF, Shipp JC: Evaluation of the rapid Dextrostix method for determination of blood glucose. *J Fla Med Assoc* 51:641–643, 1965.

Paz-Guevera AT, Hsu TH, White P: Juvenile diabetes mellitus after forty years. *Diabetes* 24:559–565, 1975.

Peacock PB, Riley CP, Lampton TD, Raffel SS, Walker JS: The Birmingham stroke, epidemiology, and rehabilitation study, in Stewart GT (ed): *Trends in Epidemiology: Application to Health Service Research and Training.* Springfield, Ill, Charles C Thomas Pub, 1972, p 281–286.

Pearce MB, Bulloch RT, Kizzler JC: Myocardial small vessel disease in patients with diabetes mellitus. *Circulation* 48(suppl IV):6, 1973.

Peck FB, Kirtley WR, Peck FB: Complete remission of severe diabetes. *Diabetes* 7:93–97, 1958.

Pedersen J: *The Pregnant Diabetic and Her Newborn: Problems and Management,* ed 2. Baltimore, Williams and Wilkins Co, 1977.

Pedersen J, Olsen S: Small vessel disease of the lower extremity in diabetes mellitus. *Acta Med Scand* 171:551, 1962.

Pehrson SL: A study of the relationship between some prediabetic stigmas, glucose tolerance in late pregnancy and the birthweight of the children. *Acta Obstet Gynecol Scand* (suppl 33) 1974, p 107–131.

Pell S, D'Alonzo CA: Acute myocardial infarction in a large industrial population: Report of a 6-year study of 1,356 cases. *JAMA* 185:831–838, 1963.

Pell S, D'Alonzo CA: Immediate mortality and five-year survival of employed men with a first myocardial infarction. *N Engl J Med* 270:915, 1964.

Pell S, D'Alonzo CA: Some aspects of hypertension in diabetes mellitus. *JAMA* 202:104–110, 1967.

Pell S, D'Alonzo CA: Diabetes in industry: Prevalence, epidemiology, and prognosis in a large employed population. *Arch Environ Health* 17:425–435, 1968.

Pell S, D'Alonzo CA: Factors associated with long-term survival of diabetics. *JAMA* 214:1833–1840, 1970.

Pennel BM, Keagle JG: Predisposing factors in the etiology of chronic inflammatory periodontal disease. *J Periodontol* 48:517–532, 1977.

Perkins RP: Failure of pyridoxine to improve glucose tolerance in gestational diabetes mellitus. *Obstet Gynecol* 50:370–372, 1977.

Persson B, Sterky G, Thorell J: Effect of low carbohydrate diet on plasma glucose, free fatty acids, glycerol, ketones and insulin during glucose tolerance tests in adolescent boys. *Metabolism* 16:714–722, 1967.

Pessi TT: Prevalence of diabetes in Nokia, a Finnish country town in 1960. *Duodecim* 80:1071–1076, 1964.

Petersen K: A profile of diabetes mellitus among the Indians of a Sioux/Assiniboine reservation. Proc 4th Joint Meet of Clin Soc and Commissioned Officers Assoc USPHS, Boston, June 1969, p 35.

Petersen KG, Schmitthenner U, Kerp L: A hyperglycemic syndrome induced in mice by a protein rich diet. *Diabetologia* 10:383, 1974.

Peterson AD, Baumgardt BR: Food and energy intake of rats fed diets varying in energy concentration and density. *J Nutr* 101:1057–1068, 1971.

Peterson CM, Jones RL, Koenig RJ, et al: Reversible hematologic sequelae of diabetes mellitus. *Ann Intern Med* 86:425–429, 1977.

Peterson DT, Reaven GM: Evidence that glucose load is an important determinant of plasma insulin response in normal subjects. *Diabetes* 20:729–733, 1971.

Petersson B, Hellman B: Long-term effects of restricted calorie intake on pancreatic islet tissue in obese-hyperglycemic mice. *Metabolism* 11:342–348, 1962.

Petrie LM, Bowdoin CD, McLoughlin CJ: Voluntary multiple health tests. *JAMA* 148:1022–1024, 1952.

Petrie LM, McLoughlin CJ, Hodgins TE: Mass screening for lowered glucose tolerance. *Ann Intern Med* 40:963–967, 1954.

Petzoldt R, Frerichs H, Selbmann HK, et al: The natural history of diabetes mellitus: Results of a retrospective study. *Diabetologia* 11:369, 1975.

Pfeiffer EF: Obesity: Islet function and diabetes mellitus. *Acta Endocrinol* 173(suppl):181, 1973.

Picard C, Preumont P, Rothschild E: Analyse des resultants de l'eruve d'hyperglycemie intraveineuse pendant la grossesse. *Bull Fed Soc Gyn Obst* 15:249, 1963.

Pillai RP: Diabetes in Malaya. *Med J Malaysia* 14:225, 1960.

Pillay RP, Hin LE: Incidence of diabetes mellitus in Malaya. *Med J Malaysia* 14:242–244, 1960.

Pimstone B, Becker D, Kernoff L: Growth and growth hormone in protein calorie malnutrition. *S Afr Med J* 46:2101–2105, 1972.

Pirart J: Diabetic neuropathy: A metabolic or a vascular disease? *Diabetes* 14:1–9, 1965.

Pirart J: Diabetes mellitus and its degenerative complications: a prospective study of 4,400 patients observed between 1947 and 1973. *Diabete Metab* 3:97–107, 1977.

Pirart J, Lauvaux JP: Diabetic retinopathy, nephropathy, neuropathy: Relation to duration and control. *Diabetologia* 11:370, 1975.

Pitchumoni CS: Pancreas in primary malnutrition disorders. *Am J Clin Nutr* 26:374–379, 1973.

Pitchumoni CS, Thomas E: Chronic cassava toxicity: Possible relationship to chronic pancreatic disease in malnourished populations. *Lancet* 2:1397–1398, 1973.

Podolsky S: Lipoatrophic diabetes and miscellaneous conditions related to diabetes mellitus, in Marble A, White P, et al (eds): *Joslin's Diabetes Mellitus*, ed 11. Philadelphia, Lea & Febiger, p 722–766.

Politzer WM, Schneider T: Incidence of diabetes mellitus in Basutoland: Possible nutritional influences. *South Afr Med J* 34:1037–1039, 1960.

Pollack AA, McCarl TJ, MacIntyre N: Diabetes mellitus: A review of mortality experience. *Arch Intern Med* 119:161–163, 1967.

Poon-King T, Henry MV, Rampersad F: Prevalence and natural history of diabetes in Trinidad. *Lancet* 1:155, 1968.

Poulsen JE: Recovery from retinopathy in a case of diabetes with Simmond's disease. *Diabetes* 2:7, 1953.

Pozefsky T, Colker JL, Langs HM, Andres R: The cortisone-glucose tolerance test: The influence of age on performance. *Ann Intern Med* 63:988–1000, 1965.

521

Pozefsky T, Santis MR, Soeldner JB, et al: Insulin sensitivity of forearm tissues in prediabetic man. *J Clin Invest* 22:1608–1615, 1973.

Price AVG, Tulloch JA: Diabetes mellitus in Papua and New Guinea. *Med J Aust,* October 1966, p 645–648.

Prior IAM: A health survey in a rural Maori community with particular emphasis on cardiovascular, nutritional and metabolic findings. *NZ Med J* 61:333–340, 1962.

Prior IAM: The price of civilization. *Nutr Today* 6:2–11, 1971.

Prior IAM: Cardiovascular epidemiology in New Zealand and the Pacific. *NZ Med J* 80:245–252, 1974.

Prior IAM: Diabetes in the South Pacific, in Hillebrand SS (ed): *Is the Risk of Becoming Diabetic Affected by Sugar Consumption?* Proc 8th Int symp of Sugar Res Fdn. Bethesda, Maryland, International Sugar Research Foundation, 1974a, p 4–13.

Prior IAM, Davidson F: The epidemiology of diabetics in Polynesians and Europeans in New Zealand and the Pacific. *NZ Med J* 65:375–383, 1966.

Prior IAM, Evans JG: Current developments in the Pacific: Atherosclerosis. Proc 2nd Int symp. New York, Springer-Verlag, 1970, p 335–342.

Prior IAM, Rose BS, Davidson F: Metabolic maladies in New Zealand Maoris. *Br Med J* 1:1065–1069, 1964.

Prior IAM, Rose BS, Harvey HPB, Davidson F: Hyperuricemia, gout, and diabetic abnormality in Polynesian people. *Lancet* 1:333–338, 1966.

Prior IAM, Stanhope JM, Evans JG, Salmond CE: The Tokelau Island migrant study. *Int J Epidemiol* 3:225–232, 1974.

Prosnitz LR, Mandell GL: Diabetes mellitus among Navajo and Hopi Indians: The lack of vascular complications. *Am J Med Sci* 253:700–705, 1967.

Proust AJ, McCracken DI: Organization and methods used in the Canberra, Goulburn and Toowoomba diabetes surveys. *Med J Aust,* November 1968, p 772–774.

Proust AJ, Smithurst BA: Epidemiology of diabetes mellitus in Australia. *Med J Aust,* November 1968, p 769–771.

Prout TE: Therapy of early diabetes: The University Group Diabetes Program, in Camerini-Davalos RA, Cole HS (eds): *Vascular and Neurological Changes in Early Diabetes.* New York and London, Academic Press, 1973, p 501.

Prout TE: The use of screening and diagnostic procedures: The oral glucose tolerance test, in Sussman KE, Metz RJS (eds): *Diabetes Mellitus,* ed 4. New York, American Diabetes Assoc, 1975, p 57–68.

Prout TE, et al: Report of the workgroup on definition and diagnosis of diabetes mellitus, in Rep of Nat Comm on Diab of the US, vol 3, part 1. US Nat Inst Hlth, Dept of HEW Publ (NIH) 76-1021, 1976, p 43–64.

Pruet EDR, Oseid S: Effect of exercise on glucose and insulin response to glucose infusion. *Scand J Clin Lab Invest* 26:277–285, 1970.

Puckett DW, et al: Psychological impact of diabetes, in Rep of Natl Comm on Diab of the US, vol 3, part 2. US Ntl Inst Hlth, Dept of HEW (NIH) 76-1022, 1976, p 259–302.

Pyke DA: Parity and the incidence of diabetes. *Lancet* 1:818–821, 1956.

Pyke DA: Aetiological factors in diabetes. *Postgrad Med J* 35:261, 1969.

Pyke DA: Diagnostic tests, in Oakley WG, et al (eds): *Clinical Diabetes and Its Biochemical Basis.* Oxford, Blackwell Scientific Publications, 1968, p 284–310.

Pyke DA: Arterial disease in diabetes, in Oakley WG, Pyke DA, Taylor KW (eds): *Clinical Diabetes and Its Biochemical Basis.* Edinburgh, Blackwell Scientific Publications, 1968, p 506–541.

Pyke DA: Coronary disease and diabetes. *Postgrad Med J* 44:966, 1968a.

Pyke DA: The geography of diabetes. *Postgrad Med J* 45(suppl):796–801, 1969.

Pyke DA: The genetics of diabetes. *Postgrad Med J* 46:604–606, 1970.

Pyke DA: Men, women, and diabetes. *Postgrad Med J* 47:54, 1971.

Pyke DA: Diabetic retinopathy. *Trans Med Soc Lond* 90:96–100, 1974.

Pyke, DA: Genetics of diabetes. *Clin Endocrinol Metab* 6:285–303, 1977.

Pyke DA, Cassar J, Todd J, Taylor KW: Glucose tolerance and serum insulin in identical twins of diabetics. *Br Med J* 4:649–651, 1970.

Pyke DA, Nelson PG: Histocompatibility antigens in diabetic identical twins. *Diabetes* 24:402, 1975.

Pyke DA, Please NW: Obesity, parity and diabetes. *J Endocrinol* 15:24–33, 1957.

Pyke DA, Roberts D St C: Retinopathy in early cases of diabetes mellitus. *Acta Med Scand* 163:489–493, 1959.

Pyke DA, Smith RBW, Nelson PG, Goetz FC, Johnson E: Serum cholesterol and blood pressure levels in diabetic identical twins. *Diabetologia* 13:426, 1977.

Pyke DA, Tattersall RB: Diabetic retinopathy in identical twins. *Diabetes* 22:613–618, 1973.

Pyke DA, Tattersall RB: Birthweight and diabetes. *Lancet* 2:638, 1976.

Pyke DA, Wattley GH: Diabetes in Trinidad. *West Ind Med J* 11:22–26, 1962.

Pyorala K, Lehtovirta E, Llumaki L: The relationship of obesity to prevalence and incidence of diabetes in Helsinki policemen. *Acta Endocrinol* 181:23–24, 1974.

Pyorala K, Reunanen A, Aromaa A: The relationship of hyperglycaemia to the risk of cardiovascular death. *Diabetologia* 11:371, 1975.

Rabb-Smith HT: Global aspects of ischaemic heart disease, in *The Enigma of Coronary Heart Disease.* London, Lloyd-Luke Ltd, 1967, p 62–83.

Rabinowitch IM: The cholesterol content of the blood plasma as an index of the progress in insulin-treated diabetics. *Can Med Assoc J* 17:171–175, 1927.

Rabinowitch IM: Simultaneous determinations of arterial and venous blood-sugars in diabetic individuals. *Br J Exp Pathol* 8:76–84, 1927a.

Rabinowitch IM: The cholesterol content of blood plasma in diabetes mellitus: A statistical study based on two thousand observations in 385 cases. *Arch Intern Med* 43:363–371, 1929.

Rabinowitch IM: Clinical and laboratory experiences with high carbohydrate–low calorie diets in the treatment of diabetes mellitus. *N Engl J Med* 204:799–809, 1931.

Rabinowitch IM: Prevention of premature arteriosclerosis in diabetes mellitus. *Can Med Assoc J* 51:300–306, 1944.

Rabinowtich IM: Diabetes mellitus. *Am J Dig Dis* 16:95–101, 1949.

523

Rabinowitch IM, Ritchie WL, McKee SH: A statistical evaluation of different methods for the detection of arteriosclerosis in diabetes mellitus. *Ann Intern Med* 7:1478–1490, 1934.

Rabinowitz D, Zierler KL: Forearm metabolism in obesity and its response to intraarterial insulin: Characterization of insulin resistance and evidence for adaptive hyperinsulinism. *J Clin Invest* 41:2173–2181, 1962.

Rabkin MT, Field RA: The impact of diabetes mellitus on the responsibilities of a general hospital. *J Chron Dis* 15:91–103, 1962.

Racic Z, Kozarevic D, Vojvodic N: Blood sugar level and coronary heart disease (CHD) incidence, in Bajaj JS (ed): *Current Topics in Diabetes Research*. Proc 9th Congr of Int Diab Fed, India, Series 400, 1976, p 181.

Raheja BS: Diet in diabetes mellitus amongst Sindhis, in Patel JD, Talwalker NG (eds): *Diabetes in the Tropics*. Bombay, Diab Assoc of India, 1966, p 548–551.

Rajasuriya K, Thenabadu PN, Munasinghe DR: Pancreatic calcification in Ceylon with special reference to its etiology. *Ceylon Med J* 15:11, 1970.

Ramachandran S, Rajapakse CNA, Yoganathan M: Diabetic nephropathy in the Tropics. *J Indian Med Assoc* 61:28–32, 1973.

Rand CG, Jackson RJD, Mackie CC: A method for epidemiologic study of early diabetes. *Can Med Assoc J* 111:1312–1314, 1974.

Ranofsky AL: Utilization of short-stay hospitals. Natl Health Survey:Series 13, No 31. DHEW (HRA) 77–1782, 1977.

Rao B, Verma N, Khare OP, et al: Isocaloric high carbohydrate diets in therapy of diabetes mellitus, in Bajaj JS (ed): *Current Topics in Diabetes Research*. Proc 9th Congr of Int Diab Fed, India, Series 400, 1976, p 84.

Rao PS, Naik BK, Saboo RV, et al: Incidence of diabetes in Hyderabad, in Patel JD, Talwalker NG (eds): *Diabetes in the Tropics*. Bombay, Diab Assoc of India, 1966, p 68–75.

Rasch R: The effect of diabetic control on kidney weight, glomerular volume and glomerular basement membrane thickness. *Diabetologia* 13:426, 1977.

Ravid M, Berkowicz M, Sohar E: Hyperglycemia during acute myocardial infarction: A six-year follow up study. *JAMA* 233:807–809, 1975.

Raychaudhuri BJ: Causes of death in diabetes. *J Indian Med Assoc* 61:10–11, 1973.

Reaven GA, Calciano R, Lucas C, Miller R: Carbohydrate intolerance and hyperlipidemia in patients with myocardial infarction without known diabetes mellitus. *J Clin Endocrinol* 23:1013–1023, 1963.

Reaven GM, Olefsky J, Farquhar JW: Does hyperglycemia or hyperinsulinemia characterise the patient with chemical diabetes? *Lancet* 1:1247–1249, 1972.

Redhead IH: Incidence of glycosuria and diabetes mellitus in a general practice. *Br Med J* 1:685–699, 1960.

Redisch W, Kuthan F, Camerini-Davalos R, Clauss RH: Vascular disease in diabetics: 1. Incidence. *Vasa* 2:40–44, 1973.

Reed AC: Diabetes in China. *Am J Med Sci* 151:577–581, 1976.

Reed D, Labarthe D, Stallones R: Health effects of westernization and migration among Chamorros. *Am J Epidemiol* 92:94–112, 1970.

Reed D, Labarthe D, Stallones R, Brody J: Epidemiologic studies of serum glucose levels among Micronesians. *Diabetes* 22:129–136, 1973.

Reichle FA, Tyson RR: Comparison of long-term results of 364 femoropoliteal or femorotibial bypasses for revascularization of severely ischemic lower extremities. *Ann Surg* 182:449–455, 1975.

Reid DD: Epidemiology in modern medicine, editorial. *Triangle* 12:1–2, 1973.

Reid DD, Brett GZ, Hamilton RJ, et al: Cardiorespiratory disease and diabetes among middle-aged male civil servants: A study of screening and intervention. *Lancet* 1:469–473, 1974.

Reid J, Fullmer SD, Pettigrew KD, et al: Nutrient intake of Pima Indian women: Relationships to diabetic mellitus and gallbladder disease. *Am J Clin Nutr* 24:1281–1289, 1971.

Reilly RW, Kirsner JB: Fiber deficiency and colonic disorders. *Am J Clin Nutr* 28:293–294, 1975.

Reinhard KR, Greenwalt NI: Epidemiological definition of the cohort of diseases associated with diabetes in Southwestern American Indians. *Med Care* 13:160–175, 1975.

Reinheimer W, Davidson PC, Albrink MJ: Effect of moderate exercise on plasma glucose, insulin, and free fatty acids during oral glucose tolerance tests. *J Lab Clin Med* 71:429–437, 1968.

Reinheimer W, Bliffen G, McCoy J, et al: Weight gain, serum lipids and vascular disease in diabetics. *Am J Clin Nutr* 20:986, 1967.

Remein QR, Wilkerson HLC: The efficiency of screening tests for diabetes. *J Chron Dis* 13:6, 1961.

Rennie IDB, Keen H, Southon A: A rapid enzyme-strip method for estimating blood sugar. *Lancet* 2:884–886, 1964.

Rennie JL: Diabetes mellitus following mumps. *Glasgow Med J* 124:203–205, 1935.

Renold AE, Burr I, Stauffacher W: On the pathogenesis of diabetes mellitus: Possible usefulness of spontaneous hyperglycemic syndromes in animals, in Cerasi E, Luft R (eds): *The Nobel Symposium #13, Pathogenesis of Diabetes Mellitus*. New York, John Wiley, 1970, p 215–236.

Renold AE, Burr IM, Stauffacher W: Experimental and spontaneous diabetes in animals: What is their relevance to human diabetes mellitus? *Proc R Soc Med* 64:613–617, 1971.

Renold AE, Soeldner JS, Steinke J: Immunological studies with homologous and heterologous pancreatic insulin in the cow. in *Etiology of Diabetes Mellitus and Its Complications*. Ciba Foundation Colloquium vol 15. Boston, Little, Brown and Co, 1964, p 122.

Renold AE, Steinke J, Soeldner JS, et al: Immunological response to the prolonged administration of heterologous and homologous insulin in cattle. *J Clin Invest* 45:702, 1966.

Reunanen A, Pyorala K, Aromaa A: Regional differences in the prevalence and incidence of diabetes mellitus in Finland. *Diabetologia* 12:416, 1976.

Reynertson RH, Tzagournis M: Clinical and metabolic characteristics. *Arch Intern Med* 132:649–653, 1973.

Rezler D: Epidemiology of diabetes in the South Moravian region. *Vnitr Lek* 14:937–945, 1968.

Richardson JF: The sugar intake of businessmen and its inverse relationship with relative weight. *Br J Nutr* 27:449–461, 1972.

Ricketts HT, Cherry RA, Kirsteins L: Biochemical characteristics of the "pre-diabetic state", in Patel JC, Talwalker NG (eds): *Diabetes in the Tropics*. Bombay, Diab Assoc of India, 1966, p 115–119.

Ries W: Feeding behavior in obesity. *Proc Nutr Soc* 32:187–193, 1973.

Rifkin H, Berkman J: Diabetes and the kidney, in Ellenberg M, Rifkin H (eds): *Diabetes Mellitus: Theory and Practice*. New York, McGraw-Hill Book Co, 1970.

Rifkin H, Ross H: Classification and natural history of genetic diabetes mellitus, in Sussman KE, Metz RJS (eds): *Diabetes Mellitus*, ed 4. New York, American Diabetes Association, 1975.

Rifkind BM: Relationship between relative body weight and serum lipid levels. *Br Med J* 2:208–210, 1966.

Rifkind, BM, Levy RI (eds): *Hyperlipidemia. Diagnosis and Therapy*. New York, Grune and Stratton, 1977.

Riley CP, Oberman A, Sheffield LT: Electrocardiographic effects of glucose ingestion. *Arch Intern Med* 130:703–707, 1972.

Rimm AA, Werner LH, Van Yserloo B, Bernstein RA: Relationship of obesity and disease in 75,532 weight-conscious women. *Public Health Rep* 90:44–54, 1975.

Rimoin DL: Ethnic variability in glucose tolerance and insulin secretion. *Arch Intern Med* 124:695–700, 1969.

Rimoin DL: Inheritance in diabetes mellitus. *Med Clin North Am* 55:807–819, 1971.

Rimoin DL: Genetic syndromes associated with glucose intolerance, in Creutzfeldt W, Kobberling J, Neel JV (eds): *Genetics of Diabetes Mellitus*. New York, Springer-Verlag, 1976, p 43–63.

Rimoin DL, Schimke RN: Endocrine pancreas, in *Genetic Disorders of the Endocrine Glands*. St Louis, CV Mosby Co, 1971, p 150–215.

Roberts HJ: Afternoon glucose tolerance testing: A key to the pathogenesis, early diagnosis and prognosis of diabetogenic hyperinsulinism. *J Am Geriatr Soc* 12:423, 1964.

Roberts SR: Comments on obesity and diabetes. *South Med J* 15:243, 1922.

Robertson WB: Diabetes, hypertension and atherosclerosis. *Postgrad Med J* December 1968 (suppl), p 939–943.

Robertson WB, Strong JP: Atherosclerosis in persons with hypertension and diabetes mellitus. *Lab Invest* 18:538–551, 1968.

Rodriguez JLM, Gaona T, Poveda P: Epidemiologia del diabete. *Minerva Med* 61:3848–3855, 1970.

Rogers WR, Holcomb B: Lengthy diabetes: Causes and effects. *Arch Intern Med* 105:746–751, 1960.

Rogot E, Goldberg ID, Goldstein H: Survivorship and causes of death among the blind. *J Chron Dis* 19:179, 1966.

Rolles CJ, Rayner PHW, Mackintosh P: Aetiology of juvenile diabetes. *Lancet* 2:230, 1975.

Rollo J: The history, nature and treatment of diabetes mellitus, in *Cases of the Diabetes Mellitus,* vol 1. London, T Gillet, C Dilley, 1798.

Romero H: Diabetes in the overall picture of Chilean Health. *Rev Med Chile* 100:464–467, 1972.

Romo M: Factors related to sudden death in acute ischemic heart disease: A community study in Helsinki. *Acta Med Scand* (suppl 547) 1972, p 5–25, 54–56.

Roon AJ, Moore WS, Goldstone J: Below-knee amputation: A modern approach. *Am J Surg* 134:153–158, 1977.

Root HF: The association of diabetes and tuberculosis: Epidemiology, pathology treatment and prognosis. *N Engl J Med* 210:1–13, 1934.

Root HF, Mirsky S, Ditzel J: Proliferative retinopathy in diabetes mellitus: Review of eight hundred forty-seven cases. *JAMA* 169:903–909, 1959.

Root HF, Pote WH Jr, Frehner H: Triopathy of diabetes. *Arch Intern Med* 94:931–941, 1954.

Rose GA, Blackburn H: Cardiovascular survey methods. WHO Monogr Series No. 56, 1968.

Rosen AJ, DePalma RG, Victor Y: Risk factors in peripheral atherosclerosis. *Arch Surg* 107:303–308, 1973.

Rosenbaum P: Juvenile diabetes mellitus at Charity Hospital: Selected experiences with 31 diabetic children on the LSU Pediatric Service from 1953–1967 are reviewed. *J La State Med Soc* 119:389–393, 1967.

Rosenbloom AL: Insulin responses of children with chemical diabetes mellitus. *N Engl J Med* 282:1228–1231, 1970.

Rosenbloom AL: The natural history of diabetes mellitus. *Public Health Rev* 2:115–154, 1973.

Rosenbloom AL: Criteria for interpretation of the oral glucose tolerance tests in children and insulin responses with normal and abnormal tolerance. *Metabolism* 22:301–305, 1973A.

Rosenbloom AL: Nature and nurture in the expression of diabetes mellitus and its vascular manifestations. *Am J Dis Child* 131:1154–1159, 1977.

Rosenbloom AL, Allen CM: Mass urine glucose screening in children (Part II). *Metabolism* 22:323–326, 1973.

Rosenbloom AL, Drash A, Guthrie R: V. Conference summary. Chemical diabetes in childhood. *Metabolism* 22:413–419, 1973.

Rosenbloom AL, Giordano B: Is there a sex difference in juvenile diabetes? *J Pediatr* 87:150–151, 1975.

Rosenbloom AL, Lezotte DC, Weber FT, et al: Diminution of bone mass in childhood diabetes. *Diabetes* 26:1052–1055, 1977.

Rosenbloom AL, Sherman L: The natural history of idiopathic hypoglycemia of infancy and its relation to diabetes mellitus. *N Engl J Med* 274:815–820, 1966.

527

Rosenbloom AL, Sherman L: Glucose tolerance testing in children with random glucosuria with symptoms suggestive of hypoglycemia and with idiopathic hypoglycemia of infancy. *Metabolism* 22:363, 1973.

Rosenman RH, Brand RJ, Jenkins CD, et al: Coronary heart disease in the Western Collaborative group study: Final follow up experience of 8 & ½ years. *JAMA* 233:872–877, 1975.

Rosenthal MI, Goldfine ID, Siperstein MD: Genetic origin of diabetes: Re-evaluation of twin data. *Lancet* 2:250–251, 1976.

Ross CW: The determination of glucose tolerance, in Harris C, Moncrieff A (eds): *Archives of Disease in Childhood,* vol 13. London, Br Med Assoc House, 1938, p 289–309.

Ross H, Johnston IDA, Welborn TA, Wright AD: Effect of abdominal operation on glucose tolerance and serum levels of insulin, growth hormone, and hydrocortisone. *Lancet* 2:563–566, 1966.

Rosselin GE, Claude JR, Eschwege EP, et al: Diabetes survey: Plasma insulin during 0–2 h oral glucose tolerance test systematically carried out in a professional group: 1. Relationship with plasma glucose, free fatty acids, cholesterol, triglycerides and corpulence. *Diabetologia* 7:34–45, 1971.

Rostlapil J: Frequency of malignant tumours in diabetes mellitus. *Acta Diabetol Lat* 11:43–45, 1974.

Rostlapil J: Juvenile diabetes in Czechoslovakia, cited by Jarrett RJ: Int Diab Fed Bull 21:22, 1976.

Rottiers RP, Mattheeuws D, Vermeulen A: Glucose assimilation and insulin secretion in low- and high-dose intravenous glucose tolerance tests in normal dogs, in Bajaj JS (ed): *Current Topics in Diabetes Research.* Proc 9th Congr of Int Diab Fed, India, Series #400, 1976, p 28–29.

Royal College of Physicians of London and the British Cardiac Society: Diabetes and coronary heart disease, in *Prevention of Coronary Heart Disease.* Report of a Joint Working Party. *J R Coll Physicians* 10:253–255, 1976.

Rubenstein AH, Horwitz DL, Steiner DF: Clinical significance of circulating proinsulin and C-peptide, in Sussman KE, Metz RJS (eds): *Diabetes Mellitus,* ed 4. New York, Comm on Prof Educ Amer Diab Assoc, 1975, p 9–14.

Rubenstein AH, Seftel HC, Miller K, et al: Metabolic response to oral glucose in healthy South African White, Indian, and African subjects. *Br Med J* 1:748–751, 1969.

Rubenstein P, Suciu-Foca N, Nicholson JF, et al: The HLA system in the families of patients with juvenile diabetes mellitus. *J Exp Med* 143:1277–1281, 1976.

Rubenstein P, Suciu-Foca N, Nicholson, JF: Genetics of juvenile diabetes mellitus. A recessive gene closely linked to HLA D and with 50 per cent penetrance. *N Engl J Med* 297:1036–1040, 1977.

Rublek S, Dlugash J, Yuceoglu YZ, et al: New type of cardiomyopathy associated with diabetic glomerulosclerosis. *Am J Cardiol* 30:595–601, 1972.

Rudnick PA, Anderson PS Jr: Diabetes mellitus in Hiroshima, Japan: A detection program and clinical survey. *Diabetes* 11:533–543, 1962.

Rudy A, Keeler CE: Studies on heredity in Jewish diabetic patients. *N Engl J Med* 221:329–332, 1939.

Rupe BD, Mayer J: Endogenous glucose release stimulated by oral sucrose administration in rats. *Experientia* 23:1009–1010, 1967.

Rushforth NB, Bennett PH, Steinberg AG, et al: Comparison of the value of the two- and one-hour glucose levels of the oral glucose tolerance test in the diagnosis of diabetes in Pima Indians. *Diabetes* 24:538–546, 1975.

Ryan JR, Balodimos MC, Chazan MB, et al: Quarter century victory medal for diabetes: A follow-up of patients one to 20 years later. *Metabolism* 19:493–501, 1970.

Ryan WG, Economou PG, Schwartz TB: Intravenous glucose tolerance test in an industrial population: Controls, subjects with coronary heart disease and relatives of diabetics. *Diabetes* 16:171–174, 1967.

Saddi R, Feingold J: Idiopathic haemochromatosis and diabetes mellitus. *Clin Genet* 5:242–247, 1974.

Sagel J, Colwell JA, Crook L, et al: Increased platelet aggregation in early diabete mellitus. *Ann Intern Med* 82:733–738, 1975.

Sagild U, Littauer J, Jespersen CS, Andersen S: Epidemiological studies in Greenland 1962–1964. *Acta Med Scand* 179:29–39, 1966.

Saiki JH, Rimoin DL: Diabetes mellitus among the Navajo. *Arch Intern Med* 122:1–5, 1968.

Sakaguchi K: *Treatment of Diabetes Mellitus* (Japanese), ed 2. Tokyo, Tohoda, 1926, p 35–36.

Sakumoto S: Epidemiology of diabetes mellitus in Okinawa, in Tsuji S, Wada M (eds): *Diabetes Mellitus in Asia.* Proc symp, Kobe, May 1970, Amsterdam, Excerpta Medica, p 98–101.

Sakumoto S, Kyoda S, Oshiro S, et al: Epidemiology of diabetes mellitus in Okinawa. *J Jpn Diabetes Soc* 14:37–39, 1970.

Salans LB, Dougherty JW: The effect of insulin upon glucose metabolism by adipose cells of different size: Influence of cell lipid and protein content, age, and nutritional state. *J Clin Invest* 50:1399, 1971.

Salans LB, Knittle JL, Hirsch J: The role of adipose cell size and adipose tissue insulin sensitivity in the carbohydrate intolerance of human obesity. *J Clin Invest* 47:153–165, 1968.

Samokhvalova MA, Romensky AA, Zhukovsky GS, et al: Statistical methods in studying the epidemiology of diabetes mellitus. *Probl Endokrinol* 20:7–12, 1974.

Sanchez MM, Cortazar J: A preliminary study of relatives of diabetics in Colombia. Proc 7th Congr of Int Diab Fed, Series 231, 1970, p 345–362.

Sanders MJ: The effect of prednisolone on glucose tolerance in respect to age and family history of diabetes mellitus. *Diabetes* 20:41, 1961.

Sandwith FM: Discussion on diabetes in Egypt. *Br Med J,* October 1907, p 1059.

Sankale M, Sow AM, Signate S: Diabetes mellitus in black Africans in Senegal. *Afr J Med Sci* 1:17–31, 1970.

Santen RJ, Willis PW III, Fajans SS: Atherosclerosis in diabetes mellitus. *Arch Intern Med* 130:833–843, 1972.

Sarker AK, Pal G, Chakravarty RN: Effect of alloxan diabetes and insulin treatment on the development of atherosclerosis in cholesterol-fed rabbits, in Patel JS, Talwalker NG (eds): *Diabetes in the Tropics.* Bombay, Diab Assoc of India, 1966, p 168–172.

529

Sarles H: An international survey on nutrition and pancreatitis. *Digestion* 9:389–402, 1973.

Sasaki A, Cho T, Suzuki T, et al: An epidemiological study on diabetes mellitus in Osaka Japan—a preliminary report. Annual Report, Center for Adult Diseases, 1964, p 3–6, 128–137.

Sasaki A, Horiuchi N, Kamodo K: A changing pattern of causes of death in Japanese diabetics in the past 15 years, in Bajaj JS (ed): *Current Topics in Diabetes Research.* Proc 9th Congr of Int Diab Fed, India, Series 400, 1976, p 182.

Sasaki A, Horiuchi N, Suzuki T: A population-based epidemiological study on diabetes mellitus in a Japanese town. Proc 8th Congr of Int Diab Fed, Belgium, Series 280, 1973, p 162.

Sasaki A, Kamodo K, Horiuchi N: A changing pattern of the causes of death in Japanese diabetics: Observations over 14 years, in Baba S, Goto Y, Fukui I (eds): *Diabetes Mellitus in Asia.* Proc 2nd symp, Kyoto, Amsterdam, Excerpta Medica, Series 390, 1975, p 98–108.

Sathe RV: The problem of diabetes mellitus in India. *J Indian Med Assoc* 61:12–16, 1973.

Satyanarayana RP, Naik BK, Saboo RV, et al: Incidence of diabetes in Hyderabad, in Patel JC, Talwalker NG (eds): *Diabetes in the Tropics.* Bombay, Diab Assoc of India, 1966, p 68–75.

Saundby R: *Lectures on Diabetes.* Bristol, John Wright, 1891.

Saundby R: Diabetes mellitus, in Allbutt C, Rolleston HD (eds): *A System of Medicine by Many Writers,* vol 3. London, MacMillan and Co, Ltd, 1908, p 167–212.

Saundby R: Diabetes mellitus among the Chinese. *Br Med J* 1:116–117, 1908a.

Savage PJ, Bennett PH, Gorden P, Miller M: Insulin responses to oral carbohydrate in true prediabetics and matched controls. *Lancet* 1:300–302, 1975.

Savage PJ, Bennion LJ, Flock EV, Bennett PH: Recovery of beta cell function in diabetes following weight reduction. *Diabetes* 26(suppl 1):414, 1977.

Schade DS, Eaton PR: Glucagon regulation of plasma ketone body concentration in human diabetes. *J Clin Invest* 56:1340–1344, 1975.

Schaefer O: Medical observations and problems in the Canadian Arctic: Part 2. Nutrition and nutritional deficiencies. *Can Med Assoc J* 81:386–393, 1959.

Schaefer O: When the Eskimo comes to town. *Nutr Today* 6:8–16, 1971.

Schaefer O: Are Eskimos more or less obese than other Canadians? A comparison of skinfold thickness and ponderal index in Canadian Eskimos. *Am J Clin Nutr* 30:1623–1628, 1977.

Schauberger G, Brinck UC, Guildner G, et al: Exchange of carbohydrates according to their effect on blood glucose. *Diabetes* 26(suppl 1):415, 1977.

Schellenberg B, Schlierf G: 24-hour pattern of blood sugar, plasma insulin and free fatty acids in patients with Type IV hyperlipoproteinemia given isocaloric diets containing 30, 43, and 79 cal % carbohydrate. *Diabetologia* 12:375–428, 1976.

Schemmel R, Nicholsen O, Tolgay Z: Dietary obesity in rats: Influence on diet, weight, age, and sex on body composition. *Am J Physiol* 216:373–379, 1969.

Schernthaner G, Ludwig H, Mayr WR, et al: Genetic factors on insulin antibodies in juvenile-onset diabetes. *N Engl J Med* 295:622, 1976.

Schernthaner G, Ludwig H, Mayr WR: Islet cell antibodies in HLA-typed juvenile diabetics, in Bajaj JS (ed): *Current Topics in Diabetes Rsearch*. Proc 9th Congr of Int Diab Fed, India, Series 400, 1976, p 144.

Schettler G: Comments on postwar dietary deprivation and their effects on diabetes, in Levine R, Pfeiffer EF (eds): *Lipid Metabolism, Obesity and Diabetes Mellitus, Impact on Atherosclcrosis.* Supplement to *Horm Metabol Res* 4:152, 1974.

Schlesinger FG, Schwarz F, Wagenvoort CA: The association of diabetes mellitus with primary carcinoma of the pancreas. *Acta Med Scand* 166:377–441, 1960.

Schliack V: Untersuchungen über die reele diabetes Haufigkeit. *Verb Dtsch Ges Inn Med* 22:1049–1053, 1952.

Schliack V: Mangelernahrung und Diabetesmorbidität, untersuchungen an 11, 194 diabetikern. *Z Klin Med* 151:382, 1954.

Schliack V: Über die Diabetes-Morbidität. *Dtsch Med Wochenschr* 90:2321–2337, 1965.

Schliack V: Epidemiology of diabetes in Eastern Europe. Proc 6th Congr of Int Diab Fed, 1969, p 684–692.

Schliack V: Zur epidemiologischen Situation auf dem Gebiet des diabetes mellitus in der DDR und speziell Berlin. *Z Aerztl Fortbild* 66:422–423, 1972.

Schliack V, Mohnike H, Rost H, et al: A brief account of the European diabetes epidemiology study group and its activities. *Diabetologia* 6:453–454, 1970.

Schliack V, Thoelke H, Zegenhagen R, Anders M: On the causes of death in 3,254 diabetics in Berlin as shown by postmortem findings. *Acta Diabetol Lat* 11:237–244, 1974.

Schlierf G, Reinheimer W, Stossberg V: Diurnal patterns of plasma triglycerides and free fatty acids in normal subjects and patients with endogenous (type IV) hyperlipoproteinemia. *Nutr Metabol* 13:80, 1971.

Schneeberg NG, Finestone I: The effect of age on the intravenous glucose tolerance test. *J Gerontol* 7:54–60, 1952.

Schneider H: 11 Jahre Diabetes—Screening im Bezirk Neubrandenburg. *Z Gesamte Inn Med* 28:355–360, 1973.

Schneider S, Aronoff SL, Tchou P, et al: Urinary protein excretion in prediabetic (PD), normal (N) and diabetic (D) Pima Indians and normal caucasians (NC). *Diabetes* 26(suppl 1):362, 1977.

Schonfeld G, Kudzma DJ: Type IV hyperlipoproteinemia. *Arch Intern Med* 132:55–62, 1973.

Schor S, Shani M, Modan B: Factors affecting immediate mortality of patients with acute myocardial infarction: A nationwide study. *Chest* 68:217–221, 1975.

Schwartz K, Mertz W: Chromium III and the glucose tolerance factor. *Arch Biochem Biophys* 85:292–295, 1959.

Schwartz TB: Who is a Diabetic?, editorial. *Ann Intern Med* 69:161–163, 1968.

Scott EM, Griffith IV: Diabetes mellitus in Eskimos. *Metabolism* 6:320–325, 1957.

Scott RC: Diabetes and the heart. *Am Heart J* 90:283–289, 1975.

Scott-Samuel A: Rising incidence of childhood diabetes. *Br Med J* 1:840, 1977.

Scow RO, Cornfield J: Quantitative relations between the oral and intravenous glucose tolerance curves. *Am J Physiol* 179:435–438, 1954.

531

Scrimshaw NS, Guzman MA: Diet and atherosclerosis. *Lab Invest* 18:623–639, 1968.

Searcy RL, Low EMY: Occult glucose intolerance incidence in a general population. *Calif Med* 106:364–367, 1967.

Seftel HC: Diabetes mellitus in urbanized Johannesburg, Africa. *S Afr Med J* 35:66, 1961.

Seftel HC: Diabetes in the Johannesburg African. *The Leech* 34:82–87, 1964.

Seftel HC: Some medical impressions of India with particular reference to diabetes mellitus and cardiovascular disease. *S Afr Med J* 38:278–282, 1964a.

Seftel HC, Isaacson C, Bothwell TH: The relationship between siderosis and diabetes in the Bantu. *S Afr J Med Sci* 25:89–98, 1960.

Seftel HC, Schultz E: Diabetes mellitus in the urbanized Johannesburg African. *S Afr Med J* 35:66–70, 1971.

Seftel HC, Walker ARP: Vascular disease in South African Bantu diabetics: Clinical notes. *Diabetologia* 2:286–290, 1966.

Seki J, Yamamoto M, Sowa E, et al: Clinical implications of body weight changes in maturity-onset diabetics, in Baba S, Goto Y, Fukui I (eds): *Diabetes Mellitus in Asia.* Proc 2nd symp of Int Diab Fed, Kyoto, Amsterdam, Excerpta Medica, 1975, p 275–279.

Seltzer CC: Genetics and obesity, in Vague J, Denton RM (eds): *Physiopathology of Adipose Tissue.* Proc 3rd Int Mtg of Endocrinology, Marseilles, 1968, p 325–344.

Seltzer CC, Jablon S: Army rank and subsequent mortality by cause: 23-year follow up. *Am J Epidemiol* 105:559–566, 1977.

Seltzer HS: Diagnosis of diabetes, in Ellenberg M, Rifkin H (eds): *Diabetes Mellitus: Theory and Practice.* New York, McGraw-Hill Book Co, 1970, p 436–507.

Seltzer HS, Fajans SS, Conn JW: Spontaneous hypoglycemia as an early manifestation of diabetes mellitus. *Diabetes* 5:437–442, 1956.

Selvaag O: Atherosclerosis obliterans. *J Oslo City Hosp* 12:14–63, 1962.

Selye H, MacLean A: Prevention of gastric ulcer formation during the alarm reaction. *Am J Dig Dis* 11:319–322, 1944.

Sen BC: Diabetes mellitus. *Indian Medical Gazette,* July 1893, p 241–246.

Serr DM, Ismajovitch B, Mashiach S, et al: Effect on insulin on perinatal mortality in gestational diabetes. *Isr J Med Sci* 8:789, 1972.

Service FJ, Molnar GD, Rosevear JW, et al: Mean amplitude of glycemic excursion, a measure of diabetic instability. *Diabetes* 19:644–655, 1970.

Sestak A: The occurrence of diabetes in children and adolescents in the Slovak Socialist Republic (SSR). *Cs Pediat* 32:193–195, 1977.

Sevel D, Bristow JH, Bank S, et al: Diabetic retinopathy in chronic pancreatitis. *Albrecht von Graefes Arch Klin Ophthalmol* 86:245–250, 1971.

Shafer SQ, Bruun B, Richter RW: Brain infarction risk factors in black New York City stroke patients. *J Chron Dis* 27:127–133, 1974.

Shafrir E: Hyperlipidemia in diabetes, in Sussman KE, Metz RJS (eds): *Diabetes Mellitus,* ed 4. New York, Am Diab Assoc, 1975.

Shah SJ, Shah SS, Tulpule AT, et al: Ischemic heart disease and diabetes in the low income group, in Patel JC, Talwalker NG (eds): *Diabetes in the Tropics.* Bombay, Diab Assoc of India, 1966, p 321–328.

Shankar PS: Incidence of diabetes in Hubli, in Patel JC, Talwalker NG (eds): *Diabetes in the Tropics*. Bombay, Diab Assoc of India, 1966, p 48–52.

Shaper AG: The pattern of diabetes in Africans in Uganda, in Oberdisse K, Jahnke K (eds): *Diabetes Mellitus*. Proc 3rd Congr of Int Diab Fed, Dusseldorf, 1958, Georg Thieme Verlag, p 664–669.

Shaper AG: Chronic pancreatic disease and protein malnutrition. *Lancet* 1:1223–1224, 1960.

Shaper AG: Observations on the incidence and nature of chronic pancreatic disease in African diabetics in Uganda, in Denob M (ed): Proc 4th Congr of Int Diab Fed. Editions Medicine et al Hygiene, Geneva, 1961, p 519.

Shaper AG: Aetiology of chronic pancreatic fibrosis with calcification seen in Uganda. *Br Med J* 1:1607, 1964.

Shaper AG, Jones KW: Serum cholesterol diet and coronary heart disease in Africans and Asians in Uganda. *Lancet* 2:534–537, 1959.

Shaper AG, Lee KT, Scott RF, et al: Chemico-anatomic studies in the geographic pathology of arteriosclerosis: Comparison of adipose tissue, fatty acids and plasma lipids in diabetics from East Africa and the US with different frequencies of myocardial infarction. *Am J Cardiol* 9:390–399, 1962.

Shapiro DJ, Truswell AS, Jackson WPU: Comparison of serum cholesterol and triglyceride concentrations in white and Bantu diabetics. *S Afr Med J* 47:1445–1450, 1973.

Sharkey TP, Troup P, Miller R, Van Kirk HC, Freeman R, Williams HH: Diabetes detection drive in Dayton Ohio. *JAMA* 144:914–919, 1950.

Sharp CL: Diabetes survey in Bedford 1962. *R Soc Med* 57:193–202, 1964.

Shaw S, Pegrum GD, Wolff S, Ashton WL: Platelet adhesiveness in diabetes mellitus. *J Clin Pathol* 20:845–847, 1967.

Sherman L, Glennon JA, Brech JA, et al: Failure of trivalent chromium to improve hyperglycemia in diabetes mellitus. *Metabolism* 17:439, 1968.

Sherwin RS: Limitations of the oral glucose tolerance test in diagnosis of early diabetes. *Primary Care* 4:255–266, 1977.

Sherwin RS, Fisher M, Hendler R, et al: Hyperglucagonemia and blood glucose regulation in normal, obese and diabetic subjects. *N Engl J Med* 294:455–461, 1976.

Shigeta Y, Oji N, Shichiri M, et al: Pathogenesis and clinical characteristics of obese diabetics in Japan, in Tsuji S, Wada M (eds): *Diabetes Mellitus in Asia*. Proc symp, Kobe, Amsterdam, Excerpta Medica, 1970, p 159–167.

Shin D, Becker B, Burgess D, et al: Histocompatibility antigens and diabetic retinopathy. *Diabetes* 26(suppl 1) 1977, p 417.

Short JJ, Johnson HJ: Glucose tolerance in relation to weight and age: A study of 541 cases. *Proc Assoc Life Ins Med Dir Am* 25:237–257, 1939.

Shurpalekar KS, Doraiswamy TR, Sundaravalli OE, et al: Effect of inclusion of cellulose in an "atherogenic" diet on the blood lipids of children. *Nature* 232:554–555, 1971.

Sievers J, Blomquist G, Biorck G: Studies on myocardial infarction in Malmo 1935–1954: 6. Some clinical data with particular reference to diabetes, menopause and heart rupture. *Acta Med Scand* 169:95, 1961.

Sievers ML: Serum cholesterol levels in Southwestern American Indians. *J Chron Dis* 21:107–115, 1968.

533

Sievers ML: Unusual comparative frequency of gastric carcinoma, pernicious anemia and peptic ulcer in Southwestern American Indians. *Gastroenterology* 65:867–876, 1973.

Silbert S: Amputation of the lower extremity in diabetes mellitus. *Diabetes* 1:297–299, 1952.

Silverstein MJ, Kadish L: Study of amputations of the lower extremity. *Surg Gynecol Obstet* 137:579–580, 1973.

Silverstone FA, Brandfonbrenner M, Shock NW, et al: Age difference in the intravenous glucose tolerance tests and the response to insulin. *J Clin Invest* 36:504–514, 1957.

Silverstone FA, Solomons E, Rubricius J: The rapid intravenous glucose tolerance test in obstetrical patients with a family history of diabetes. *Diabetes* 12:398, 1963.

Silwer H: Incidence of diabetes mellitus in a Swedish County: Survey of diabetics in the County of Kristianstad, in Silwer H, Oscarsson PN (eds): *Incidence and Coincidence of Diabetes Mellitus and Pulmonary Tuberculosis in a Swedish County,* Suppl 335. *Acta Med Scand,* 1958, p 5–22.

Simon M, Vongsavanthong S, Hespel JP, et al: Diabetet et Hemochromatose (I and II). *Sem Hop Paris* 49:2125, 1973.

Simonds JF: Psychiatric status of diabetic youth matched with a control group. *Diabetes* 26:921–925, 1977.

Simpson NE: Diabetes in the families of diabetics. *Can Med Assoc J* 98:427–432, 1968.

Simpson NE: Heritabilities of liability to diabetes when sex and age at onset are considered. *Ann Hum Genet* 32:283–303, 1969.

Sims EAH, Horton ES: Endocrine and metabolic adaption to obesity and starvation. *Am J Clin Nutr* 21:1455–1470, 1968.

Singal DP, Blajchman MA: Histocompatibility (HL-A) antigens, lymphocytotoxic antibodies and tissue antibodies in patients with juvenile diabetes. *Diabetes* 22:429–432, 1973.

Singer R, Elias H: Diabetes mellitus und Kriegskost in Wien. *Dtsch Med Wochenschr* 46:561, 1920.

Sinnett P, Buck L: Coronary heart disease in Papua New Guinea: Present and future. *Papua New Guinea Med J* 17:242–247, 1974.

Siperstein MD: The glucose tolerance test, in Stollerman GH (ed): *Advances in Internal Medicine.* Chicago, Year Book Medical Publishers, Inc, 1975, p 297.

Siperstein MD, Foster DW, Knowles HC Jr, Levine R, et al: Control of blood glucose and diabetic vascular disease. *N Engl J Med* 296:1060–1063, 1977.

Siperstein MD, Raskin P, Burns H: Electron microscopic quantification of diabetic microangiopathy. *Diabetes* 22:514–524, 1973.

Siperstein MD, Unger RM, Madison LL: Studies of muscle capillary basement membranes in normal subjects, diabetic and prediabetic patients. *J Clin Invest* 47:1973, 1968.

Sipple HL, McNutt KW: *Sugars in Nutrition.* New York, Academic Press, 1974.

Sirtori CR, Biasi G, Vercellio G: Diet, lipids and lipoproteins in patients with peripheral vascular disease. *Am J Med Sci* 268:325–332, 1974.

Sisk CW, Burnham CE, Stewart J, et al: Comparison of the 50 and 100 gram oral glucose tolerance test. *Diabetes* 19:852–862, 1970.

Sitnikova AM: The effect of age on the association between the presence and the extent of adiposity and disturbance of glucose tolerance. *Probl Endokrinol* 20:3–6, 1974.

Skillern PG, Rynearson EH: Medical aspects of hypoglycemia. *J Clin Endocrinol* 13:587, 1953.

Skipper E: Diabetes mellitus and pregnancy. *Q J Med* 2:353–380, 1933.

Skouby AP: Vascular lesions in diabetics with a special reference to the influence of treatment. *Acta Med Scand* 155(suppl 317):1–46, 1956.

Slama G, Candui P, Tchobroutsky G: Severe visceral neuropathy with cachexia in ten patients with less than 10 years of insulin dependent diabetes and no or minimal microangiopathy. *Diabetes* 26(suppl 1):417, 1977.

Sloan NR: Ethnic distribution of diabetes mellitus in Hawaii. *JAMA* 183:123–128, 1963.

Slome C, Gampel B, Abramson JH, et al: Weight, height and skinfold thickness of Zulu adults in Durban. *S Afr Med J* 34:505–509, 1960.

Smith C, Falconer DS, Duncan LJP: A statistical and genetical study of diabetes: 2. Heritability of liability. *Ann Hum Genet* 35:281–299, 1972.

Smith CS, Hudson FP: Mortality in juvenile diabetes mellitus over 25 years. *Arch Dis Child* 51:297, 1976.

Smith JAW: Association of diabetes and coeliac disease. *Arch Dis Child* 50:668, 1975.

Smith ME, Becker B: Ocular complications in diabetes, in Fajans SS (ed): *Diabetes Mellitus.* Dept of HEW Publ (NIH) 76-854, 1976, p 213–226.

Smith RBW, Kiddle GB, Prior IAM: Early and late observations after acute myocardial ischaemic episodes with particular reference to glucose tolerance. *N Z Med J* 67:486–492, 1968.

Smith SR, Edgar PJ, Pozefsky T, et al: Insulin secretion and glucose tolerance in adults with protein-calorie malnutrition. *Metabolism* 24:1073–1084, 1975.

Smithurst BA: Epidemiological survey of diabetes in Toowoomba Queensland. *J Chron Dis* 22:153, 1969.

Smithurst BA, Gout WMG: Toowoomba diabetic survey. A community followup in 1970. *Med J Aust* 1:234–238, 1973.

Smithurst BA, Wallace DC, Proust AJ: The Toowoomba and Goulburn diabetes surveys. *Med J Aust* 2:775–777, 1968.

Snapper I: *Chinese Lessons to Western Medicine: A Contribution to Geographical Medicine from the Clinics of Peiping Union Medical College.* New York, Interscience Publishers, Inc, 1941.

Society of Actuaries: Build and blood pressure study, Vol 1. Chicago, Society of Actuaries, 1959.

Soeldner JS: The intravenous glucose tolerance test, in Fajans SS, Sussman KE (eds): *Diabetes Mellitus: Diagnosis and Treatment,* vol 3. New York, Amer Diab Assoc, 1971, p 107–113.

Soeldner JS, Christacopoulos PD, Gleason RE: Mean retinal circulation time as determined by fluorescein angiography in normal, prediabetic, and chemical-diabetic subjects. *Diabetes* 25(Suppl 2):903–908, 1976.

535

Soler NG, Bennett MA, Pentecost BL, et al: Myocardial infarction in diabetics. *Q J Med* 44:125–132, 1975.

Soler NG, Malins JM: Prevalence of glucosuria in normal pregnancy: A quantitative study. *Lancet* 1:619–621, 1971.

Soler NG, Pentecost BL, Bennett MA, et al: Coronary care for myocardial infarction in diabetics. *Lancet* 1:475, 1974.

Sonnet J, Brisbois P, Bastin JP: Chronic pancreatitis with calcifications in Congolese Bantus. *Trop Geogr Med* 18:97–113, 1966.

Sorge F, Schwartzkopff W, Neuhaus GA: Insulin response to oral glucose in patients with a previous myocardial infarction and in patients with peripheral vascular disease: Hyperinsulinism and its relationships to hypertriglyceridemia and overweight. *Diabetes* 25:586–594, 1976.

Sorokin M: Hospital morbidity in the Fiji Islands with special reference to the saccharine disease. *S Afr Med J* 49:1481, 1975.

Sorsby A: Prevention of blindness: Present prospects. *Health Trends* 5:7–9, 1973.

Soskin S: Use and abuse of the dextrose tolerance test. *Postgrad Med* 10:108–116, 1951.

Sotto LS, Heimback DP, Seigner AW: Unsuspected prediabetic state and pregnancy. *Am J Obstet Gynecol* 76:425, 1958.

South African Medical Journal: Sugar, editorial. *S Afr Med J* 40:21, 1966.

South African Medical Journal: Diabetes in South Africa, editorial. *S Afr Med J* 43:1485, 1969.

South African Medical Journal: Sugar intake, obesity, and coronary heart disease, editorial. *S Afr Med J* 43:1513–1514, 1969a.

South African Medical Journal: Whither Sugar Consumption?, editorial. *S Afr Med J* 46:1651–1652, 1972.

Southgate DAT, Branch WJ, Hill MJ, Drasar BS, et al: Metabolic response to dietary supplements of bran. *Metabolism* 25:1129–1130, 1976.

Sowton E: Cardiac infarction and the glucose tolerance test. *Br Med J* 1:84–86, 1962.

Spellacy WN, Buhi WC, and Birk SA: Vitamin B_1 treatment of gestational diabetes mellitus. *Am J Obstet Gynecol* 127:599–602, 1977.

Spellberg MA, Leff WA: The incidence of diabetes mellitus and glycosuria in inductees. *JAMA* 129:246–250, 1945.

Spence JC: Some observations on sugar tolerance with special reference to variations found at different ages. *J Med* 14:314–326, 1921.

Spencer H: Diabetes mellitus in children. Studies of the height and weight of forty-five patients. *Am J Dis Child* 36:502–507, 1928.

Sperling M, Drash A: Evolution of diabetes mellitus from hypoglycemia. *Am J Dis Child* 121:5–9, 1971.

Spiegelman M, Marks HH: Age and sex variations in the prevalence and onset of diabetes mellitus. *Am J Public Health* 36:26–33, 1946.

Spier P: *Tin Lizzie.* New York, Doubleday, 1975.

Spiro RG: Biochemistry of the renal glomerular basement membrane in diabetes mellitus. *N Engl J Med* 288:1337, 1973.

536

Stamler J: Epidemiology of coronary heart disease. *Med Clin North Am* 57:1–46, 1973.

Stamler J: Atherosclerotic coronary heart disease, in Sussman KE, Metz RJS (eds): *Diabetes Mellitus*, ed 4. New York, Amer Diab Assoc, 1975, p 229–242.

Stamler J, Berkson DM, Levinson J, Lindberg HA, et al: Relationship between glycemia after oral glucose and status with respect to other coronary risk factors and clinical coronary disease. *Circulation* 36:241–242, 1967.

Stamler J, Berkson DM, Lindberg HA: Risk factors: Their role in the etiology and pathogenesis of the atherosclerotic disease, in Wissner RW, Geer JC (eds): *The Pathogenesis of Atherosclerosis*. Baltimore, Williams and Wilkins Co, 1972, p 67–69.

Stamler J, Shekelle RB, Schoenberger JA, Shekelle S: Glycemia and its relationship to other CHD risk factors and ECG abnormalities in 35,000 employed Chicagoans, read at *Am* Heart Assoc Conf, Cardiovascular Disease Epidemiology, New Orleans, 1973.

Stare FJ: Discussion of sugar consumption and diabetes in Marabou. Int Sugar Fdn symp, Sweden. Bethesda, Md, International Sugar Foundation, 1973, p 53.

Stavljenic A, Skrabalo Z: Oral glucose tolerance test: Whole capillary and venous blood, plasma and serum (own experience), in Gutsche H, Holler HD: *Diabetes Epidemiology in Europe*. Stuttgart, Georg Thieme, 1975, p 63–69.

Steel JM, Awan AM, Mngola EN: Diabetic retinopathy in Kenya. *Trop Doct* 7:12–14, 1977.

Steel JM, Mngola EN: Diabetes in Kenya. *Trop Doct* 4:184–187, 1974.

Stein GM, Nebbia AA: A chairside method of diabetic screening with gingival blood. *Oral Surg* 5:607–612, 1969.

Stein HJ, West KM, Robey JM, et al: The high prevalence of abnormal glucose tolerance in Cherokee Indians of North Carolina. *Arch Intern Med* 116:842–845, 1965.

Stein SP, Charles E: Emotional factors in juvenile diabetes mellitus: A study of early life experience of adolescent diabetics. *Am J Psychiatry* 128:700–704, 1971.

Steinberg AG: Heredity and diabetes. *Diabetes* 7:244, 1958.

Steinhausen HC, Borner S, Koepp P: The personality of juvenile diabetics. In Laron Z (ed): Psychological Aspects of Balance of Diabetes in Juveniles, 3rd International Beilinson Symposium, Herzlia, 1975 Part II. S Karger, New York, 1977. p 1–7.

Sterky G: Diabetic schoolchildren. *Acta Paediatr Scand* 144(suppl):1–39, 1963.

Sterky G: Growth patterns in juvenile diabetes. *Acta Paediatr Scand* 177(suppl 1):80–82, 1967.

Sterky G, Larsson Y, Persson B: Blood lipids in diabetic and nondiabetic schoolchildren. *Acta Paediatr Scand* 52:11, 1963.

Sterne J, Hirsch C, Pele MF: Effects of an exclusive glucose diet in the goldfish. *Diabetes* 16:113–117, 1968.

Stewart MS, et al: Polyol accumulations in nervous tissues of rats with experimental diabetes and galactosemia. *J Neurochem* 14:1057, 1967.

Stewart WK, Robertson PC: Detection of diabetes mellitus under population survey conditions (Forfar Community Survey 1962). *Lancet* 2:184–187, 1963.

Stocks AE, Martin FIR: Insulin sensitivity and vascular disease in maturity onset diabetics. *Br Med J* 4:396–398, 1969.

537

Stocks AE, Powell LW: Carbohydrate intolerance in idiopathic haemochromatosis and cirrhosis of the liver. *Q J Med* 42:733–749, 1973.

Stocks P: Diabetes mortality in 1861–1942 and some of the factors affecting it. *J Hyg* 43:242–247, 1944.

Stone DB, Connor WE: The prolonged effects of a low cholesterol, high carbohydrate diet upon the serum lipids in diabetic patients. *Diabetes* 12:127, 1963.

Stoudt HW, Damon A, McFarland RA: Skinfolds, body girths, biacromial diameter and selected anthropometric indices of adults. US National Center for Health Statistics, Dept of HEW Publ (HRA) 74-1281, Series 11, No. 35, 1974.

Stout RW: The role of insulin in the development of atherosclerosis, in Camerini-Davalos RA, Cole HS (eds): *Vascular and Neurological Changes in Early Diabetes.* New York, Academic Press, 1973, p 41–48.

Stout RW, Bierman EL, Brunsell JD: Atherosclerosis and disorders of lipid metabolism in diabetes, in Vallance-Owen J (ed): *Diabetes: Its Physiological and Biochemical Basis.* Baltimore, University Park Press, 1975.

Strandness DE, Priest RE, Gibbons GE: Combined clinical and pathologic study of diabetic and nondiabetic peripheral arterial disease. *Diabetes* 13:366, 1964.

Strauss FG, Argy WP, Schreiner GE: Diabetic glomerulosclerosis in the absence of glucose intolerance. *Ann Intern Med* 75:239–242, 1971.

Striker C: Special report on diabetes in Costa Rica, Guatemala and Mexico. *Proc Am Diab Assoc* 5:40–49, 1945.

Strom A: The influence of wartime on health conditions in Norway. *Akademisk Tryk-Central* Oslo, 1954, p 33–34.

Studer PP, Muller WA, Renold AE: Alterations of retinal capillaries by long-term streptozotocin diabetes, in Bajaj JS (ed): *Current Topics in Diabetes Research.* Proc 9th Congr of Int Diab Fed, India, Series 400, 1975, p 125.

Suarez J: Diabetes in Puerto Rico. *Puerto Rico J Public Health* 5:325–331, 1928–1930.

Suciu-Foca N, Rubinstein O: Intra-HLA recombinations in juvenile diabetes mellitus. *Lancet* 1:371–372, 1976.

Sujono S, Sukaton U: Complications of diabetes mellitus in Indonesia as observed at the General Hospital in Djakarta, in Tsuji S, Wada M (eds): *Diabetes Mellitus in Asia.* Proc symp Kobe, Amsterdam, Excerpta Medica, 1970, p 195–197.

Sukhatme PV: On the trend of obesity in advanced countries, in Ostman J, Milner RDG (eds): *Diabetes.* Proc 6th Congr of Int Diab Fed, Stockholm, 1967, p 704–714.

Sultz HA, Hart BA, Zielzny M: Is mumps virus an etiologic factor in juvenile diabetes mellitus? Preliminary report. *J Pediatr* 86:654–656, 1975.

Sultz HA, Schlesinger ER, Mosher WE: The Erie County survey of long-term childhood illness: II. Incidence and prevalence. *Am J Public Health* 58:491–498, 1968.

Summers ROC, Soler NG, FitzGerald MG: Retinopathy at diagnosis in young diabetics. *Diabetologia* 5:202, 1969.

Sundberg A, Grönberg A: Diabetes mellitus and pernicious anaemia. *Acta Med Scand* 166:147–150, 1960.

Susser M: *Causal Thinking in the Health Sciences: Concepts and Strategies of Epidemiology.* New York, Oxford University Press, 1973.

Sussman KE (ed): *Juvenile Type Diabetes and Its Complications: Theoretical and Practical Considerations.* Springfield, Ill, Charles C Thomas Co, 1971, p 6, 7, 16.

Sussman KE, Stimmler L, Birenboim H: Plasma insulin levels during reactive hypoglycemia. *Diabetes* 15:1–4, 1966.

Sutherland H, Stowers JM, Fisher PM: Gestational diabetes. *Br Med J* 1:639–640, 1974.

Swan DC, Davidson P, Albrink MJ: Effect of simple and complex carbohydrates on plasma non-esterified fatty acids, plasma-sugar and plasma-insulin during oral carbohydrate tolerance tests. *Lancet* 1:63–65, 1966.

Sweeney JWS: Dietary factors that influence the dextrose tolerance test. *Arch Intern Med* 40:818–830, 1927.

Szabo AJ, Stewart MD, Joron GE: Factors associated with increased prevalence of diabetic retinopathy: A clinical survey. *Can Med Assoc J* 97:286–292, 1967.

Takazakura E, Nakamoto Y, Hayakawa H, et al: Onset and progression of diabetic glomeruloscerosis. *Diabetes* 24:1–9, 1975.

Tan MH, Williams RF, Soeldner JS, et al: Serum insulin response to slow-rise glucose infusion in "genetic prediabetics" (offspring of 2 diabetic parents). *Diabetes* 26:490–499, 1977.

Tandon DL, Wahi PL, Rastogi GK: Peripheral vascular disease in diabetes mellitus. *Indian J Med Res* 61:1187–1193, 1973.

Tansey MJB, Opie LH, Kennelly BM: High mortality in obese women diabetics with acute myocardial infarction. *Br Med J* 25:1624–1626, 1977.

Tarui S, Ikura Y, Nonaka K, et al: The progression of retinopathy in two different ways in Japanese diabetic patients in Rodriguez RR, Vallance-Owen J (eds): *Diabetes.* Proc 7th Congr of Int Diab Fed, Buenos Aires, Series 209, 1970, p 140.

Taton J, Pometta D, Camerini-Davalos RA, et al: Genetic determinism to diabetes and tolerance to glucose. *Lancet* 2:1360, 1964.

Tattersall RB: Mild familial diabetes with dominant inheritance. *Q J Med* 43:339–357, 1974.

Tattersall RB, Fajans SS: A difference between the inheritance of classical juvenile-onset and maturity-onset type diabetes of young people. *Diabetes* 24:44–53, 1975.

Tattersall RB, Pyke DA: Diabetes in identical twins. *Lancet* 2:1120–1125, 1972.

Tattersall RB, Pyke DA: Growth in diabetic children: Studies in identical twins. *Lancet* 2:1105–1109, 1973.

Tattersall RB, Pyke DA: Splanchnic glucose production and its regulation in healthy monozygotic twins of diabetics. *Clin Sci Mol Med* 45:721–722, 1973a.

Taylor E, Adnitt PI, Jennings AM: An analysis of diabetic retinopathy. *Q J Med* 42:305–315, 1973.

Taylor E, Dobrel JH: Proliferative retinopathy: Site and size of initial lesions. *Br J Ophthalmol* 54:11, 1970.

Taylor KW: Viruses in experimental and human diabetes. *Postgrad Med J* 50(suppl 3):546–548, 1974.

Tejada C, Strong JP, Montenegro R, et al: Distribution of coronary and aortic atherosclerosis by geographic location, race and sex, in McGill HC Jr (ed): *The Geographic*

Pathology of Atherosclerosis, vol 18. Baltimore, Williams and Wilkins Co, 1968, p 509–526.

Terkildsen AB, Christensen NJ: Reversible nervous abnormalities in juvenile diabetics and recently diagnosed diabetics. *Diabetologia* 7:113–117, 1971.

Terra GJA: The significance of leaf vegetables, especially of cassava in tropical nutrition. *Trop Geogr Med* 16:97–108, 1964.

Terry MC: Taste-blindness and diabetes in the colored population of Jamaica. *J Hered* 41:306–307, 1950.

Teuscher A: Lack of correlation between postprandial plasma glucose determination and weight, age and heredity in 500 subjects with diabetes risk, in Gutsche H, Holler HD (eds): *Diabetes Epidemiology in Europe.* Stuttgart, George Thieme, 1975, p 166–167.

Teuscher A, Zuppinger K, Luscher R, et al: Incidence of juvenile diabetes in Canton of Bern. *Schweiz Med Wochenschr* 105:1218–1223, 1975.

Teuscher A, Zuppinger K, Moser H: Frequency of juvenile diabetes in Switzerland, in Bajaj JS (ed): *Current Topics in Diabetes Research.* Proc 9th Congr of Int Diab Fed, India, Series 400, 1976, p 182.

Thannhauser SJ, Pfitzer H: Über experimentelle hyperglykamic beim Menschen durch intravenose Zuckeringjektion. *Munch Med Woschnschr.* 50:2155–2158, 1913.

Thomas PK: The morphological basis for alterations in nerve conduction in peripheral neuropathy. *Proc R Soc Med* 64:295–298, 1971.

Thomas PK, Ward JD: Diabetic neuropathy, in Keen H, Jarrett J (eds): *Complications* of Diabetes. London, Edward Arnold Pub Co, 1975, p 151–178.

Thomsen AC: *The Kidney and Diabetes Mellitus.* Copenhagen, Munksgaard, 1965.

Thomsen V: Studies of trauma and carbohydrate metabolism with special reference to the existence of traumatic diabetes. *Acta Med Scand* (Suppl 1) 91:1–416, 1938.

Tibblin G, Wilhelmsen L, Werko L: Risk factors for myocardial infarction and death due to ischemic heart disease and other causes. *Am J Cardiol* 35:514–522, 1975.

Tibell B: Peripheral arterial insufficiency: An epidemiologic study of 2,243 hospital admissions caused by arteriosclerosis obliterans, diabetes mellitus, thromboangitis obliterans and arterial embolism. *Acta Orthop Scand* 139:(Suppl):1–54, 1971.

Tillotson JL, Kato H, Nichaman MZ: Epidemiology of coronary heart disease and stroke in Japanese men living in Japan, Hawaii, California. *Am J Clin Nutr* 26:177–184, 1973.

Tipton IH, Schroeder HA, Perry HM Jr, et al: Trace elements in human tissue: 3. Subjects for Africa, the near and Far East and Europe. *Health Phys* 11:403–451, 1965.

Tjokroprawiro A: Diabetes mellitus in Indonesia. *Int Diab Fed Bull* 21:18–19, 1976.

Toepfer WWW, Mertz W, Roginski EE, et al: Chromium in foods in relation to biological activity. *Food Chem* 21:69, 1973.

Tokuhata GK, Miller W, Digon E, et al: Diabetes mellitus: An underestimated health problem. *J Chron Dis* 28:23–25, 1975.

Tokuhata GK, et al: Report of the workgroup on mortality. National Commission on Diabetes, vol 3 part 1. US Dept of HEW Publ (NIH) 76-1021, 1976.

Tolstoi E: The effect of an exclusive meat diet lasting one year on the carbohydrate tolerance of two normal men. *J Biol Chem* 83:747–752, 1929.

Toole JF, Janeway R, Choi K, et al: Transient ischemic attacks due to atherosclerosis. *Arch Neurol* 32:5–12, 1975.

Trenchard PM, Jennings RD: Diurnal viariation in glucose tolerance and its reversal by lengthened fasting. *Br Med J* 2:640–642, 1974.

Treuting TF: The role of emotional factors in the etiology and course of diabetes mellitus: A review of the recent literature. *Am J Med Sci* 244:93–109, 1962.

Tripathy BB, Kar BC: Observation on clinical pattern of diabetes mellitus in India. *Diabetes* 14:404–412, 1965.

Tripathy BB, Kar BC: Possible role of nutrition on the pattern of diabetes in the tropics, in Patel JC, Talwalker NG (eds): *Diabetes in the Tropics.* Bombay, Diab Assoc of India, 1966, p 446–452.

Tripathy BB, Moharana SN, Roy BB, et al: Population survey for detection of frank and latent diabetes in one part of Cuttack, Orissa. *J Indian Med Assoc* 54:55–61, 1970.

Tripathy BB, Panda NC, Tej SC: Diabetes among the undernourished: Epidemiological and clinical observations, in Bajaj JS (ed): *Current Topics in Diabetes Research.* Proc 9th Congr of Int Diab Fed, India, Series 400, 1976, p 171.

Tripathy BB, Tej SC, Panda NC: Epidemiology of diabetes mellitus in urban and rural population of Orissa, India, Proc 8th Congr of Int Diab Fed, Belgium, Series 280, 1973, p 162–163.

Trousseau A: Lectures on Clinical Medicine, ed 3. London, New Sydenham Society from 1868 edition).

Trowell HC: *Non-infective Disease in Africa: The Peculiarities of Medical Noninfective Diseases in the Indigenous Inhabitants of Africa South of the Sahara.* London, Edward Arnold Pub Co, 1960, p 304–311.

Trowell H: Dietary fibre, coronary heart disease and diabetes mellitus: Part 1. Historical aspect of fibre in the food of western man. *Plant Foods for Man* 1:11–16, 1973.

Trowell H: Fibre and obesity. *Lancet* 1:95,1974.

Trowell H: Diabetes mellitus death-rates in England and Wales 1920–1970 and food supplies. *Lancet* 2:998–1002, 1974a.

Trowell H: Incidence of diabetes in children. *Lancet* 2:1510, 1974b.

Trowell H: Dietary-fiber hypothesis of the etiology of diabetes mellitus. *Diabetes* 24:762–765, 1975.

Trowell H: Definition of dietary fiber and hypothesis that it is a protective factor in certain diseases. *Am J Clin Nutr* 29:417–418, 1976.

Trowell H: Difficulties surround fiber. *JAMA* 236:252, 1976a.

Trowell H: Food and dietary fibre. *Nutr Rev* 35:6–11, 1977.

Trowell H, Painter N, Burkitt D: Aspects of the epidemiology of diverticular disease and ischemic heart disease. *Am J Dig Dis* 19:864–873, 1974.

Troxler RG, Traval JF, Lancaster MC: Interpretation of an abnormal oral glucose tolerance test encountered during multiphasic laboratory screening. *Aviation, Space, Environmental Medicine* 46:729–735, 1975.

Truett J, Cornfield J, Kannel W: A multivariate analysis of the risk of coronary heart disease in Framingham. *J Chron Dis* 20:511–524, 1967.

Truswell AS: The role of sugar in modern nutrition in Marabou. Int Sugar Fdn symp, Sweden. Bethesda, Md, International Sugar Foundation, 1973, p 12.

Truswell AS, Mann JI: Epidemiology of serum lipids in Southern Africa. *Atherosclerosis* 16:15–29, 1972.

Truswell AS, Mann JI, Campbell GD: Serum-lipids in Sugar-cane cutters. *Lancet* 1:602, 1971.

Tsai SH: Clinical studies on cardiovascular disease of diabetes in Taiwan. *J Formosan Med Assoc* 62:1, 1964.

Tsai SH: Discussion on sugar consumption in Taiwan, in Tsuji S, Wada M (eds): *Diabetes Mellitus in Asia.* Proc of Kobe, symp 1970, p 104.

Tsai S: Epidemiology of diabetes mellitus in Taiwan. *J Jpn Diab Soc* 14:33–35, 1971.

Tsuji S: The pathophysiological significance of diabetes mellitus in Asia, in Tsuji S, Wada M (eds): *Diabetes Mellitus in Asia.* Proc symp Kobe, Amsterdam, Excerpta Medica, 1970, p 1–2.

Tsuji S: Discussion of sugar consumption and diabetes, in Tsuji S, Wada M (eds): *Diabetes Mellitus in Asia.* Proc symp, Kobe, Amsterdam, Excerpta Medica, 1970a, p 104.

Tsuji S, Baba S, Matsuoka Y, et al: A five-year follow up of diabetes in a Japanese farm land, in Patel JC, Talwalker NG (eds): *Diabetes in the Tropics.* Bombay, Diab Assoc of India, 1966, p 83–93.

Tsuji S, Wada M (eds): *Diabetes Mellitus in Asia, 1970.* Amsterdam, Excerpta Medica, 1970.

Tulloch JA: The prevalence of diabetes in Jamaica. *Diabetes* 10:286, 1961.

Tulloch JA: *Diabetes Mellitus in the Tropics.* Edinburgh, E & S Livingstone Ltd, 1962.

Tulloch JA: The occurrence of diabetes in the tropics. *Scott Med J* 7:64–73, 1962.

Tulloch JA: The incidence of glycosuria and diabetes mellitus among hospital outpatients in Uganda. *East Afr Med J* 41:572–580, 1964.

Tulloch JA: Diabetes in Africa, in Duncan LJ (ed): *Diabetes Mellitus.* Edinburgh, Edinburgh Univ Press, 1966, p 115–124.

Tulloch JA, MacIntosh D: "J" type diabetes. *Lancet* 2:119–121, 1961.

Tunbridge RE, Allibone EC: The intravenous dextrose tolerance test. *Q J Med* 9:11, 1940.

Turner RC, Mann JI, Simpson RD, et al: Fasting hyperglycemia and relatively unimpaired meal responses in mild diabetes. *Clin Endocrinol* 6:253–264, 1977.

Tustison WA, Bowen AJ, Crampton JM: Clinical interpretation of plasma glucose values. *Diabetes* 15:775–777, 1966.

Tzagournis M: Atherosclerosis and diabetes mellitus, in Kryston LJ, Shaw RA (eds): *Endocrinology and Diabetes.* New York, Grune and Stratton, 1975, p 391–401.

Tzagournis M, Seidensticker JF, Hamwi GJ: Serum insulin, carbohydrate and lipid abnormalities in patients with premature coronary heart disease. *Ann Intern Med* 67:42–47, 1967.

Ueda H, et al: The incidence of myocardial infarction in hospitalized patients and the risk factors of myocardial infarction: Committee report of the Japanese Public Health Ministry. *Jpn Heart J* 16:465–479, 1975.

Ueda K, Omae T, Hirota Y, et al: Epidemiological and clinico-pathological study on renal diseases observed in the autopsy cases in Hisayama population, Kyushu Island Japan. *J Chron Dis* 29:159–173, 1976.

Umezawa K, Maruyama H, Yasuda M, et al: Evidence for the decrease of body muscle mass in obese diabetics by means of height, weight and upper arm circumference measurements, in Howard A (ed): *Recent Advances in Obesity Research. 1.* Proc 1st Int Congr on Obesity, London. London, Newman Publishing Co, Ltd, 1974, p 138–140.

Unger RH: The Banting Memorial Lecture 1975: Diabetes and the Alpha Cell. *Diabetes* 25:136–151, 1976.

Unger RH, Madison LL: A new diagnostic procedure for mild diabetes mellitus. *Diabetes* 7:455–461, 1958.

Unger RH, Madison LL: Comparison of response to intravenously administered sodium tolbutamide in mild diabetic and nondiabetic subjects. *J Clin Invest* 37:627–630, 1958a.

Unger RH, Madison LL: Diagnosis: Intravenous tolbutamide test, in Danowski TS (ed): *Diabetes Mellitus: Diagnosis and Treatment.* New York, Amer Diab Assoc, 1964, p 41–45.

University Group Diabetes Study Program (UGDP): A study of the effects of hypoglycemic agents on vascular complications in patients with adult-onset diabetes. *Diabetes* 19(suppl 2):784–815, 1970.

UGDP: A study on the effects of hypoglycemic agents on vascular complications in patients with adult-onset diabetes: 1. Design methods and baseline results. *Diabetes* 19(suppl 2):747–784, 1970.

UGDP: Effects of hypoglycemic agents on vascular complications in patients with adult-onset diabetes: 3. Clinical implications of UGDP resluts. *JAMA* 218:1400–1410, 1971.

UGDP: A study of the effects of hypoglycemic agents on vascular complications in patients with adult-onset diabetes: 5. Evaluation uf phenformin therapy. *Diabetes* 24(suppl 1):65, 1975.

UGDP: A study of the effects of hypoglycemic agents on vascular complications in patients with adult-onset diabetes: 6. Supplementary report on nonfatal events in patients treated with tolbutamide. *Diabetes* 25:1129–1153, 1976.

Uram JA, Friedman L, Kline OL: Influence of diet on glucose tolerance. *Am J Physiol* 192:521–524, 1958.

US Bureau of Labor Bulletin: Causes of death by occupation. *Bull US Bureau of Labour Statistics* 507:1–128, 1930.

US Dept of HEW: *Diabetes Source Book.* Public Hlth Serv Publ No. 1168, 1969.

US Dept of HEW: *Ten State Nutrition Survey 1968–1970.* Publ 72-8131 (HSM), vol 3. p 44.

US National Center for Health Statistics: *Skinfold Thickness of Youths 12–17 Years, United States.* Dept of HEW Publ (HRA) 74-1614, Series 11, No. 132, January 1974.

543

US National Center for Health Statistics: *Height and Weight of Children: Socioeconomic status, United States.* Dept of HEW Publ (HSM) 73-1601, Series 11, No. 119, 1972.

US National Office of Vital Statistics: *Mortality by Marital Status.* Special Rp, Selected Studies, No. 39, 1956, p 305.

US Public Health Service: *The Magnitude of the Chronic Disease Problem in the United States. Natl Health Survey 1935–1936.* Sickness and Medical Care Series Bull No. 6, 1938.

US Public Health Service: *Diabetes Control. A Public Health Program Guide.* Publ No. 506, 1967, revised 1969.

Vacca JB, Henke WJ, Knight WA Jr: Exocrine pancreas in diabetes mellitus. *Ann Intern Med* 61:242–247, 1964.

Vague J: The degree of masculine differentiation of obesities: A factor determining predisposition to diabetes, atherosclerosis, gout, and uric calculus disease. *Am J Clin Nutr* 4:20–34, 1965.

Vague J: Implications of lipid metabolism, obesity and diabetes mellitus on atherosclerosis. *Horm Metab Res* (suppl 4) 1974, p 153–158.

Vague J, Vague PH, Boyer J, Cloix ND: Antropometry of obesity, diabetes, adrenal and beta-cell functions, in Rodriguez RR, Vallance-Owen J (eds): *Diabetes.* Proc 7th Congr of Int Diab Fed, Buenos Aires, 1970, p 517–525.

Vague P, Melis C, Vialettes B, Mercier P: Increased frequency of the Lewis negative blood group in the diabetic population. *Diabetologia* 13:437, 1977.

Vaishnava H, Bashin RC, Galati PD: Diabetes mellitus with onset under 40 years in North India. *J Assoc Physicians India* 22:879–888, 1974.

Vaishnava H, Cheriyan PT, Gupta SC, et al: Ischemic heart disease and diabetes mellitus, in Patel JD, Talwalker NG (eds): *Diabetes in the Tropics.* Bombay, Diab Assoc of India, 1966, p 293–301.

Vaishnava H, Hagroo AA: Diabetes in the young, editorial. *J Assoc Physicians India* 22:915–918, 1974.

Vaishnava H, Hagroo AA, Verma NPS, et al: Lipolysis in ketosis-resistant growth onset diabetics, in Bajaj JS (ed): *Current Topics in Diabetes Research.* Proc 9th Congr of Int Diab Fed, India, Series 400, 1976, p 81.

Vaisrub S: Intravascular factors in diabetic retinopathy. *JAMA* 233:1303, 1975.

Vaisrub S: Nature and nurture in diabetic glomerulopathy, editorial. *JAMA* 236:1387–1388, 1976.

Valenstein ES, Kakolewski JW, Cox VC: Sex differences in taste preference for glucose and saccharin solutions. *Science* 156:942–943, 1967.

Vallance-Owen J: Causation of diabetes. *Proc R Soc Med* 55:207–210, 1962.

Vallance-Owen J: Synalbumin insulin antagonism. *Diabetes* 13:241, 1964.

Valleron AJ, Aboulker JP, Papoz L, Rathery M: Reproducibility of borderline fasting to 2 hr oral glucose tolerance test, in Gutsche H, Holler HD (eds): *Diabetes Epidemiology in Europe.* Stuttgart, Georg Thieme, 1975, p 109–111.

Valleron AJ, Eschwege E, Rathery M: Epidemiological definition of unequivocal normal and diabetic glucose tolerance, in Bajaj JS (ed): *Current Topics in Diabetes Research.* Proc 9th Congr of Int Diab Fed, India, Series 400, 1976, p 183.

Van de Putte I, Vermylen C, Decraene P, et al: Segregation of HLA B7 in Juvenile-onset diabetes mellitus. *Lancet* 2:251, 1976.

Van der Linden SJL, Mastboom JL: Insulin treatment of latent and potential diabetics during pregnancy. *J Obstet Gynaecol* 78:924, 1971.

Van der Westhuizen J, Mbizvo M, Jones JJ: Unrefined carbohydrate and glucose tolerance. *Lancet* 2:719, 1972.

VanSoest PJ, McQueen RW: The chemistry and estimation of fibre. *Proc Nutr Soc* 32:123, 1973.

van't Laar A: Comparison of the 50 and 100 gram oral glucose tolerance test in patients with borderline glucose tolerance. *Diabetologia* 8:71, 1972.

Vannasaeng S, Inthuprapa M, Tandhanand S: Diabetes mellitus in Siriraj Hosp, in Bajaj JS (ed): *Current Topics in Diabetes Research.* Proc 9th Congr of Int Diab Fed, India, Series 400, 1976, p 108.

Vartiainen I: War time and the mortality in certain diseases in Finland. *Ann Acad Sci Fenn* 35:234–240, 1946.

Vartiainen I: The inheritance of craving for sugar in rats. *Ann Acad Sci Fenn* 56:137–153, 1976.

Vartiainen I, Vartiainen O: Studien über den Diabets mellitus in Finland: 3. Das Vorkommen des diabetes. *Acta Med Scand* 119:364–379, 1944.

Vecchio TJ: Predictive value of a single diagnostic test in unselected populations. *N Engl J Med* 274:171–173, 1966.

Venkateschwara RS, Choudhurani CPD, Satyanarayana D: Pancreatic calculi and diabetes (in Hyderbad), in Patel JC, Talwalker NG (eds): *Diabetes in the Tropics.* Bombay, Diab Assoc of Ind, 1966, p 234.

Verdonk CA, Palumbo PJ, Gharib H, et al: Diabetic microangiopathy in patients with pancreatitic diabetes mellitus. *Diabetologia* 11:395–400, 1975.

Verdy M. Gagnon MA, Caron D: Birth weight and adult obesity in children of diabetic mothers. *N Engl J Med*, March 1974, p 576.

Verdy M, Roussy J, Tetreult L, et al: Study of the factors regulating the disposal of repeated glucose injections. *Metabolism* 20:273–276, 1971.

Vernet A, Fabre J, Mulli JC: Factors of arterial and renal complication in diabetes. *Schweiz Med Wochenschr* 105:296–303, 1975.

Vieira FJP: Considerations in the incidence of diabetes mellitus among the American Indians. *Rev Assoc Med Bras* 20:447–449, 1974.

Vieira Filho JP: Diabetes mellitus and fasting glycemias in Caripuna Palikur Indians. *Rev Ass Med Brasil* 23:175–178, 1977.

Vihert AM, Zhdanov VS, Matove ED: Atherosclerosis of the aorta and coronary vessels of the heart in cases of various diseases. *Atherosclerosis* 9:179–192, 1969.

Vinke B, Nagelsmit WF, Van Buchem FSP: Some statistical investigations on sufferers from diabetes mellitus, in Oberdisse K, Jahnke K (eds): *Diabetes Mellitus.* Proc 3rd Congr of Int Diab Fed, Dusseldorf. Stuttgart, Springer-Verlag, 1958, p 660–664.

Vinke B, Nagelsmit WF, Van Buchem FSP, Smid LJ: Some statistical investigations in diabetes mellitus. *Diabetes* 8:100–104, 1959.

Viskum K: The prognosis of conservatively treated diabetic gangrene. *Acta Med Scand* 185:319–322, 1969.

Viswanathan M, Mohamed U, Krishnamoorthy M, et al: Diabetes in the young: Study of 166 cases, in Patel JD, Talwalker NG (eds): *Diabetes in the Tropics.* Bombay, Diab Assoc of India, 1966, p 277–281.

Viswanathan M, Moses SGP, Krishnamoorthy M: Prevalence of diabetes in Madras, in Patel JC, Talwalker NG (eds): *Diabetes in the Tropics.* Bombay, Diab Assoc of India, 1966, p 29–32.

Viswanathan M, Snehalatha C, Swaminathan G, et al: Effect of a calorie restricted, high carbohydrate, high protein, low fat diet, serum lipid levels in diabetes: A follow up study, in Bajaj JS (eds): *Current Topics in Diabetes Research.* Proc 9th Congr of Int Diab Fed, India, Series 400, 1976, p 84–85.

Viton A, Pignalosa F: Trends and forces of world sugar consumption: Commodity Bulletin Series 32, Food and Agriculture Organization of the United Nations, Rome, 1961, p 54–56.

Vladutiu AO: Bisalbuminemia and diabetes? *JAMA* 236:2393, 1976.

Vogelberg KH, Berchtold P, Berger H: Primary hyperlipoproteinemias as risk factors in peripheral artery disease documented by arteriography. *Atherosclerosis* 22:271–285, 1975.

von During A: Urasche and Heilung des diabetes mellitus, Hanover, ed 2. 1875. Urasche und Heilung der Zuckerkrankheit, Hanover, ed 5. 1905.

von Euler U, Larsson Y: Glucose tolerance tests in children: A methodological study. *Scand J Clin Lab Invest* (suppl 64) 1962, p 62–70.

von Knorre G, Bode H: Fettsucht und Diabetesmorbiditat—eine prospective 5 Jahres Studie (summary in Eng. p 9). *Z Gesamte Inn Med* 31: 6–9, 1976.

von Kruger HU: Reihenuntersuchungen auf Diabetes mellitus bei Kindern. *Z Deutsch Gesundh* 20:781–782, 1965.

von Schneider H, Bartels H, Burrman H, et al: Untersuchung zur Haufigkeit von Glucosetoleranzstorungen der über Funfundvierzigjahrigen der Landgemeinde Furstenwerder/Uckermark. *Z Alternsforsch* 23:23–28, 1970.

Vracko R, Bendett EP: Manifestations of diabetes mellitus: Their possible relationship to an underlying cell defect. *Am J Pathol* 75:204, 1974.

Vuayagopal P, Saraskwathi DK, Devi K, Kurup PA: Fibre content of different dietary starches and their effect on lipid levels in high fat–high cholesterol diet fed rats. *Atherosclerosis* 17:156–160, 1973.

Wada M, Shigetta Y: Cardiovascular complications in Japanese diabetics. In Patel JC, Talwalker NG (eds): *Diabetes in the Tropics.* Bombay, Diab Assoc of India, 1966, 302–305.

Wada S, Toda S, Omori Y, et al: The clinical features of diabetes mellitus in Japan as observed in a hospital outpatient clinic. *Diabetes* 13:485–491, 1964.

Wadsworth MEF, Jarrett RJ: Incidence of diabetes in the first 26 years of life. *Lancet* 2:1172, 1974.

Wagner R, White P, Goban IK: Diabetic dwarfism. *Am J Dis Child* 63:667, 1942.

Wahlberg F: Intravenous glucose tolerance in myocardial infarction, angina pectoris and intermittent claudication. *Acta Med Scand* (suppl 453) 1966, p 1–93.

Wahlberg F, Thomasson B: Glucose tolerance in ischaemic cardiovascular disease, in Dickens F, Randle RJ, Whelen WJ (eds): *Carbohydrate Metabolism and its Disorders*. London, Academic Press, 1968.

Wahren J, Felig P, Cerasi E, et al: Splanchic glucose production and its regulation in healthy monozygotic twins of diabetics. *Clin Sci* 44:493–504, 1973.

Wainwright J: Diabetic retinopathy and nephropathy (postmortem incidence). *S Afr Med J*, January 1969, p 83–85.

Waitzkin L: Unknown diabetes mellitus among apparently healthy men with "nonspecific" 'T' wave abnormalities—in a mental hospital. *Diabetes* 16:711–727, 1967.

Wakisaka A, Aizawa M, Matsuura N, et al: HLA and juvenile diabetes mellitus in the Japanese. *Lancet* 2:970, 1976.

Wales A: The role of the combination of sucrose and milk in diabetes mellitus. *Am J Clin Nutr* 29:689–690, 1976.

Wales JK: Plasma lipid levels, carbohydrate tolerance and complications in untreated maturity onset diabetes, in Bajaj JS (ed): *Current Topics in Diabetes Research*. Proc 9th Congr of Int Diab Fed, India, Series 400, 1976, p 108.

Walker ARP: Nutritional, biochemical and other studies on South African populations. *S Afr Med J* 40(suppl):64–75, 1966.

Walker ARP: Prevalence of diabetes mellitus. *Lancet* 1:1163, 1966a.

Walker ARP: Studies on glycosuria, glucose tolerance and diabetes in South African populations. *S Afr Med J* 40:814, 1966b.

Walker ARP: Sugar intake, obesity and coronary heart disease. *S Afr Med J* 43:1513–1514, 1969.

Walker ARP: Problems in studying the epidemiology of coronary heart disease in unsophisticated populations. *Am Heart J* 80:725–728, 1970.

Walker ARP: Biological and disease patterns in South African inter-racial populations as modified by rise in privilege. *S Afr Med J* 46:1127–1134, 1972.

Walker ARP: Studies on sugar intake and overweight in South African black and white schoolchildren. *A Afr Med J* 48:1650–1654, 1974.

Walker ARP: Sugar intake and diabetes mellitus. *S Afr Med J* 51:842–851, 1977.

Walker ARP, Bernstein RE, duPlessis I: Hyperinsulinaemia from glucose dose in South African Indian children. *S Afr Med J* 46:1916, 1972.

Walker ARP, Mistry SD, Seftel HC: Studies in glycosuria and diabetes in non-white populations of the transvaal: Part 2. Indians. *S Afr Med J* 37:1217–1220, 1963.

Walker ARP, Seftel HC: Coronary heart-disease, strokes and diabetes in South African Indians. *Lancet* 2:786–787, 1962.

Walker ARP, Walker FB: The bearing of race, sex, age, and nutritional state on the precordial electrocardiograms of young South African Bantu and Caucasian subjects. *Am Heart J* 77:441–459, 1969.

Walker JB: The detection of latent diabetes. *Postgrad Med J* 35:302–307, 1959.

Walker JB: Ten year follow up of diabetes in an English Community in Gutsche H, Holler HD (eds): *Diabetes Epidemiology in Europe*. Stuttgart, Georg Thieme, 1975, p 2–7.

Walker JB, Kerridge D: *Diabetes in an English Community: A Study of its Incidence and Natural History.* Leicester, University Press, 1961.

Wallach V: Notizen zur diabetessterblichkeit in Frankfurt. *Dsch Med Wochenschr* 19:779, 1893.

Waller BF, Palumbo PJ, Connolly DC: Distribution of coronary artery disease in diabetic and nondiabetic hearts, abstract. *Diabetes* 25(suppl 1):346, 1976.

Walsh CH, Malins JM, Soler NG: Diabetes mellitus and primary hyperparathyroidism. *Postgrad Med J* 51:446–449, 1975.

Walsh CH, O'Regan J, O'Sullivan DJ: Effect of different periods of fasting on oral glucose tolerance. *Br Med J* 2:691–693, 1973.

Walsh CH, Wright AD, Allbutt E, Pollock A: The effect of cigarette smoking on blood sugar, serum insulin and nonesterified fatty acids in diabetic and non diabetic subjects. *Diabetologia* 13:491–494, 1977.

Waltman S, Ostreich C, Krupin T, et al: Quantitative vireous fluorophotometry: A sensitive technique for measuring early disruption of the blood retinal barrier in young diabetics. *Diabetes* 26(suppl 1):361, 1977.

Wang S: Diabetes mellitus: An analysis of 347 cases (Chinese inpatients): 1. Incidence symptoms, examinations and complications. *Chin Med J* 51:9–32, 1937.

Wapnick S, Wicks AC, Kanengoni E, et al: Can diet be responsible for the initial lesion in diabetes? *Lancet* 2:300–301, 1972.

Ward JD: Improvement in motor nerve conduction following treatment in newly diagnosed diabetics. *Adv Metab Disord* 2(suppl 2):569–573, 1973.

Ward JD, Barnes CG, Fisher DJ: Improvement in nerve conduction following treatment in newly diagnosed diabetics. *Lancet* 1:428–430, 1971.

Wardle EN, Piercy DA, Anderson J: Some chemical indices of diabetic vascular disease. *Postgrad Med J* 49:1–9, 1973.

Warren R, Recrod EE: *Lower Extremity Amputations for Arterial Insufficiency.* Boston, Little, Brown and Co, 1967.

Warren S: The pathology of diabetes in children. *JAMA* 88:99, 1927.

Warren S, Corfield A: Mortality from diabetes. *Lancet* 1:1511–1512, 1973.

Warren S, LeCompte PM, Legg MA: Spontaneous diabetes in animals, in Warren S, LeCompte PM, Legg MA (eds): *The Pathology of Diabetes Mellitus,* ed 4. Philadelphia, 1966a, p 441–445.

Warrier CBC: Clinical aspects of pancreatic diabetes mellitus in Calicut, in Patel JC, Talwalker NG (eds): *Diabetes in the Tropics.* Bombay, Diab Assoc of India, 1966, p 239.

Watkins PJ, Blainey JD, Brewer DB, et al: The natural history of diabetic renal disease: A follow up study of a series of renal biopsies. *Q J Med* 41:437–456, 1972.

Watkins PJ, Page MMcB, Washbourne J: Diagnostic value of continuous heart rate monitoring in diabetic neuropathy. *Diabetologia* 12:425–426, 1976.

Watkins PJ, Parsons V, Bewick M: The prognosis and management of diabetic nephropathy. *Clin Nephrol* 7:243–249, 1977.

Watson BA: An analysis of 583 glucose tolerance tests. *Endocrinology* 25:845–852, 1939.

Weaver JA, Bhatia SK, Boyle D, et al: Cardiovascular state of newly discovered diabetic women. *Br Med J* 1:783–786, 1970.

Webb SR, Loria RM, Madge GE, et al: Susceptibility of mice to group B Coxsackie virus is influenced by the diabetic gene. *J Exp Med* 143:1239–1248, 1976.

Weber HW, Wicht CL: The peripheral angiopathy of diabetics: A plethysmographic and histopathological study. *S Afr J Lab Clin Med* 8:83–93, 1962.

Weerasinghe HD: Epidemiology of diabetes mellitus. *Ceylon Med J,* September 1967, p 168–175.

Weil WB Jr: Skeletal maturation in juvenile diabetes mellitus. *Pediatr Res* 1:470–478, 1967.

Weil WBJ: Mortality factors in Diabetes, letter. *J Soc Occup Med* 18:606, 1976.

Weinblatt E, Shapiro S, Frank CW: Prognosis of women with newly diagnosed coronary heart disease—A comparison with course of disease among men. *Am J Public Health* 63:577–593, 1973.

Weinsier RL, Seeman A, Herrera MG, et al: High- and low-carbohydrate diets in diabetes mellitus: Study on effects of diabetic control, insulin secretion and blook lipids. *Ann Intern Med* 80:332–341, 1974.

Weinstein B: Diabetes: A regional survey in British Guiana (Preliminary report). *West Indian Med J* 11:88–93, 1962.

Weisse AB, Abiuso PD, Thind IS: Acute myocardial infarction in Newark, N J. *Arch Int Med* 137:1402–1405, 1977.

Weitz R, Laron Z: Height and weight of children born to mothers with diabetes mellitus. *Isr J Med Sci* 12:195–198, 1976.

Welborn TA, Cullen KJ, Balazs N: Diabetes detection in mass health examinations: Three-year experience from Busselton. *Med J Aust* 2:133–137, 1972.

Welborn TA, Cumpston GN, Cullen KJ, et al: The prevalence of coronary heart disease and associated factors in an Australian rural community. *Am J Epidemiol* 89:521–536, 1969.

Welborn TA, Curnow DH, Wearne JT, et al: Diabetes detected by blood sugar measurement after a glucose load: Report from the Busselton survey 1966. *Med J Aust* 2:778–783, 1968.

Welch RJ: Causes of blindness in addition to MRA registers for 1967. Proc Conf of MRA for Blindness, US Dept of HEW (NIH), Bethesda, Md, 1969, p 23–26.

Welsh GW: Studies of abnormal glucose metabolism in pregnancy. *Diabetes* 9:446, 1960.

West KM: Comparison of the hyperglycemic effects of glucocorticoids in human beings: The effect of heredity on responses to glucocorticoids. *Diabetes* 6:168–175, 1957.

West KM: Normal kidneys and retinae after 35 years of diabetes. *Ann Intern Med* 47:1256–1259, 1957a.

West KM: Response of the blood glucose to glucocorticoids in man: Determination of the hyperglycemic potencies of glucocorticoids. *Diabetes* 8:22–28, 1959.

West KM: Response to cortisone in prediabetes: Glucose and steroid-glucose tolerance in subjects whose parents are both diabetic. *Diabetes* 9:379, 1960.

West KM: Oral carbohydrate tolerance tests. *Arch Intern Med* 113:641–648, 1964.

West KM: Laboratory diagnosis of diabetes: A reappraisal. *Arch Intern Med* 117:187–191, 1966.

West KM: Epidemiology of diabetes, in Fajans SS, Sussman KE (eds): *Diabetes Mellitus: Diagnosis and Treatment,* vol 3. New York, Amer Diab Assoc, 1971, p 121–129.

West KM: Epidemiologic evidence linking nutritional factors to the prevalence and manifestations of diabetes. *Acta Diabetol Lat* 9(suppl 1):405–428, 1972.

West KM: Epidemiology of adiposity, in Vague J, Boyer J (eds): *The Regulation of the Adipose Tissue Mass.* Series 315, Proc 4th Int Mtg of Endocrinology, Marseilles, 1973, p 201–207.

West KM: Diet therapy of diabetes: An analysis of failure. *Ann Intern Med* 79:425–434, 1973a.

West KM: Diabetes in American Indians and other native populations of the new world. *Diabetes* 23:841–855, 1974.

West KM: Epidemiologic observations on 13 populations of Asia and the Western hemisphere, in Hillebrand SS (ed): *Is the Risk of Becoming Diabetic Affected by Sugar Consumption?* Proc 8th Symp of Int Sugar Res Fdn. Bethesda, Md, International Sugar Research Foundation, 1974a, p 33–43.

West KM: Substantial differences in diagnostic criteria used by diabetic experts. *Diabetes* 24:641, 1975.

West KM: Diabetes in American Indians, in Bennett PH, Miller M (eds): *Epidemiology of Diabetes, Advances in Metabolic Diseases.* New York, Academic Press, 1977 (in press).

West KM et al: Diabetes in nineteen Oklahoma Indian tribes. *Diabetes* 23(suppl 1):385, 1974.

West KM, Johnson PC: Metabolism and relative hypoglycemic potencies of four sulfonylureas in man. *Diabetes* 9:454–458, 1960.

West KM, Kalbfleisch JM: Glucose tolerance, nutrition, and diabetes in Uruguay, Venezuela, Malaya, and East Pakistan. *Diabetes* 15:9–18, 1966.

West KM, Kalbfleisch JM: Diabetes in Central America. *Diabetes* 19:656–663, 1970.

West KM, Dalbfleisch JM: Influence of nutritional factors on prevalence of diabetes. *Diabetes* 20:99–108, 1971.

West KM, Kalbfleisch JM: Sensitivity and specificity of five screening tests for diabetes in ten countries. *Diabetes* 20:289–296, 1971a.

West KM, Kalbfleisch JM: Diabetes and cardiovascular disease, in *Nutritional Evaluation of the Population of Central America and Panama.* Institute of Nutrition of Central America and Panama, and Interdepartmental Committee on Nutrition for National Development. US Dept of HEW Publ (HSM) 72-8120, 1972, p 50–60.

West KM, Mako ME: Effect of prediabetes, preobesity, and dietary sugar on insulin secretion, abstract. *Diabetes* 25(suppl 1):389, 1976.

West KM, Oakley EL, Sanders ME, et al: Nutritional factors in the etiology of diabetes, in Keen H (ed): *Epidemiology of Diabetes.* Geneva, World Health Organization, 1978.

West KM, Rockwell DA, Wulff JA: Value of the skin-surface glucose test as a screening procedure for diabetes. *Diabetes* 12:50–52, 1963.

West KM, Sanders ME, McCulloch EL, Robinson RP, et al: Does sugar consumption increase risk of diabetes and obesity? *Diabetes* 25(suppl 1):342, 1976.

West KM, Stein JH, Sanders TJ: Dextrostix estimates of blood glucose in mass screening for diabetes. *Am J Public Health* 56:2059–2064, 1966.

West KM, Wells RG, Burk BT: Case history of a diabetes detection program: Reappraisal of roles and methods of voluntary community programs, in *Early Disease Detection*. Miami, Halos and Assoc, 1970, p 32–41.

West KM, Wood DA: The intravenous glucose tolerance test. *Am J Med Sci* 238:25–37, 1959.

West KM, Wulff JA, Reigel DG, et al: Oral carbohydrate tolerance tests. *Arch Intern Med* 113:641, 1964.

Westlund K: *Incidence of Diabetes Mellitus in Oslo Norway 1925 to 1954*, report 11. Life Insurance Companies Institute for Medical Statistics at the Oslo City Hospitals. *Br J Prev Soc Med* 20:3, 105–116, 1966.

Westlund K: *Mortality of Diabetics*, report 13. Life Insurance Companies Institute for Medical Statistics at the Oslo City Hospitals. The Norwegian Research Council for Science and the Humanities, Oslo. Printed in Denmark, by PJ Schmidts Bogtrykkeri, Vojens, 1969, p 69–70.

Westlund K, Nicholaysen R: Ten-year mortality and morbidity related to serum cholesterol. *Scand J Clin Lab Invest* 30(suppl 127):3–24, 1972.

Whichelow MJ, Wiggelsworth A, Cox BD, Butterfield WMH, et al: Critical analysis of blood sugar measurements in diabetes detection and diagnosis. *Diabetes* 16:219–226, 1967.

White KL: Opportunities and need for epidemiology and health statistics in the United States, in White KL, Henderson MM (eds): *Epidemiology as a Fundamental Science: Its Uses in Health Services Planning, Administration, and Evaluation*. New York, Oxford University Press, 1976, p 66–83.

White P: The child with diabetes. *Med Clin North Am* 49:1069–1079, 1965.

White P: Life cycle of diabetes in youth: 50th anniversary of the discovery of insulin (1921–1971). *J Am Med Wom Assoc* 27:203–315, 1972.

White P: Diabetes mellitus in pregnancy: Symposium on management of the high-risk pregnancy. *Clinics in Perinatology* 1:331–347, 1974.

White P, Graham CA: The child with diabetes, in Marble A, White P, et al (eds): *Joslin's Diabetes Mellitus*, ed 11. Philadelphia, Lea & Febiger, 1971, p 339–360.

Whitehouse FW, Jurgensen C, Block MA: The later life of the diabetic amputee: Another look at fate of the second leg. *Diabetes* 17:520–521, 1968.

Whyte HM: Behind the adipose curtain: Studies in Australia and New Guinea relating to obesity and coronary heart disease. *Am J Cardiol* 15:66–80, 1965.

Wicks ACB, Castle WM, Gelfand M: The effect of time on the prevalence of diabetes on the urban African of Rhodesia. *Diabetes* 22:733–737, 1973.

Wicks ACB, Clain DJ: Chronic pancreatitis in African diabetics. *Am J Dig Dis* 20:1–8, 1975.

Wicks ACB, Jones JJ: Ethnic differences in coronary heart disease. *S Afr Med J* 3:362, 1973.

Wicks ACB, Jones JJ: Insulinopenic diabetes in Africa. *Br Med J* 1:773–776, 1973a.

Wicks ACB, Jones JJ: Diabetes mellitus in Rhodesia: A comparative study. *Postgrad Med J* 50:659–663, 1974.

551

Wicks ACB, Lowe RF, Jones JJ: Alcohol: A cause of diabetes in Rhodesia. *S Afr Med J* 48:1114–1117, 1974.

Widmer LK, Greensher A, Kannel WB: Occlusion of peripheral arteries: A study of 6400 working subjects. *Circulation* 30:836–842, 1964.

Wikramanayake PR: Diabetes as it exists in Ceylon. *Int Diab Fed Report*. Amsterdam, Excerpta Medica Foundation, 1968, p 70–76.

Wilansky DL, Shochat G: The course of latent diabetes. *Ann NY Acad Sci* 148:844–858, 1968.

Wilcox HB: Diabetes in infants and young children. *Arch Pediatrics* 25:655–668, 1908.

Wilder RM: Necropsy findings in diabetes. *South Med J* 19:241–248, 1926.

Wilder RM: The unknown diabetic and how to recognize him. *JAMA* 138:349, 1948.

Wilkerson HLC, Hyman H, Kaufman M, et al: Diagnostic evaluation of oral glucose tolerance tests in nondiabetic subjects after various levels of carbohydrate intake. *N Engl J Med* 262:1047, 1960.

Wilkerson HLC, Krall LP: Diabetes in a New England town: A study of 3,516 persons in Oxford Mass. *JAMA* 135:209, 1947.

Wilkerson HLC, O'Sullivan JB: A study of glucose tolerance and screening criteria in 752 unselected pregnancies. *Diabetes* 12:313, 1963.

Williams JL, Dick GF: Decreased dextrose tolerance in acute infectious diseases. *Arch Intern Med* 1:801–818, 1932.

Williams RH: Etiologic, pathophysiologic and clinical inter-relationships in diabetes. *Johns Hopkins Med J* 136:25–37, 1975.

Williamson JR, Rowold E, Hoffman P, et al: Influence of fixation and morphometric technics on capillary basement-membrane thickening prevalence data in diabetes. *Diabetes* 25:604–613, 1976.

Williamson JR, Vogler NJ, Kilo C: Estimation of vascular basement membrane thickness. *Diabetes* 18:567, 1967.

Williamson RT: Diabetes mellitus and its treatment. Edinburgh and London, 1898 (publisher unknown).

Williamson RT: Geographic distribution of diabetes mellitus. *Medical Chronicle* (Manchester) 1:234–252, 1909.

Williamson RT: Remarks on the etiology of diabetes mellitus. *Br Med J* 1:139–141, 1918.

Willis T: *Of the Diabetes or Pissing Evil*. Pharmaceutice Rationalis. London, T Dring, C Harper, J Leight, 1679, chap 3, part 1.

Wilson D: Distribuicao do diabetes melito segundo as racas. *Arq Hig Saude Pub* 29:111–114, 1964.

Wilson DE, Schriebman PH, Day VC, et al: Hyperlipidemia in an adult diabetic population. *J Chron Dis* 23:501–506, 1970.

Wilson JMcG, Junger G: Principles and practices of screening for disease. Geneva, Switzerland, WHO. Public Health Papers No. 34, 1968.

Wilson MA: The influence of diet prescriptions and instruction materials on the diabetic patient's dietary adherence. *W Va Med J* 61:193–196, 1965.

Wilson RB, Martin JM, Hartroft WS: Failure of insulin therapy to prevent cardiovascular lesions in diabetic rats fed an atherogenic diet. *Diabetes* 18:225–231, 1969.

Wingerd J, Duffy TJ: Oral contraceptive use and other factors in the standard glucose tolerance test. *Diabetes* 26:1024–1033, 1977.

Winterbotham HJ: Diabetes mellitus at Mabuiag Island, Torres Straits, 1960. *Med J Aust* 1:780–781, 1961.

Wise JK, Hendler R, Felig P: Obesity: Evidence of decreased secretion of glucagon. *Science* 178:513–514, 1972.

Wise PH, Edwards FM, Craig RJ, Evans B, et al: Diabetes and associated variables in the South Australian Aboriginal. *Aust NZ J Med* 6:191–196, 1976.

Wise PH, Edwards FM, Thomas DW, et al: Hyperglycaemia in the urbanized Aboriginal: The Devenport Survey. *Med J Aust* 2:1001–1006, 1970.

Woldman EE, Segal AJ: Relation of fibrosis of the pancreas to fatty liver and/or cirrhosis: An analysis of one thousand consecutive autopsies. *JAMA* 169:1281–1283, 1959.

Wolf PA, Dawber TR, Thomas HE, Colton T, Kannel WB: Epidemiology of stroke. *Adv Neurol* 16:5–19, 1977.

Wolf S: Animal model. Sekoke: Diabetes of nutritional origin in carp. (Animal model of human disease, diabetes mellitus). *Am J Pathol* 85:805–808, 1976.

Woodrow JC: HL-A and its association with clinical disease. *Proc R Soc Med* 68:802–804, 1975.

Woodrow JC, Cudworth AG: HL-A8 and W15 in diabetes mellitus. *Lancet* 1:803, 1975.

Woods SC, Vassel JF, Kaestner E, et al: Conditioned insulin secretion associated with meals in rats. *Diabetes* 25(suppl 1):390, 1976.

Woodyatt RT: Some milder forms of diabetes with special reference to mild diabetes in the elderly persons with arteriosclerosis. *South Med J* 18:145–176, 1924.

Woolf N: Diabetes and atherosclerosis. *Acta Diabetol Lat* 8:14, 1971.

World Health Organization: *Manual of the International Statistical Classification of Diseases, Injuries and Causes of Death,* vol 1, rev 6. Geneva, Switzerland, WHO, 1948. (9th ed., ICD, 1977).

World Health Organization: Medical certification of causes of death: Instructions to physicians. *Bull WHO* (suppl 3) 1952.

World Health Organization: *Statistical Yearbook,* 1956.

World Health Organization: *Statistical Yearbook:* Epidem vital statist Report 17:47, 51, 307–330, 1964.

World Health Organization McDonald GW, Butterfield WJH, et al (eds): *Diabetes Mellitus. Report of a WHO Expert Committee.* Technical Report Series No 310, Geneva, WHO, 1965.

World Health Organization: World Health Statistics report 27, Geneva, WHO, 1974, p 196–197.

Wright HB, Taylor B: The incidence of diabetes in a sample of the adult population in South Trinidad. *West Indian Med J* 7:123, 1958.

Wylie CM, Carpenter JO: Comparison of hospital admissions for cerebrovascular disease in Michigan and North Carolina. *J Community Health* 2:21–30, 1976.

Wyse BM, Dulin WE: The influence of age and dietary conditions on diabetes in the Db mouse. *Diabetologia* 6:268–273, 1970.

553

Yanko L, Ungar H, Michaelson IC: The exudate lesions in diabetic retinopathy with special regard to the hard exudate. *Acta Ophthalmol* 52:150–160, 1974.

Yefimov AS, Limanskaya GF, Cheban A, et al: Classification and frequency of diabetic angiopathy depending on the clinical characteristics of diabetes and the preceding treatment. *Vrach Delo* 12:28–32, 1972.

Yodaiken R, Joffe B, Simms F: Capillaries of South African diabetics: 3. Pancreatic diabetics, in Rodriguez RR, Vallance-Owen J (eds): *Diabetes.* Proc 7th Congr of Int Diab Fed, Buenos Aires, Series 209, 1970, p 157.

Yodaiken RE, Pardo V: Diabetic capillaropathy. *Hum Pathol* 6:455–464, 1975.

Yokote M: Retinal and renal microangiopathy in carp with spontaneous diabetes mellitus, in Camerini-Davalos RA, Cole HS (eds): *Vascular and Neurological Changes in Early Diabetes.* New York, Academic Press, 1973, p 299–307.

Yoon JW, Notkins AL: Virus-induced diabetes mellitus: 6. Genetically determined host differences in the replication of encephalomyocarditis virus in pancreatic beta cells. *J Exp Med* 143:1170–1185, 1976.

Yoshida T: The finding of autopsy in Japanese diabetes. *Jpn Diabetes* 4:3, 1961.

Yoshikawa K: Experimental diabetes produced by repeated intra-peritoneal injections of glucose. *Tohoku J Exp Med* 49:25, 1954.

Young FG: The endocrine approach to the problem of diabetes (The Banting Memorial Lecture). *Proc Am Diab Assoc* 10:11–22, 1950.

Younger D, Hadley WB: Infection and diabetes, in Marble A, White P, et al (eds): *Joslin's Diabetes Mellitus,* ed 11. Philadelphia, Lea & Febiger, 1971, p 621–636.

Yssing M: Long-term prognosis of children born to mothers diabetic when pregnant, in Camerini-Davalos RA, Cole HS (eds): *Early Diabetes in Early Life.* Academic Press, New York, 1975, p 575–586.

Yudkin J: Evolutionary and historical changes in dietary carbohydrates. *Am J Clin Nutr* 20:108–115, 1957.

Yudkin J: Dietary fat and dietary sugar in relation to ischemic heart disease and diabetes. *Lancet* 2:4–5, 1964.

Yudkin J: Sugar as a food: An historical survey, in Yudkin J, Edelman J, Hough L (eds): *Sugar: Chemical, Biological and Nutritional Aspects of Sucrose.* London, Butterworth's, 1971, p 11–17.

Yudkin J: Sugar and disease. *Nature* 239:197–199, 1972.

Yudkin J: Infant feeding and diabetes. *Lancet* 1:268, 1973.

Yudkin J, Edelman J, Hough L (eds): *Sugar: Chemical Biological and Nutritional Aspects of Sucrose.* London, Butterworths, 1971.

Yuen KK, Kahn HA: The association of female hormones with blindness from diabetic retinopathy. *Am J Ophthalmol* 81:820–822, 1976.

Zalme E, Knowles HC: A plea for plasma sugar. *Diabetes* 14:165–166, 1965.

Zaragoza N, Rivier D, Bringolf M, et al: Study of nutritional obesity in the rat. *Diabetologia* 6:69–70, 1970.

Zaragoza N, Rivier D, Felber JP: Study in vivo and in vitro of obesity with intolerance to glucose and insensitivity to insulin in rat rendered obese by a hyperlipid diet. *Diabetologia* 5:59–60, 1969.

Zawalich WS, Dye ES, Rognstad R, Pagliara AS, Matschinsky FM: Starvation induced alterations of islet cell sensitivity. *Diabetes* 26(suppl 1):379, 1977.

Zdanov VS, Vihert AM: Atherosclerosis and diabetes mellitus. Atherosclerosis of the Aorta and Coronary Arteris in Five Towns. *Bull WHO* 53:547–553, 1976.

Zetterstrom B, Gjotterberg M: The diagnosis of retinopathy of fluorescein angiography in latent diabetes. *Acta Ophthalmol* 52:1–12, 1974.

Zhukovsky GS, Zybina VD, et al: Effect of various factors on diabetes mellitus morbidity in the population of Ulan-Ude (Russian, Eng. summary). *Probl Endokrinol* 22:3–6, 1976.

Ziegler E: Statistical studies on the relationship between current sugar consumption and mortality of diabetes. *Helv Paediatr Acta* 11: 360–365, 1967.

Ziegler E, Chiumello G, Marko HH: The effect of the carbohydrate pattern of three isocaloric mixed breakfasts on the postprandial concentrations of plasma glucose, insulin, growth hormone and free fatty acids in normal man. *Int J Vitam Nutr Res* 43:212–226, 1973.

Ziemann H: Discussion on diabetes in Cameroons. *Br Med J*, October, 1907, p 1061.

Zimmet P, Guinea A, Taft P, et al: The high prevalence of diabetes mellitus on a Pacific Island. *Diabetologia* 12:428, 1976.

Zimmet P, Seluka A, Collins J, et al: Diabetes mellitus in an urbanized, isolated Polynesian population. *Diabetes* 26:1101–1108, 1977.

Zimmet P, Whitehouse S: Bimodality in glucose tolerance—the phenomenon and its possible significance. *Diabetologia* 13:441, 1977.

Zonana J: Diabetes mellitus: Considerations on genetic counseling, in New MI, Fisher RH (eds): *Diabetes and Other Endocrine Disorders During Pregnancy and in the Newborn.* New York, Alan R Liss Inc, 1976, p 1–12.

Zubiran S, Chavez A: Estudio epidemiologico de la diabetes en la ciudad de Mexico. *Rev Invest Clin* 16:367, 1964.

Zuidema PJ: Calcification and cirrhosis of the pancreas in patients with deficient nutrition. *Doc Med Geog Trop* 7:229–251, 1955.

Zuidema PJ: Cirrhosis and disseminated calcification of the pancreas in patients with malnutrition. *Trop Geogr Med* 11:70–74, 1959.

Zumoff B, Hellman L: Aggravation of diabetic hyperglycemia by chlordiazepoxide. *JAMA* 237:1960–1961, 1977.

Zybina VD, Zhukovsky GS, et al: A study of diabetes mellitus morbidity in Ulan-Ude (Russian, Engl. summary). *Probl Endokrinol* 21:11–18, 1975.

Index